Robotics in General Surgery

Keith Chae Kim
Editor

Robotics in General Surgery

Springer

Editor
Keith Chae Kim, M.D., F.A.C.S.
Metabolic Medicine and Surgery Institute
Florida Hospital Celebration Health
Celebration, FL, USA

ISBN 978-1-4614-8738-8 ISBN 978-1-4614-8739-5 (eBook)
DOI 10.1007/978-1-4614-8739-5
Springer New York Heidelberg Dordrecht London

Library of Congress Control Number: 2013949142

Printed on acid-free paper

Springer is part of Springer Science+Business Media (www.springer.com)

There are many people who have been instrumental in the publication of this book and others who have been essential in creating the circumstances that led me to embrace robotic surgery. Thank you.

I dedicate this book to Ella, Alex, Jennifer, John, Cathy, Sofia, and Young, and especially to my parents, Sun Tok Kim, my mother, and Kwi Hyon Kim, my father, who have taught me through their actions that hard work and perseverance have no equal.

Preface

Robotic surgery will prove to be the most significant advance in surgery for this generation of surgeons and the next few generations to come. The current platform, the da Vinci system, is the product of an evolution from the US Department of Defense's efforts to produce telerobotic capabilities in order to provide injured frontline soldiers with advanced surgical care from remote locations to commercial efforts to provide enhanced dexterity to facilitate complex surgeries while maintaining minimally invasive techniques. The enhanced dexterity, based on an anthropomorphic model whereby the robotic system is designed to mimic the human hand in its range and freedom of movements, is fairly advanced and has allowed both average surgeons to adopt minimally invasive techniques and skilled surgeons to push the envelope in the complexity of minimally invasive procedures. The robotic approach has permeated essentially every specialty in general surgery.

More importantly, however, the robotic platform has introduced two new dynamics between the patient and the surgeon that will have a far greater impact. First, the system is based on a master–slave relationship in which the surgeon is remote from the patient and performs the operation by controlling a patient cart slave that is docked to the patient. Second, the console represents a digital interface between the surgeon and the patient. In these aspects, we are just starting to scratch the surface of the possibilities.

The master–slave configuration allows for telepresence as was dramatically demonstrated by Professor Marescaux and colleagues in "Operation Lindbergh," a transatlantic cholecystectomy. This capability will not only have a profound impact on providing sophisticated and complex care to remote locations from a command center but will also dramatically facilitate professional education and collaborative surgery. Experts will be able to have a global presence without having to leave their operating rooms and will be able to demonstrate surgery as well as assist or take over surgeries being performed in remote locations by linking their console to the remote patient cart. Additionally, the master–slave platform will eventually allow for the manipulation of wireless "slave" components that will form the foundation of the future of endoscopy, interventional radiology, and natural orifice interventions.

The digital interface, which allows for the collection and manipulation of data that can be used for diagnostic or interventional purposes, represents an even greater potential. Even in the relatively early stages, imaging technology is being used to identify structures and provide a road map to the surgical anatomy in real time. The future will see the digital interface between patient and surgeon evolve to facilitate image-guided surgery, computer-aided surgery, as well as pre-performed surgery in simulation models that is reproduced by a computer-driven system on the actual patient.

This textbook, the first comprehensive overview of the role of robotic surgery in general surgery, is intended as a "how-to" reference of robotically performed procedures in general surgery. Additionally, in recognition of the importance of understanding the evolution of robotic surgery thus far, and the impact that it will have on the future of surgery, this book provides a historical perspective of robotic surgery as well as an overview of the emerging technology and future robotic platforms.

Celebration, Florida, USA Keith Chae Kim, M.D., F.A.C.S.

Contents

Contributors

Abbas E. Abbas, M.D. Department of Surgery, Ochsner Clinic Foundation, New Orleans, LA, USA

Haidar Abdul-Muhsin, M.D. Florida Hospital—Celebration Health, Global Robotics Institute, Celebration, FL, USA

Sami Alasari, M.D. Department of Surgery, Yonsei University College of Medicine, Seoul, South Korea

Matthew Albert, M.D., F.A.C.S., F.A.S.C.R.S. Center for Colon and Rectal Surgery, Florida Hospital, Altamonte, FL, USA

Mehran Anvari, M.B.B.S., Ph.D., F.R.C.S., F.A.C.S. Department of Surgery, McMaster University, Hamilton, ON, Canada

St. Joseph's Healthcare Hamilton, Hamilton, ON, Canada

Sam Atallah, M.D., F.A.C.S., F.A.S.C.R.S. Center for Colon and Rectal Surgery, Florida Hospital, Winter Park, FL, USA

Hossein Bagshahi, M.D. Department of Surgery, Harris Methodist Hospital, Fort Worth, TX, USA

Reshape Bariatric and General Surgery of Fort Worth, Fort Worth, TX, USA

Nilanjana Banerji, Ph.D. Neuroscience and Spine Clinical Service Line, Abbott Northwestern Hospital, Minneapolis, MN, USA

David L. Bartlett, M.D. Department of Surgery and Surgical Oncology, University of Pittsburgh Medical Center, Pittsburgh, PA, USA

Lorena Bejarano-Pineda, M.D. Division of Transplantation, Department of Surgery, University of Illinois Hospital and Health Sciences System, Chicago, IL, USA

Eren Berber, M.D., F.A.C.S. Department of General Surgery, Cleveland Clinic, Cleveland, OH, USA

Jamin V. Brahmbhatt, M.D. Department of Urology, Winter Haven Hospital and University of Florida, Winter Haven, FL, USA

Ayesha S. Bryant, M.D., M.S.P.H. Division of Cardiothoracic Surgery, University of Alabama at Birmingham, Birmingham, AL, USA

Luciano Casciola, M.D. Division of General, Minimally Invasive and Robotic Surgery, Department of Surgery, San Matteo degli Infermi Hospital, Spoleto, Italy

Graziano Ceccarelli, M.D. Division of General, Minimally Invasive and Robotic Surgery, Department of Surgery, San Matteo degli Infermi Hospital, Spoleto, Italy

Robert James Cerfolio, M.D., F.A.C.S., F.C.C.P. Division of Cardiothoracic Surgery, University of Alabama at Birmingham, Birmingham, AL, USA

Gyu Seog Choi, M.D., Ph.D. Colorectal Cancer Center, Kyungpook National University Medical Center, Daegu, South Korea

WoongYoun Chung, M.D., Ph.D. Department of Surgery, Yonsei University College of Medicine, Seoul, South Korea

Myriam J. Curet, M.D. Intuitive Surgical International, Sunnyvale, CA, USA

Department of Intuitive Surgery, Stanford University, Sunnyvale, CA, USA

Michele Diana, M.D. Department of Digestive and Endocrine Surgery, IRCAD (Research Institute against Digestive Cancer), Strasbourg, France

Martin J. Dib, M.D. Department of Surgery, Beth Israel Deaconess Medical Center, Boston, MA, USA

Brian Dunkin, M.D., F.A.C.S. Department of Surgery, The Methodist Hospital, Houston, TX, USA

Daniel H. Dunn, M.D. Esophageal and Gastric Care Program, Virginia Piper Cancer Institute, Abbott Northwestern Hospital, Minneapolis, MN, USA

Mark R. Dylewski, M.D. Department of Cardiac Vascular and Thoracic Surgery, Baptist Health of South Florida, Miami, FL, USA

Angela Echeverria, M.D. Department of Surgery, University of Arizona, Tucson, AZ, USA

Randy Fagin, M.D. Texas Institute for Robotic Surgery, Hospital Corporation of America, Austin, TX, USA

Intuitive Surgical International, Sunnyvale, CA, USA

Carlos A. Galvani, M.D. Department of Surgery, University of Arizona, Tucson, AZ, USA

Robert Ganz, M.D., F.A.S.G.E. Department of Gastroenterology, Abbott Northwestern Hospital, Bloomington, MN, USA

Anthony M. Gonzalez, M.D. Bariatric Surgery, Baptist Health Medical Group, Miami, FL, USA

Ahmet Gudeloglu, M.D. Department of Urology, Winter Haven Hospital and University of Florida, Winter Haven, FL, USA

Eric M. Haas, M.D. Division of Minimally Invasive Colon and Rectal Surgery, Department of Surgery, The University of Texas Medical School at Houston, Houston, TX, USA

Colorectal Surgical Associates, Ltd, LLP, Houston, TX, USA

Monika E. Hagen, M.D., M.B.A. Intuitive Surgical International, Sunnyvale, CA, USA

Department of Digestive Surgery, University Hospital Geneva, Geneva, Switzerland

Woo Jin Hyung, M.D., Ph.D. Department of Surgery, Yonsei University College of Medicine, Seoul, Republic of Korea

Mehraneh D. Jafari, M.D. Department of Surgery, Irvine School of Medicine, University of California, Orange, CA, USA

Eric M. Johnson, M.D. Department of Surgery, Abbott Northwestern Hospital, Minneapolis, MN, USA

Kourtney Kemp, M.D. Specialists in General Surgery, Maple Grove Hospital, Maple Grove, MN, USA

Tara Kent, M.D., F.A.C.S. Department of Surgery, Beth Israel Deaconess Medical Center, Boston, MA, USA

Keith Chae Kim, M.D., F.A.C.S. Metabolic Medicine and Surgery Institute, Florida Hospital Celebration Health, Celebration, FL, USA

Seon Hahn Kim, M.D. Ph.D. Department of Surgery, Korea University Anam Hospital, Seoul, Republic of Korea

Jung Myun Kwak, M.D., Ph.D. Department of Surgery, Korea University Anam Hospital, Seoul, Republic of Korea

Richard Lazzaro, M.D. North Shore LIJ Health System, Lenox Hill Hospital, New York, NY, USA

Jandee Lee, M.D., Ph.D. Department of Surgery, Eulji University College of Medicine, Seoul, South Korea

Kang Hong Lee, M.D., Ph.D. Department of Surgery, Hanyang University College of Medicine, Seoul, South Korea

Sean Lee, M.D. Division of Metabolic and Weight Loss Surgery, Duke University Medical Center, Durham, NC, USA

Sam Leon, M.D. Minnesota Gastroenterology, Minneapolis, MN, USA

Henry J. Lujan, M.D., F.A.C.S., F.A.S.C.R.S. Deparment of Surgery, Jackson South Community Hospital, Miami, FL, USA

Jacques Marescaux, M.D., F.A.C.S., (Hon) F.R.C.S., (Hon) J.S.E.S. Department of Digestive and Endocrine Surgery, IRCAD (Research Institute against Digestive Cancer), Strasbourg, France

John J. Meehan, M.D., F.A.C.S. University of Washington School of Medicine, Seattle Children's Hospital, Seattle, WA, USA

Byung Soh Min, M.D., Ph.D. Department of Surgery, Yonsei University College of Medicine, Seoul, South Korea

A. James Moser, M.D., F.A.C.S. Institute for Hepatobiliary and Pancreatic Cancer, Beth Israel Deaconess Medical Center, Boston, MA, USA

José Oberholzer, M.D. Division of Transplantation (MC 958), University of Illinois Hospital and Health Sciences System, Chicago, IL, USA

Carlos M. Ortiz-Ortiz, M.D. Department of General Surgery, Florida Hospital—Celebration, Celebration, FL, USA

Sijo J. Parekattil, M.D. Department of Urology, Winter Haven Hospital and University of Florida, Winter Haven, FL, USA

Eduardo Parra-Davila, M.D., F.A.C.S., F.A.S.C.R.S. Departments of General Surgery, Colorectal, Bariatric, Florida Hospital—Celebration, Celebration, FL, USA

Vipul Patel, M.D. Florida Hospital—Celebration Health, Global Robotics Institute, Celebration, FL, USA

Alberto Patriti, M.D., Ph.D. Division of General, Minimally Invasive and Robotic Surgery, Department of Surgery, San Matteo degli Infermi Hospital, Spoleto, Italy

Rodrigo Pedraza, M.D. Division of Minimally Invasive Colon and Rectal Surgery, Department of Surgery, The University of Texas Medical School at Houston, Houston, TX, USA

Colorectal Associates, Ltd, LLP, Houston, TX, USA

Alessio Pigazzi, M.D., Ph.D. Division of Colorectal Surgery, Department of Surgery, Irvine Medical Center, University of California, Orange, CA, USA

Gustavo Plasencia, M.D., F.A.C.S., F.A.S.C.R.S. Department of Surgery, Jackson South Community Hospital, Miami, FL, USA

Jorge Rabaza, M.D. South Miami Hospital, Baptist Health Medical Group, Miami, FL, USA

M. Shirin Sabbaghian, M.D. Division of Surgical Oncology, Department of Surgery, University of Pittsburgh Medical Center, Pittsburgh, PA, USA

Avanish Saklani, M.S., F.R.C.S. Colorectal Division, Surgical Oncology, Tata Memorial Centre, Parel, Mumbai, India

Julia Samamé, M.D. Department of Surgery, University of Arizona, Tucson, AZ, USA

Brad Snyder, M.D. Department of Surgery, Memorial Hermann Texas Medical Center, Houston, TX, USA

Giuseppe Spinoglio, M.D. Department of General and Oncological Surgery, City Hospital SS. Antonio e Biagio, Alessandria, Italy

Hubert Stein, DIPL.-ING, BMT Clinical Development Engineering, Intuitive Surgical Inc., Sunnyvale, CA, USA

Ranjan Sudan, M.D. Department of Surgery, Duke University Medical Center, Durham, NC, USA

Halit Eren Taskin, M.D. Endocrine Surgery Division, Cleveland Clinic, Cleveland, OH, USA

Department of General Surgery, Cleveland Clinic, Cleveland, OH, USA

Allan Tsung, M.D. Division of Hepatobiliary and Pancreatic Surgery, Department of Surgery, University of Pittsburgh Medical Center Liver Cancer Center, Montefiore Hospital, Pittsburgh, PA, USA

Ivo G. Tzvetanov, M.D. Division of Transplantation, Department of Surgery, University of Illinois Hospital and Health Sciences System, Chicago, IL, USA

Victor Wilcox, M.D. Department of Surgery, Houston Methodist Hospital, Houston, TX, USA

Erik B. Wilson, M.D. Department of Surgery, The University of Texas Health Science Center, Houston, TX, USA

Yanghee Woo, M.D. Division of GI/Endocrine Surgery, Center for Excellence in Gastric Cancer Care, Columbia University Medical Center, New York, NY, USA

Department of Surgery, Columbia University College of Physicians and Surgeons, New York, NY, USA

Department of Surgery, New York Presbyterian Hospital, New York, NY, USA

Vicky D. Woodruff, Ph.D. Department of Surgery, University of Texas Health Science Center, Houston, TX, USA

Anusak Yiengpruksawan, M.D., F.A.C.S. Department of Surgery, The Valley Minimally Invasive and Robotic Surgery Center, The Valley Hospital, Ridgewood, NJ, USA

Part I

Overview of the Robotic System

History of Robotic Surgery

1

Haidar Abdul-Muhsin and Vipul Patel

Introduction

Human dreams and fantasies to develop a "robot" roots back deep in history, as old as ancient civilizations. History of robotic development is an interesting example of how a myth can transform to reality, how fiction becomes the seeds of historical inventions and achievements that serves humanity for decades.

As we go through the history of robotic development, we realize how difficult it is to attribute this development to a certain person or a certain era. This is not due to lack of historical resources but because robot creation was the result of interaction of multiple civilizations, cultures, and sciences.

"Robota" is a Czech term that described compulsory work. In its original Czech, *robota* means forced labor of the kind that serfs had to perform on their masters' lands and is derived from the term *rab*, meaning "slave." Despite the existing debate in Czech literature regarding the first person who invented this term, the most reliable references point that this term appeared first when Karel Capek used it in his play "Rossum's Universal Robot" (RUR) in 1921. It was used to describe the artificial people in his play. The idea came from his brother Joseph Capek who advised him to use this term to describe these characters. Ironically, 5 years earlier, when he wrote "Opilec," Joseph described the artificial people as "automats" and not robots.

Karel Capek in RUR wanted to warn against the rapid growth of the modern world and thus described the evolution of the robots with increasing capabilities that eventually revolted against their human makers [1]. He envisioned that these robots would revolt 40 years after the time the play was created, which is nearly in the 1960s. This coincided with the first appearance of the industrial robot later on. However, The Robots described in Capek's play were not robots, as we know them now, a mechanical device that sometimes resembles a human. They were not machines, but rather live creatures that may be mistaken for humans.

RUR quickly became famous and was influential early in the history of its publication. Two years after its first spread, it had been translated into 30 languages. This fact played a major role in the widespread popularity of this term.

Many years later Isaac Asimov, a science fiction writer, used the term "Robotics" to describe the field of study of robotics in 1942. This usage further popularized the use of this term and resulted in the widespread of robots in subsequent artistic works with multiple roles that varied from friendly roles to hostile or comedian ones [2]. Asimov outlined the three rules of robotics in his books Runaround and I, Robot that were published between 1938 and 1942.

H. Abdul-Muhsin, M.D. • V. Patel, M.D. (✉)
Florida Hospital–Celebration Health, Global Robotics Institute, 410 Celebration Place, Suite 200, Celebration, FL 34747, USA
e-mail: vpatel2171@aol.com; Haidar.AbdulMuhsin@flhosp.org

K.C. Kim (ed.), *Robotics in General Surgery*, DOI 10.1007/978-1-4614-8739-5_1,

These rules were:

1. A robot may not injure a human being.
2. A robot must obey orders given by humans except when doing so conflicts with the first law.
3. A robot must protect its own existence as long as this does not conflict with the first and second laws.

These literary sources led our imagination to build stereotypes for robots. However, in order to study history of robots, we need to define what do we mean by "robot" from the scientific point of view.

The first scientific definition of the robot did not appear until lately in 1972 when the Robot Institute of America set a definition for the robot which was "A reprogrammable, multifunctional manipulator designed to move materials, parts, tools, or specialized devices through various programmed motions for the performance of a variety of tasks."

Looking at history with this meaning in mind, we can find that human trials to build a "robot" extend into the deepest roots of human civilizations and represent a continuum of developments that led to the current status of robotics.

Robots in Ancient History

One of the first known automated machines ever built was in 1300 BC, when Amenhotep made the statue of king Memnon that was able to produce sounds. In Ancient China (1023–957 BC), Yan Shi (engineer) presented King Mu of Zhou with a life-size, human-shaped mechanical figure. In the fifth century BC, King-shu Tse in China designed a flying magpie and a horse that was able to jump.

One century afterward, Aristotle looked at automation from a philosophical point of view. In his famous "politics" book, he mentioned that "if every tool, when ordered, or even of its own accord, could do the work that befits it then there would be no need either of apprentices for the master workers or slaves for the lords." In this description, he imagined the future role of automation and robotics.

In the fourth century (428–347 BC), the Greek mathematician Archytas of Tarentum designed a mechanical bird that was made of wood and could fly by propelling steam. One century later (250 BC), Ctesibius of Alexandria designed the "clepsydra" which meant the water thief in Greek. Clepsydra was a water clock with moveable figures on it. Initially this water clock was used as a timer only and was later on modified into an ordinary clock. This was followed by the landmark efforts of Heron of Alexandria (10–70 AD) who made numerous innovations in the field of automata. He made the first vending machine and he utilized his steam-driven engine, as known as aeolipile, to make many machines including one that was supposed to speak.

The Arabic Muslim inventor, Al Jazari (1136–1206), designed and constructed several automatic machines and invented the first programmable robot. For entertainment purposes, he made a "robotic band," a boat with automated humanoid musicians.

The sketches of Leonardo da Vinci that were discovered in the 1950s demonstrated the first record of a humanoid robot design and showed a presentation of a mechanical knight. This work could possibly present an extension of his famous anatomical study of human body proportions in his Vitruvian man sketches. This inspired the current surgical robot makers to name their robot after this genius Italian architect and inventor.

Da Vinci ideas inspired Gianello Torriano who created a robotic mandolin-playing lady in 1540. This was followed by many European innovators like Jacques Vaucanson 1738 (the creator of the loom) who constructed a mechanical duck that could eat, drink, move its wings, and digest grains. Pierre Jaquet-Droz made the first android in 1772. He made a child robot and called it the writer. This robot was able to write complete phrases. It was programmable to make movements to draw each letter of the alphabet. This allowed it to write whatever the user wants. In collaboration with his son, Henri-Louis, he developed two other androids using the same principle. The first one could draw and the second one could play different musical pieces. It actually could play musical instruments like a flute.

In 1801, Joseph Jacquard modified the loom by making it automatic by following a set of preordered commands. These commands were in the form of holes punched into cardboard.

History of Robotic Technology in Surgery

The development of contemporary robots was mainly driven by the need for "telepresence." Telepresence is a term used to describe the sensation that a person is in one location while being in another. It was needed to let automated machines perform certain tasks in hazardous or unwanted environments for human being and probably in a more accurate method.

This was first made possible in 1951 when Raymond Goertz, while working for the Atomic Energy Commission, designed the first teleoperated master–slave manipulator in order to handle hazardous radioactive materials. This presented the first example for successful implementation of telepresence.

Inspired by the science fiction stories of Isaac Asimov, George Devol, and Joseph Engelberger developed the first commercial robot. They established a company and called it Universal Automation. They were successful in producing a programmable robot that can replace a human worker. Their first robot was called "Unimate" and was produced in 1961. The Unimate robot was able to store commands and had six degrees of freedom. It was able to precisely conduct potentially hazardous tasks like handling molten die casting and perform spot welding. This robot was used for the first time by General Motors to work in their car assembly. This highlighted the past need for telepresence where the machine was used for potentially dangerous chores that were previously performed by humans.

The Unimate presented a huge commercial success. For manufacturers it performed repetitive tasks with a great degree of precision, no fatigue, and without need for human labor. It simply meant less spending. After many years of success, the company was acquired by Westinghouse and continued production until today. The usage of this robot has diffused into many other factories and resulted in widespread use of robots since its introduction. Moreover, it has extended into many other countries that started production of their own robots.

Several years later (1978) PUMA (Programmable Universal Machine for Assembly) was developed by Victor Scheinman at Unimation. This device utilized electric motors and was a smaller version of the Unimate robot. It had more variable usages and multitasking abilities. This by itself resulted in more spread of the robot. This spread reached fields beyond industry including medicine.

In the strict sense of the word, the robotic systems currently used in surgery are not actually robots but remote performers that use end effectors or instruments. The systems capable of performing such tasks are called "telemanipulators" and it works using the master–slave style. These master–slave systems do not perform tasks automatically but obey orders through the voice or hand of the surgeon.

PUMA was used for the first time in 1985 in the field of medicine when it was used to direct a needle to undergo a brain CT-guided biopsy [3]. This stereotactic brain biopsy achieved an accuracy of 0.05 mm. With this accuracy of execution, this first robot-assisted surgical procedure paved the road for robot-assisted surgery. Soon afterward, it was used to resect an astrocytoma of the thalamus.

The fixed anatomical landmarks in neurosurgery and orthopedic surgery facilitated the quick use and distribution of the robot-assisted techniques. This robot was developed to become the prototype of "NeuroMate" that is currently FDA approved (1999).

The first robot-assisted surgical procedure was performed in 1983 with the use of "Arthrobot," which was designed to assist in orthopedic procedures. In 1988 the "ROBODOC" production of integrated surgical systems was used in total hip arthroplasty to allow precise preoperative planning [4]. This robot is computer guided to precisely drill the femoral head to insert the hip replacement prosthesis. This approach gained FDA approval in August 2008 after multiple clinical trials [5–7]. Similar designs have been used in knee replacement surgery using the "ACROBOT" and temporal bone surgery "RX-130."

In 1988 at Imperial College in London, a group of researchers started the first application of robot in urology with the PUMA to aid in performing one of the most commonly performed urological procedures, transurethral resection of the prostate [8].

The successor for this robot was the surgeon-assistant robot for prostatectomy "SARP." This was motorized rather than using the manual frame in the previous robot. It was used successfully on 1991 in London, UK. This was perhaps the world's first robotic surgery on the prostate. Further development on "SARP" led to the creation of "PROBOT," "URobot," and "SPUD," which are abbreviation for prostate robot, urology robot, and Surgeon Programmable Urological Device, respectively.

The PROBOT worked through a computer-generated 3D image of the prostate. Once the surgeon determines the boundaries of resection area using this 3D model, the system starts using these data to calculate the area of resection and executes the procedure without further intervention from the surgeon. This system had four degrees of freedom and rapidly rotating blade [9, 10]. Despite the initial encouraging result with PUMA, Westinghouse stopped the manufacturing of this device secondary to concerns of safety during surgery.

The SARP and PROBOT devices (from Imperial College, London) were further developed to develop the URobot in 1991. This device was utilized for multiple purposes including transurethral HIFU (high-intensity focused ultrasound), brachytherapy, needle prostate biopsy, and laser resection of the prostate [11, 12]. Collaboration with Dornier Asia Medical Systems led to the creation of the SPUD device (Surgeon Programmable Urological Device).

Robotics in Visceral Surgery

The mobility of the visceral organs in visceral surgery presented an obstacle toward the use of a programmable device to achieve a certain surgical task. The main place where robots could play a part was when used as a telemanipulator that are completely operated by a surgeon. This indirectly meant the usage of telemanipulation in laparoscopy.

Despite the fact that the concept of laparoscopy dates back to more than a decade ago (G Kelling 1901 and HC Jacobaeus in 1911), this approach was not deemed possible until after 1969 when Smith and Boyle invented the charge coupling device. This new technology allowed the conversion of light into an analog signal that can be transmitted into a digital image. This new technique not only allowed laparoscopic intervention but was also a key step toward telepresence through the interposition of a technological interface.

In the 1980s the National Aeronautics and Space Administration (NASA) joined with the Ames Research Center to start the development of a head-mounted virtual reality display to allow users to immerse themselves in large data sets that were transmitted from aerospace missions. This resulted in the head-mounted display (HMD) that immersed the user in a 3D virtual environment using tiny television monitors attached to a helmet. This was developed by Michael McGreevy and Stephen Ellis and later was enhanced by the addition of a 3D audio by Scott Fischer (computer scientist). By coupling this technology with the data glove that was originally developed by Jaron Lanier, they allowed the users to see their own interaction with the virtual world [13, 14].

In parallel Dr. Joseph Rosen, a plastic surgeon at Stanford University, began to experiment with Philip Green from Stanford Research Institute (SRI) to develop a dexterity- enhancing surgical telemanipulator.

Joe Rosen and Scott Fischer later produced the idea of telepresence surgery. Their vision was to design a surgical system that could be used to perform remote surgical operations in space that could be achieved by combining HMD at NASA and the robotic telepresence system at SRI.

Many of the initially designed features of Green's Telepresence System were at the time unworkable from an engineering standpoint [15]. The HMD was subsequently replaced with monitors, and the data gloves were replaced with handles for controllers at the surgeon's console. Since the imperative at this time was for space and/or military application for acute surgical care, the end effectors were substantially similar to open surgical instruments. By 1989, Richard Satava, a military surgeon, joined this team.

While Jacques Perrisat of Bordeaux was presenting on the technique of laparoscopic cholecystectomy at the Society of American Gastrointestinal and Endoscopic Surgeons (SAGES) in Atlanta, the team of investigators began to consider developing a system that could be applied to minimally invasive laparoscopic surgery.

Satava looked for further funding and presented a videotape of a bowel anastomosis using the telepresence surgery system to the Association of Military Surgeons of the United States. The results of demonstrating this technology resulted in a Defense Advanced Research Projects Agency (DARPA) grant for further investigation and development in July of 1992. In addition, Satava became the program manager for Advanced Biomedical Technologies to aid funding of technologically advanced projects. By 1995, the robotic system had progressed to a prototype mounted into an armored vehicle (the Bradley 557A) that could "virtually" take the surgeon to the front lines and immediately render surgical care to the wounded, called MEDFAST (Medical Forward Area Surgical Team) [15].

Vascular surgeon Jon Bowersox performed the first telesurgery experiment, an ex vivo intestinal anastomosis using this system for demonstration. This was later developed to be used for vascular anastomosis [16]. This demonstrated the delicate ability of this system.

ZEUS

In 1993, Yulyn Wang developed a software for control of motion of robotic systems and founded a company called Computer Motion. Wang succeeded in developing the first FDA-approved robotic device for use in laparoscopic surgery. The system, Automated Endoscopic System for Optimal Positioning (AESOP), consisted of a table-mounted articulating arm that was used to control the movements of the camera during laparoscopic surgery and provided 7 degrees of freedom of movement [17]. Originally the AESOP was manipulated by hand or foot controls, but the later version was capable of utilizing voice commands and incorporated voice control of endoscopic and OR room lights (HERMES) [18].

Wang became interested in complete robotic surgery and obtained DARPA funding to develop a modular robotic system to be integrated with AESOP. HERMES was the integrated operating room control system that allowed the complete integration of Computer Motion's robotic system [19]. In 2001, Computer Motion, the ZEUS robotic system, developed a device combining both the AESOP and HERMES. This was a master–slave configuration that allowed the surgeon to control a robotic slave device that was docked to the patient remotely from a console.

The ZEUS robotic system, similar to the AESOP, had an endoscope holder arm that was voice controlled, along with two other operating arms that provided four degrees of freedom and were able to hold a variety of instruments. These instruments were manipulated with joysticks from the surgeon console. The computer system that interfaced the surgeon console with the operating robotic arms allowed filtration of surgeon tremor and scaling of movements by a factor of 2–10. The surgical field was visualized through a regular 2D screen or through polarized glasses with a different axis for each eye that allowed for 3D images [20]. This system was used for the first time in a full laparoscopic procedure for fallopian tube anastomosis at the Cleveland Clinic in 1998 [21]. One year later, it was used for coronary bypass by Reichenspurner [22].

In 2001, in a dramatic demonstration of telepresence surgery, Jacques Marescaux utilized this platform to perform a robot-assisted cholecystectomy on a patient in Strasbourg, France, who was separated from the surgeon in New York by 4000 km [23]. This procedure was nicknamed "Operation Lindberg" and lasted for 54 min and had no technical complications.

In almost a parallel path, another group in California, using as the foundation the early works funded by the US Department of Defense on telerobotic surgery, as well as licensed technologies from MIT, IBM, and SRI, set about to develop a surgical robotic system for civilian use. In 1995 Intuitive Surgical International was founded, and this group was eventually able to develop the first FDA-approved fully robotic system for use in minimally invasive surgery, which remains today as the only system in use in minimally invasive general surgery.

References

1. Capek K. The meaning of R.U.R. Saturday Rev 21 July 1923; 136:79.
2. Hockstein NG, Gourtin CG, Faust RA. History of robots: from science fiction to surgical robotics. J Robot Surg. 2007;1:113–8.
3. Kwoh YS, Hou J, Jonekheere EA, Hayall S. A robot with improved absolute positioning accuracy for CT guided stereotactic brain surgery. IEEE Trans Biomed Eng. 1988;35:153.
4. Cowley G. Introducing "Robodoc". A robot finds his calling in the operating room. Newsweek. 1992; 120:86.
5. Nishihara S, Sugano N, Nishii T, Tanaka H, Nakamura N, Yoshikawa H, Ochi T. Clinical accuracy evaluation of femoral canal preparation using the ROBODOC system. J Orthop Sci. 2004;9(5):452–61.
6. Honl M, Dierk O, Gauck C. Comparison of robotic-assisted and manual implantation of a primary total hip replacement. A prospective study. J Bone Joint Surg Am. 2003;85(A(8)):1470–8.
7. Zipper SG, Puschmann H. Nerve injuries after computer assisted hip replacement: case series with 29 patients. Z Orthop Ihre Grenzgeb. 2005;143(4):399–402. German.
8. Harris SJ, Arambula-Cosio F, Mei Q, et al. The Probot—an active robot for procedures. Proc Inst Mech Eng H. 1997;211:317–25.
9. Davies BL, Hibberd RD, Coptcoat MJ, Wickman JEA. A surgeon robot prostatectomy—a laboratory evaluation. J Med Eng Technol. 1989;13:273–7.
10. Paul HA, Bargar WL, Mittlestadt B, et al. Development of a surgical robot for total hip arthroplasty. Clin Orthop Relat Res. 1992;285:57.
11. Ho G, Ng WS, Teo MY. Experimental study of transurethral robotic laser resection of the prostate using the laser Trode lightguide. J Biomed Opt. 2001;6: 244–51.
12. Ho G, Ng WS, Teo MY, Kwoh CK, Cheng WS. Computer- assisted transurethral laser resection of the prostate (CALRP): theoretical and experimental motion plan. IEEE Trans Biomed Eng. 2001;48(10): 1125–33.
13. Patel V. Robotic urologic surgery. 1st ed. London: Springer; 2007.
14. Sackier JM, Wang Y. Robotically assisted laparoscopic surgery: from concept to development. Surg Endosc. 1994;8:63–6.
15. Parekattil SJ, Moran ME. Robotic instrumentation: evolution and microsurgical applications. Indian J Urol. 2010;26(3):395–403. doi:10.4103/0970-1591.70580.
16. Bowersox JC, Shah A, Jensen J, Hill J, Cordts PR, Green PS. Vascular applications of telepresence surgery: initial feasibility studies in swine. J Vasc Surg. 1996;23(2):281–7.
17. Unger SW, Unger HM, Bass RT. AESOP robotic arm. Surg Endosc. 1994;8:1131.
18. Oddsdottir M, Birgison G. AESOP: a voice-controlled camera holder. In: Ballantyne GH, Marescaux J, Giulianotti PC, editors. Primer of robotic and telerobotic surgery. Philadelphia, PA: Lippincott Williams and Wilkins; 2004. p. 35–41.
19. Wang YSJ. Robotically enhanced surgery: from concept to development. Surg Endosc. 1996;8:63–6.
20. Kalan S, Chauhan S, Coelho RF, et al. History of robotic surgery. JRS. 2010;4(3):141–7.
21. Falcone T, Goldberg J, Garcia-Ruiz A, Margossian H, Stevens L. Full robotic for laparoscopic tubal anastomosis: a case report. J Laparoendosc Adv Surg Tech A. 1999;9:107–13.
22. Reichenspurner H, Damiano RJ, Mack M, et al. Use of the voice-controlled and computer-assisted surgical system ZEUS for endoscopic coronary artery bypass grafting. J Thorac Cardiovasc Surg. 1999; 118(1):11–6.
23. Marescaux J, Leroy J, Rubino F, et al. Transcontinental robot-assisted remote telesurgery: feasibility and potential applications. Ann Surg. 2002;235(4):487–92.

Introduction to the Robotic System

2

Monika E. Hagen, Hubert Stein, and Myriam J. Curet

Historical Overview

The da Vinci® Surgical System (Intuitive Surgical Inc., Sunnyvale, CA, USA) is currently the most frequently used computer-enhanced endoscopic instrument control system capable of laparoscopic surgery. The US Food and Drug Administration (FDA) has cleared this system for use in urological surgical procedures, general laparoscopic surgical procedures, gynecologic laparoscopic surgical procedures, transoral otolaryngology surgical procedures restricted to benign and malignant tumors classified as T1 and T2, general thoracoscopic surgical procedures, and thoracoscopically assisted cardiotomy procedures. Additionally, the system is approved to be employed with adjunctive mediastinotomy to perform coronary anastomosis during cardiac revascularization (as of July 2012).

The design of the da Vinci® is the result of a long developmental process which integrated many ideas and technologies to produce a functional system. Much of the early work on telerobotic surgery was funded by the US Department of Defense, with the aim of providing injured soldiers with a frontline surgical suite controlled by surgeons operating from a safe remote location. Although at the time this proved impractical with the technology available, several prototypes showed promise and Intuitive Surgical International was founded in 1995 to license and develop this technology for civilian use. The ultimate goal of the company was to produce a reliable, intuitive system which would deliver the benefits of minimally invasive surgery to patients while preserving the benefits of open surgery to surgeons. The goal was to enable many difficult surgeries (such as cardiac surgery) to be performed through small incisions and also achieve better results for procedures already performed through ports. The technology specifically aimed to address port-access limitations in dexterity, intuitiveness, visualization, and ergonomics through advances in telepresence and stereoscopic capture as well as display.

After securing venture capital, the relevant technologies were licensed from MIT, IBM, and SRI International and a team of engineers set to work on producing a prototype. Initial efforts using off-the-shelf and custom-built components that were passed on from SRI yielded a device

M.E. Hagen, M.D., M.B.A.
Intuitive Surgical International, Sunnyvale, CA, USA

Department of Digestive Surgery, University Hospital Geneva, 14, rue Gabrielle-Perret-Gentil, Geneva 1211, Switzerland
e-mail: monikahagen@aol.com

H. Stein, DIPL.-ING. B.M.T.
Clinical Development Engineering, Intuitive Surgical Inc., 1266 Kifer Road, Sunnyvale, CA 94107, USA
e-mail: Hubert.Stein@intusurg.com

M.J. Curet, M.D. (✉)
Intuitive Surgical International, Sunnyvale, CA, USA

Department of Surgery, Stanford University School of Medicine, Stanford, CA, USA
e-mail: myriam.curet@intusurg.com

K.C. Kim (ed.), *Robotics in General Surgery*, DOI 10.1007/978-1-4614-8739-5_2,

called "Lenny," which was used in animal trials to inform further design. These trials clearly demonstrated the promise of seven-degrees-of-freedom manipulators as well as the need for a mobile patient-side manipulator platform. The next major design iteration was called "Mona," and featured exchangeable sterile components, which allowed human trials to proceed in 1997. The experience gleaned from these trials enabled the design to be refined further into the first generation "da Vinci®" Surgical System platform that is still in use today. In December 1998, the first commercial version was delivered to the Leipzig University Heart Center in Germany.

Further product developments were delayed due to a legal battle with Computer Motion Inc. (Santa Barbara, CA, USA) over intellectual property rights. In 2003, Intuitive Surgical Inc. merged with Computer Motion Inc., and their Zeus telepresence system, which was the competitive product to the da Vinci Surgical System, was discontinued. Refinement of the original da Vinci design continued with the addition of a fourth manipulator arm and expansion of the instrument families. These changes were fully integrated into the simplified and streamlined "da Vinci® S" model, which takes less time to set up and has improved range of motion manipulators; the latest product iteration is the "da Vinci® Si" (released in 2009), which features improvements to the vision and control system and ergonomic improvements and allows two surgeons to share control of manipulators (dual-console mode). This allows all four manipulators to be controlled simultaneously during complex operations and greatly improves the training paradigm for computer-enhanced surgery.

System Overview

The da Vinci® Surgical System is built following an anthropomorphic principle or a humanoid concept. That means that the motion capabilities of the system are designed to mimic those of its human operator. The mechanical components of the system have physical limitations of reach and range of motion. Whenever possible, these limits are designed to meet or exceed the way the human hand and arms work. For instance, the EndoWrist® instrument wrist will run out of ability to flex when the user's wrist is most flexed. In addition, the systems are designed to offer hand–eye alignment which means that the EndoWrist instruments move in the same way with respect to the camera as the hands of the surgeon move with respect to the surgeon's eye. The orientations of the instrument tips mimic the surgeon's hand alignment inside the master controller joysticks. These two properties establish a strong sense of eye-hand coordination and natural, intuitive motion, promulgating the illusion that the robotic instruments are his/her fingers. The EndoWrist instruments that are inserted into the patient move around a fixed point in the body wall that is established by a mechanical remote center concept. This enables the system to maneuver instruments and endoscopes into and within the surgical site while exerting minimal force on the patient's body wall.

Three different commercial models currently exist: the da Vinci Standard System represents the first generation of the da Vinci® Surgical System and was marketed in Europe in late 1998. This model is no longer commercialized, but it is still in use and being supported by Intuitive Surgical. The next generation of da Vinci® Surgical Systems is the da Vinci® S which offers a newer and slimmer robotic arm design that facilitates the surgical cart setup and enables a greater reach within the abdomen when compared to the earlier version. It also contains a superior vision system with HD, a streamlined user interface and some other soft- and hardware innovations. The most current model is the da Vinci® Si Surgical System which was launched in April 2009. The da Vinci® Si introduces several enabling features, including dual-console capability (two surgical consoles can be attached to a single surgical cart) to support training and collaboration during minimally invasive surgery (for details, see Chap. 33), enhanced high-definition 3D vision, improved ergonomics, an updated user interface for streamlined setup and OR turnover, and extensibility for digital OR integration.

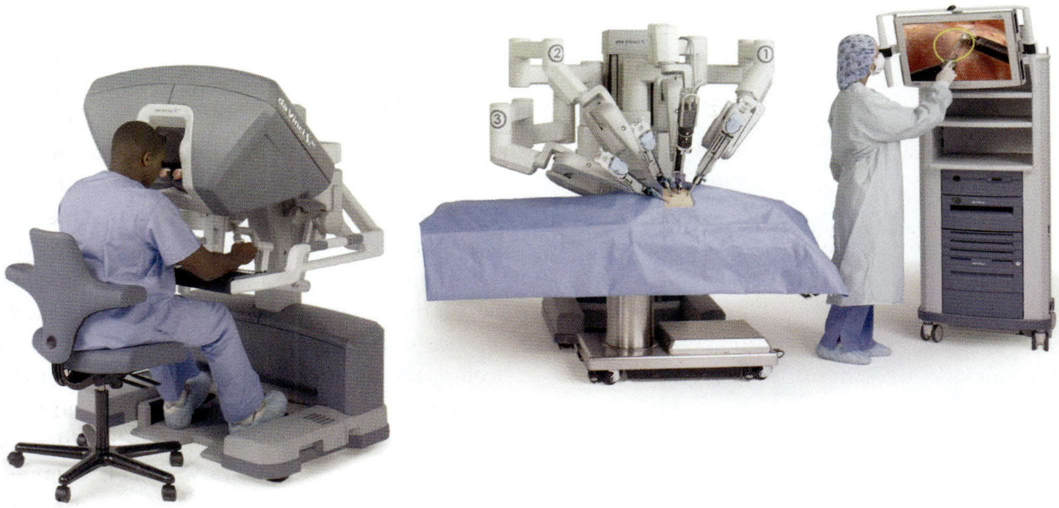

Fig. 2.1 The da Vinci® Surgical System with its main components (courtesy of Intuitive Surgical, Inc.)

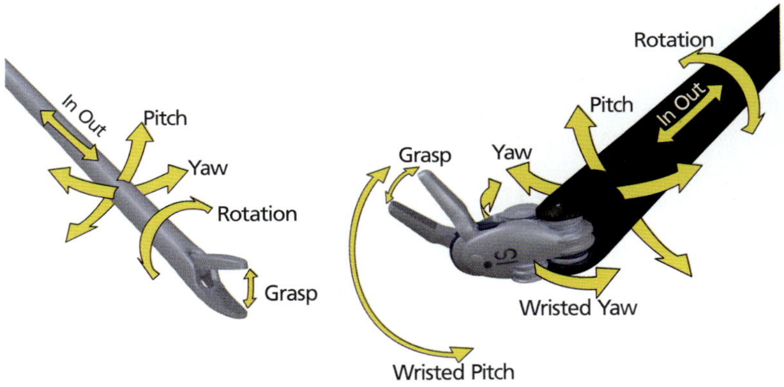

Fig. 2.2 Range of motion of robotic instruments (courtesy of Intuitive Surgical, Inc.)

All above-mentioned systems have three major components: the surgeon's console, the surgical cart, and the vision cart (Fig. 2.1).

The shared core technology of all systems offers the following distinguished features:

- Physical separation of the surgeon from the patient by operating at a console rather than at the patient's side
- A three-dimensional stereoscopic image (HD for the S and Si model) with up to ten times magnification
- Wrist action of the robotic instruments providing seven degrees of freedom (compared with five degrees of freedom for standard laparoscopic instruments), a range of motion greater than the human hand and with intuitive control (Fig. 2.2)
- Software features such as tremor elimination and optional motion scaling up to 3:1

The following description of the main da Vinci® components are based on the da Vinci® Si Surgical System.

The da Vinci® Surgical System: The Surgical Console

The surgical console is the workplace of the robotic surgeon and contains the following core elements: master controllers, stereo viewer,

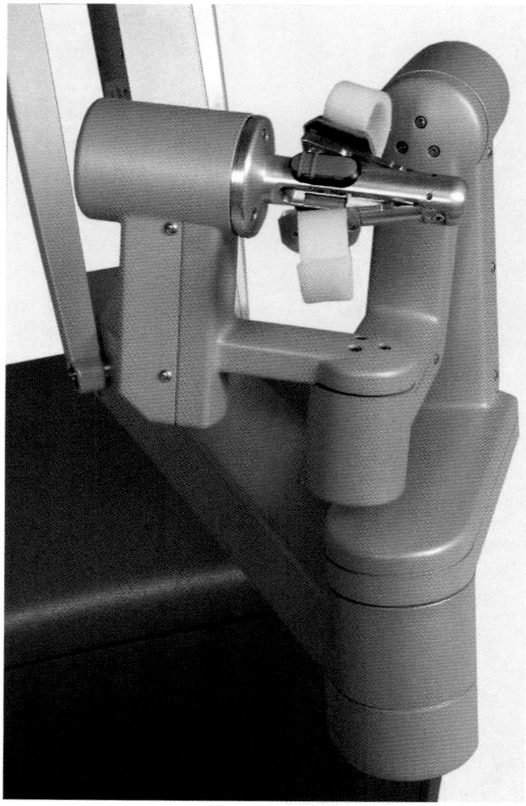

Fig. 2.3 Master controllers (courtesy of Intuitive Surgical, Inc.)

touchpad for preference and feature selection, left-side pod for ergonomic controls, right-side pod for power and emergency stop, and a footswitch panel for operative mode selection and energy actuation.

The *master controllers* (Fig. 2.3) or masters are the joysticks of the robotic surgeon. Two fingers of each hand are placed inside the Velcro straps to control the movements of the patient cart instruments.

The masters are built essentially like a human arm, with a wrist portion (orienting platform) and the elbow/shoulder joints for positioning. The wrist portion orients the instrument tip in the surgical environment. The elbow and shoulder joints move the instrument to the appropriate location in the surgical field and can be scaled to a 3:1 (fine), 2:1 (normal), or 1.5:1 (quick) ratio. The master controllers also possess finger clutches, which decouple the master from control of its instrument to allow for ergonomic repositioning of the master controllers during surgery. Research on learning curves has indicated that appropriately frequent use of master clutching appears to be a crucial part of mastering the da Vinci Surgical System as it results in workspace and ergonomic optimization.

The *stereo viewer* provides the video image to the surgeon including the image of the surgical site and extended system information. With the head in the viewer, the surgeon can view the 3D image in full-screen mode or can choose to swap to TilePro™ mode, which displays the 3D image along with up to two auxiliary images. Icons and text messages are overlaid on the video to provide extended information to the surgeon. The system provides 2-way audio communications with the patient cart operator by a microphone located under the viewport and a pair of speakers located in the headrest.

The *touchpad* is the main control interface at the Surgeon Console for system functions. The touchpad home screen provides system status, including instrument arm selection, and control selections. In dual-console mode, the surgeon can use the touchpad to assign robotic arm control between the two consoles. The center of the touchpad provides three quick setting buttons indicating settings for scope angle, zoom level, and motion scaling.

The *left-side pod* provides the ergonomic adjustment controls for the Surgeon Console. Choosing the correct ergonomic setup is particularly important in order to avoid unnecessary physical strain during the surgical procedure and time should be taken to do so before the actual procedure starts. The *right-side pod* provides Power and Emergency Stop buttons (Fig. 2.4).

The *footswitch panel* (Fig. 2.5) is located at the base of the console directly beneath the surgeon and provides the interface for various system functions without removing the head from the stereo viewer.

The footswitch panel features two groups of footswitches. The three switches on the left control system function such as camera control,

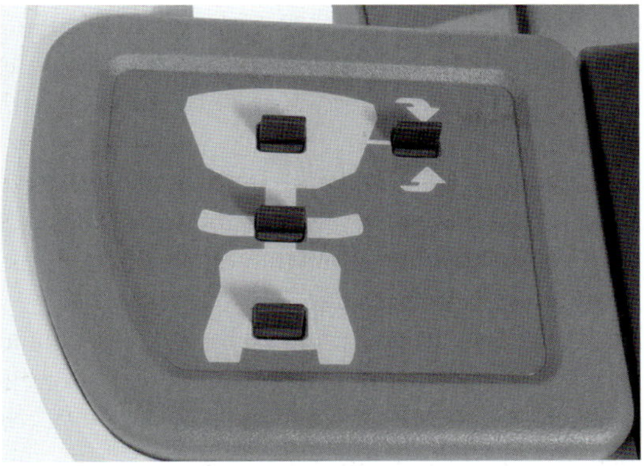

Fig. 2.4 *Left-side* and *right-side* pod (courtesy of Intuitive Surgical, Inc.)

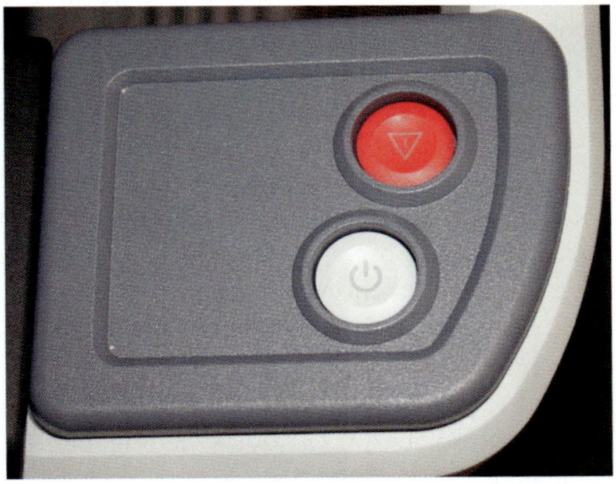

Fig. 2.5 Food switch panel (courtesy of Intuitive Surgical, Inc.)

master clutch, and arm swap. The four pedals on the right side of the footswitch panel are used for energy activation and are arranged as a left pair of pedals and a right pair of pedals. Cautery, ultrasonic shears, suction/irrigation, and other advanced instrumentation are available for control.

The da Vinci® Si Surgical console can be augmented for training by attaching the da Vinci® simulator to its back. For details see Chap. x: simulation. Additionally, up to two surgical consoles can be attached to a single surgical cart for dual-console surgery, which is particularly useful for teaching purposes.

The da Vinci® Surgical System: The Patient Cart

The patient cart (Fig. 2.6) is the operative component of the da Vinci Si System, and its primary function is to support the instrument arms and camera arm. It contains five main components: the setup joints, instrument arms, camera arm, EndoWrist instruments, and an endoscope.

The *setup joints* enable movements of the instrument and the camera arm to position them for sterile draping and docking of the system to the patient. Clutch buttons are used by the patient-side assistants to free the setup joints, which is applied in some cases to readjust instrument arms if needed during the procedure. To help ensure patient safety, any actions of the patient cart operator will always preclude simultaneous telepresence actions from the Surgeon Console operator.

While the *instrument arms* hold the EndoWrist instruments, the camera arm holds the endoscope during surgery. As described above, all arms can be controlled within their range of motion by the surgeon from the surgical console. The setup is performed by the bedside assistant using the clutch buttons to release the setup joints.

EndoWrist instruments are installed onto the instrument arms after the system is docked to ports that are inserted into the patient. Most instruments offer 7 degrees of freedom and ±90 degrees of articulation in the wrist. The arsenal of instruments includes advanced energy instruments (monopolar cautery shears, hooks, spatulas,

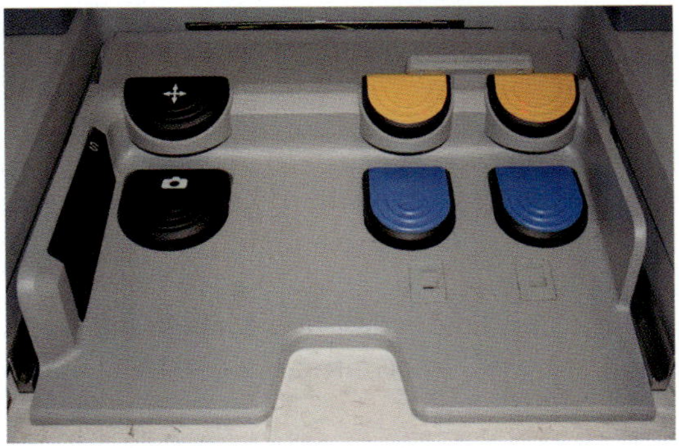

Fig. 2.6 Patient cart (courtesy of Intuitive Surgical, Inc.)

bipolar shears, bipolar graspers, Harmonic™ ACE, PK™ dissecting forceps, and laser), different types of forceps, needle drivers, retractors, and other specialized instruments such as clip appliers, probe graspers, and cardiac stabilizers. The most common instruments have a diameter of 8 mm. A selection of 5 mm instruments is available for use with smaller access ports.

Most instruments contain the following elements:

- A tip that represents the appropriate end effector for a specific surgical task such as different type of graspers, dissectors, cautery tips, and scalpels
- An articulating wrist designed to mimic the wrist of the human hand (some instruments are not wristed as required by the underlying technology, such as the Harmonic™ ACE which is a long ultrasonic horn that cannot be bent)
- A shaft that represents the rotating "arm" of the instrument and through which the motive force is transferred from the robotic arms to the wrist tips
- Release levers which are the mechanism for removal of the instrument
- An instrument housing which is the portion of the instrument that engages with the sterile adapter of the instrument arm

The EndoWrist instruments are reposable, which means that the main component needs to be replaced after a certain number of surgeries.

The *da Vinci® Si HD Vision System* uses a 12 mm or 8.5 mm 3D rod lens endoscope with either a straight (0°) or angled (30°) tip. Light from the illuminator is sent down the shaft of the endoscope via fiber optics and projected onto the surgical site. The video image of the surgical site captured by the endoscope is sent back through the left and right channels to the camera head. The camera head connects to the camera control unit, as well as the illuminator. In keeping with the anthropomorphic principle, the endoscope contains two separate optical chains and focusing elements, and the camera head contains two separate cameras. When displayed on two monitors to the left and right eye of the surgeon, a true and natural 3D image is recreated.

The da Vinci® Surgical System: The Vision Cart

The vision cart (Fig. 2.7) houses the system's central processing and vision equipment. It includes a 24″ touch screen monitor used to control system settings and view the surgical image.

It also provides adjustable shelves for optional ancillary surgical equipment such as insufflators and electrosurgical generators. The da Vinci® Si core on the vision cart is the system's central connection point where all system, auxiliary equipment, and audiovisual connections are routed. The core also is the "brain" of the system where all computer calculations are processed to control

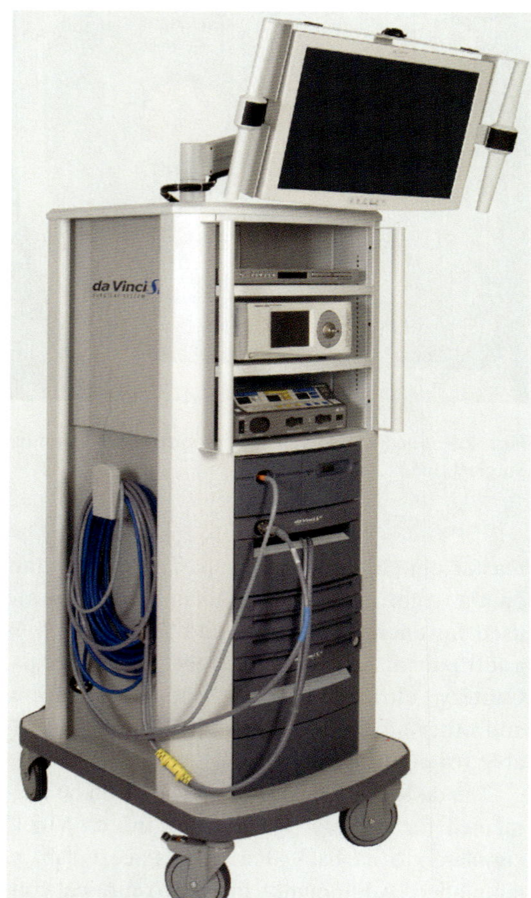

Fig. 2.7 Vision cart (courtesy of Intuitive Surgical, Inc.)

the motions of the instruments inside the body. An integrated illuminator on the vision cart provides lighting for the surgical field. A camera control unit on the vision cart is connected to the camera and controls the acquisition and processing of the image from the camera.

Conclusion

The da Vinci Surgical System is a success story of visionary concepts brought into wide clinical adoption to improve clinical outcomes through the interdisciplinary work of many different specialties. However, this is just the beginning of an exciting journey that might change the surgical landscape sustainably. New robotic platforms for the use in surgical specialties will emerge down the line and distinct new features will enable more procedures to be performed with the help of computer-enhanced systems. Further technology adopted into currently existing or new robotic platforms will evolve and transform these systems into surgical cockpits that hold the promise of becoming the central workstation of surgical care. Integrated diagnostics and real-time imaging will enhance training, diagnostic assessment, and therapeutic treatment in unforeseen new ways for the benefit of many patients in the years to come.

Overview of General Advantages, Limitations, and Strategies

3

Erik B. Wilson, Hossein Bagshahi, and Vicky D. Woodruff

For centuries surgical technique remained relatively unchanged despite an improved understanding of medicine. Only 30 years ago, the general surgeon's work spanned the abdomen, chest, neck, and soft tissues, but in the late 1980s, minimally invasive surgery (MIS) segmented general surgery into sub-specializations and challenged the general surgeon to learn new skill sets to take advantage of the innovative tech tools. More recently, the explosion of robotic technology is poised to repeat further segmentation and challenges the surgeon to adopt an even more advanced skill set to keep pace with more advanced technology that overcomes obstacles as rapidly as they are encountered [1]. This is especially so for single incision or no incision procedures. Robotic technology now enjoys a presence in cardiology, electrophysiology, neurology, gynecology, urology, bariatric, pediatrics, orthopedics, and radiosurgery. This introduction reviews general advantages and limitations related to technical and clinical aspects, strategies of robotics, and the future of robotics.

E.B. Wilson, M.D. (✉)
Department of Surgery, The University of Texas Health Science Center, 6431 Fannin Street MSB4.162, Houston, TX 77030, USA
e-mail: erik.b.wilson@uth.tmc.edu

H. Bagshahi, M.D.
Department of Surgery, Harris Methodist Hospital, of Fort Worth, 800 Fifth Avenue, Suite 404, Fort Worth, TX 76104, USA

Reshape Bariatric and General Surgery of Fort Worth, 800 Fifth Avenue, Suite 404, Fort Worth, TX 76104, USA
e-mail: hbagshahi@gmail.com

V.D. Woodruff, B.A., B.S., Ph.D.
Department of Surgery, University of Texas Health Science Center, 6431 Fannin Street, Suite 4.294, Houston, TX 77030, USA
e-mail: vicky.woodruff@uth.tmc.edu

Technical Advantages of Robotics

In general, the development of robotic surgery with Intuitive Surgical's da Vinci platform has successfully built on the advantages of laparoscopic surgery and overcome its fundamental limitations allowing completion of complex and advanced surgical procedures with increased precision in a minimally invasive approach [2–4]. Technical advantages of robotics are plenteous and embrace mechanical improvements, surgery via telecommunication systems, and safe simulation systems that allow skill training prior to actual human procedures.

Improved mechanical advantages include enhanced stabilized three-dimensional stereoscopic vision of the operative field, boost visual sharpness, and depth perception beyond the standard laparoscopic monitor. Additionally, the ability to digitally zoom without sacrificing clarity provides greater confidence in preciseness of surgical dissection and reconstruction. The increased maneuverability of articulating wrist instruments created additional degrees of freedom from five movements to seven, improving the surgeons' dexterity and allowing greater precision in the

K.C. Kim (ed.), *Robotics in General Surgery*, DOI 10.1007/978-1-4614-8739-5_3,

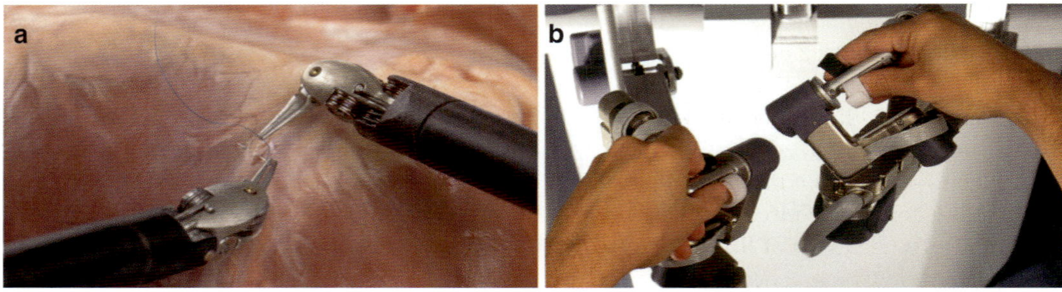

Fig. 3.1 Freedom of (**a**) movement and (**b**) instrumentation

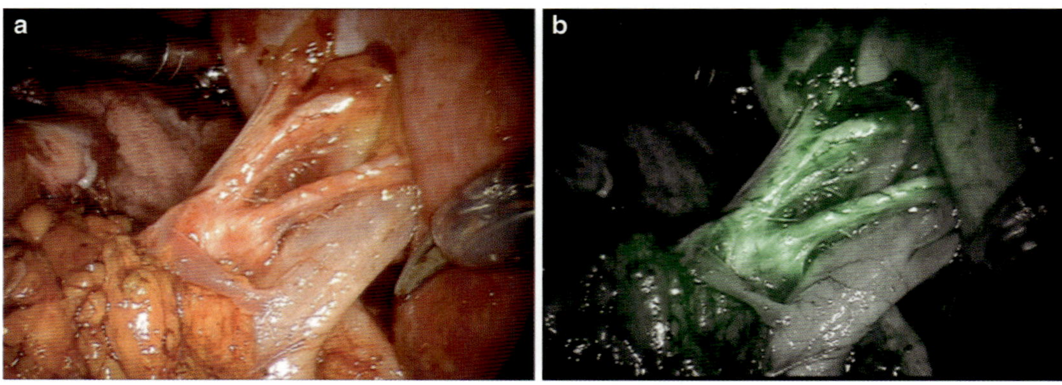

Fig. 3.2 (**a**) White light and (**b**) fluorescent imaging

surgical field, which more closely mimics open surgery (Fig. 3.1a, b). Coupled with this technology, hand stabilization eliminates surgeon tremor and allows for refinement of scaled movements.

This gives the surgeon the capability of adjusting the degree of precision of his or her motions from bold to very fine. One of the newest additions to the platform is a new integrated fluorescence imaging capability that provides real-time, image-guided identification of key anatomical landmarks using near-infrared technology (Fig. 3.2a, b). This allows the surgeon to visualize the end perfusion of the tissue of interest.

Linking the robot to a telecommunication device creates two new revolutionary applications. The SOCRATES system achieves a "telepresence" surgery with "telerobotic" and "telementoring" capability [5, 6]. In a telerobotic procedure, the surgeon, operating from a console miles away from the slave robot, guides the procedure via fiber-optic cable. In 2001, the first major transatlantic surgery via telerobotic presence was a cholecystectomy performed by robot in Strasbourg, France, by surgeons in New York, NY [7, 8]. Since then, many telerobotic operations have been performed allowing surgeons to operate where their skills are needed without being in the direct presence of the patient. Proponents of telerobotic surgery tout the beneficial delivery of surgical care in medically underserved areas [9, 10]. However, the cost of a surgical robot (>$1 million) is beyond the financial ability of many medically underserved areas, but when finances are not limiting, robotic surgery presents the potential for delivering surgical care to patients who have no direct access to a surgeon [11, 12]. In telementoring, two surgeons located a distance away "share" the view of the surgical field and control the robotic system, communicating via microphones. This system has advantages for teaching surgical skills to fellows, junior surgeons, and advanced medical students all around the world by expert colleagues [13–15].

A robotic simulation system provides a medium for anyone to acquire or refine their surgical skills, thus reducing the learning curve and surgical error [5]. Utilizing the 3D, virtual reality of the simulator, visual simulations, and soft tissue models recreate the textures of human tissues through forced feedback haptics [15, 16]. Image-guided simulations of the anatomy of the actual patient allow for practice of planned reconstructions prior to the actual procedure [17–19]. Since all surgical movements in both simulation sessions and actual surgery are automatically captured as objective precise data measurements by the robotic system, they can be utilized as a means for establishing surgical proficiency criteria, measuring quality improvement in surgical skill; provide hospitals quality measures on surgeons; and as best practice for educational instruction. In due course, simulation training may be integrated into surgical course work and licensing of surgeons to provide an objective means for assessment of surgical effectiveness.

Clinical Advantages

Clinical advantages for robotic surgery touch the patient, the surgical institution, and the healthcare insurer. Due to greater precision, smaller incisions, lack of fatigue during extended operative procedures, reduction of blood loss, less pain, quicker healing time, and a reduction of complications, benefits such as reduced duration of hospital stays, transfusions, and use of pain medications are common. Patients undergoing robotic procedures typically return to normal activity faster and experience very low mortality and morbidity events [1]. The advantage of multiple robotic arms that do not become fatigued, hold instruments steady, and provide constant strength in holding selected tissue opens greater surgical opportunity to the morbidly obese patient or patient with difficult anatomy (usually due to scaring or altered anatomy from prior abdominal surgeries) and allows multiple teams of surgeons to seamlessly and effortlessly transition during extended procedures, making wider range of procedures more realistic.

Technical and clinical advantages of robotics have been well documented, and safety has been substantially established with many series of cases reporting favorable outcomes [20–23]. Robotic technology is expected to play an increasingly important role in the future of surgery.

Limitations in Robotics: Technical and Clinical

Technical limitations form the drawback for the majority of resistance to robotic surgery. Near the top of the list is the decreased tactile feedback sense. It remains that the robot is still a self-powered, computer-controlled device not intended to act independently from human surgeons or to replace them [1, 3, 11]. Although true "feel" of tissues has yet to be realized, there are some crude haptics that occur if the instruments bump or hit each other (usually due to poor trocar placement or planning), transmitting a tactile sensation back to the surgeon's console finger apparatus. Otherwise, the surgeon must maintain visual contact through the monitor to guide the instrumentation and ensure appropriate and safe manipulation is preserved. It has been our experience that with time working with the robot, it may become possible for visual cues to become so strong a faux tactile sensation can be realized.

The size of the available robotic instruments becomes a real limitation in certain surgical specialties. For example, the trocar and instrument size in relation to the pediatric patient may prevent its advantage in this population. In otorhinolaryngology and head and neck surgery, this small area of accessibility also limits the use of robotics.

More minor technical limitations include the bulkyness of the robot, extended time to set it up in position for activity, and difficulty traversing wide fields. While bulkyness may be a valid issue in a small operating space, the time to set up can through practice be reduced to less than 5 min. Traversing multiple quadrants has been addressed through alternate positioning of the robot at the head of the patient and a specific five or six trocar placement system that avoids patient repositioning (cite book1).

Clinical Limitations

Although rapidly overcoming technical limitations, robotic surgical technology has yet to achieve its full potential due to substantial clinical limitations. Undoubtedly, the greatest clinical limitation is the cost of the robot system. Two studies comparing robotic procedures with conventional operations showed that although the absolute cost for robotic operations was higher, the major part of the increased cost was attributed to the initial cost of purchasing the robot [24, 25]. Coming in at over $2 million, $500–$1,500/case in disposable costs, maintenance cost upward to $100,000/year, and robotic instruments limited to a fixed number of uses (unrelated to instrument wear), the cumulative cost is prohibitive to most healthcare organizations. Even in the USA, surgical robots are chiefly limited in availability to hospital systems and large academic centers. Factors such as more wide spread acceptance, decreased operative times, complications, and hospital stay will contribute to the cost-effectiveness. Conversely, further technical advances may at first drive prices even higher. Although there is research and development currently underway to develop indefinitely reusable instruments, until then the robot remains a major capital expense to the bottom line. It has been estimated that the sum of these costs each year is approximately 10 % of the capital acquisition cost [24, 25]. The cost factor also becomes prohibitive to the spread of telerobotic technology to underserved areas that need it most. Studies to determine the cost over time vs. reduction of morbidities and mortalities and associated collateral costs are needed to better evaluate the long-term cost/benefit ratio. Ultimately, it is felt that competition and marketing of various robotic systems such as the Amadeus from Titan Medical, Inc. (Canada), the ARAKNES robot from SSSA BioRobotics Institute and Surgical Robotics S.p.a.'s Surgenius (both from Italy), the DLR system (Germany), and Mazor Robotics Ltd's SpineAssist (Israel) may drive costs down.

Another major limitation is that performance of robotic procedures requires specialized training. A chief complaint is the steep learning curve to become proficient in the needed technical skills. While a hybrid laparoscopic and robotic approach has been suggested, nothing can substitute time logged on the simulator or the actual robot [1]. However, the majority of hospitals, fellowships, and residency programs in the USA do not provide formal training in robotic surgery skills. This glaring deficit of development in surgical technology needs to be addressed as robotics is likely to reshape the way we practice surgery.

A review of residency programs in the USA shows an inadequate emphasis on training in robotic surgery [11]. A 2002 survey reported 23 % of surgical program directors have plans to incorporate robotics into their programs [26]. Sadly, the same survey group also reported that although 57 % of surgical residents indicated a high interest in robotic surgery, 80 % did not have a robotic training program at their institution [27]. Currently, individual hospitals bear the burden of ensuring competency to perform robotic procedures. There is a glaring need for standardized credentials to be developed and required to obtain robotic surgical privileges.

In conjunction with training, documentation and publishing of clinical randomized controlled trials comparing robotic-assisted procedures with laparoscopic or open techniques are needed to inform data-driven decisions for the surgeon, hospital administrator, and medical education institutions in regard to cost, training, and clinical effectiveness of robotics.

Robotic surgery, while still in a relatively early stage, is on a continuous journey that will have substantial implications for the future of surgery. This emerging technology allows surgeons to perform operations that were not so long ago, impossible, tedious, visually and physically challenging, replete with complications, and not amenable to minimal access techniques. The future of robotics is yet to be fully written but is already holding great promise.

Future of Robotics

The future of robotics is poised to include earth, under the sea, and space—the great frontier. In 2005, studies were already underway by the National Aeronautics and Space Administration

(NASA) for robotic application in emergency surgery on astronauts in a submarine to simulate conditions in space [28]. The project is called NEEMO 7. Additionally, testing telerobotic capabilities, the Pentagon also invested $12 million in a project using a "trauma pod" surgical robot. The system tests the ability to evacuate wounded soldiers under enemy fire and then operate on them [11, 29]. To address the size limitations of instruments and versatility, the University of Nebraska Medical Center has led a multicampus effort to provide collaborative research on mini-robotics among surgeons, engineers, and computer scientists [30].

Although surgical robotics is growing, the market is yet to be fully matured. Concerns regarding costs, standardization for evaluating surgeon skill level, robotic education to the medical student, and other challenges remain; however, as more industry investments are made and more competition develops for robotic systems, robotics will become the primary mechanism for surgical interaction with the patient. The digital platform will allow for infinite opportunities to produce learning avenues, a higher quality surgeon, and make surgery safer, better, faster, and ultimately cheaper.

References

1. Wilson EB. The evolution of robotic general surgery. Scand J Surg. 2009;98(2):125–9.
2. Wilson EB, Snyder B, Yu S, et al. Robotic bariatric surgery outcomes with laparoscopic biliopancreatic diversion and gastric bypass. Presentation. Washington, DC: American Society of Metabolic and Bariatric Surgery; 2008.
3. Yu SC, Clapp BL, Lee MJ, et al. Robotic assistance provides excellent outcomes during the learning curve for laparoscopic Roux-en-Y bypass: result from 100 robotic assisted gastric bypasses. Am J Surg. 2006;192(6):746–9.
4. Stephen W, Eubanks MD, Eubanks S (editor), Lee L, Swanstrom MD (editor), Soper NJ (editor). Mastery of endoscopic and laparoscopic surgery. 2nd ed. Lippincott Williams & Wilkins; 2004.
5. Gomez G. Emerging technology in surgery: informatics, electronics, robotics. In: Townsend CM, Beauchamp RD, Evers BM, Maddox KL, editors. Sabiston textbook of surgery. 17th ed. Philadelphia, PA: Elsevier Saunders; 2004.
6. Ballantyne GH. Robotic surgery, telerobotic surgery, telepresence, and telementoring. Review of early clinical results. Surg Endosc. 2002;16:1389–402. Abstract.
7. Marescaux J, Leroy J, Gagner M, et al. Transatlantic robot-assisted telesurgery. Nature. 2001;413:379–80. Abstract.
8. Marescaux J, Rubino F. Robot-assisted remote surgery: technological advances, potential complications, and solutions. Surg Technol Int. 2004;12:23–6. Abstract.
9. Marescaux J, Leroy J, Rubino F, et al. Transcontinental robot-assisted remote telesurgery: feasibility and potential applications. Ann Surg. 2002;235:487–92. Abstract.
10. Anvari M, McKinley C, Stein H. Establishment of the world's first telerobotic remote surgical service: for provision of advanced laparoscopic surgery in a rural community. Surg Laparosc Endosc Percutan Tech. 2002;12:17–25. Abstract.
11. Morris B. Robotic surgery: applications, limitations, and impact on surgical education, MBBCH (Hons). Med Gen Med. 2005;7(3):72.
12. Ballantyne GH. The pitfalls of laparoscopic surgery: challenges for robotics and telerobotic surgery. Surg Laparosc Endosc Percutan Tech. 2002;12:1–5. Abstract.
13. Bove P, Stoianovici D, Micali S, et al. Is telesurgery a new reality? Our experience with laparoscopic and percutaneous procedures. J Endourol. 2003;17: 137–42. Abstract.
14. Marescaux J, Rubino F. Telesurgery, telementoring, virtual surgery, and telerobotics. Curr Urol Rep. 2003;4:109–13. Abstract.
15. Suzuki S, Suzuki N, Hayashibe M, et al. Tele-surgical simulation system for training in the use of da Vinci surgery. Stud Health Technol Inform. 2005;111: 543–8. Abstract.
16. Satava RM. Virtual reality, telesurgery, and the new world order of medicine. J Image Guid Surg. 1995;1:12–6. Abstract.
17. Weiss H, Ortmaier T, Maass H, Hirzinger G, Kuehnapfel U. A virtual-reality-based haptic surgical training system. Comput Aided Surg. 2003;8:269–72. Abstract.
18. Marescaux J, Solerc L. Image-guided robotic surgery. Semin Laparosc Surg. 2004;11:113–22. Abstract.
19. Hattori A, Suzuki N, Hayashibe M, Suzuki S, Otake Y, Tajiri H, Kobayashi S. Development of navigation function for an endoscopic robot surgery system. Stud Health Technol Inform. 2005;111:167–71. Abstract.
20. Tieu K, Allison N, Snyder B, Wilson T, Toder M, Wilson E. Robotic-assisted Roux-en-Y gastric bypass update from 2 high-volume centers. Surg Obes Relat Dis. 2012;9(2):284–8.
21. Weinstein GS, O'Malley Jr BW, Magnuson JS, Carroll WR, Olsen KD, Daio L, Moore EJ, Holsinger FC. Transoral robotic surgery: a multicenter study to assess feasibility, safety, and surgical margins. Laryngoscope. 2012;122(8):1701–7.
22. Hu Y, Zhang J, Li C, Cheng S, Wang L, Zhang J. Robotics and Biomimetics. In: ROBIO 2008. IEEE International Conference on 1 Jan 2009. 2008.
23. Yi O, Yoon JH, Lee Y-M, Sung T-Y, Chung K-W, Kim TY, Kim WB, Shong YK, Ryu J-S, Hong SJ. Meta-

analysis of observational studies on the safety and effectiveness of robotic gynaecological surgery. Br J Surg. 2010;97:1772–178.
24. Morgan JA, Thornton BA, Peacock JC, et al. Does robotic technology makes minimally invasive cardiac surgery too expensive? A hospital cost analysis of robotic and conventional techniques. J Card Surg. 2005;20:246–51. Abstract.
25. Lotan Y, Cadeddu JA, Gettman MT. The new economics of radical prostatectomy: cost comparison of open, laparoscopic and robot assisted techniques. J Urol. 2004;172:1431–5. Abstract.
26. Donias HW, Karamanoukian RL, Glick PL, Bergsland J, Karamanoukian HL. Survey of resident training in robotic surgery. Am Surg. 2002;68:177–81. Abstract.
27. Patel YR, Donias HW, Boyd DW, et al. Are you ready to become a robo-surgeon? Am Surg. 2003;69:599–603.
28. National Aeronautics and Space Administration (NASA). Behind the scenes: NEEMO 7: NASA Extreme Environment Mission Operations expedition. http://spaceflight.nasa.gov/shuttle/support/training/neemo/neemo7/. Accessed 7 Sep 2005.
29. Pentagon invests in using robots to operate on wounded soldiers. USA Today. http://www.usatoday.com/news/washington/2005-03-28-trauma-pod_x.htm. Accessed 2 May 2013.
30. Dmitry Oleynikov, Stephen Platt, Shane Farritor. Before they did their research, they did their research. Retrieved 050613 from: http://www.nebraska.edu/docs/newfrontiers/ResearchAd.pdf

Part II

Surgical Techniques: *Esophagus*

Robotic Assisted Minimally Invasive Esophagectomy

4

Abbas E. Abbas and Mark R. Dylewski

Introduction

The esophagus is an organ that traverses three body cavities, hence the difficulty and possible morbidity associated with esophagectomy. Resecting the esophagus always requires accessing the peritoneal space, in addition to either a direct approach to the intrathoracic esophagus as in trans-thoracic esophagectomy (TTE) or an indirect dissection of this portion of the esophagus as in transhiatal esophagectomy (THE). Multiple approaches have arisen for this operation but no one technique has been universally accepted as the standard. In fact, with the advent of minimally invasive techniques in the latter part of the twentieth century, there have been even more techniques described for esophagectomy. The most-commonly performed procedures for esophagectomy include:

1. *Ivor Lewis TTE procedure*: which incorporates a laparotomy for gastric mobilization and tubularization followed by a right thoracotomy for completion of the esophageal resection and creation of an intrathoracic esophagogastric anastomosis.
2. *THE*: this also includes a laparotomy as described for TTE in addition to a cervicotomy. Mobilization of the intrathoracic esophagus is done through the hiatus and the neck, mostly in a blunt fashion. The anastomosis is made at the neck.
3. *McKeown esophagectomy (MKE)* or the "3-hole esophagectomy": attempts to provide a more radical approach to the procedure. A right thoracotomy is made for dissection of the entire thoracic esophagus and mediastinal lymph nodes. This is followed by a laparotomy as described above and a cervicotomy. The gastric conduit is delivered to the neck as in THE where a cervical esophagogastrostomy is performed. This approach allows the potential for a three-field lymphadenectomy of the entire lymph node basin of the esophagus, in the neck, thorax, and abdomen. It also allows removal of most of the esophagus, leaving only a short proximal segment to complete the anastomosis.
4. *Left thoracotomy or left thoracoabdominal approach*: this is less commonly used than the above-mentioned procedures. It allows resection of only the distal esophagus. The stomach is mobilized either through an incision in the left diaphragm or through an extension of the thoracotomy across the costal margin. After the specimen is resected, the esophagogastrostomy is performed in the left chest.

A.E. Abbas, M.D.
Department of Surgery, Ochsner Clinic Foundation, 1514 Jefferson Highway, New Orleans, LA 70121, USA
e-mail: aabbas@ochsner.org

M.R. Dylewski, M.D. (✉)
Department of Cardiac Vascular and Thoracic Surgery, Baptist Health of South Florida, 6200 SW 72nd Street, Suite 604, Miami, FL 33143, USA
e-mail: markd@baptisthealth.net

K.C. Kim (ed.), *Robotics in General Surgery*, DOI 10.1007/978-1-4614-8739-5_4,

Table 4.1 Published reports on robotic esophagectomy

Horgan et al. [1]	2003	1	Hybrid	RATS + laparoscopy	THE
Dapri et al. [2]	2006	2	Hybrid	RATS + Laparoscopy	MKE
Gutt et al. [3]	2006	1	Hybrid	Robotic laparoscopy	THE
Kernstine et al. [4]	2007	14	Mix of hybrid (6) and totally robotic (8)	RATS + laparotomy, laparoscopy, RALS	MKE
Kim et al. [5]	2010	21	Hybrid	RATS + Laparoscopy	MKE
Sutherland et al. [6]	2011	36	Hybrid	Robotic laparoscopy	THE
Puntambekar et al. [7]	2011	32	Hybrid	RATS + Laparoscopy	MKE
Weksler et al. [8]	2011	17	Hybrid	RATS + laparoscopy	ILE

RATS robotic assisted thoracoscopic surgery, *RALS* robotic assisted laparoscopic surgery, *THE* transhiatal esophagectomy, *MKE* McKeown esophagectomy, *ILE* Ivor Lewis esophagectomy

Each of the above procedures except perhaps for the left thoracotomy approach has been described in a "minimally invasive" fashion. Thoracoscopy and laparoscopy may replace thoracotomy and laparotomy, and in the hands of surgeons experienced in these techniques, may offer results that are equivalent to those achieved by their traditional open counterparts while still providing all the established benefits of minimally invasive surgery.

More recently, robotic technology has entered the arena of minimally invasive surgery. The benefits of dexterous dissection and manipulation in a confined space make it ideal for esophageal dissection in the mediastinum. In the abdomen, the ability of the surgeon to handle and manipulate the stomach with excellent visualization allows the safe creation of the conduit. Robotic surgery has allowed fine dissection of lymph nodes with better precision than traditional endoscopic techniques.

The first published report of a robotic-assisted esophagectomy is that by Horgan et al. [1] who described a transhiatal approach. Table 4.1 summarizes several published reports for robotic esophagectomy. Most reported series have described hybrid techniques with robotic-assisted thoracoscopy in addition to laparotomy or laparoscopy [2, 4, 5]. Others have described a robotic-assisted THE with cervical esophago-gastrostomy [3, 6]. Few reports have described totally robotic laparoscopic and thoracoscopic approach [4].

Debating the merits of each approach is beyond the scope of this chapter, which focuses on the applicability of robotics to esophagectomy. The preferred approach by both authors is that of the totally endoscopic robotic-assisted three-field approach, or a robotic MKE procedure. The technique described is that employed in the vast majority of our patients with esophageal cancer or end-stage benign esophageal disease.

Technique

1. Anesthesia (Fig. 4.1):

   All patients are done under general anesthesia with endotracheal intubation. A 8 mm single lumen endotracheal tube is utilized through which a right-sided bronchial blocker is placed. This blocker is used for the thoracic portion of the procedure, after which it is simply removed and the remainder of the case is done with double lung ventilation. Esophagogastroscopy is performed by the surgeon to confirm location of the tumor and clear the esophagus and stomach of any retained contents. It is important to avoid excessive insufflation of the stomach, which would hinder the abdominal exposure and may affect mucosal integrity. A nasogastric tube is then passed and connected to low intermittent wall suction to keep the stomach decompressed. There is no need for placement of an epidural catheter as most patients can be easily managed

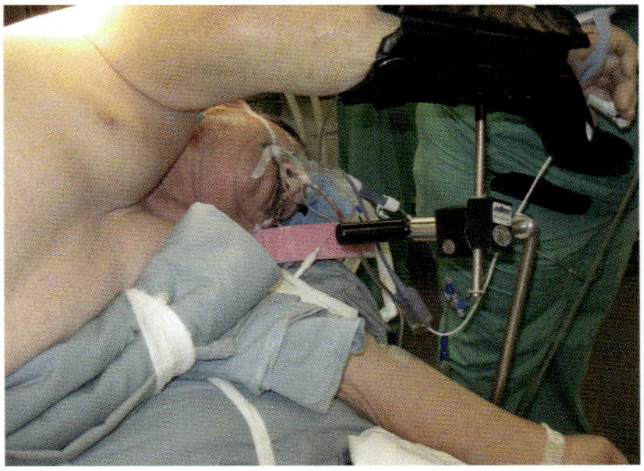

Fig. 4.1 Patient intubated with right bronchial blocker and nasogastric tube

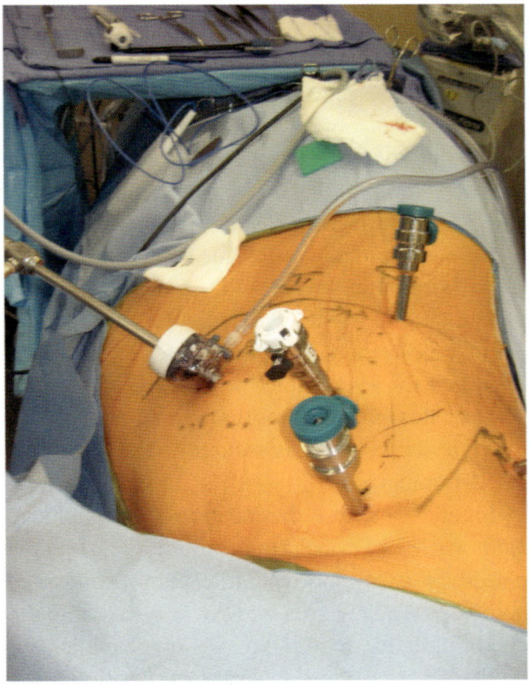

Fig. 4.2 Right thoacoscopic ports

with routine parenteral non-opioids. Early extubation is strongly recommended.

2. Right Robotic Assisted Thoracoscopic Surgery (RRATS):

The patient is then placed in the left lateral position with slight flexion and slight anterior tilting. A total of four ports are placed (Fig. 4.2).

The first is a 12 mm port at the seventh intercostal space (ICS), just anterior to the anterior axillary line. A 5 or 10 mm thoracoscope is placed and after ensuring intrathoracic placement of the port, carbon dioxide insufflation of the pleural space is administered to a maximum pressure of 10 mmHg. The standard thoracoscope is then utilized to assist in proper placement of the other three ports. A 8.5 mm port is placed for the robotic camera at the sixth ICS, mid-axillary line. It is important to avoid placing this port too far posteriorly. Ideally this port will be at the mid-point of the thoracic esophagus, about 2 in. below the azygous vein arch. Following this an 8 mm port is placed in the third ICS, mid-axillary line for the right arm and am 8 mm port is placed in the ninth intercostal space at the mid-axillary line also (this one can be slightly more posterior). Before placing the latter three ports, it is helpful to pass a needle percutaneously at the proposed sites and using the thoracoscope to confirm adequacy of location. The standard guideline of ensuring at least a hand's breadth between ports is important to avoid arm-collision.

For the thoracic dissection, the right arm (#1) will alternate using the robotic harmonic scalpel and the bipolar Maryland dissector while the left arm (#2) will use mainly the Caudier forceps for retraction. The assistant at the bedside will assist in providing suction and in passing the stapler. The lung is retracted anteriorly and the inferior pulmonary ligament is divided. The mediastinal pleura are then divided longitudinally both anterior and posterior to the esophagus up to the level of the azygous vein arch. The vein is then dissected free and divided using the endo-GIA stapler with a vascular load. Above the divided vein, it is important not to divide the pleura and to let it remain as a "tent" to overlie the eventual conduit. This may help wall off any cervical anastomotic leakage from the chest. The esophagus is then dissected circumferentially to include all the lymphatics and fatty tissue in-between the azygous vein, aorta and pericardium. The harmonic scalpel is helpful in dividing the aortic esophageal branches. This dissection must include a complete mediastinal nodal dissection.

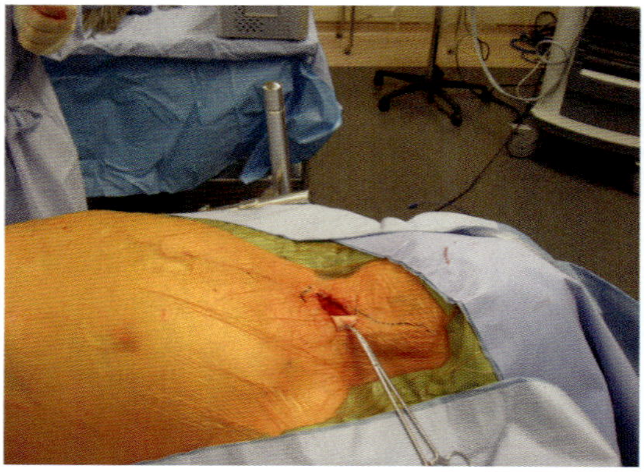

Fig. 4.3 Left cervicotomy and delivery of penrose drain

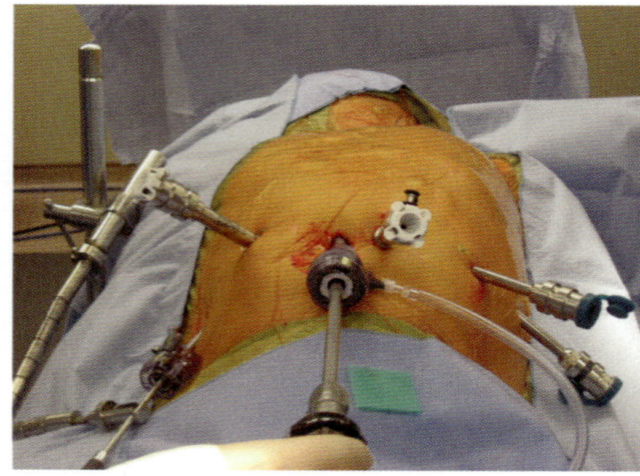

Fig. 4.4 Laparoscopic ports

Stations 7, 8 and 9 are left on the esophagus, while stations 2 and 4 are removed separately. After completing the dissection of the thoracic esophagus in its entirety, a penrose drain is placed to encircle it at both the thoracic inlet and outlet of the esophagus. These drains help in identifying the esophagus in the next stages of the operation. A flexible 19 F drain is then placed along the posterior esophageal gutter. This drain may be secured to the pleura with an absorbable suture to avoid its dislodgement with ventilation. The instruments are then removed and the robot is undocked.

3. Left Cervicotomy:

The patient is then positioned supine and a foam roll is placed under the left shoulder as well as under the left flank. A 4 cm incision is made along the inferior anterior border of the left sternocleidomastoid muscle. A careful circumferential dissection of the cervical esophagus is then made with care to avoid injuring the left recurrent laryngeal nerve. This dissection is carried down to the level of the Penrose drain, which was previously placed at the thoracic inlet. This drain is then partially delivered through the wound (Fig. 4.3).

4. Robotic Assisted Laparoscopic Surgery (RALS):

Following this, standard laparoscopic technique is used to establish a pneumoperitoneum. The authors prefer a Verres needle through the umbilicus. We then proceed to place a 12 mm port just above the umbilicus and again use a laparoscope to aid in correct placement of the robotic ports using a percutaneous needle before committing to the location of the port. Four other ports are placed. An 8.5 mm port for the camera at the left paramedian line, about 1 in. above the level of the umbilicus and below the lowest point of the greater curve of the stomach. Two 8 mm ports are placed in the left flank (#3) and the left midclavicular line (#2), at about the same horizontal level. A 13 mm port (#1) is placed at the right midclavicular line, about 7 cm below the costal margin. The preferred approach for liver retraction is used. The author places a flexible retractor through a 5 mm port in the right flank, which is secured to the table with a self-retainer.

Figure 4.4 shows the location of the abdominal ports. Before docking the robot, the patient is placed in a reverse Trendelenburg position to help keep the omentum and bowel away from the operating field.

The #3 arm is used mainly for retraction using atraumatic double fenestrated robotic clamp. The #2 arm or right hand will alternate the Harmonic scalpel and any other instruments such as the Bipolar Maryland dissector or a needle holder as the need arises. The #1 arm will mainly use the Caudier forceps to assist in dissection. Dissection is begun by dividing the gastrohepatic ligament and the peritoneum along the edges of the diaphragmatic hiatus. It is helpful to delay complete division of the phrenoesophageal ligament until the end of the gastric mobilization to avoid loss of pneumoperitoneal pressure and also avoid creating a pneumothorax. The short gastric vessels are then divided using the Harmonic scalpel. After visualizing and confirming the location of the right gastroepiploic arcade, the greater omentum is divided just lateral to the right gastroepiploic vessels along the entire length of the arcade. This requires division of several omental branches and it is important to always confirm that the main vessels are not injured during this procedure especially in cases with excessive omental fat. The attachments of the hepatic flexure are divided to allow exposure of the duodenum. Gentle "kocherization" of the duodenum is then done. This promotes a tension-free gastric outlet. The pylorus at this stage is identified and can be approached according to the surgeon's preference regarding gastric drainage. These preferences range from no gastric drainage procedure to pyloroplasty and certainly all the techniques are possible at this time. One of the authors (MD) prefers to inject Botox while the other author (AEA) performs a pyloromyotomy using bipolar cautery. At this time, the stomach is retracted anteriorly to expose retro-gastric adhesions, which are divided until the left gastric pedicle is identified. A complete dissection is done of the lymphatic and nodal tissue down to the trifurcation of the celiac artery. The artery is divided using the stapler at its most proximal point. A separate dissection of nodal tissue around the celiac trunk and hepatic artery is then undertaken.

At this point the stomach has been completely mobilized and the phrenoesophageal ligament is divided to deliver the penrose drain into the abdomen. The stomach is then ready for tailoring of the conduit. It is important at this point to pull back the nasogastric tube until its tip is in the thoracic esophagus. The assistant using the endo-GIA stapler divides the stomach. The conduit is fashioned as a long 5 cm tube extending from the incisura to the fundus. It is important to avoid the common mistake of stapling too close to the esophagogastric junction (EGJ) as this precludes an adequate lateral margin at the EGJ and may predispose to local recurrence. The initial angle

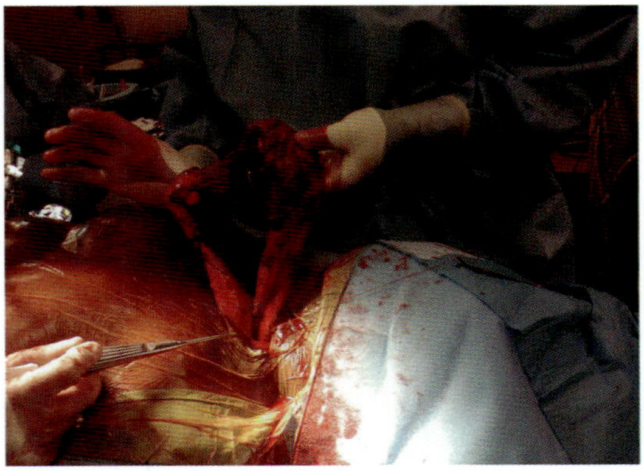

Fig. 4.5 Delivery of the specimen from the neck

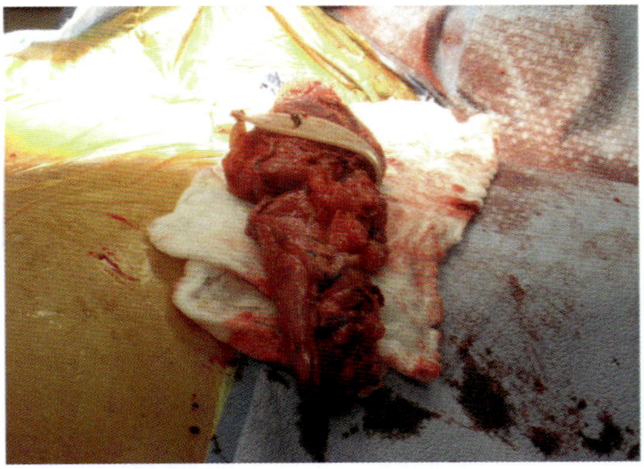

Fig. 4.6 Resected specimen

for division of the stomach may be easier from the right subcostal 13 mm port. After completing the conduit, the distal end of the specimen and the proximal end of the conduit are connected with a silk stitch.

The assistant is then asked to deliver the esophagogastric specimen from the neck along with the attached conduit (Figs. 4.5 and 4.6).

During this procedure the surgeon remains at the console to ensure that the conduit does not twist and is free of tension. It is also important to close the diaphragmatic hiatus posterior to the conduit to avoid visceral herniation. This is done with interrupted silk sutures. The robot is then undocked and the surgeon returns to the table to

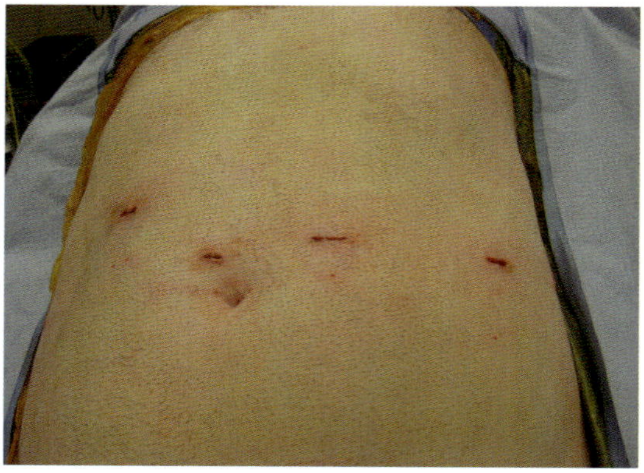

Fig. 4.7 Incisions upon completion

divide the proximal esophagus and complete the cervical anastomosis and perform a laparoscopic feeding jejunostomy. Figure 4.7 shows the abdominal incisions after closure.

Postoperative Management

Patients typically remain in the hospital until their thoracic and nasogastric drains are removed. This is usually achieved by postoperative day 4. They are discharged on jejunal tube feedings. A gastrografin swallow study is done as an outpatient procedure at postoperative day 10–14. When leakage is ruled out, the patient is allowed small amounts of food and drink. These rations are progressively increased over a period of 2 months while simultaneously decreasing the tube feeding.

Complications

The most common postoperative complications are the same as those encountered after open esophagectomy. They may be classified according to onset into early and late complications.

Early Complications

Anastomotic Leaks

These usually present after the fifth postoperative day. They range from mild to severe. Once identified, endoscopy is performed to evaluate the extent of the dehiscence and rule out gastric tip necrosis. The leak is treated according to the extent of the anastomotic dehiscence. In cases of disruption less than 50 % of the circumference of the anastomosis, conservative management with simple drainage, stent placement or passage of a percutaneous sump catheter through the defect into the gastric conduit. The cervical skin incision is always opened to allow drainage of any infection. Cases with complete disruption of the anastomosis are treated the same as those with gastric necrosis.

Gastric Tip Necrosis

This is a rare but lethal complication related to ischemia of the gastric conduit. This usually requires taking down of the anastomosis, resecting the ischemic portion and diversion of the esophagus with a cervical esophagostomy. The remaining healthy portion of the stomach is returned to the abdomen. The patient usually also requires decortications. It is necessary to identify these cases early to avoid the onset of sepsis.

Chylothorax

When identified, this complication should be treated surgically. After esophagecotmy it is almost always caused by complete division of the main thoracic duct and can seldom be treated conservatively with fasting and TPN. Delayed repair may predispose to malnutrition, infection and dehydration. Ligation of the thoracic duct can usually be performed by means of a reoperative right robotic-assisted approach. Injecting 100 cm^3 of cream or olive oil in the jejunostomy tube helps in identifying the source of chyle leak.

Vocal Cord Paralysis

Although this complication is usually temporary and secondary to retraction, it may impact on the patient's ability to clear pulmonary secretions. If necessary patients are referred for medialization of the cords.

Delayed Gastric Emptying

Precautions to avoid this devastating complication include performing a gastric drainage procedure such as pyloroplasty or pyloromyotomy, creating a narrow straight conduit to avoid pooling of contents, and avoiding a twist or kink of the conduit at the time of pulling up of the conduit through the hiatus. Medical management includes prokinetic agents such as metoclopramide or erythromycin. If the condition does not improve, endoscopic pyloric balloon dilation or pyloric Botox injection can be attempted.

Late Complications

Anastomotic Stricture

Typically patients present with late onset dysphagia. This may occur up to a year after surgery. Usually this can be managed endoscopically by endoscopic dilation. Refractory strictures may be amelriorated with temporary self-expanding covered stents, placed for 4–6 weeks. In severe cases, surgical strictureplasty is performed.

Hiatal Hernia

When the hiatus is not closed at the time of surgery, there is a risk of visceral herniation. Surgical repair may be approached by means of a thoracotomy on the side of the herniation or laparotomy. Minimally invasive repair is usually not possible.

Outcomes After Ramie

Totally robotic esophagectomy has not been reported frequently. Kernstine et al. [4] reported on 14 patients with a median age of 64 years who underwent robotic esophagectomy, 8 of who were completely robotic MKE while 6 were hybrid procedures. Total operating room time was 11.1 ± 0.8 h (range, 11.3–13.2 h). Complications included death ($n=1$), thoracic duct leak ($n=1$), severe pneumonia ($n=1$), anastomotic leak ($n=2$) and bilateral vocal cord paresis ($n=1$). Mean total operating time was 11.1 h.

Kim et al. reported on 21 patients who underwent hybrid RATS/laparoscopic MKE in the prone position [5]. One patient had a positive margin; major complications included anastomotic leakage ($n=4$), vocal cord palsy ($n=6$), and intra-abdominal bleeding ($n=1$).

Weksler et al. reported on 11 cases of robot assisted Ivor Lewis procedures [8]. In comparison with their series of traditional MIE, robotic thoracoscopic MIE did not offer clear advantages.

Dunn et al. reported on 40 patients underwent transhiatal RE [9]. Five patients were converted from robotic to open. Complications included anastomotic stricture ($n=27$), recurrent laryngeal nerve paresis ($n=14$), anastomotic leak ($n=10$), pneumonia ($n=8$), pleural effusion ($n=18$) and death ($n=1$).

The authors present their own series of totally endoscopic robotic McKeown procedures.

Author AEA's series includes 33 patients (3 females, 10 %) with median age of 62 who underwent totally endoscopic robotic assisted McKeown esophagogastrectomy in an 18 month period from January 2011 to July 2012. Indication for surgery was esophageal adenocarcinoma ($n=26$, 79 %), squamous cell carcinoma ($n=3$, 9 %), end-stage achalasia ($n=2$, 6 %), giant esophageal diverticulum ($n=1$, 3 %), and complicated eosinophilic esophagitis ($n=1$, 3 %).

For the 29 cases of esophageal cancer, neoadjuvant or definitive chemoradiation was administered in 15 cases ($n=51.7$ %) and pathologic stage was Stage 0 ($n=3$, 10.3 %), IA ($n=8$, 27.6 %), IB ($n=3$, 10.3 %), IIB ($n=4$, 13.8 %), IIIA ($n=9$, 31 %), IIIB ($n=2$, 6.9 %). Stage 0 related to complete pathologic response after neoadjuvant therapy, which occurred in 3 of 15 patients (20 %).

Mean duration of surgery was 310 min (range, 270–340 min) with no cases of conversion to open procedure. The mean number of lymph nodes with the specimen in all cases was 16 (7–44). The median length of hospital stay was 7 days (range, 4–31 days).

Complications are summarized in Table 4.2. Short-term complications after surgery occurred in 13 patients (39 %). Complications included mild anastomotic leak ($n=2$, 6 %), vocal cord paresis ($n=2$, 6 %) and chylothorax requiring reoperation ($n=2$, 6 %). One patient died of mesenteric ischemia on day 12 after surgery. Patients in the series were followed for a mean of 160.7 days (range, 12–492 days). Two patients have

Table 4.2 Complications after RAMIE. Author AEA series of 33 MKE procedures

Short-term	
Atrial arrhythmia	15 %
UTI	9 %
Pneumonia	9 %
Wound infection	6 %
Anastomotic leak	6 %
Vocal cord paresis	6 %
Delerium tremens	6 %
Chylothorax	6 %
ARDS	3 %
Pulm embolism	3 %
Renal failure	3 %
Mesenteric ischemia	3 %
Death	3 %
Long-term	
Anastomotic stricture	15 %
Delayed gastric emptying	3 %

developed metastatic disease (lung, peritoneum), five developed anastomotic stricture (15 %) and one patient (3 %) developed delayed gastric emptying (DGE). Strictures and DGE were managed successfully by endoscopic balloon dilation. All patients on follow-up are tolerating oral diet.

Author MD performed the procedure on 20 patients with mean age of 63 years, 17 males. Fourteen patients had Stage IIIA disease. Mean operative time was 303 min and conversion to open surgery was necessary in one patient due to adhesions. Average hospital stay was 9 days. Ninety-day mortality was 10 %. Leak rate was 15 % and vocal cord paresis was 5 %.

Summary

As we have seen with most other traditional operations, esophagectomy has also been shown to be feasible in a minimally invasive fashion. Robotic assistance offers the same benefits normally expected when applied in other procedures. In the case of esophagectomy, these benefits may be magnified in terms of minimizing the usual severe insult to the patient from an operation that invades three body cavities. It is also advantageous due to the ability to perform a superior oncologic procedure in terms of meticulous mediastinal and periceliac nodal dissection; areas that are not easily exposed by traditional endoscopic or even open surgery.

However, it is not the goal of the authors to convey that a robotic esophagectomy is a minor procedure. It requires advanced skills, usually greater than those needed for other thoracic operations. It remains a major operation with a mortality rate of up to 10 %, in addition to the risk for all complications that are seen with esophagectomy by other means. It will be important to provide long-term follow-up for this procedure in order to truly assess its value in managing esophageal cancer.

References

1. Horgan S, et al. Robotic-assisted minimally invasive transhiatal esophagectomy. Am Surg. 2003;69(7):624–6.
2. Dapri G, Himpens J, Cadiere GB. Robot-assisted thoracoscopic esophagectomy with the patient in the prone position. J Laparoendosc Adv Surg Tech A. 2006;16(3):278–85.
3. Gutt CN, et al. Robotic-assisted transhiatal esophagectomy. Langenbecks Arch Surg. 2006;391(4):428–34.
4. Kernstine KH, et al. The first series of completely robotic esophagectomies with three-field lymphadenectomy: initial experience. Surg Endosc. 2007;21(12):2285–92.
5. Kim DJ, et al. Thoracoscopic esophagectomy for esophageal cancer: feasibility and safety of robotic assistance in the prone position. J Thorac Cardiovasc Surg. 2010;139(1):53–9.e1.
6. Sutherland J, et al. Postoperative incidence of incarcerated hiatal hernia and its prevention after robotic transhiatal esophagectomy. Surg Endosc. 2011;25(5):1526–30.
7. Puntambekar SP, et al. Robotic transthoracic esophagectomy in the prone position: experience with 32 patients with esophageal cancer. J Thorac Cardiovasc Surg. 2011;142(5):1283–4.
8. Weksler B, et al. Robot-assisted minimally invasive esophagectomy is equivalent to thoracoscopic minimally invasive esophagectomy. Dis Esophagus. 2012;25(5):403–9.
9. Dunn DH, et al. Robot-assisted transhiatal esophagectomy: a 3-year single-center experience. Dis Esophagus. 2013;26(2):159–66.

Robotic Assisted Operations for Gastroesophageal Reflux

5

Daniel H. Dunn, Eric M. Johnson, Kourtney Kemp, Robert Ganz, Sam Leon, and Nilanjana Banerji

Introduction

Despite the fact that the management of patients with gastroesophageal reflux disease (GERD) has become complex with more precise diagnostic evaluations, surgical treatment options still remain limited. Medical management with proton pump inhibitors is the mainstay as well as the first line of treatment. All patients with a diagnosis of GERD are initially tried on medical management. In general, only those who fail treatment are offered surgical options for definitive treatment. Those patients with large sliding hiatus hernias, paraesophageal hernias, severe regurgitation, atypical laryngopharyngeal symptoms or pulmonary complications from reflux are exceptions to this fairly simple treatment algorithm.

For over a half-century, hiatus hernia repair and fundoplication have been implemented as the only surgical procedures for GERD. However, the results of such operative approaches continue to be unsatisfactory in the estimation of many gastroenterologists. Patients are told to avoid operation at all costs. Recurrence rates of 25 % in 5 years are common. Reoperation for recurrent symptoms or complications of the hiatus hernia repair and Nissen fundoplication is similarly frequent. However, no other surgical procedures have been developed to replace fundoplication for the surgical management of GERD [1].

As with many other surgical procedures, over time, the operative management for GERD has evolved into a minimally invasive approach. Laparoscopic approach (as compared to the open procedures) has resulted in fewer post-operative complications such as wound infections and pneumonia. Hospital length of stay (LOS) has been reduced to an average of 1–1.5 days. Symptom relief and re-operation rates have improved. Additionally, patients have benefited

D.H. Dunn, M.D. (✉)
Esophageal and Gastric Care Program, Virginia Piper Cancer Institute, Abbott Northwestern Hospital, 2545 Chicago Avenue, Minneapolis, MN 55404, USA
e-mail: docdunn3@comcast.net

E.M. Johnson, M.D.
Department of Surgery, Abbott Northwestern Hospital, 2545 Chicago Avenue, Minneapolis, MN 55407, USA
e-mail: embjohnson@comcast.net

K. Kemp, M.D.
Specialists in General Surgery, Maple Grove Hospital, 9825 Hospital Drive, Suite 105, Maple Grove, MN 55369, USA
e-mail: kkemp@sgsmn.com

R. Ganz, M.D., F.A.S.G.E.
Department of Gastroenterology, Abbott Northwestern Hospital, 5705 West Old Shakopee Road, Bloomington, MN 55437, USA
e-mail: rganz@mngastro.com

S. Leon, M.D.
Minnesota Gastroenterology, 5705 West Old Shakopee Road, #150, Bloomington, MN 55437, USA

N. Banerji, Ph.D.
Neuroscience and Spine Clinical Service Line, Abbott Northwestern Hospital, Minneapolis, MN, USA
e-mail: Nilanjana.Banerji@allina.com

K.C. Kim (ed.), *Robotics in General Surgery*, DOI 10.1007/978-1-4614-8739-5_5,

from less post-operative pain and have been able to return to work in 1–2 weeks. Short and long-term results have improved, as our understanding of gastroesophageal reflux has improved [2, 3].

Robotic technology has been available for many years but it was not until use of the robot for prostatectomy was reported in 1988 that the robot really had a place in the surgical management of diseases. However, the predominant use of robotic procedure is for urologic operations. The adoption of this technology by other surgical specialties has been considerably restricted because of the relatively narrow operative field required by robotic instrumentation. As a consequence, pelvic anatomy and operative interventions for pelvic malignancies are ideally suited for robotic technology. Similar limited field of operations are also encountered in esophageal operations and are consequently ideal for the use of robotic procedures. Thus, robotic procedures for hiatus hernia repair, Nissen fundoplication, Heller myotomy and trans-hiatal esophagectomy with an abdominal approach without thoracoscopy or thoracotomy have been performed safely with reasonable success [4, 5].

The robotic surgical procedures described in this chapter were performed with the da Vinci robotic instrument (Intuitive Surgical, Palo Alto, CA) for management of paraesophageal hiatus hernias, giant hernias, and recurrent hiatus hernias as well as the more standard anatomy seen with most patients with gasroesophageal reflux. The operations described here are hiatus hernia repair with and without mesh, Nissen fundoplication, partial posterior fundoplication or the 270° wrap (Toupet) procedure, and the anterior fundoplication of Dor, and Collis gastroplasty.

Pre-operative Diagnostic Evaluations

Most patients with GERD undergo a period of self-medication with over the counter treatments for management of typical symptoms of heartburn or regurgitation for many years, before they present themselves to their primary physician. Primary care physicians are well versed in the initial management of GERD. It is usually only those patients who are resistant to standard medical treatments or escalate to manifestation of uncontrolled and/or additional symptoms of regurgitations, nighttime reflux, cough, or hoarseness are referred to the gastroenterologist. The gastroenterologist usually initiates the diagnostic evaluation protocol for patients who develop severe GERD-related complications or have uncontrolled or atypical symptoms.

Esophagogastroduodenoscopy

Esophagogastroduodenoscopy (EGD) is usually the first diagnostic procedure performed in the diagnostic work-up for complicated GERD. The endoscopy gives valuable information regarding the anatomy of the esophagus and gastroesophageal junction. The presence and size of hiatus hernia and presence and degree of esophagitis can be classified by the Hill and LA grading systems. Barrett's esophagus can be documented and strategy for treating or surveillance can be established. Long-term risk assessment can be discussed with the patient. Strictures, eosinophilic esophagitis, Cameron erosions and esophageal cancer can be diagnosed before beginning a long-term approach to treatment.

pH Monitoring

The 48-h pH-monitoring test (Bravo) is used to obtain objective data regarding the degree of acid reflux. Either 24- or 48-h tests can be used; however, the 48-h test is generally considered more reliable. The percentage of time of esophageal acid exposure to $pH<4.0$ is recorded as a DeMeester score (normal <14.72). Patients with high DeMeester scores are considered positive for significant reflux.

pH-monitoring is not used in every patient. In general, patients with very large hernias or large paraesophageal hernias may be considered operative candidates whether or not they had significant GERD or abnormal Bravo tests. Likewise pH-monitoring is not used in patients with known

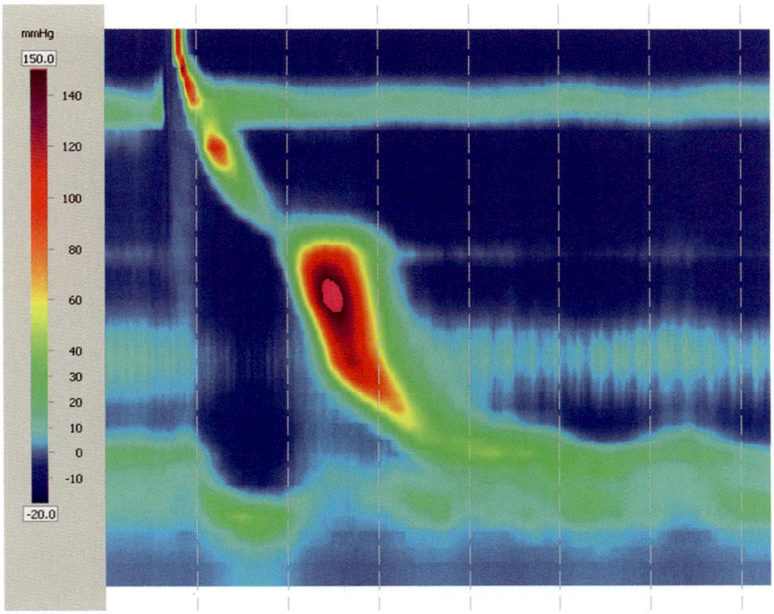

Fig. 5.1 High-resolution manometry of a typical patient with GERD showing normal esophageal motility and decreased lower esophageal sphincter pressure

Barrett's esophagus. pH-monitoring is particularly helpful in making a diagnosis of gastroesophageal reflux in patients with atypical symptoms or patients who do not respond to medical management.

pH-monitoring using multichannel intraluminal impedence-ph (MII-pH) monitoring has gained acceptance in several GI laboratories [6]. The MII-pH monitoring can distinguish non-acid as well as acid reflux thereby facilitating correlation of the reflux episodes with symptoms. Most GI laboratories choose one method and use that method exclusively. At our Institution the preferred diagnostic procedure of gastroenterologists is the Bravo pH monitoring test.

Manometry

Esophageal manometry is used to determine esophageal motor function as well as lower esophageal sphincter pressure and relaxation with swallowing. Manometry is used in most patients with typical symptoms of heartburn. In patients with dysphagia, regurgitation, atypical symptoms or abnormal findings on endoscopy such as a dilated esophagus, stricture or esophageal diverticulum, manometry is critical. A typical picture of a low resting mean pressure of the lower esophageal sphincter and normal esophageal motility is usually observed in most of patients with typical GERD symptoms (Fig. 5.1).

Preferably, a team of gastroenterologists with a special interest in GERD should evaluate the outcomes of these studies.

In our clinical experience, a group of patients thought to have a clear diagnosis of GERD was confirmed to have achalasia on manometry, with high-resolution manometry (HRM) showing typical pictures of failed swallows, low peristaltic pressures, or no peristalsis (Fig. 5.2).

One particular patient had been treated for GERD for many years, had done reasonably well on PPI's, and had a very large paraesophageal hiatus hernia with 70 % of her stomach in the chest. She had regurgitation as a predominant symptom along with heartburn. A diagnostic EGD procedure indicated esophagitis. However, review of the HRM was indicative of a combination of type II and III achalasia. Based on the

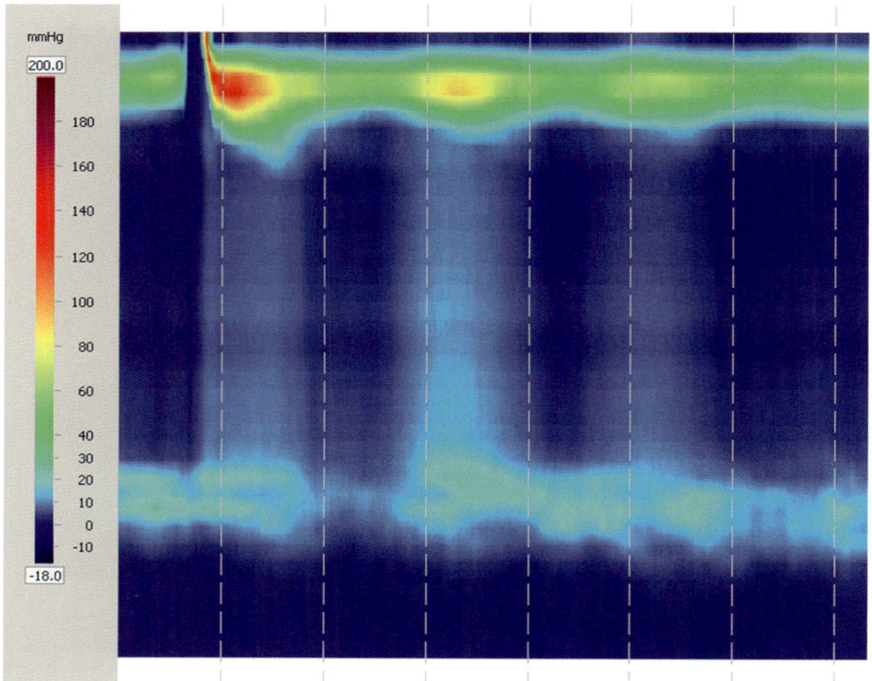

Fig. 5.2 High-resolution manometry of typical patient with Classic Achalasia showing poor to no peristalsis, the common cavity affects and high resting lower esophageal sphincter pressure without relaxation

manometry results, this patient was treated for achalasia with a Heller myotomy and Dor fundoplication.

If patients have significant esophageal dysmotility on HRM and symptoms of dysphagia without anatomic obstruction, in our practice we selectively use this information to perform a partial 270° fundoplication (Toupet procedure) (Fig. 5.3). A loose wrap may function just as well for these patients since a partial wrap has been shown to be as durable as a loose full wrap in several studies [7–9].

Operative Procedure

There is an obvious difference in the operative time required for patients undergoing robotic-assisted procedures vs. laparoscopic procedures for management of gastroesophageal reflux with robotic surgery requiring a longer time for completion in comparison to the same procedures performed laparoscopically. In addition, the room time (defined as "time in to time out") is significantly longer with the robotic procedure. In our experience, there exists a learning curve for surgeons, and the room time as well as operative time decreases as the operative team gains experience. The pre-operative time, i.e. time from a patient entering the room to incision time, makes up most of the extra time for the robotic procedure. The operating table needs to be turned away from the anesthesiologist and the logistics of tube and monitoring placement is time consuming. It is best to have an anesthesia team during the initial period of implementation of these procedures, as the set up for esophageal surgery is different from robotic pelvic operations. The docking time from first incision to the surgeon beginning on the console decreases with experience. In our experience, following the first 10–15 cases the docking time stabilizes in the range of 10–15 min.

For experienced laparoscopic surgeons who perform anti-reflux operations frequently the

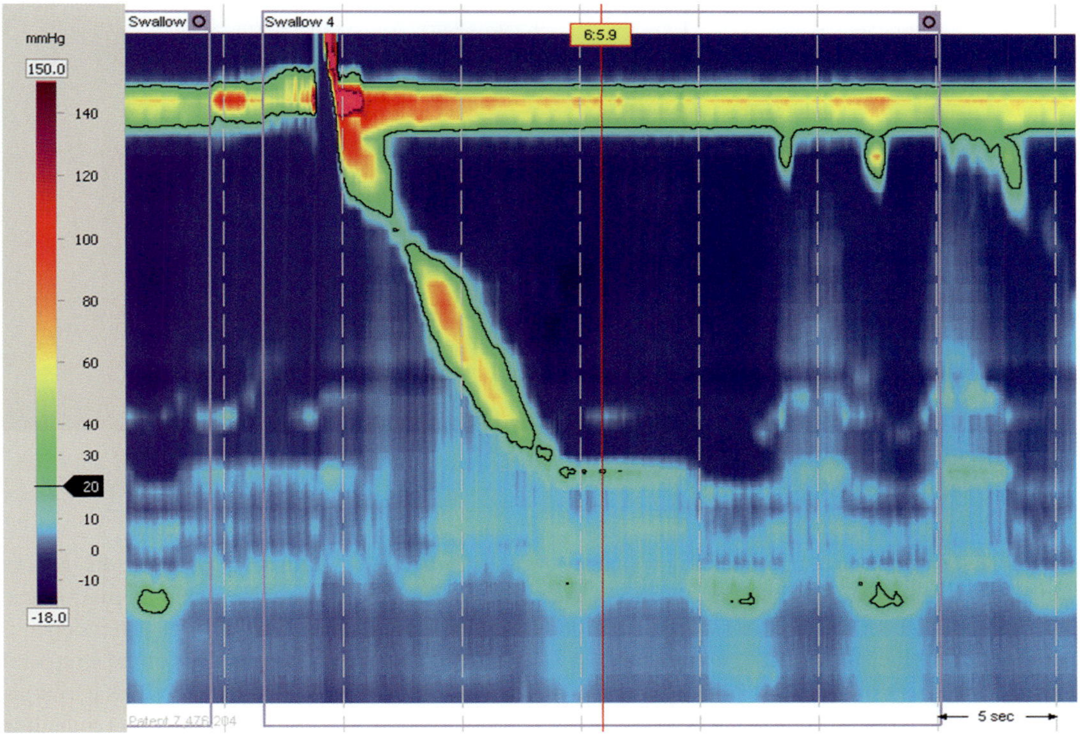

Fig. 5.3 High-resolution manometry of patient with GERD showing poor esophageal motility with hiatus hernia and low lower esophageal sphincter pressure

adjustment to using robotic technology is not challenging. Surgeons should be well versed in laparoscopic fundoplication procedures before performing robotic assisted fundoplications. A robotic general surgeon experienced with anti-reflux operations should proctor the first robotic case. Each robotic program must determine the credentialing criteria for privileging surgeons for these procedures. If possible, the first several cases should be performed with an experienced laparoscopic surgeon as an assistant. After the surgeon and operating room team have gained experience, the procedure can be performed assisted by surgical technologists, residents, or physician assistants. As mentioned previously, operative time decreases with experience. The learning curve for using the robotic technology is in the first 10–15 cases for experienced laparoscopic surgeons.

The operation begins with the laparoscopic placement of the ports. The configuration of the port placement is different from the laparoscopic procedure. Placement of the camera port is critical. The typical position of 12 cm caudad and 2 cm to the patient's left of the xiiphoid for women or small men and 15 cm caudad and 2 cm to the left for large women or men does not always function efficiently. The body habitus is important and with experience the distance from the xiphoid to the camera port becomes shorter. This distance is especially important for patients with large hiatus hernias because of the mediastinal dissection needed to reduce the contents of the hernia sac. The position of the robotic arms is determined by the position of the camera port. This distance is constant, again demonstrating the importance of the first trocar placement for the camera. The 8 mm trocars for the arms of the robot are placed 4 cm cephalad to the 12 mm camera port and 8 cm to either side of the camera port.

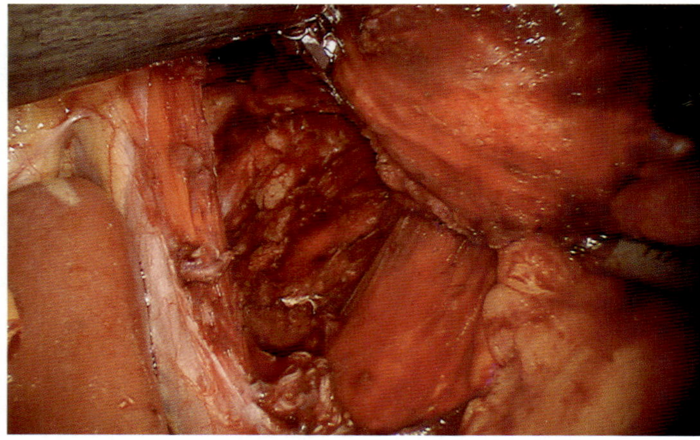

Fig. 5.4 Dissection of the hiatus in-patient with GERD and moderate hiatus hernia

The liver retractor port is placed at a convenient position beneath the right costal margin. We use a standard liver retractor from this position; however, a Nathanson retractor can be used in a sub-xiphoid position. The last port is placed in a convenient left lateral subcostal position. This port is used by the assistant for retraction and passing needles as well as for the stapler for patients who are having a Collis gastroplasty.

Once all the ports and the liver retractor are placed, the robot is brought into the field. The patient is placed into a reverse Trendelenburg position and the camera port and two robotic arms are attached to the appropriate trocars. In our surgical practice, we do not routinely use the third arm of the robot. The operating surgeon then goes to the console and initiates the robotic part of the operation.

Dissection of the hiatus with the robot is similar to a laparoscopic approach. The advantage of robotic technology is that the camera can be positioned and secured in place by the operator. If necessary, the camera can literally be placed through the hiatus to gain better visualization for large paraesophageal hernias. This placement is important for maximum mobilization of the esophagus in the mediastinum, so that an adequate length of esophagus, usually 3 cm below the diaphragm, can be obtained for the wrap (Fig. 5.4).

Once the hiatus is dissected and the esophagus circumferentially mobilized preserving the anterior and posterior vagus nerves, the short gastric arteries are taken down to mobilize the greater curvature of the stomach for a Nissen fundoplication. The number of short gastrics taken depends on the amount of fundus needed for the wrap or if a Collis gastroplasty is indicated. The harmonic scalpel is used for all of the dissection including the mediastinum, mobilization of the esophagus and takedown of short gastric arteries.

The next step is taking the gastroesophageal fat pad and separation of the anterior vagus nerve from the esophagus and GE junction (Fig. 5.5).

Removing the fat pad clears the distal esophagus and cardia of excess tissue, which might interfere with an exact placement of the wrap, but more importantly with this procedure the GE junction can be better visualized. As the anterior vagus is preserved after it is mobilized from the esophagus with the GEJ fat pad the wrap can be brought underneath the vagus and this sling can serve to hold the wrap in place so that it does not slip (Fig. 5.6). The hiatus is then repaired with primary closure of figure of eight stitches with pledgets for reinforcement, if necessary (Fig. 5.7).

Bridging grafts, whether biologic or synthetic have a high failure rate and multiple complications associated with their use. Most of the time, a primary closure is possible. We use an onlay graft only if the closure needs reinforcement with GoreTex suture and U clips (Fig. 5.8a, b).

Following repair of the hiatus, the esophagus is examined to determine if a standard Nissen

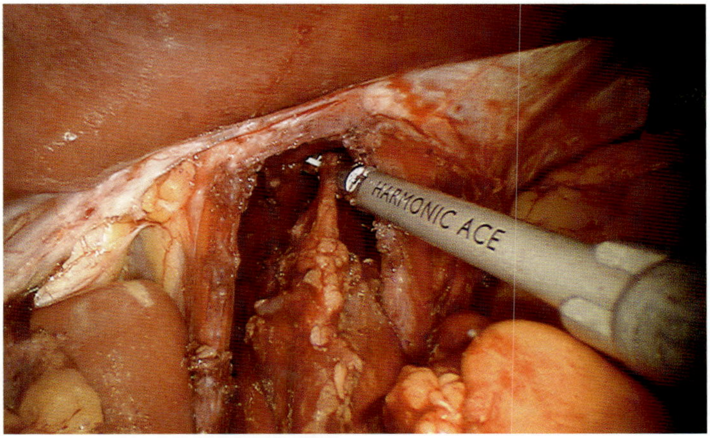

Fig. 5.5 Dissection of the Anterior Vagus Nerve showing the development of a sling, which will hold the fundoplication in place

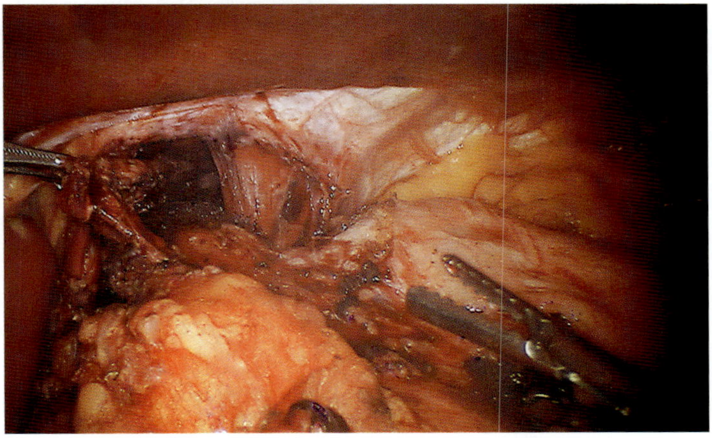

Fig. 5.6 Takedown of the gastroesophageal fat pad to clearly identify the junction of the longitudinal esophageal muscle and the serosa of the stomach

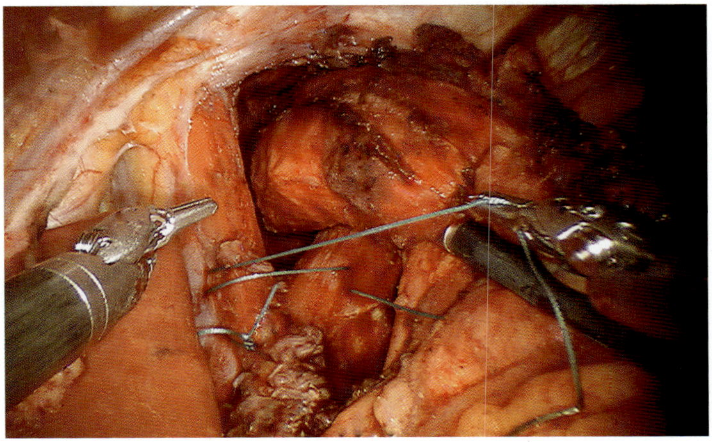

Fig. 5.7 Primary closure of the hiatus with figure of 8 suturing, without use of onlay or pledgets as reinforcement

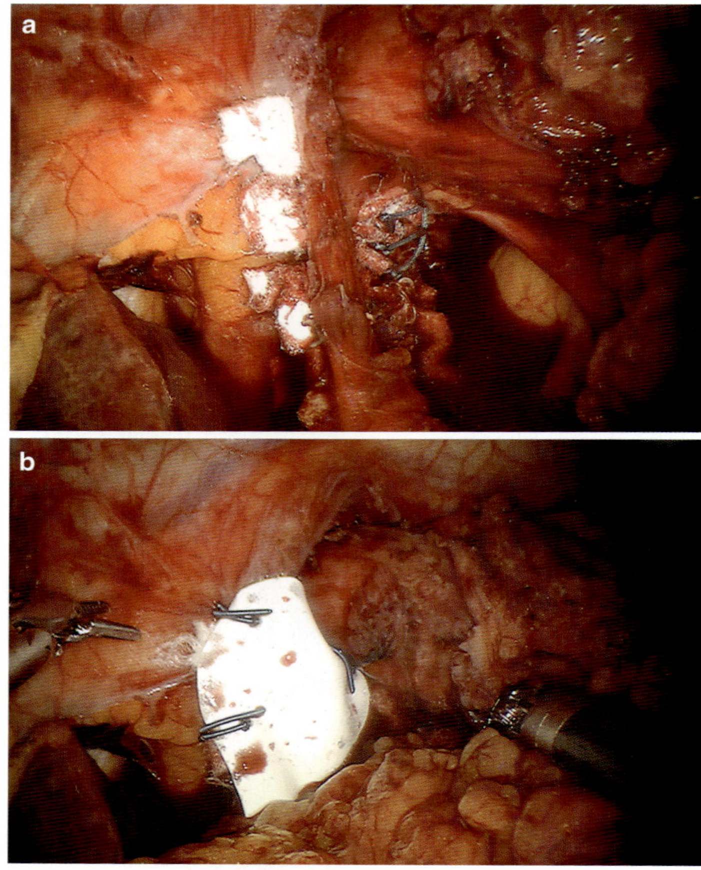

Fig. 5.8 (**a** and **b**) Hiatus Hernia repair with primary closure and reinforcement with an onlay Gore-Tex graft

fundoplication can be performed. If the esophagus can be brought down to at least 3 cm below the diaphragmatic hiatus without tension, a 3 stitch Nissen fundoplication over a 50–56 fr. dilator is performed. We often will tack the wrap to the diaphragm at the end of the procedure (Figs. 5.9, 5.10, and 5.11). The robot is then undocked and the liver retractor removed, followed by evacuation of the pneumoperitoneum and incision closure.

Partial Fundoplication (The Toupet Procedure)

The principal indications for our patients undergoing a 270° fundoplication (or the Toupet procedure) were dysphagia or esophageal dysmotility diagnosed on HRM. Partial fundoplication is no different from the full wrap until the actual suturing of the wrap. The reduction and repair of hernia as well as mobilization of the esophagus and greater curvature of the stomach are all similar to the standard Nissen fundoplication. In the Toupet procedure, the fundus is brought around behind the esophagus and sutured with three stitches to the esophagus at 10 o'clock position. Left side of the fundic wrap is sutured to 2 o'clock position on the esophagus. This leaves the anterior esophagus open and approximately 270° of the posterior esophagus wrapped (Figs. 5.12 and 5.13).

Dor (Anterior) Fundoplication

We have had minimal experience in using the anterior fundoplication i.e. the Dor fundoplication for patients having GERD as their indication

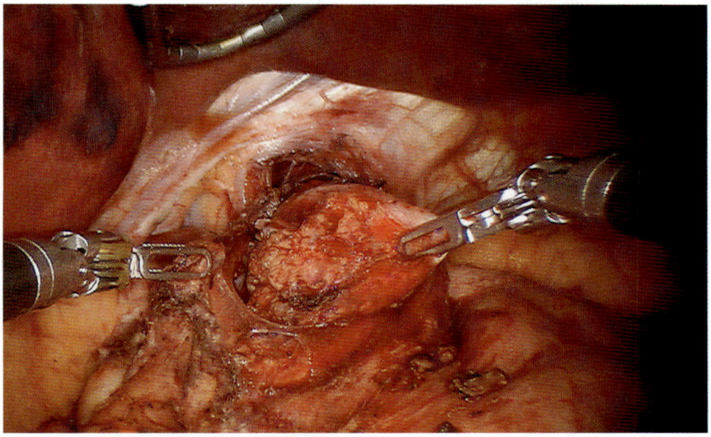

Fig. 5.9 Mobilizing the fundus and bringing it around the back of the esophagus under vagus nerve sling and mobilized gastroesophageal fat pad

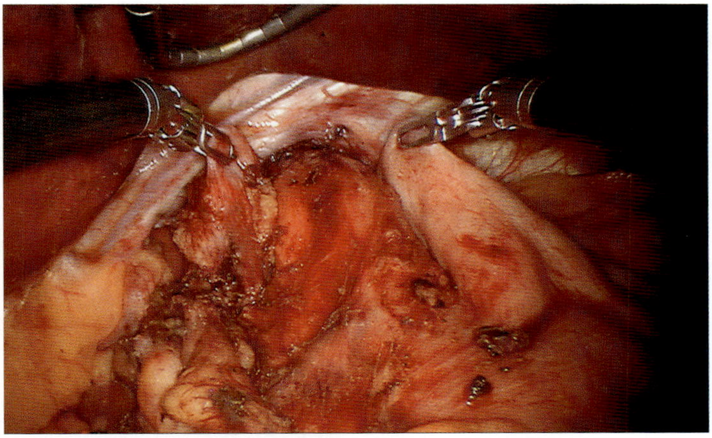

Fig. 5.10 Preparing the fundoplication for suturing to the esophagus

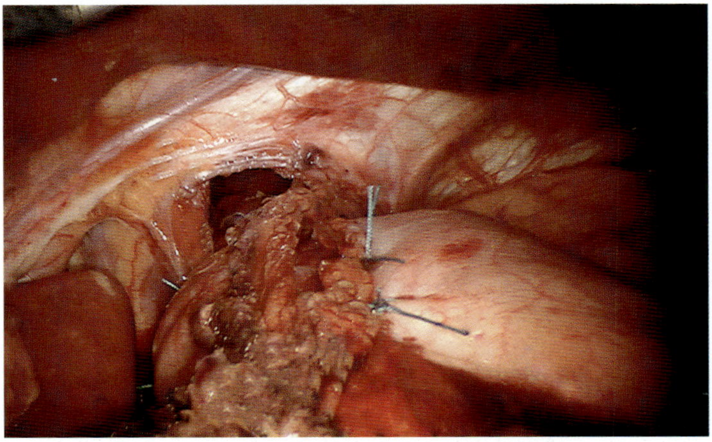

Fig. 5.11 Completed 360° Nissen fundoplication

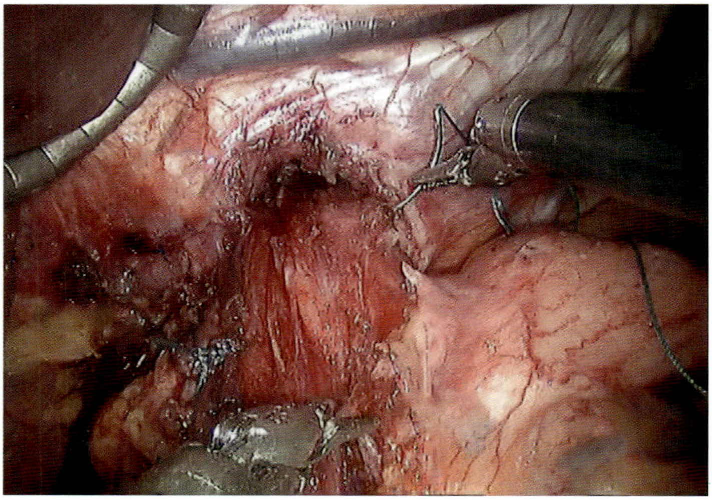

Fig. 5.12 270° fundoplication for patients with esophageal dysmotility or patients who refuse a 360° fundoplication because of unwanted side effects

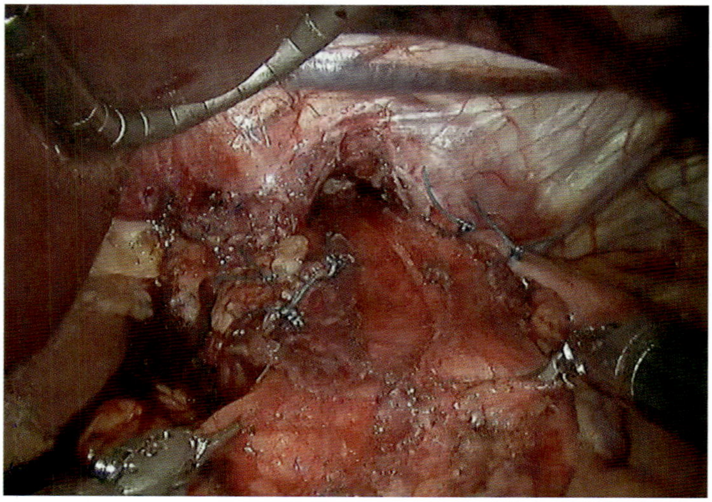

Fig. 5.13 Toupet, the 270° fundoplication

for operation. We have used the anterior fundoplication almost exclusively for patients with achalasia. The Dor fundolplication has been an effective procedure for the reduction of symptomatic GERD following esophageal myotomy. The Dor fundoplication has been suggested as an alternative for a full Nissen fundoplication (Figs. 5.14 and 5.15).

Several studies have shown similar results comparing an anterior wrap to a 360° wrap, with fewer side effects for the anterior fundoplication in comparison to the full fundoplication [10].

Collis Gastroplasty

Our surgical practice has used the Collis gastroplasty procedure for the past 3 years almost exclusively for the management of patients with large paraesophageal hiatus hernia or giant sliding hernia with foreshortened esophagus. The esophagus is mobilized as much as possible and the hiatus is closed. The gastroesophageal junction must be at least 3 cm below the diaphragm without tension; otherwise a Collis gastroplasty is performed. This is especially important in patients with a BMI > 35. To perform the Collis, a

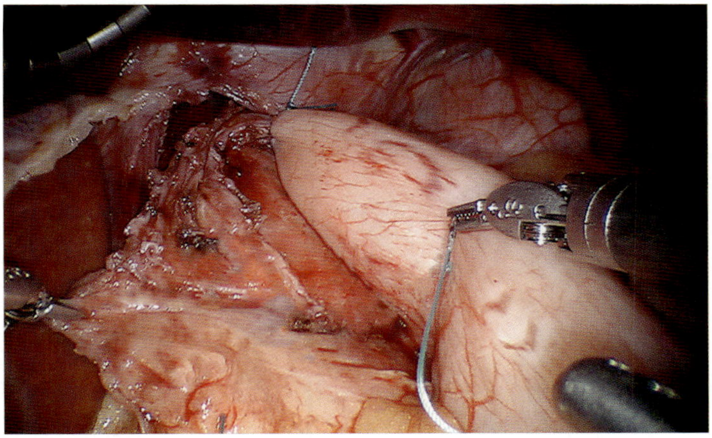

Fig. 5.14 Anterior 180° fundoplication or Dor fundoplication. For this case the anterior fundoplication was performed with a Heller myotomy

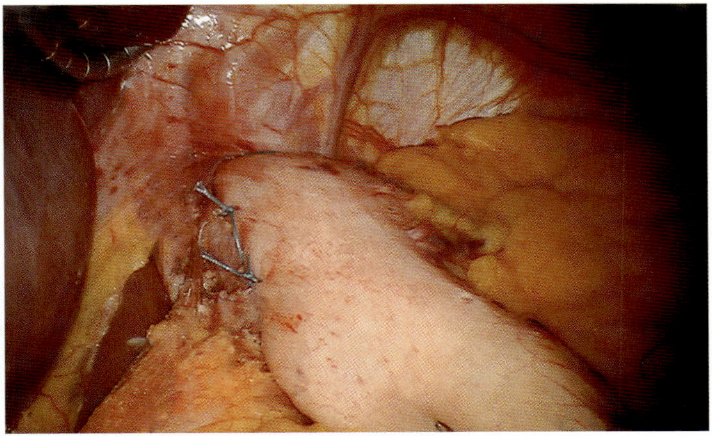

Fig. 5.15 Completed 180° anterior fundoplication

second surgeon, surgical resident, or physician assistant is required because the procedure requires stapling of the cardia of the stomach. A wedge resection of the cardia using one of the GIA stapling devices is used to lengthen the esophagus (Fig. 5.16a).

A 46–50 fr. dilator is placed into the esophagus to prevent narrowing of the "neo-esophagus" (Fig. 5.16b).

We have used the Echelon stapler with a green load of both 60 and 45 mm. In our experience, the 45 mm is much easier to manipulate in the upper abdomen. It is used through the assistant's port in the lateral upper abdomen. The standard 8 mm trocar is changed to a 12 mm trocar to accommodate the stapler. The amount of cardia removed depends on the anatomy. A relatively small wedge of cardia can be removed and accomplish the lengthening procedure.

The first two staple lines are directed at the dilator that is positioned nest to the lesser curvature of the stomach (Fig. 5.17). The third staple line is parallel to the esophagus and held against the dilator (Fig. 5.18a, b). After the wedge resection is performed (Fig. 5.19), the remaining fundus is wrapped around the neo-esophagus (Figs. 5.20 and 5.21). A Nissen fundoplication is then performed which allows a tension free wrap with reduced chance for recurrence due to herniation or a slipped Nissen (Fig. 5.22).

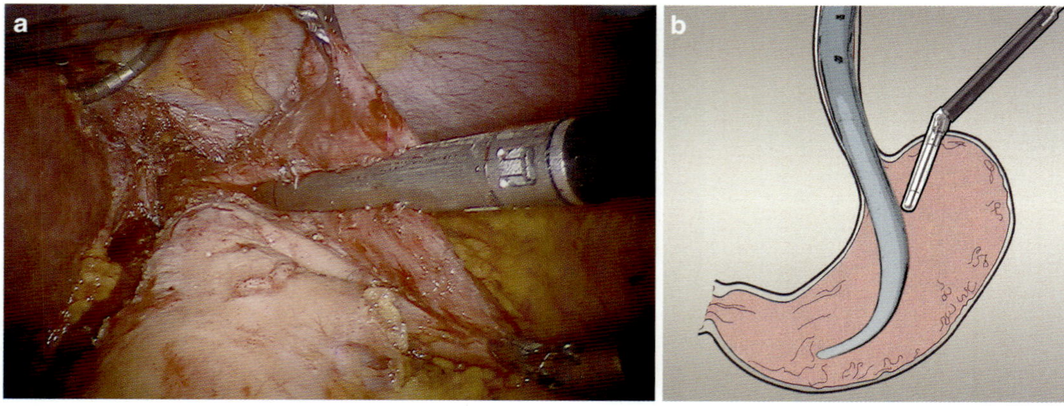

Fig. 5.16 Collis Gastroplasty—Photographs and corresponding illustrations of resecting a wedge of the gastric cardia and creating a neo-esophagus to lengthen the esophagus and prevent undue cephalad tension on the fundoplication. (**a** and **b**) Illustration of the first cut across the gastric cardia in the beginning of the lengthening of the esophagus

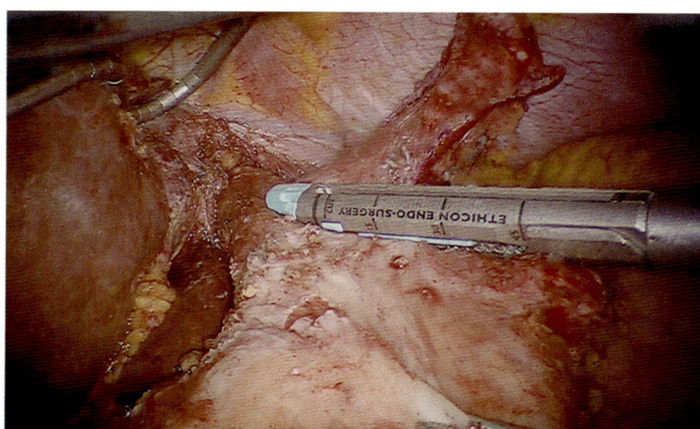

Fig. 5.17 Collis Gastroplasty—Photographs and corresponding illustrations of resecting a wedge of the gastric cardia and creating a neo-esophagus to lengthen the esophagus and prevent undue cephalad tension on the fundoplication. The "second cut" using an Echelon 45 mm green load to create a neo-esophagus. Illustration showing the "second cut" ending at the point where the stapler is at the edge of the dilator to prevent narrowing of the Neo-esophagus

Re-operative Robotic Procedures for Recurrent Gastroesophageal Reflux, Recurrent Hiatus Hernia, Incarcerated Hiatus Hernia and Esophageal Dysmotility

Re-operative procedures for recurrent hiatus hernia can be challenging. For a majority of cases, these procedures can be performed using robotic technology. There are some important aspects of these re-operative procedures that need to be emphasized.

It is prudent to note that tactile sensation is not possible with the robot. Haptic memory allows surgeons to successfully tie knots with the robot without being able to feel the tension. Surgeons can experience what it feels like when the knot or suture is tight, thereby allowing them to keep the suture intact. This also allows them to gauge how much pressure or pull they can exert while

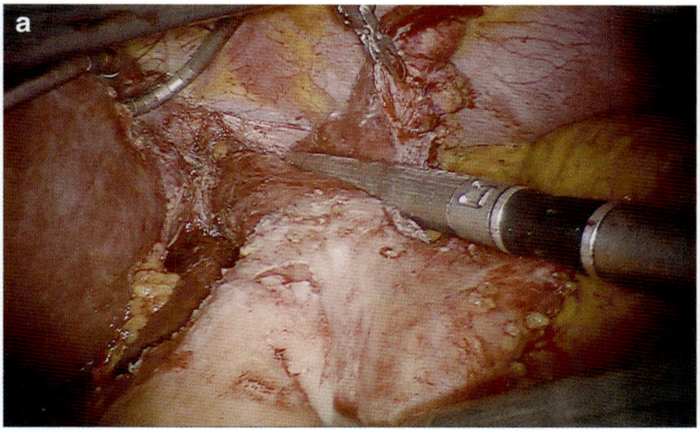

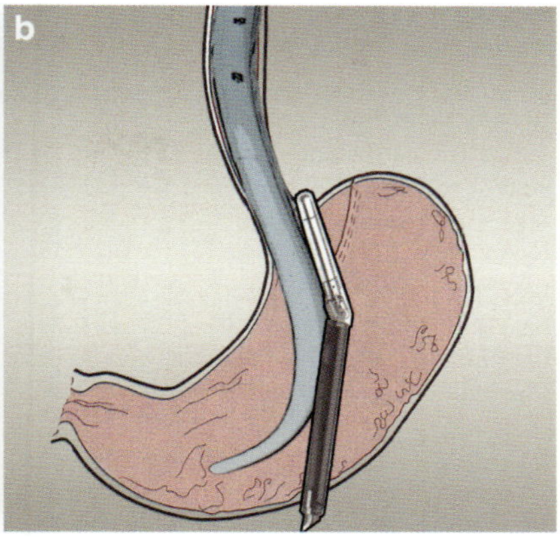

Fig. 5.18 Collis Gastroplasty—Photographs and corresponding illustrations of resecting a wedge of the gastric cardia and creating a neo-esophagus to lengthen the esophagus and prevent undue cephalad tension on the fundoplication. (**a** and **b**) The "third cut" using an Echelon 45 mm green load to finish the creation of the neo-esophagus. Accompanying illustration showing the completed segmental resection of a portion of the cardia of the stomach leaving the remaining fundus for the fundoplication

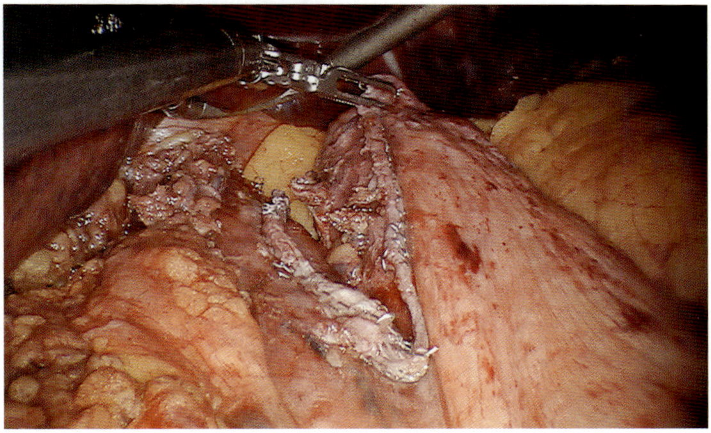

Fig. 5.19 Collis Gastroplasty—Photographs and corresponding illustrations of resecting a wedge of the gastric cardia and creating a neo-esophagus to lengthen the esophagus and prevent undue cephalad tension on the fundoplication. Completed wedge resection for esophageal lengthening with illustration

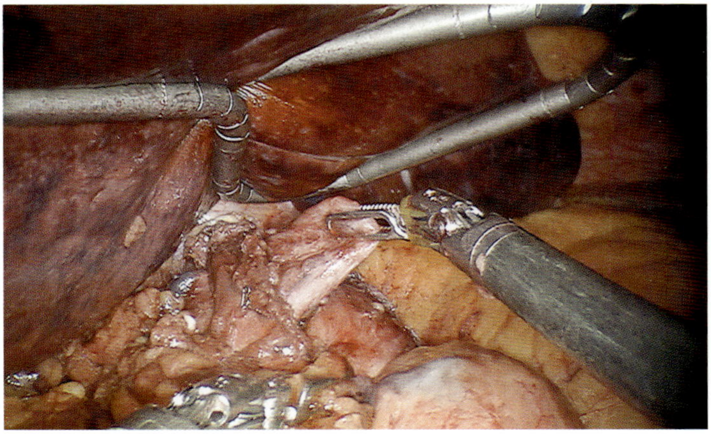

Fig. 5.20 Collis Gastroplasty—Photographs and corresponding illustrations of resecting a wedge of the gastric cardia and creating a neo-esophagus to lengthen the esophagus and prevent undue cephalad tension on the fundoplication. Bringing the fundus around the esophagus and under the anterior vagus nerve after the segmental gastric resection

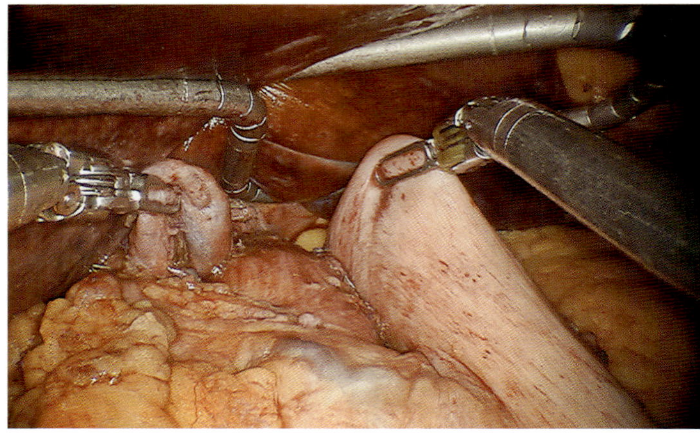

Fig. 5.21 Collis Gastroplasty—Photographs and corresponding illustrations of resecting a wedge of the gastric cardia and creating a neo-esophagus to lengthen the esophagus and prevent undue cephalad tension on the fundoplication. Bringing the *right* and *left portions* of the fundus in apposition for finishing the fundoplication

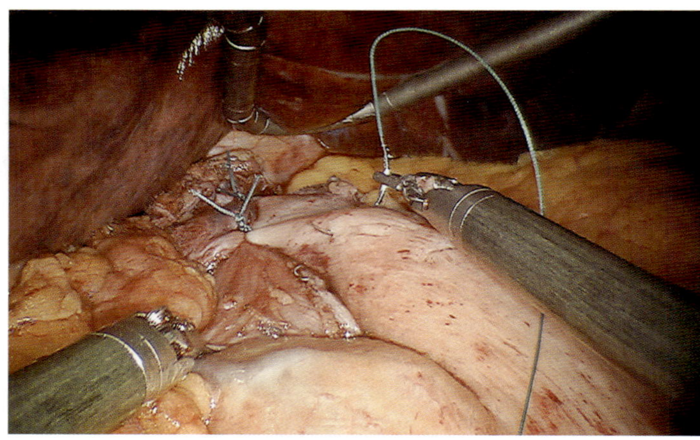

Fig. 5.22 Collis Gastroplasty—Photographs and corresponding illustrations of resecting a wedge of the gastric cardia and creating a neo-esophagus to lengthen the esophagus and prevent undue cephalad tension on the fundoplication. Final stitch of Collis gastroplasty and 3 stitch Nissen fundoplication

dissecting tissue. The challenge with re-operative robotic surgery is that during a repeat procedure surgeons are not able to assess the tensile strength of the structures that they are dissecting. Therefore, it is much more likely to tear tissue during a re-operation. If the wrap has migrated into the chest through the hiatus, dissection can be extremely difficult and the ability to have tactile sensation may be more important than benefits of the robot (Fig. 5.23). In these instances, a laparoscopic approach might be preferred.

Obese patients (BMI > 35) who have recurrence should be considered for gastric bypass. In this situation the Nissen or Toupet is taken down and a gastric bypass performed in the standard fashion. Since short gastrics are usually taken with a Nissen fundoplication, care must be taken to preserve the left gastric branches to the fundus. If gastric bypass is not an option or the recurrent symptoms are of an obstructive nature, then reoperations should include a Collis gastroplasty, even if it appears that there is minimal tension on the esophagus after hernia reduction and repair.

Patients, who have unremitting dysphagia following Nissen fundoplicaton and manifest preoperatively unrecognized esophageal dysmotility, should have a takedown of the Nissen. For a redo

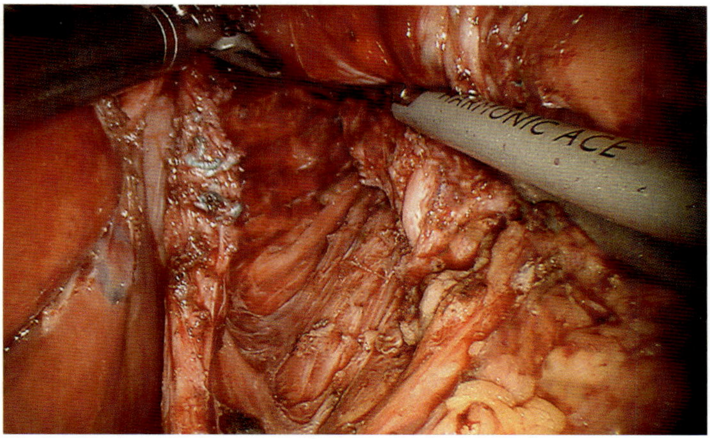

Fig. 5.23 Re-do hiatus hernia repair and takedown of Nissen fundoplication showing posterior vagus nerve, aorta and *right* and *left crus*

of this type, use of the robot is particularly advantageous because of the precise nature of dissection of the wrap as well as importance of adequate visualization (Figs. 5.24 and 5.25).

The same procedure should be performed for a Nissen that is too tight. Attempting to loosen the Nissen in this situation has the risk of still being too taut after the second operation. Therefore a partial fundoplication is a more reasonable approach in these instances (Fig. 5.26).

The ability to visualize anatomy with high definition optics used with robotic technology and articulated instruments for dissection in the chest is a definite advantage over the standard laparoscopic technology (Fig. 5.27).

These operations are often tedious and time consuming compared to a standard Nissen. In our opinion, the benefits of improved ergonomics of the robotic console cannot be matched with laparoscopic techniques (Fig. 5.28).

Outcomes of Robotic Assisted Operations for Gerd at Abbott Northwestern Hospital

Over a 4 year period from June 2007 to December 2011 175 patients, with 59 (33.72 %) men and 116 (66.28 %) women, have undergone robotic-assisted operations for symptomatic GERD management in the general surgery program of Abbott Northwestern Hospital (ANW) using the da Vinci Computer-Enhanced Robotic Surgical System (Table 5.1). Patients presenting with recurrent hiatus hernias, large sliding hiatus hernias, paraesophageal hiatus hernias and patients with recurrent hiatus hernia or other complications of previous hiatus hernia repairs are included in this cohort. Mean age of the patients was 51.61 ± 14.67 years (median 52; range 19–86) and average pre-operative BMI was 30.40 ± 5.16 (median 30; range 20–47).

A majority of the patients were referred from Minnesota Gastroenterology (MNGI) group. Prior to the first visit with the surgeons, patients were evaluated in a gastroenterology clinic for esophageal disorders. Ninety-five percent of patients was evaluated by a gastroenterologist. Diagnostic work-up included EGD, Bravo (48 h pH probe), high-resolution manometry (HRM) and UGI X-rays. Patient response to medical therapy was noted. All patients with heartburn as their major symptom had failed medical management.

For further outcome evaluations, patients were separated into two groups, namely, (a) patients with symptomatic GERD diagnosed with large (paraesophageal or sliding) hernias ($n = 70$) and (b) patients with symptomatic GERD with small or no evident hernias ($n = 105$) (Table 5.1). Eighty-one percent of patients who had small

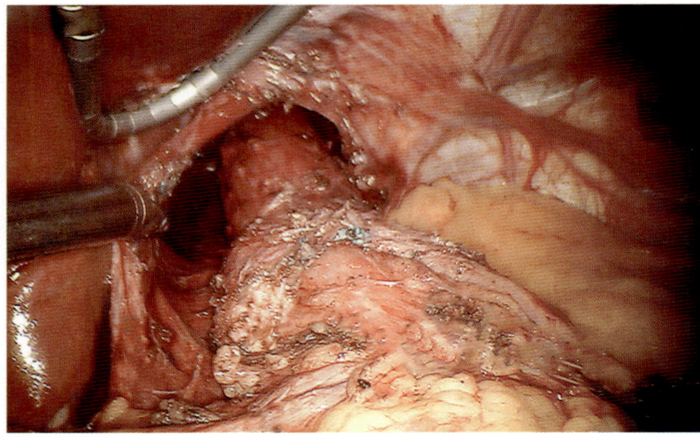

Fig. 5.24 Dehisced Nissen fundoplication

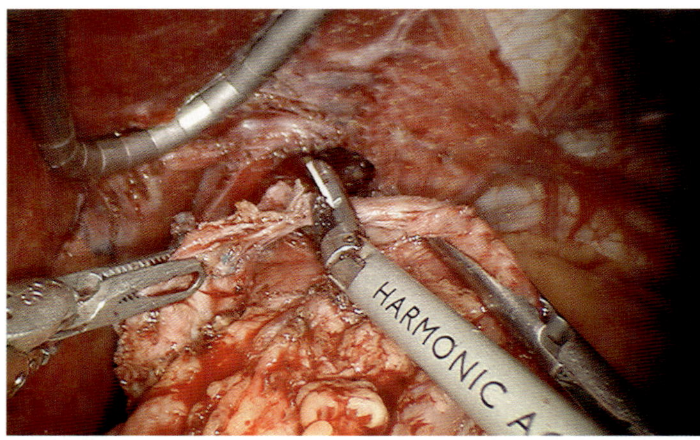

Fig. 5.25 Takedown of dehisced Nissen fundoplication

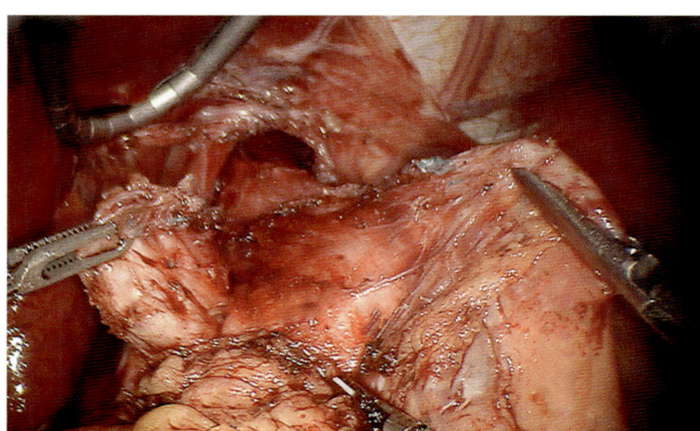

Fig. 5.26 Re-do Nissen fundoplicaton unwrapped

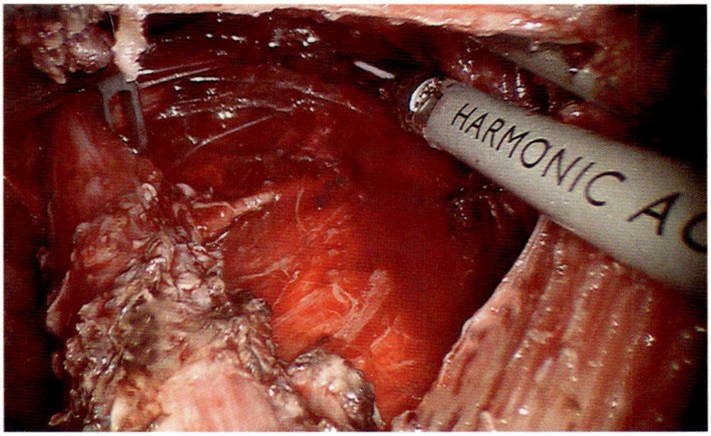

Fig. 5.27 *Left* and *right diaphragmatic crura*, aorta before re-do hiatus hernia repair and re-do Nissen fundoplication

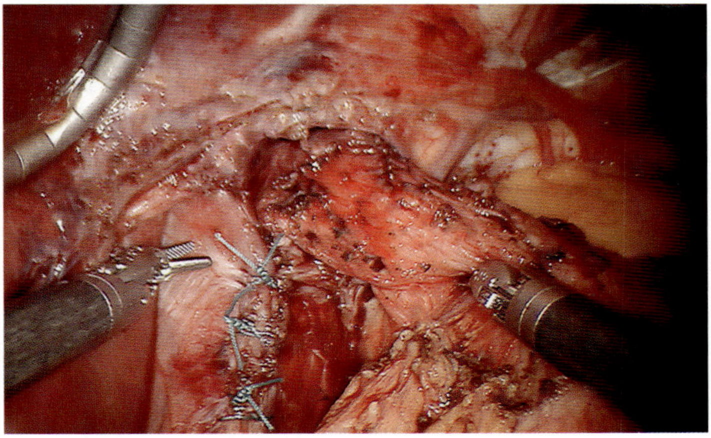

Fig. 5.28 Re-do Hiatus hernia repair

hernias or no hernias had typical symptoms of heartburn, regurgitation or aspiration. Patients with paraesophageal or large sliding hernias were more likely to have atypical symptoms with 44.3 % presenting with cough, recurrent aspiration, sore throat, hoarseness, dysphagia or substernal chest pain. In this group, typical symptoms were present in 32.8 % cases. Presenting symptom information was not available for 22.9 % GERD patients with large hernias and 3.8 % GERD patients with small hernias (Table 5.1).

In our case series, 91.4 % of patients with large hernias or paraesophageal hernias had a BMI>30 and 57.1 % had BMI>35. In comparison, 52.4 % of patients with small hernias had a BMI>30 and 18.1 % had BMI > 35 (Table 5.1). Early in our experience we did not have a limit on the BMI for patients undergoing an anti-reflux procedure. It is apparent from our data and other published reports that the operative time, rate of hiatus hernia recurrence, and reoperations is increased in those patients with BMI>35 [10].

Table 5.1 Characteristics and presenting symptoms for 175 patients undergoing robotic-GERD management procedures

	Large hiatal hernias ($n=70$)	Small hiatal hernias ($n=105$)
Age (years)	56±24	49±26
Pre-operative BMI		
<30	6 (8.6 %)	50 (47.6 %)
30–35	24 (34.3 %)	36 (34.3 %)
>35	40 (57.1 %)	19 (18.1 %)
Pre-operative PPI therapy	32 (45.7 %)	92 (87.6 %)
Presenting symptoms		
Typical symptoms[a]	23 (32.8 %)	85 (81.0 %)
Atypical symptoms[b]	31 (44.3 %)	16 (15.2 %)
Undetermined[c]	16 (22.9 %)	4 (3.8 %)

[a]Typical symptoms included are heartburn, regurgitation, sore throat, nighttime regurgitation and aspiration
[b]Atypical symptoms are cough, chest pain, esophageal spasm, dysphagia and bronchospasm
[c]Presenting symptoms were not documented for 20 patients

Table 5.2 Surgical outcomes in 175 patients

	Large hiatal hernias ($n=70$)	Small hiatal hernias ($n=105$)
Room time (mins)[a]	188±70	190±58
Operative time (mins)[b]	135±42	120±54
Mesh repairs	16 (22.9 %)	29 (27.6 %)
Median EBL (range) (ml)	34 (10–150)	30 (10–100)
Collis gastroplasty	18 (25.7 %)	8 (7.6 %)
Conversion to open	1 (1.4 %)	2 (1.9 %)
Transfusions	0	0
LOS (days)	2.4±0.9	1.9±0.5
Reoperations	3 (4.3 %)	11 (10.5 %)
30-day symptom reduction	64 (91.4 %)	90 (81.7 %)
30-day symptom relief	59 (84.3 %)	82 (78.1 %)

EBL estimated blood loss, *LOS* length of stay
[a]Room time is defined as time from patient entering the room until the time when the patient leaves the room
[b]Operating time is from first incision to all incisions closed at the end of the procedure. It includes "docking time, time on the DaVinci console, undocking, and closing incisions"

These patients are generally referred for gastric bypass or asked to lose weight to attain a BMI<35. Patients with large hernias or paraesophageal hernias are more likely to have BMI>35 than those patients whose primary symptom is heartburn.

Operative time was defined as time from incision to skin closure and room time was measured from time when a patient entered the room to he/she leaving the room. The room time included anesthesia time, which is invariably longer than the anesthesia time for laparoscopic operations for GERD. The patient must be turned, which puts anesthesiologists at the foot of the bed. The ventilator tubing must be stretched and secured the length of the patient. An arterial line is frequently used because of the difficulty in monitoring the patient in this position. The operative time also includes the docking time, which is the time needed for placing the robotic ports and docking the robot. In our experience, the room time and operative time between patient with large and small hernias were comparable with no statistically significant difference between room times (unpaired t-test, $p=0.84$) or operative times (unpaired t-test, $p=0.05$) (Table 5.2).

We found that there were other factors that lengthened the operative time. Patients with BMI >35 had a longer mean operative time at 146 min compared to 120 min for patients with BMI < 30. Presence of large hiatus hernias and paraesophageal hernias, which included more involved hiatus hernia repairs often times with, mesh increased mean operative time by 37 min. All reoperations were associated with increased operative times. In this group, there was a wide variation in the range of operative times depending on the number of recurrences and type of procedure done for the previous operation(s).

In the two groups of patients presenting with large and small hernias, mesh repairs were performed in 22.9 % ($n=16$) and 27.6 % ($n=29$), respectively (Table 5.2). The repair of the diaphragmatic hiatus is controversial and without any strong evidence to recommend a standard approach. With any hiatus dissection, even without a hiatus hernia, the takedown of the phrenoesophageal attachments will unavoidably disrupt the hiatal opening. This can be repaired with primary closure without mesh or reinforcing synthetic pledgets. However, several surgery-based repair approaches have been recommended when the hiatus hernia is large and the hiatus dilated. While these recommendations are not specific for patients operated on with robotic technology, the repair of the hiatus with placement of sutures can be much more precise in our experience. We utilize figure of eight sutures with reinforcing pledgets as our preferred method. Additionally, if the closure is tenuous we recommend the use onlay biologics or goretex. Grafts that bridge the gap in the hiatus have not worked well in our experience.

Total estimated blood loss for the procedures was in an acceptable range for our cohort of 175 patients (Table 5.2).

Eighteen patients with large paraesophageal hiatal hernias at presentation were treated with Collis gastroplasty. A review of data indicated that increased use of Collis gastroplasty resulted in an improvement of outcomes for our patients with large paraesophageal hiatus hernia and foreshortened esophagus. While there are several who espouse negligible need for performing such esophageal lengthening procedures, there is little doubt that Collis gastroplasty in selected patients reduces the incidence of recurrent hiatus hernia [11, 12]. Collis gastroplasty has significantly reduced the re-operation rate and hiatus recurrence rate for our patients undergoing anti-reflux procedures. We routinely use Collis gastroplasty for re-do Nissen fundoplication with the assumption that recurrent symptoms following anti-reflux operations is largely due to recurrent hernias resulting from undue tension at the diaphragmatic hiatus. Of the 26 combined fundoplication and Collis gastroplasty operations we have performed, there has been only one recurrent hernia.

There were no major intra-operative complications related exclusively to the use of the robot or to the changes in the position of the anesthesiologist relative to the patient as well as any of the monitoring equipment. Three patients had to be converted to open procedures for difficult exposure or dissection (Table 5.2). There was one post-operative death. This was a cardiac death in an elderly patient with a prolonged operation for a large paraesophageal hiatus hernia. On post-operative day 1, the patient had a cardiac event from which he did not recover. One patient had DVT, which required heparinization but no pulmonary complications were evident.

In our patient population, robotic assisted anti-reflux procedures did not decrease the hospital length of stay (LOS) compared to laparoscopic anti-reflux procedures. Patients undergoing laparoscopic Nissen fundoplication and hiatus hernia repair had a mean LOS of 1.1 days [13]. The longer stay with the robotic procedures was due in part to the gradually increasing comorbidities of our more recent patients and the increase in the numbers of patient with large hernias and paraesophageal hernias. The mean LOS for individuals undergoing Nissen procedures without a paraesophageal hiatus hernia repair was 1.9 days whereas Nissens with a paraesophageal hiatus hernia repair had a mean LOS of 2.4 days (Table 5.2). Interestingly, a statistically significant difference was noted in the LOS between GERD patients with large (paraesophageal or sliding) hernias as compared to patient with small or no hernias (unpaired t-test; $p<0.0001$).

Fourteen (8.0 %) patients required reoperations and all reoperations were performed with the robotic technology (Table 5.2). Three patients who had paraesophageal hernias developed recurrent hernias and became symptomatic. Of the 11 remaining reoperations (for patients with small hernias), two required reoperations within the first week after their first procedure. One patient, with a BMI>35, had immediate incarceration and obstruction of the fundoplication through the hiatus within 5 days of operation. A second patient was readmitted to the hospital for unrelenting chest pain and dysphagia 7 days following operation and a takedown of the fundoplication was required. Another fundoplication was not performed and the hiatus hernia repair was left intact.

There were six patients who underwent reoperation for symptomatic reflux and/or recurrent hernia within 2–10 months of their first operation. Of these patients, two had significant esophageal dysmotility that was either unrecognized preoperatively or the severity of the condition underestimated. Of the recurrent hernias, one individual had mesh repair and Nissen fundoplication, four patients had primary hiatus hernia repair and Nissen fundoplication, and one patient had a primary hiatus hernia repair with a Collis gastroplasty. Six of the ten patients who had recurrent hernia as an indication for reoperation had BMI>35.

Early symptomatic relief was achieved in 80.6 % (141 of 175) of our patients. Long-term relief and need for continued PPIs and other reflux medications is currently being evaluated. The patients who had regurgitation or atypical symptoms such as cough, sore throat or hoarseness had slightly better symptomatic relief than those who had mostly heartburn as their main symptom. Patients who had large symptomatic hernias either paraesophageal or sliding type hernias also had improvement in some of the less well defined symptoms of chest discomfort, chest pain, chest pressure and dysphagia.

Discussion

Laparoscopic fundoplication is considered the gold standard surgical management option for GERD [14]. It is an operation, which in experienced hands has a negligible mortality, very low operative morbidity, and excellent short-term results [15]. However, discouraging long-term (>5 year) outcomes have prevented gastroenterologists from recommending fundoplications solely for (a) patients with intolerable symptoms or paraesophageal hernias which may be causing obstructive symptoms, (b) patients bleeding from Cameron erosions, or (c) those who might be having episodes of torsion of the herniated stomach. Patients whose main symptoms are related to regurgitation are not helped by medical management and thus present to operative intervention more often because of lack of alternative medical management options. Fundoplication is very effective for the management of patients with regurgitation.

The average length of stay in the hospital for patients having laparoscopic fundoplication is 1 day. The hospital stay may be extended to 2 days for elderly patients or patients with significant co-morbidities. Patients having more extensive operations such as large paraesophageal hernias or upside-down stomachs in the chest may require additional days in the hospital.

Generally, laparoscopic equipments are relatively sturdy, inexpensive and re-usable. The instruments are adaptable to a multitude of different laparoscopic procedures and the same cameras can be utilized in all laparoscopic operations. In other words, laparoscopy is a relatively economical way to perform a variety of general surgical procedures including fundoplication. This raises the question, why should we use robotic technology for operations performed effectively with laparoscopic techniques?

Robotic technology was first put to use in operations for prostate cancer. For this oncologic operation, robotic-procedures have proven advantages over open procedures with less operative blood loss, easier post-operative recovery, less post-operative pain, comparable oncological parameters, and decreased LOS [16]. Within a relatively short period of time robotic prostatectomy has become the standard for surgical management of prostate cancer. Currently, ~75 % of patients having operative procedures performed for management of prostate cancer undergo robotic assisted prostatectomy. This has been a major change in practice for urologists who have traditionally performed most procedures with open techniques. Accepting and adapting to robotic procedures was daunting for most and the early results indicated that the adaptation to a minimally invasive approach resulted in a significant number of complications. The learning curve for robotic prostatectomy was steep. The early results suggested that surgeons should be proctored for at least ten cases and a high level of proficiency was reached only at completion of ~50 procedures. Nevertheless, at present time, most surgeons consider robotic assisted prostatectomy as a major advance in patient care.

The adoption of robotic technology by the gynecological specialty has been a considerably simpler and safer process for patients and the transition from laparoscopic to robotic techniques in gynecology has proven to be remarkably straightforward. The learning curve for gynecologists using robotic technology has not been as steep and the number of cases to gain proficiency has been fewer. Consequently, gynecologic operations for benign disease have now overtaken the lead in numbers of patients having robotic-assisted operations. The operative blood loss, improved oncologic parameters, post-op pain, LOS and overall easier recovery have caused many gynecologic oncologists to adopt robotic technology [2].

Other surgical specialties notably cardiovascular, pediatric urology and thoracic surgery have had increasing numbers of cases and surgeons performing their operations robotically. Again, for many of these specialties the transition from open procedures to robotic was accompanied by a steep learning curve due to the lack of prior exposure to the use of laparoscopic technology. During the initial period of adoption of robotic technology, with the steep learning curve came increased morbidity for the patients. Robotic assisted operations for general gastro-esophageal management procedures have not increased as one might expect for procedures such as fundoplication, Heller myotomy, trans-hiatal esophagectomy and low-anterior resection or abdominal perineal resection [2, 17]. The lack of interest in performing robotic assisted operations could be due to many factors. The learning curve is thought to be quite steep. In actuality, for an experienced laparoscopic surgeon, robotic assisted operations are not difficult to learn and are somewhat easier to perform than the same laparoscopic operation. The surgeon is supported in the operative process by high definition optics and the three-dimensional vision in the robotic technology, which provides better visualization than laparoscopic technology. Suturing with complete dexterity is very similar to that for an open operation that is impossible to duplicate with the commonly used endo-stitch. During laparoscopic procedures, it is difficult for many surgeons to utilize laparoscopic needle drivers. Very few surgeons have completely mastered this technique.

The other advantage of robotic surgical-procedures is from an ergonomic viewpoint. The ergonomics of performing these operations, especially with difficult paraesophageal hiatus hernia repairs, is ideal. The arms are at rest at the surgeon's side with minimal movement. The shoulders are in a natural position without any strain. The head is positioned on a cushion with comfortable viewing ports for the camera. Much of the positioning of camera and instruments and all of the energy usage is accomplished with the surgeon's feet. Essentially, at the end of the day, the mere ergonomic advantages of operating with the robot can make it worthwhile even without the other obvious benefits, such as better visualization and more precise dissecting and suturing.

Robotic surgery is not for the casual user. It requires frequent usage, as do more complicated operations, no matter how they are performed. Recent discussions of the detrimental musculoskeletal and visual effects that are a result of poor ergonomic positioning and techniques for laparoscopic general surgical procedures require a serious look at the present state of laparoscopic surgery [18]. Surgeons who are considering devoting a major portion of their operative time in performing laparoscopic procedures should consider robotic technology for these same operations.

The cost of developing a robotic program is significant for any hospital system. There is no doubt that robotic technology is necessary for a well-developed prostate cancer program. It is also necessary for a cutting edge gynecologic oncology program and by patient demand it is becoming quite necessary for benign gynecologic procedures. The new robotic assisted operations for head and neck cancers, especially those procedures performed for tonsillar cancers and posterior pharynx and tongue cancers, has allowed patients to avoid the more disfiguring operations traditionally performed by head and neck surgeons. This leaves general surgeons with little of the burden of justifying the cost of a robotic general surgical program. The short-term results for the patients in our series are similar to our experience with the laparoscopic approach. The long-term results are unknown at this time. Perhaps the benefits for the surgeon mentioned above will be bolstered by a lower hiatus hernia recurrence rate, fewer patients on anti-reflux medications and result in fewer ergonomically caused injuries for the surgeon.

Conclusion

Robotic technology has become essential for the performance of complicated minimally invasive operations for many surgical specialties. The technology will find its place in the operative armamentarium of many more specialties and surgeons. The role of robotic technology for general surgeons is yet to be defined but the advances that have been made and some of the newer procedures performed such as single port cholecystectomy portend a bright future for the robotic technology.

Acknowledgment The authors are grateful to Gary Edelburg for procuring images incorporated in this chapter.

References

1. Broeders JA, Mauritz FA, Ahmed Ali U, Draaisma WA, Ruurda JP, Gooszen HG, Smout AJ, Broeders IA, Hazebroek EJ. Systematic review and meta-analysis of laparoscopic Nissen (posterior total) versus Toupet (posterior partial) fundoplication for gastro-oesophageal reflux disease. Br J Surg. 2010;97(9):1318–30.
2. Anderson JE, Chang DC, Parsons JK, Talamini MA. The first national examination of outcomes and trends in robotic surgery in the United States. J Am Coll Surg. 2012;215(1):107–14.
3. Niebisch S, Fleming FJ, Galey KM, Wilshire CL, Jones CE, Litle VR, Watson TJ, Peters JH. Perioperative risk of laparoscopic fundoplication: safer than previously reported-analysis of the American college of surgeons national surgical quality improvement program 2005 to 2009. J Am Coll Surg. 2012;215(1):61–8.
4. Dunn DH, Johnson EM, Morphew JA, Dilworth HP, Krueger JL, Banerji N. Robot-assisted transhiatal esophagectomy: a 3-year single-center experience. Dis Esophagus. 2013;26(2):159–66.
5. Mi J, Kang Y, Chen X, Wang B, Wang Z. Whether robot-assisted laparoscopic fundoplication is better for gastroesophageal reflux disease in adults: a systematic review and meta-analysis. Surg Endosc. 2010;24(8):1803–14.
6. Vela MF, Camacho-Lobato L, Srinivasan R, Tutuian R, Katz PO, Castell DO. Simultaneous intraesophageal impedance and pH measurement of acid and non-acid gastroesophageal reflux: effect of omeprazole. Gastroenterology. 2001;120(7):1599–606.
7. Hafez J, Wrba F, Lenglinger J, Miholic J. Fundoplication for gastroesophageal reflux and factors associated with the outcome 6 to 10 years after the operation: multivariate analysis of prognostic factors using the propensity score. Surg Endosc. 2008;22(8):1763–68.
8. Shaw JM, Bornman PC, Callanan MD, Beckingham IJ, Metz DC. Long-term outcome of laparoscopic Nissen and laparoscopic Toupet fundoplication for gastroesophageal reflux disease: a prospective, randomized trial. Surg Endosc. 2010;24(4):924–32.
9. Varin O, Velstra B, De Sutter S, Ceelen W. Total vs. partial fundoplication in the treatment of gastroesophageal reflux disease: a meta-analysis. Arch Surg. 2009;144(3):273–78.
10. Raue W, Ordemann J, Jacobi CA, Menenakos C, Buchholz A, Hartmann J. Nissen versus Dor fundoplication for treatment of gastroesophageal reflux disease: a blinded randomized clinical trial. Dig Surg. 2011;28(1):80–6.
11. Whitson BA, Hoang CD, Boettcher AK, Dahlberg PS, Andrade RS, Maddaus MA. Wedge gastroplasty and reinforced crural repair: important components of laparoscopic giant or recurrent hiatal hernia repair. J Thorac Cardiovasc Surg. 2006;132(5):1196–202.
12. Oelschlager BK, Petersen RP, Brunt LM, Soper NJ, Sheppard BC, Mitsumori L, Rohrmann C, Swanstrom LL, Pellegrini CA. Laparoscopic paraesophageal hernia repair: defining long-term clinical and anatomic outcomes. J Gastrointest Surg. 2012;16(3):453–59.
13. Graber J, Dunn D, Johnson E, Alden P, Bretzke M, Markman J. Laparoscopic gastric fundoplication for treatment of gastroesophageal reflux disease (GERD). Results from 150 consecutive cases. Minn Med. 2002;85(1):38–42.
14. Salminen P. The laparoscopic Nissen fundoplication–a better operation? Surgeon. 2009;7(4):224–27.
15. Peters MJ, Mukhtar A, Yunus RM, Khan S, Pappalardo J, Memon B, Memon MA. Meta-analysis of randomized clinical trials comparing open and laparoscopic anti-reflux surgery. Am J Gastroenterol. 2009;104(6):1548–61.
16. Bivalacqua TJ, Pierorazio PM, Su LM. Open, laparoscopic and robotic radical prostatectomy: optimizing the surgical approach. Surg Oncol. 2009;18(3):233–41.
17. Zhang P, Tian JH, Yang KH, Li J, Jia WQ, Sun SL, Ma B, Liu YL. Robot-assisted laparoscope fundoplication for gastroesophageal reflux disease: a systematic review of randomized controlled trials. Digestion. 2010;81(1):1–9.
18. Glickson J. Surgeons experience more ergonomic stress in the OR. Bull Am Coll Surg. 2012;97(4):20–6.

Achalasia

6

Julia Samamé, Mark R. Dylewski,
Angela Echeverria, and Carlos A. Galvani

Introduction

Idiopathic achalasia, although rare, is the most common primary motility disorder of the esophagus [1]. This chronic condition is characterized by an incomplete or absent relaxation of the lower esophageal sphincter (LES) and lack of peristaltic contraction of the esophageal body that results in difficulty swallowing ultimately with dilation of the esophagus [2]. The etiology remains unclear, but studies suggest that the dysfunction results from degeneration of ganglion cells in the myoenteric plexus of Auerbach with loss of postganglionic inhibitory neurons. These neurons, by the secretion of vasoactive intestinal peptide (VIP) and nitric oxide mediate LES relaxation. Therefore, there is an unopposed acetylcholine stimulation of the sphincter with increase of the LES pressure [1]. The triggering event that leads to ganglion degeneration is not known, but because this process is associated with an inflammatory response including lymphocytes infiltration it would seem to most likely implicate an autoimmune, viral or chronic degenerative destruction in genetically susceptible individuals [3]. Rarely, a mutation in the chromosome 12 is implicated in the development of achalasia as a familial form inherited on autosomal recessive mode, known as Allgrove's syndrome or "4A syndrome" which combines achalasia, alacrymia, autonomic disturbance, and corticotropin insensitivity [4, 5].

The disease appears to have a stable incidence but rising prevalence (1.63/100,000 and 10.82/100,000 respectively) as was shown in a recent population-based study [6]. There is no gender predominance and can occur at any age, but the highest observance is in the seventh decade with a second smaller peak of incidence at 20–40 years of age. Although achalasia is uncommon among children, when it appears it affects mainly teenagers and it is usually sporadic [7].

Clinical Findings

Up to 90 % of patients with achalasia present with dysphagia, mostly for solids but it can also be for liquids [4]. Regurgitation of undigested food is the second most frequent manifestation, presenting in approximately 60 % of patients. This symptom is more common during nighttime

J. Samamé, M.D. • A. Echeverria, M.D.
Department of Surgery, University of Arizona,
1501 N. Campbell Avenue, Tucson, AZ 85724, USA
e-mail: jsamame@surgery.arizona.edu;
aechev@gmail.com

M.R. Dylewski, M.D.
Department of Cardiac Vascular and Thoracic Surgery, Baptist Health of South Florida, 6200 SW 72nd Street, Suite 604, Miami, FL 33143, USA
e-mail: MarkD@Baptisthealth.net

C.A. Galvani, M.D. (✉)
Department of Surgery, University of Arizona,
1501 N. Campbell Avenue, P.O. Box 245066,
Tucson, AZ 85712, USA
e-mail: cgalvani@surgery.arizona.edu

K.C. Kim (ed.), *Robotics in General Surgery*, DOI 10.1007/978-1-4614-8739-5_6,

while in supine position, exposing patients to an increased risk of aspiration. Consequently, bouts of aspiration pneumonia may be elicited. About 40 % of the patients will complain of heartburn, typically produced by the bacterial fermentation and thus, acidification of retention food. As a result, reflux symptoms that are unresponsive to reflux therapy may suggest achalasia. Chest pain is present in 40–50 % of cases, commonly among young patients who have been symptomatic for a short period and who often have vigorous achalasia [8, 9].

There are occasions when this disease is associated with weight loss but many patients have normal or less commonly, excess weight owing to changes in eating habits, including slow eating, stereotactic movements with eating, and avoidance of social functions that include meals [4]. Pseudoachalasia can be indistinguishable from primary achalasia on routine clinical evaluation. For that reason, in aging patients who present with shorter durations of symptoms and greater weight loss, further workup is recommended [10].

Preoperative Evaluation

Barium Swallow

The first diagnostic test in all patients with dysphagia should be a barium swallow, as up to 95 % of them will have positive findings. The typical features of achalasia are: the classic tapering at the level of the gastroesophageal junction ("bird beak") and a dilated esophagus body along with undigested food particles. With the progression of the disease, a sigmoid-shaped esophagus could be seen. Another finding of this contrasted study is a delayed emptying of the esophagus [2].

Upper Endoscopy

After a barium swallow has been performed, an upper endoscopy should be performed to rule out other causes of esophageal obstruction such as malignancy, which is known to be more prevalent in achalasia patients [11]. The endoscope is advanced through the gastroesophageal junction without increased resistance, a feature that distinguishes primary from secondary achalasia or benign strictures. Although retained food and saliva are often observed, a normal endoscopy should not rule out the diagnosis of achalasia because up to 40 % of patients will have a negative study [3, 4].

Esophageal Manometry

This study is considered the gold standard diagnostic modality for achalasia. The classic findings are aperistalsis of the esophageal body with low-amplitude simultaneous waves, a LES with an elevated resting pressure, and absent or partial relaxation of the sphincter after swallowing. However, 55 % of patients will have either normal or low pressure. The manometry is also useful for the post-treatment evaluation of patients after balloon dilation or Heller myotomy [12]. Recently, the introduction of esophageal topography in conjunction with high-resolution esophageal manometry has led to the development of the Chicago Classification of esophageal motility disorders. The ability to outline the exact location of contractions is the strength of esophageal topography and may benefit in the diagnosis of vigorous achalasia, in which spastic contractions are noted in the distal esophageal segment [13].

Ambulatory pH Monitoring

This test should be performed preoperatively in patients who have undergone pneumatic balloon dilation or surgical myotomy to determine if abnormal reflux is already present. In patients with a positive score, it is essential to distinguish between true reflux and false reflux due to stasis and fermentation of food. After procedure, this test should be repeated to assess development of new abnormal reflux [12].

Indications for Surgery

Those patients who meet the diagnostic criteria for achalasia (manometric, endoscopic, radiographic) and who are good surgical candidates should undergo a minimally invasive surgical treatment.

The aim of the therapy is to relieve the resistance at the level of the LES and to improve esophageal emptying. For many years, the therapy of choice to accomplish this was the pneumatic balloon dilatation. In 1991, the introduction of minimally invasive techniques for the treatment of achalasia with high successful rates has brought about a shift in the actual practice, where laparoscopic Heller myotomy is consider the standard treatment option. This remarkable change in the treatment algorithm was followed by documentation that laparoscopic treatment outperforms endoscopic modalities, and should be continued with the incorporation of robotic-assisted approach in the spectrum of minimally invasive achalasia treatment options (Fig. 6.1) [12, 14–16].

Surgical Technique

Perioperative Considerations

Preoperatively, patients are advised to ingest only clear liquids 2–3 days before surgery. Premedication with prophylactic anti-reflux is strongly recommended. Pneumatic compression stockings are placed routinely. In order to minimize aspiration risk during induction of anesthesia, the airway can be secured either after a rapid sequence induction with cricoid pressure or with fiberoptic bronchoscope assistance while the patient is awake. If possible, an orogastric tube (OG-Tube) is placed to fully decompress the esophagus and the stomach. The anesthesiologist is advised not to force the OG-Tube if resistance is found. In older patients with several comorbidities, a Foley catheter is set and usually removed after the surgery. Intraoperative monitoring will be guided by the American Society of Anesthesiologists (ASA) recommendations.

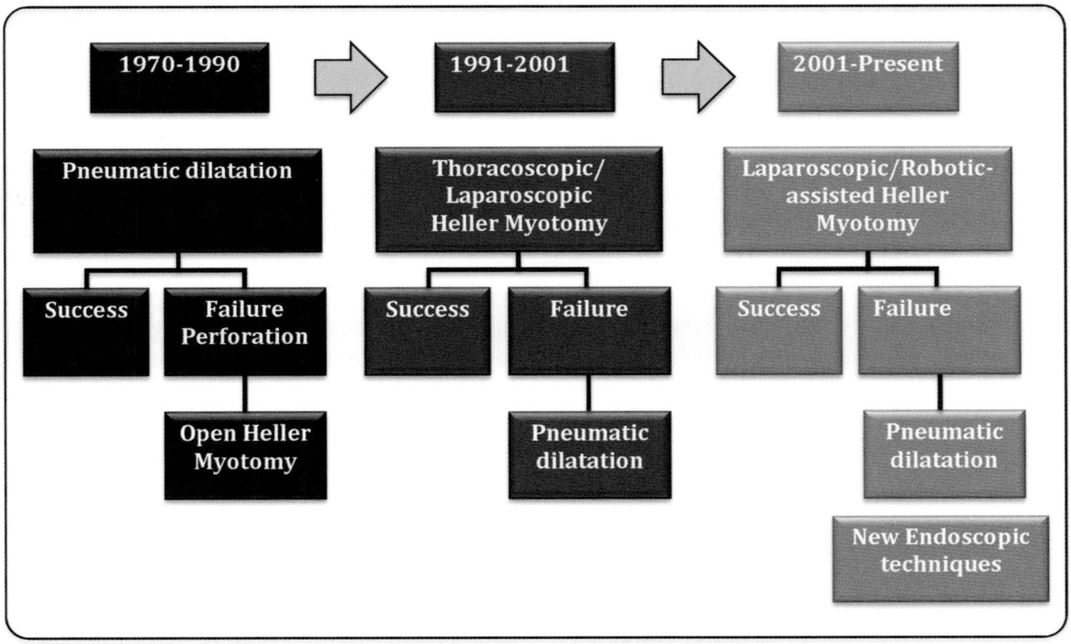

Fig. 6.1 Evolution of the treatment algorithm for Achalasia

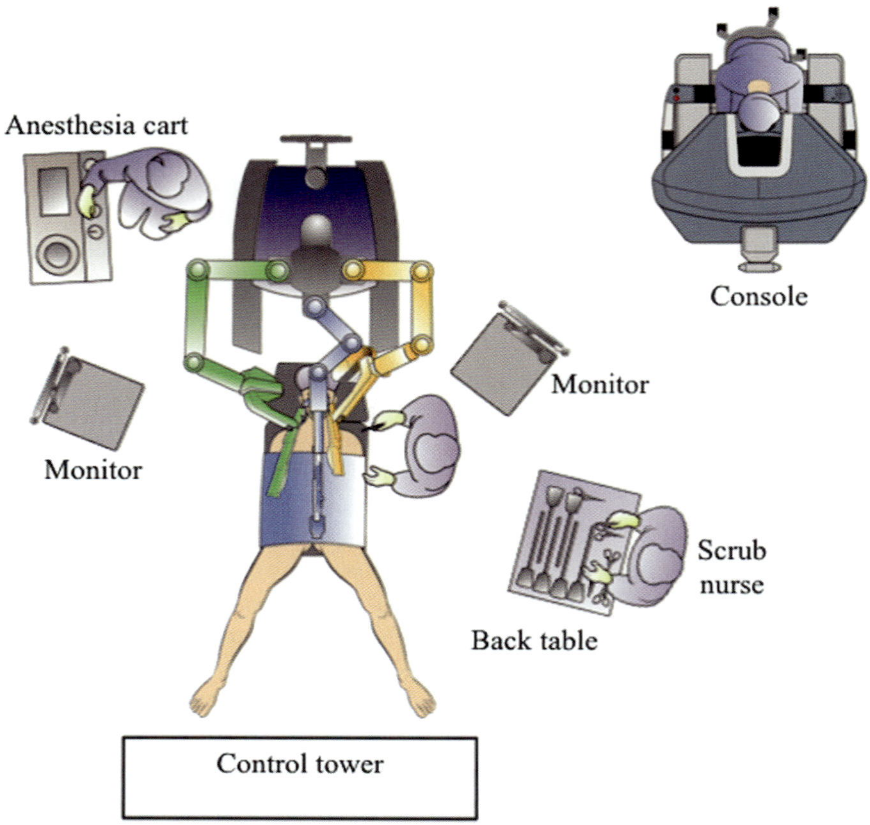

Fig. 6.2 Operating room set-up

Patient Position

Once under general endotracheal anesthesia, the patient is placed in a modified lithotomy position over a "bean bag." Its use prevents the patient from moving down the table when in steep reverse Trendelenburg is needed. The beanbag is then inflated and a 4-in. tape is used to secure the patient to the table. The legs and pressure points are cushioned appropriately. The skin of the abdomen is prepped and draped from the nipple line to the pubis. The exposure of the chest is required in the eventuality of conversion to thoracotomy. The bedside component of the robot is positioned over the patient's left shoulder. The operating room set up is shown in Fig. 6.2.

Trocar Placement

The positioning of the trocar is the same used in every advanced esophageal procedure. The first trocar is placed through a gasless optical technique in the periumbilical area, utilizing a bladeless 12-mm trocar with an optical tip that eliminates blind entry to the abdominal cavity. This 12-mm trocar is required for the 30° robotic camera system. Its positioning left to the midline allows better visualization of the gastroesophageal junction (GEJ). Pneumoperitoneum is induced. Two 8-mm trocar ports are then placed, one each at the left and right mid-clavicular line subcostal margin. The size of these trocars is specific for the robotic system. An additional

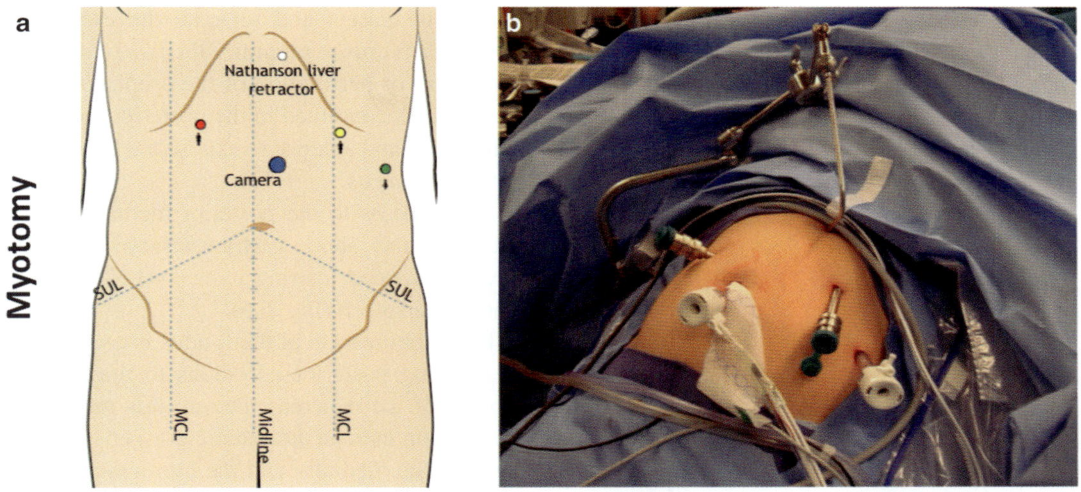

Fig. 6.3 Trocar placement for robot-assisted Heller myotomy. Four trocars technique. (**a**) Arm 1 (*red*), hook cautery, harmonic scalpel. Arm 2 (*yellow*), Cadiere grasper. Arm 3 (*green*), Cadiere grasper. (**b**) Corresponding trocars placement for four trocars technique

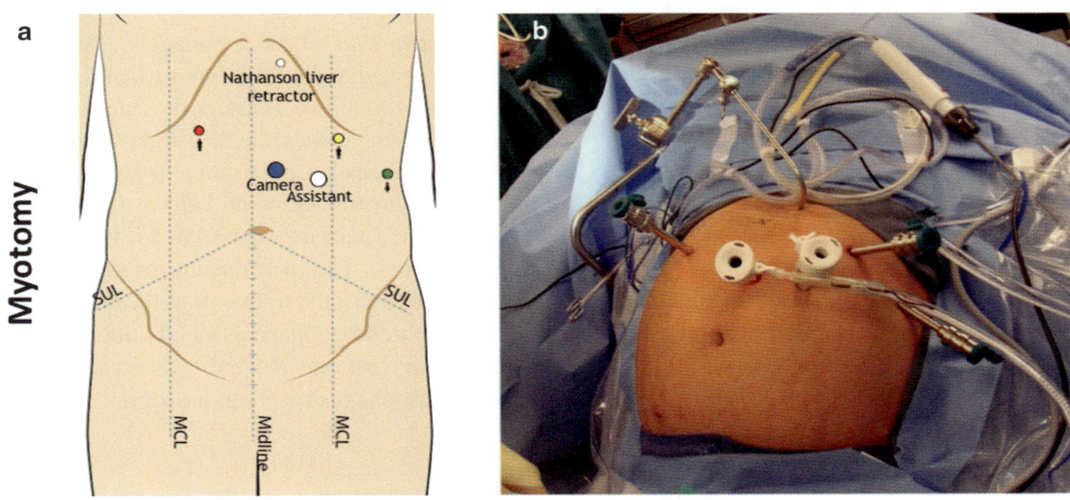

Fig. 6.4 Trocar placement for robotic-assisted Heller myotomy. Five trocars technique. (**a**) Arm 1 (*red*), hook cautery, harmonic scalpel. Arm 2 (*yellow*), Cadiere grasper. Arm 3 (*green*), Cadiere grasper. (**b**) Corresponding trocars placement for five trocars technique

10/12-mm trocar is placed at the left lateral abdominal wall to assist with suction and passage of sutures. A 5-mm incision is made in the subxiphoid area, and the left lobe of the liver is retracted using the Nathanson liver retractor, allowing exposure of the anterior part of the stomach and the hiatus (Fig. 6.3a, b).

With a 5-trocar technique, an additional 12-mm trocar is inserted. In this case, the third robotic arm is used for retraction and the assistant can use the fifth trocar for suction, passing of sutures or cutting. This technique is ideal when a well-trained assistant in robotic approach is not available (Fig. 6.4a, b).

Once the trocars are in place, the nursing personnel approximate the robotic surgical cart into position and the arms are attached to the three specific trocars. A Cadiere Forceps is placed in

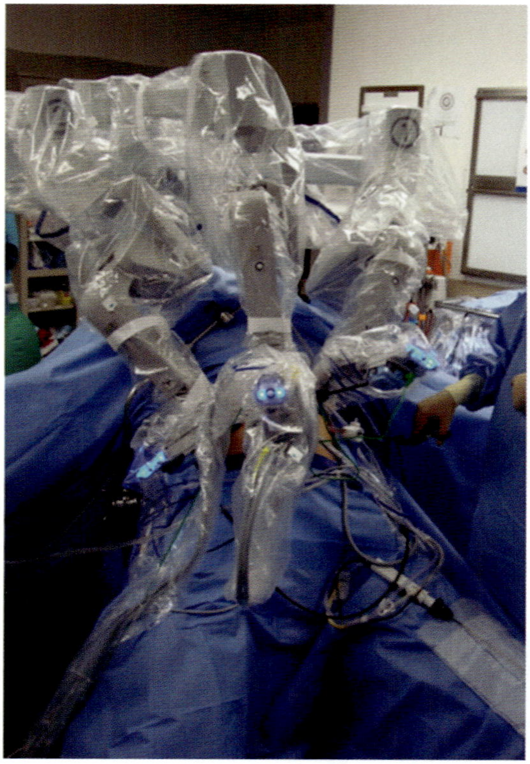

Fig. 6.5 Surgical arm cart in position to start the procedure

the surgeon's left hand and in the right hand; the articulated hook cautery or the harmonic scalpel is positioned (Fig. 6.5).

The assistant surgeon is situated on the patient's left side. During the case, the assistant is in charge of cutting, suction and retraction. Also, if needed, the assistant switches the robotic instruments for the operating surgeon. For that reason, basic training in laparoscopic surgery and robotics is essential.

Dissection of the Lower Third of the Esophagus and the Division of the Short Gastric Vessels

The procedure starts by dividing the peritoneum overlying the left crus of the diaphragm utilizing the harmonic scalpel. The phrenoesophageal membrane is transected as well. A blunt technique is used to dissect and separate the esophagus from the left crus to minimize the risk of inadvertent injury or perforation of the esophagus. The dissection is continued in the posterior mediastinum lateral and anterior to expose the lower third of the esophagus.

Once access to the posterior mediastinum is obtained, the short gastric vessels are then carefully divided, starting at the level of the lower pole of the spleen (Fig. 6.6).

Full mobilization of the fundus is carried out, by dividing posterior adhesions to the anterior capsule of the pancreas. During this maneuver, the surgeon uses an atraumatic grasper to retract the stomach medially and the harmonic scalpel, which allows performing this part of the operation in a bloodless fashion. The left side of the esophagus is identified, by dissecting the left crus from the esophagus. Only the anterior part of the esophagus is dissected, respecting the posterior attachments of the esophagus. After that, attention is centered on the exposure of the right crus. At this time, the assistant provides traction of the stomach, meanwhile the surgeon, using an atraumatic grasper and harmonic scalpel divides the gastrohepatic ligament below the hepatic branch of the vagus nerve and extends the dissection upwards. The peritoneum overlying the anterior surface of the right crus of the diaphragm and the phrenoesophageal membrane is transected. The right crus is identified and separated from the esophagus by blunt dissection.

Heller Myotomy

After passing a #44F bougie through the mouth by the anesthesia team, the removal of the fat pad is accomplished to better expose the GEJ. The placement of the bougie helps with the performance of the myotomy. The assistant retracts the GEJ caudally with the atraumatic grasper to increase the length of the intra-abdominal esophagus. It is important at this point of the dissection to identify and preserve the anterior branch of the vagus nerve (Fig. 6.7).

After its identification, the vagus nerve is dissected upwards in an extension of approximately

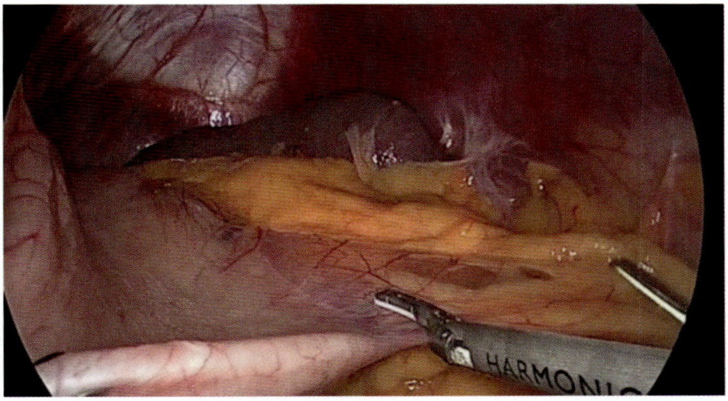

Fig. 6.6 Mobilization of fundus and division of short gastric vessels

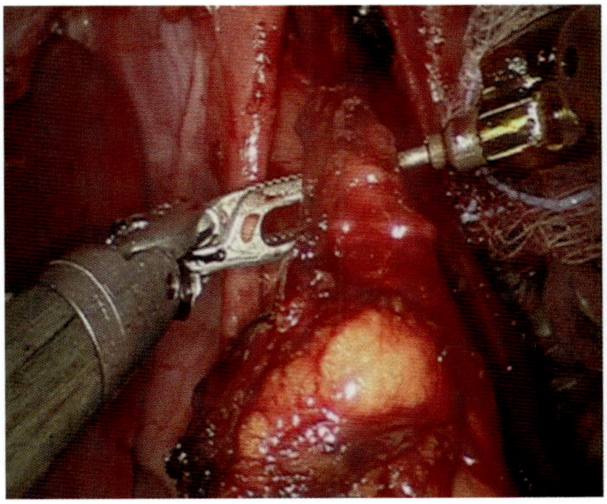

Fig. 6.7 Identification of the anterior branch of the vagus nerve

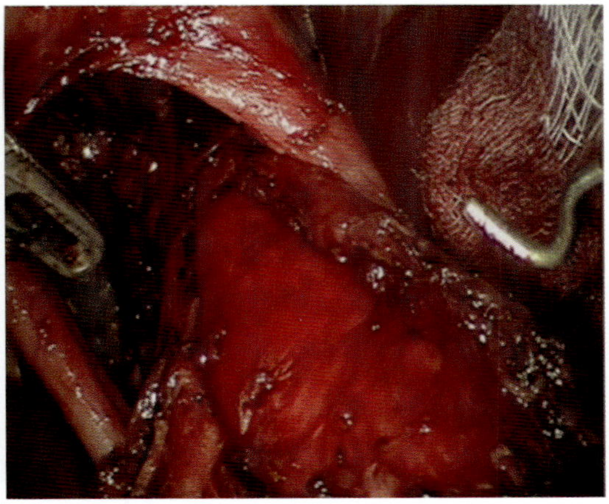

Fig. 6.8 Myotomy

10 cm, divorcing it clearly from the esophageal wall and moving it to the right side. The myotomy is started out just above the GEJ on the 12 o'clock position using the articulated hook electrocautery. Methodical marking of the area is performed by scoring the esophagus with the back of the hook electrocautery for about 6–7 cm above the GEJ. The submucosal plane is reached in one point by dividing the longitudinal and circular muscle layer (Fig. 6.8).

This is followed by extending the myotomy a minimum of 6 cm proximally and for about 2 cm distally into the stomach. During the proximal extension of the myotomy it is important to provide counter-traction of the circular fibers with the Cadiere grasper in order to divide them with the articulated hook safely. The myotomy on the gastric side, is carried down in a "Hockey stick" configuration to transect the sling fibers of the stomach wall. Failure to achieve adequate proximal dissection of the esophagus with a subsequent short myotomy is the most common reason for failure.

Creation of the Partial Fundoplication (Dor)

The preferred antireflux procedure is the Dor fundoplication, which is an anterior 180° fundoplication. This operation is chosen because other

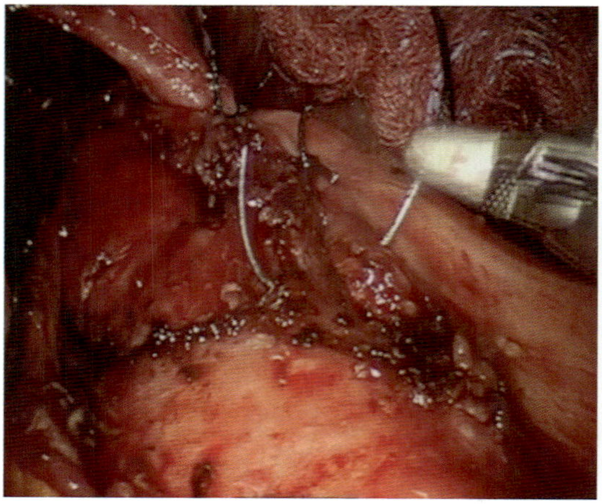

Fig. 6.9 Dor fundoplication, first row of sutures. The first stitch comprises the crura, fundus and muscular layer of the esophagus. The second and third stitches incorporate the esophageal and the gastric wall only

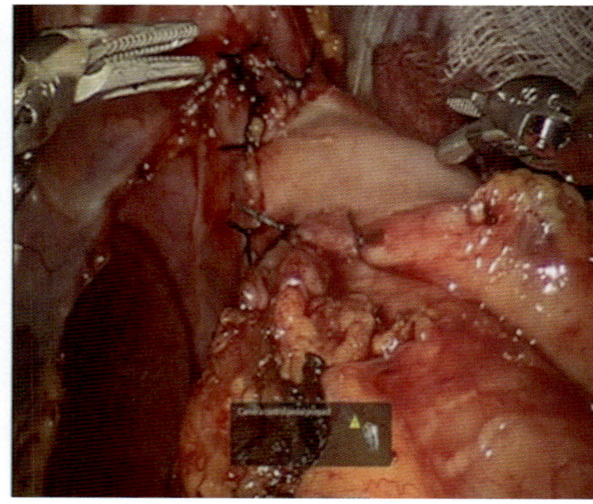

Fig. 6.10 Dor fundoplication, second row of sutures. The first stitch comprises the stomach, the right edge of the myotomy, and the right pillar. Repair completed with a second and a third stitches between the greater curvature of the stomach and the right side of the esophageal muscle

than being an effective antireflux repair, it covers the exposed mucosa. The Dor technique involves two rows of sutures, each composed of three stitches. The first row of sutures includes the gastric fundus, the crura and the left side of myotomy (Fig. 6.9).

After passing a 2-0 silk 15 cm stitch to the surgeon, the assistant grabs the fundus and pulls up toward the left crus. The first stitch is a triangular one, positioned between the fundus, the left pillar and the left side of the myotomy. Two additional stitches incorporate the gastric wall and the left side of the myotomy. Subsequently, the assistant folds the stomach over the exposed mucosa and the second row of sutures is created by placing stitches between the stomach and the right edge of the myotomy (Fig. 6.10).

The first stitch is placed between the stomach, the right edge of the myotomy, and the right pillar. Finally, the second and the third stitches are placed between the greater curvature of the stomach and the right side of the esophageal muscle. Avoiding inclusion of the right pillar in the second and third stitches of the fundoplication is vital, since this could represent a reason for postoperative dysphagia. Two supplementary stitches are placed between the gastric fundus and the rim of the hiatus completing the fundoplication. The purpose of these last stitches is to further decrease the tension of the fundoplication and to prevent the lateral rotation of the wrap.

Outcome Evaluation

Table 6.1 shows the results of the three largest series from centers where this technique is used [17–19].

Overall, excellent or good results are consistently obtained in more than 90 % of patients, with no intraoperative esophageal perforations in any of the series. Operative times ranged between 119 and 140.55 min including the robotic set-up time. In two of these series, a significant decrease in the average time was noticed after 30 cases revealing the importance of the learning curve and the experience of the operating room team in order to reduce the robot set-up time. The mean length of hospital stay is 1.5 days in all three series with no significant differences from laparoscopic Heller procedures.

Two out of fifty-nine patients in the study published by Horgan et al., 3/73 patients in our series and 1/104 in the study of Melvin et al., required postoperative endoscopic treatment with complete relief of symptoms after the procedure.

Table 6.1 Robotic-assisted Heller myotomy outcomes [17–19]

Author (year)	Patients (*n*)	Average OT (min)	Perforation rate (%)	Excellent/good results (%)	Additional tto (%)
Horgan (2005)	59	149	0	92	3.4
Melvin (2005)	104	140.55	0	100	1
Galvani (2011)	73	119	0	96	4

OT operative time, *min* minutes, *tto* treatment

Comments

Laparoscopic Heller myotomy using the standard technique has evolved into an extremely safe and accepted procedure offering better long-lasting results in terms of controlling symptoms in the treatment of Achalasia. However, it is impossible for even experienced laparoscopic surgeons to overcome some well-known disadvantages related to laparoscopic surgery that transform this procedure into a technically challenging one with a considerable learning curve [20]. This method provides a two-dimensional image, which eliminates perception of depth and the projection of the image on a screen also interrupts the natural eye-hand-target working axis. The necessity of the use of long instruments through fixed entry points in the abdominal wall limits the degree of freedom of motion and promotes friction on the instruments. The dependence on the camera operator during the surgery, the poor ergonomic positioning of the surgeon and the need for specialized training, may explain in part why, in most laparoscopic series, the rate of intraoperative esophageal perforation ranged from 1 to 16 %.

Robotic technology has emerged as a suitable alternative in the field of minimally invasive surgery to overcome some of these technical impediments. As it relates to the surgical treatment of achalasia, several reports including our own experience have documented that robotic-assisted Heller myotomy is safer, has 0 % rate of esophageal perforation and is associated with higher quality of life indices when compared with laparoscopic approach [17, 18]. Published in 2010, these same concepts were reinforced by the first systematic review and meta-analysis comparing the robotic surgical system versus laparoscopic Heller myotomy [16].

Several factors may play a role in decreasing the morbidity of the procedure. The robotic system provides a three-dimensional vision support allowing the isolation and division of each individual muscle fiber. The increase of dexterity and the elimination of tremors also contribute to a precise dissection and give a clear view of the submucosal plane, subsequently reducing the risk of perforation. The freedom of movements of the wristed instruments enables the adjustment of the angle of work according to the direction of the fibers from circular to oblique at the GEJ; the Achilles' heel of the laparoscopic myotomy is that the surgeon must operate in a narrow field around the thoracic esophagus. This not only lengthens the intra-abdominal portion of the esophagus but also admits for proper extension of the myotomy. Even though this technique is not exempt from the learning curve as calculated in 30 cases, it is extremely shorter compared with the more than 200 procedures required in order to achieve proficiency with laparoscopic approach. Moreover, there is mounting evidence that the learning curve is necessary when performing laparoscopic myotomy to reduce hospital stay and complication rates, while in the case of the robotic approach, the learning curve only affects the time consumed for the robotic system set-up but has no impact on the occurrence of intraoperative complications [4, 17–19].

The evidence provided thus far is sufficient to consider robotic-assisted Heller myotomy an excellent minimally invasive treatment option for Achalasia. Benefits include a shorter and easier learning curve, reduced morbidity, and excellent outcomes in term of symptoms relief and better quality of life without losing efficacy, at least at short-term follow-up.

Pearls and Pitfalls of the Operative Technique

- Complete mobilization of the fundus of the stomach by dividing the short gastric vessels, adequate extension of the myotomy (6 cm into the distal esophagus and 2–3 cm into the gastric wall) and the addition of a fundoplication (Dor or Toupet) are crucial maneuvers in order to obtain optimal results.
- The robotic system is especially valuable during the myotomy portion of the surgical procedure as well as facilitating intra-corporeal knot tying.
- If while performing the myotomy bleeding occurs from the muscle edges, it is very important to avoid using the electrocautery. Applying compression is sufficient enough for the bleeding to subside.
- If the myotomy was difficult, every effort should be made to identify unrecognized injuries by using upper endoscopy.
- If an esophageal perforation is recognized during surgery it can generally be easily repaired at that time by fine absorbable sutures. After repair, the surgeon can elect to buttress the repair with a Dor fundoplication as opposed to a Toupet.
- In patients that are found to have a hiatal hernia at the time of surgery, a Toupet fundoplication is preferred due to the need of posterior dissection required in these patients.
- It is important to avoid using the body of the stomach while performing the fundoplication since this could potentially lead to a tight wrap with the resultant postoperative dysphagia.
- Although prior endoscopic treatment leads to a more difficult myotomy with longer operative times, otherwise equivalent outcomes to the untreated patients are achieved.

References

1. Goldblum JR, Whyte RI, Orringer MB, Appelman HD. Achalasia. A morphologic study of 42 resected specimens. Am J Surg Pathol. 1994;18(4):327–37.
2. Beck WC, Sharp KW. Achalasia. Surg Clin North Am. 2011;91(5):1031–7.
3. Eckardt AJ, Eckardt VF. Treatment and surveillance strategies in achalasia: an update. Nat Rev Gastroenterol Hepatol. 2011;8(6):311–9.
4. Francis DL, Katzka DA. Achalasia: update on the disease and its treatment. Gastroenterology. 2010;139:369–74.
5. Mostafa RM, Moustafa YM, Hamdy H. Interstitial cells of Cajal, the Maestro in health and disease. World J Gastroenterol. 2010;16(26):3239–48.
6. Sadowski DC, Ackah F, Jiang B, Svensons LW. Achalasia: incidence, prevalence and survival. A population-based study. Neurogastroenterol Motil. 2010;22(9):e256–61.
7. Sonnenberg A. Hospitalization for achalasia in the United States 1997-2006. Dig Dis Sci. 2009;54:1680–5.
8. Patti MG, Pellegrini CA, Horgan S, Arcerito M, Omelanczuk P, Tamburini A, et al. Minimally invasive surgery for achalasia: an 8-year experience with 168 patients. Ann Surg. 1999;230(4):587–93. discussion 593–4.
9. Perreta S, Fisichella PM, Galvani G, Gorodner MV, Way LW, Patti MG. Achalasia and chest pain: effect of laparoscopic Heller myotomy. J Gastrointest Surg. 2003;7(5):595–8.
10. Moonka R, Patti MG, Feo CV, Arcerito M, De Pinto M, Horgan S, et al. Clinical presentation and evaluation of malignant pseudoachalasia. J Gastrointest Surg. 1999;3(5):456–61.
11. Sandler RS, Nyren O, Ekbom A, Eisen GM, Yuen J, Josefsson S. The risk of esophageal cancer in patients with achalasia. A popular-based study. JAMA. 1995;274(17):1359–62.
12. Gorodner MV, Galvani C, Patti MG. Heller myotomy. J Op Tech Gen Surg. 2004;6(1):23–38.
13. Bredenoord AJ, Fox M, Kahrilas PJ, Pandolfino JE, Schwizer W, Smout AJ, International High Resolution Manometry Working Group. Chicago classification criteria of esophageal motility disorders defined in high-resolution esophageal pressure topography. Neurogastroenterol Motil. 2012;24 Suppl 1:57–65.
14. Patti MG, Fisichella PM, Perreta S, Galvani C, Gorodner MV, Robinson T, et al. Impact of minimally invasive surgery on the treatment of esophageal achalasia: a decade of change. J Am Coll Surg. 2003;196(5):698–703.
15. Bresadola V, Feo CV. Minimally invasive myotomy for the treatment of esophageal achalasia: evolution of the

surgical procedure and the therapeutic algorithm. Surg Laparosc Endosc Percutan Tech. 2012;22(2):83–7.

16. Maeso S, Reza M, Mayol JA, Blasco JA, Guerra M, Andradas E, et al. Efficacy of the Da Vinci surgical system in abdominal surgery compared with that of laparoscopy: a systematic review and meta-analysis. Ann Surg. 2010;252(2):254–62.
17. Horgan S, Galvani C, Gorodner MV, Omelanczuk P, Elli F, Moser F, et al. Robotic-assisted Heller myotomy versus laparoscopic Heller myotomy for the treatment of esophageal achalasia: multicenter study. J Gastrointest Surg. 2005;9(8):1020–30.
18. Melvin WS, Dundon JM, Talamini M, Horgan S. Computer-enhanced robotic telesurgery minimizes esophageal perforation during Heller myotomy. Surgery. 2005;138(4):553–9.
19. Galvani CA, Gallo AS, Dylewski MR. Robotic-assisted Heller myotomy for esophageal achalasia: feasibility, technique, and short-term outcomes. J Robot Surg. 2011;5:163–6.
20. Bloomston M, Serafini F, Boyce HW, Rosemurgy AS. The "learning curve" in videoscopic Heller myotomy. JSLS. 2002;6(1):41–7.

Part III

Surgical Techniques: *Thoracic*

Complete Port-Access Robotic-Assisted Lobectomy Utilizing Three-Arm Technique Without a Transthoracic Utility Incision

7

Mark R. Dylewski, Richard Lazzaro, and Abbas E. Abbas

Introduction

Anatomical lobectomy with systematic mediastinal lymphadenectomy is the "gold standard" for the treatment of early-stage non-small cell lung carcinoma [1]. Traditionally, a lobectomy has been performed through a large posterolateral thoracotomy. Since the initial introduction of minimally invasive thoracoscopic surgery in the early 1990s [2–4], the procedure has rapidly demonstrated its potential for the treatment of benign and malignant disease of the chest cavity. Video-assisted thoracoscopic surgery for major lung resection has been proven to be an acceptable approach to the treatment of early-stage lung cancer. The safety, feasibility, and oncological effectiveness have been demonstrated in single and multi-institutional series [5, 6]. When compared to traditional open lobectomy, the VATS lobectomy technique is associated with shorter hospital stay, decreased postoperative pain, preservation of pulmonary function, and fewer overall complications [7]. However, the routine adoption of VATS lobectomy has been slow particularly for larger tumors and more advanced surgically treatable disease. The reasons for the lack of adoption of VATS lobectomy are multifactorial and have been outlined by Mack [8]. He cited oncological control, limitations in instrumentation, operative times, and experience as aspects influencing adoption of the VATS platform. The features of the VATS platform such as counterintuitive orientation, two-dimensional imaging, reduced depth perception, and limited instrument maneuverability have made many surgeons feel awkward during VATS lobectomy elevating concerns about sound oncological principles. These concerns, in conjunction with the fear of sudden hemorrhage and the inability to rapidly control bleeding, have made many thoracic surgeons hesitant to adopt minimally invasive major lung resection. Consequently, most published series advocate selecting patients with early-stage I NSCLC for VATS lobectomy and the use of a facilitating non-rib-spreading utility thoracotomy [9, 10]. This strategy was adopted as a result of the technical limitations of the VATS platform. This approach provides access for conventional surgical instrumentation in order to facilitate safe dissection of hilar structures and eventual extraction of lung tissue.

In an effort to overcome limitations of conventional minimally invasive instruments, robotic systems have been designed. The advent of advanced three-dimensional video optics,

M.R. Dylewski, M.D. (✉)
Department of Cardiac Vascular and Thoracic Surgery, Baptist Health of South Florida, 6200 SW 72nd Street, Suite 604, Miami, FL 33143, USA
e-mail: markd@baptisthealth.net

R. Lazzaro, M.D.
North Shore LIJ Health System, Lenox Hill Hospital, 100 E 77th Street, New York, NY 10075, USA

A.E. Abbas, M.D.
Department of Surgery, Ochsner Clinic Foundation, 1514 Jefferson Highway, New Orleans, LA 70121, USA
e-mail: aabbas@ochsner.org

K.C. Kim (ed.), *Robotics in General Surgery*, DOI 10.1007/978-1-4614-8739-5_7,

superior range of motion blended with computerized, intuitive integration of the surgeon's fundamental skills, has created a new opportunity for surgeons to offer a powerful alternative for their thoracic surgical patients. Since the demonstration of feasibility and safety of robotic-assisted thoracic surgery by several authors [11–13], the procedure is increasingly being utilized in the field of thoracic surgery for its potential advantages. Early investigations of robotic-assisted lobectomy have shown that the operative morbidity and mortality is low and many of the same advantages seen with utilization of VATS lobectomy can be realized with robotic-assisted pulmonary resection [14]. While robotics has great promise in the field of pulmonary surgery, many authors have raised concerns about the inherent higher costs of the procedure, the increased operating room times, and the steep learning curve over conventional minimally invasive techniques [15, 16]. It is our experience that these drawbacks to robotic surgery can be mitigated by refinements to the robotic surgical technique, developing specialty-specific team approaches, and standardization of operating room practices in an effort to optimize the utilization of the robotic system for maximum efficiency. In fact a retrospective analysis presented at CRSA 2012 by the lead author of 176 robotic-assisted lung lobectomies that compared to 76 VATS lobectomies performed between 2005 and 2011, lobectomies performed using robotic assistance reduced direct cost by $560 dollars per case. The majority of cost saving occurred as a result of reduced length of hospital stay and lower overall nursing care cost. The da Vinci surgical system (Intuitive Surgical, Sunnyvale, CA) represents the ideal tool for dissection of the pulmonary vascular and for the performance of a systematic lymph node dissection. An improvement in robotic minimally invasive surgery over the conventional platforms has made the adaptability of minimally invasive lobectomy easier as well as provided a greater probability of achieving complete oncological resection [17]. For the reasons outlined above, we believe that the trend in robotic-assisted thoracic surgery will surpass the adoption of VATS and mirror that of other robotic surgical subspecialties.

The technique outlined in the following chapter is an established technique for completing a total endoscopic three-arm robotic video-assisted anatomical lobectomy and systematic lymph node dissection that is performed through a port-only approach. Once the lobectomy specimen is detached from the hilar structures, it is removed from the chest cavity from a subcostal para-diaphragmatic location without the use of a traditional utility thoracotomy. We will report our 5-year experience utilizing this technique and discuss the indications for the procedure, contraindications, technical aspects of robotic video-assisted pulmonary surgery, and the perioperative outcomes.

Technique

All robotic-assisted pulmonary resections are performed under general anesthesia with an endotracheal tube capable of maintaining one-lung ventilation. Fiberoptic bronchoscopy is utilized to confirm correct positioning. Monitoring consists of pulse oximetry, electrocardiography, end-tidal CO_2, and pneumatic blood pressure measurements. The patient is positioned in the lateral decubitus position. To ensure free movement of instruments passed through the para-diaphragmatic assistant port, it is critical that the top of the patient's ipsilateral hip and lower rib cage are in a parallel plane. If this cannot be accomplished with flexion of the operating table alone, the beanbag can be placed underneath the hip for additional flexion. After placing the patient in the lateral decubitus position, the surgeon should define the anatomy of the lower rib cage by marking the position of anterior aspect of the 10th, 11th, and 12th ribs. The position of the para-diaphragmatic assistant port is placed anterior and inferior to the 10th rib along the anterior axillary line. After confirming the location of the assistant port, the anterior robotic operating port should be positioned at least 10 cm superiorly to the assistant port along the anterior axillary line (Fig. 7.1a).

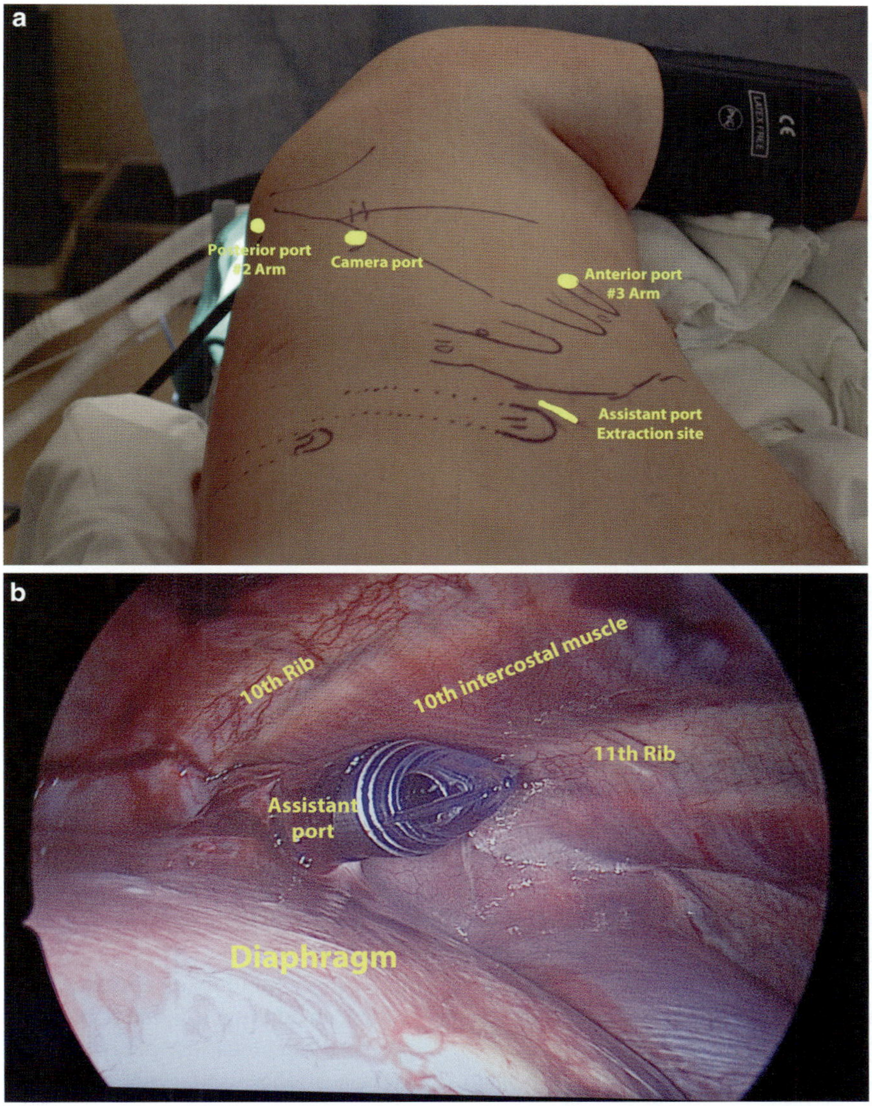

Fig. 7.1 (**a**) Layout of the external anatomy of the lower chest wall. (**b**) Introduction of 12-mm assistant port at confluence of anterior 10th intercostal muscle and diaphragm. (**c**) Port placement for three-arm robotic assisted lobectomy. (*Asterisk*) When optional posterior #3 arm port is utilized, the #1 arm is placed in the anterior port side. (**d**) Port placement in relationship to the major oblique fissure. (**e**) Docking for a three-arm robotic-assisted lobectomy

The initial access to the chest cavity is achieved by placing a 5-mm port in the anterior axillary location approximately at the level of the 5th intercostal space. A pneumothorax is induced with CO_2 (pressure/flow 8 mmHg and 8 ml/s). Using a 5-mm 30° laparoscopic camera focus on the anterior aspect of the diaphragm where the diaphragmatic muscles intertwine with the 10th intercostal muscles. The 12-mm assistant port is placed under direct visual assistance. The port enters the chest at the confluence of the muscle fibers of the diaphragm and the anterior 10th intercostal muscle (Fig. 7.1b).

Utilizing the 5-mm thoracoscope, placed through the 12-mm assistant port, two additional

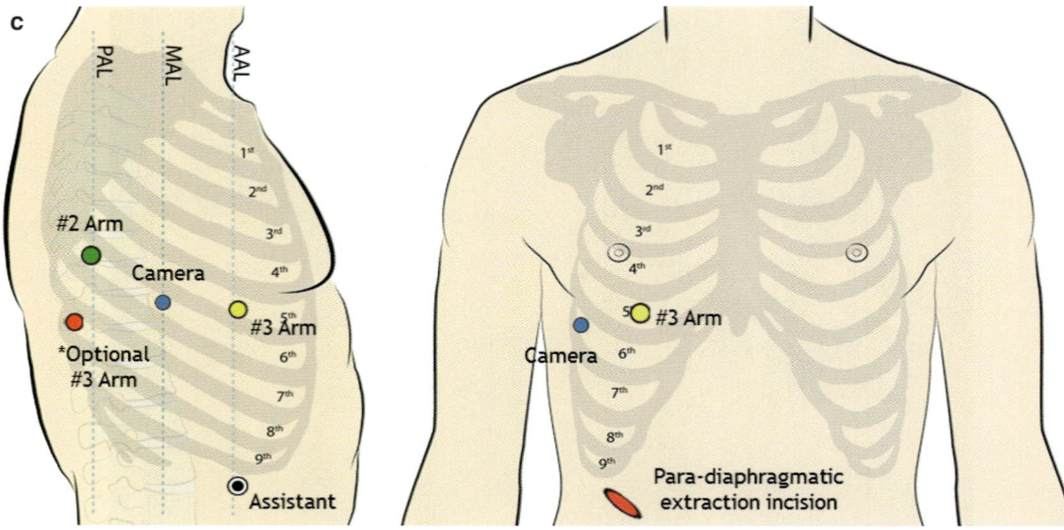

Fig. 7.1 (continued)

trocars are positioned along the major pulmonary fissure between either the 6th or 7th interspace. Successful complete port-access robotic-assisted pulmonary surgery is dependent on proper placement of the midaxillary camera and posterior thoracic port. Port placement is based on the relationship of the major pulmonary fissure to the internal chest wall rather than external landmarks (Fig. 7.1c, d).

For this reason, initial placement of a low-lying camera will provide the best vantage point in order to visualize the pulmonary fissure and chest wall simultaneously, thus facilitating accurate port placement.

It is important to maintain 10 cm or a handbreadth of space between each port. The camera trocar (8 mm) is positioned in the midaxillary location one interspace below the major oblique fissure. *A good rule of thumb is to utilize the anterior sternal-xiphoid junction as a landmark to confirm proper positioning for the midaxillary camera port.* The initial 5-mm port is replaced with a (8 mm) trocar in the anterior axillary location. A larger port (12 mm) can be placed in the anterior axillary location if a secondary access is needed for stapling. When utilizing a 12-mm anterior axillary port, the robotic 8-mm port needs to be introduced through the 12-mm port. The posterior (5 mm or 8 mm) trocar is positioned one or two interspace below the superior aspect of the oblique fissure within the corresponding rib space. As a result of the paraspinous muscles, the posterior intercostal space is restrictive. The superior and inferior movements of the robotic instruments can be significantly affected by the inflexible paraspinous musculature and narrow ribs space. Improper positioning of the posterior port will hinder instrument movement. Limiting the size of the posterior operating port to (8 mm or less), when possible, is recommended to minimize postoperative pain. If elected, an additional 5-mm port can be placed in the posterior location approximately the 8th interspace and used with a 5-mm retracting grasper. Three or four robotic arms are then docked to their respective trocars (Fig. 7.1e).

A 0° 3D (8 mm) camera is placed in the midaxillary port. The 5-mm lung grasping forceps are placed in the right robotic arm, and a bipolar dissector forceps (Intuitive Surgical, Inc., Sunnyvale, CA) is placed in the left robotic arm. The bipolar cautery is utilized for precise dissection and isolation of the pulmonary vascular structures. Avoidance of an access thoracotomy incision maintains positive pressure within the chest cavity with CO_2 insufflation. When the CO_2 pressure is maintained below 10 mmHg, hemodynamic side effects are minimal and can be

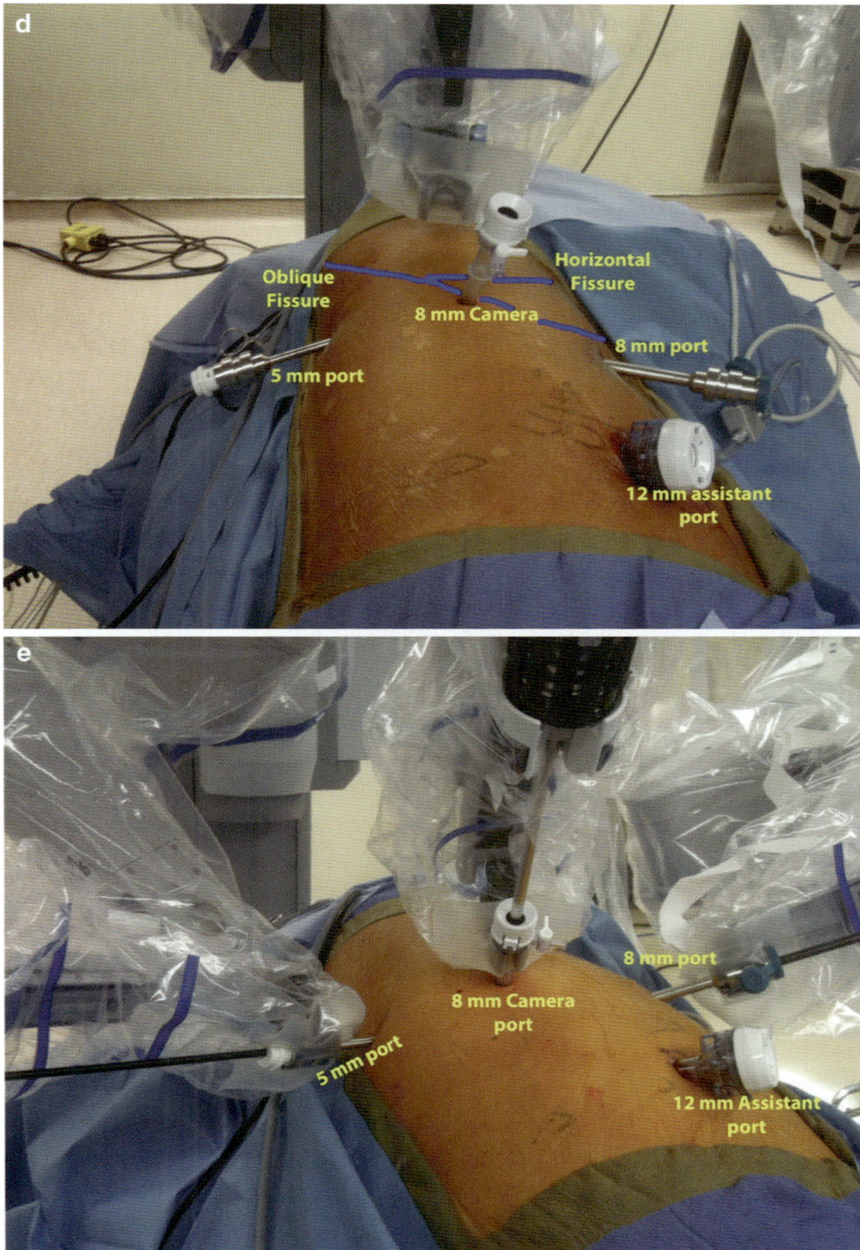

Fig. 7.1 (continued)

addressed with minor adjustments by the anesthesiologist.

We prefer the three-arm robotic technique with docking of the #3 robotic arm to the anterior port. As the #3 robotic arm is a five-joint arm, which is uniquely different from the mirror image arms #1 and #2. Instruments held with robotic arm #3 have an increased range of motion compared to the other two robotic arms. The #3 arm can be utilized to hold the primary dissecting instrument. For right-sided procedures, the robotic arms #2 and #3 are utilized, with #3 positioned anteriorly as noted, and #2 is placed posteriorly. For left-side procedures, robotic arms #2 and #3 are utilized; robotic arm #3 is positioned anteriorly, and #2 is placed posteriorly. When utilizing the four-arm robotic technique, it is necessary to use the #3 robotic arm for retraction assistance, and arms #1 and #2 are positioned anterior or posterior depending on the laterality of the case. When utilizing a four-arm robotic technique, it is necessary to dock the #3 arm posteriorly for retraction assistance only. The #1 and #2 arms become the primary dissecting instruments. One of the main disadvantages to the four-arm technique is the increased likelihood of external instrument conflict particularly in patients with small chest cavities. Utility access can be achieved through the subcostal assistant trocar for retraction, suctioning, and access for passage of staplers. With rare exceptions, all stapling can be provided through the subcostal accessory port. By utilizing the accessory port in this manor, instrument exchange, as well as the need to undock and re-dock the arms to the ports, substantially reduces the overall operating room time. As experience with this technique is gained, this arrangement requires only one bedside operative assistant and surgical technician. Following the initial trocar positioning and docking of the robot, the primary operating surgeon remains unsterile at the surgical console until it is time to extract the lung specimen from the chest cavity.

Hilar and Mediastinal Lymph Node Dissection

Once the indications for lung resection are met, the procedure begins with mediastinal and hilar lymph node dissection based on the disease process. The lymph node dissection begins with division of the inferior pulmonary ligament. A 0° scope is placed in direct upright position with minimal rotation from the horizon. Proper camera port placement allows for visualization from the base of the pulmonary ligament to the apex of the chest. Complete visualization of the anterior, posterior, and superior aspects of the hilum is attained, allowing for precise anatomic dissection. Exposure of the ligament is achieved by lifting the lower lobe superiorly with "passive" retraction. "Passive" retraction is best achieved by utilizing the full length of the shaft of the instruments to "push" the lung as needed around the chest cavity rather than to grasp and "pull" the lung where needed. Utilizing a 3×3 rolled gauze held by a robotic instrument can improve the surgeon's ability to manipulate the lung for exposure. The console surgeon should not attempt to "actively" grab the lung in an effort to reduce iatrogenic parenchymal trauma. Instead "passive" retraction should be used to push the lung upward until the ligament is visualized and the bedside assistant can grab the base of the ligament to provide exposure of the ligament for bimanual robotic dissection. While the bedside assistant maintains gentle cephalad traction on the lung, the inferior ligament is divided with electrocautery. Level 8 and 9 lymph nodes are removed during this maneuver. As the dissection progresses towards the superior aspect of the ligament, the ligament divides into anterior and posterior veils which envelope the hilum. Dividing these veils anteriorly and posteriorly to the suprahilar area allows for a circumferential release of the mediastinal pleura from the hilum. During the dissection of the posterior veil, the lung is rotated anteriorly and held in position with an external atraumatic grasper by the bedside assistant via the assistant port. Next, the console surgeon proceeds with a subcarinal lymphadenectomy.

Before forfeiting the posterior hilar exposure, additional maneuvers can be performed to facilitate division of an incomplete oblique fissure. On the right side, thorough dissection of the junction between the right upper lobe bronchus and bronchus intermedius should be completed. The landmark to identify is the posterior aspect of the descending pulmonary artery. On the left side, exposure of the main pulmonary artery and the origin of the ascending posterior pulmonary artery and superior segmental artery should be thoroughly dissected free of adjacent tissue. If these steps are performed correctly, a plane beneath the posterior oblique fissure can be easily created once the descending artery is exposed from within the mid-oblique fissure. During the dissection of the oblique fissure and isolation of the individual arteries, N1 lymph nodes are removed and collected for examination. Throughout the process of the lymph node dissection, a frozen section examination is performed on any suspicious hilar (N1) and mediastinal (N2) lymph nodes to determine a clinically appropriate anatomical resection. Following the hilar dissection and removal of the subcarinal lymph nodes, dissection should be carried cephalad to the hilum. On the right side, levels 2, 3, and 4 lymph nodes are resected. On the left, level 5 and 6 para-aortic lymph nodes are resected.

Dissection and Division of Hilar Structures

The major oblique fissure is separated, and the arteries to the designated lobe are isolated and individually divided. The bipolar dissector forceps are utilized to meticulously divide the pulmonary parenchyma when necessary. With the use of the high-definition, three-dimensional camera, the surgeon can visualize the thin visceral pleural layer between the fissures and avoid violating the parenchyma of the uninvolved lobe. Careful attention to this maneuver is important to avoid excessive bleeding that may interfere with identification of vascular structures. Blunt dissection through the lung parenchyma should be avoided. Division of the pulmonary vein prior to division of the arteries to the corresponding lobe is not recommended because of the risk of engorgement of the pulmonary parenchyma. Such engorgement will lead to increased bleeding during dissection of the hilar structures and lung parenchyma. In circumstances where there is an incomplete fissure, we recommend initially dividing the posterior parenchymal bridge. This is accomplished by exposing the common descending branch of the pulmonary artery within the mid-oblique fissure. Following the identification of the ascending posterior segmental artery to the upper lobe and the superior segmental artery to the lower lobe, dissection with a blunt dissector is performed beneath the posterior parenchymal bridge. A tissue stapler is passed through the assistant trocar and utilized to divide the posterior parenchymal bridge. The order of the hilar structures divided for the right upper lobe is as follows: ascending posterior artery, right upper lobe bronchus, and common truncus anterior artery. Dividing the right upper lobe bronchus facilitates isolation of the truncus anterior branch of the pulmonary artery. The venous structures are typically divided last in order to avoid engorgement of the corresponding lobe. *In situations where dissection through the fissure is difficult, a fissure-less technique can be utilized. However, the authors recommend performing isolation of all major vessels prior to dividing the pulmonary vein to the respective lobe. This will facilitate rapid division of the major arterial supply and limit the risk of lobar engorgement.* In the case of a middle lobectomy, the segmental pulmonary arterial branches to the respective lobe are individually isolated and divided with a vascular stapler. When performing a lower lobectomy, isolation and division of the common descending pulmonary artery is performed when feasible.

When performing a left upper lobectomy, separation of the oblique fissure is initially performed. The order of the hilar structures divided for a left upper lobe is as follows: lingual arteries, ascending posterior artery, left superior pulmonary vein, apical and anterior arterial branches, and left upper lobe bronchus. Division of the left superior pulmonary vein will facilitate exposure of the apical and anterior arterial branches during a left upper lobectomy. For lower lobectomies, the common descending pulmonary artery is divided before the inferior pulmonary vein. The vein and arteries are stapled with a 45-mm vascular tissue stapler, and bronchi are stapled and divided with a 45-mm medium thick tissue stapler.

Extraction of the Specimen

Once the anatomical resection is completed, the specimen is placed in a 5×8-cm Lapsac (Cook Group Inc., Bloomington, IN). The Lapsac string is then pulled out through the subcostal trocar (Fig. 7.2a, b).

A small 2–3-cm subcostal incision is created at the tip of the 11th rib. Once the anterior aspect of the 11th rib is identified, the edge of the diaphragm is separated from its attachments to the anterior 10th intercostal muscle fibers as they insert into the anteroinferior aspect of the tenth rib. The extraction of the specimen from the chest cavity is *not* performed through a traditional transthoracic approach. It is removed through a para-diaphragmatic, subcostal approach. Repair of the diaphragm is accomplished using 0-vicryl on CT1 needle (Fig. 7.2c).

The suture is passed initially through the upper posterior edge of the divided oblique muscles. It is then run as a semi-purse-string alone the open edge of the diaphragm from superior to inferior. The suture is then run through the inferior posterior edge of the divided oblique muscles. Tying the suture will reapproximate the diaphragm to the anterior tenth intercostal musculature. After a final inspection of the thorax, paravertebral blocks are performed using 0.5 % bupivacaine with epinephrine for analgesia. A single 24 F Blake drain is placed and has been found to be sufficient for closed chest drainage in this patient population.

Result

A review of our complete experience from December 2006 through September 2010 identified 200 consecutive patients who underwent a robotic video-assisted lung resection [14]. The patient characteristics are listed in Table 7.1. Of the study cohort, 154 patients underwent an anatomical lobectomy, four patients required a bilobectomy, one patient had a pneumonectomy, and 35 patients underwent a formal segmentectomy. Three patients underwent a sleeve lobectomy. Three patients underwent an en bloc chest wall or diaphragm resection concurrently with lobectomy. Robotic video-assisted lung resection was successfully completed in 197 (98.5 %) patients. Three patients required conversions to a muscle-sparing mini-thoracotomy for either bleeding, central tumor invasion, or completion of a sleeve lobectomy. Every type of lobectomy was performed (Table 7.1).

Segmental resections were limited to the posterior apical segments of the right upper lobe and the lingual or superior segment of the lower lobes. The median number of lymph node stations removed totaled 5.0 (range 4–8). The results of our series are listed in Table 7.2.

Mean and median operative times were 100 and 90 min, respectively (range 30–279 min). The total operative room times were measured from patient entering to exiting the operating room. Mean and median total operating room times were 180 and 175 min, respectively. The majority of patients were admitted from the postoperative recovery room directly to a standard floor bed with continuous cardiac and pulse oximetry monitoring. No patient required an epidural catheter or PCA for postoperative pain control. The median length of stay in the ICU was 0 (range 0–15). Fifteen patients required a stay in the ICU during their postoperative hospital stay. Thirteen patients during the first half of the series required an ICU stay, and two patients required an ICU stay in the last half of the series. In our series, the most common cause for the patient to require transfer to ICU was respiratory failure and pneumonia.

Learning Curve

Although, there is no standard definition for a learning curve, the traditional method of measure is to plot the average time verses number of cases. As the surgeon gains experience, the curve should begin to plateau. The learning curve is then set to that number of cases required for the surgeon to reach the plateau. Unfortunately, operative time alone cannot be the single criteria

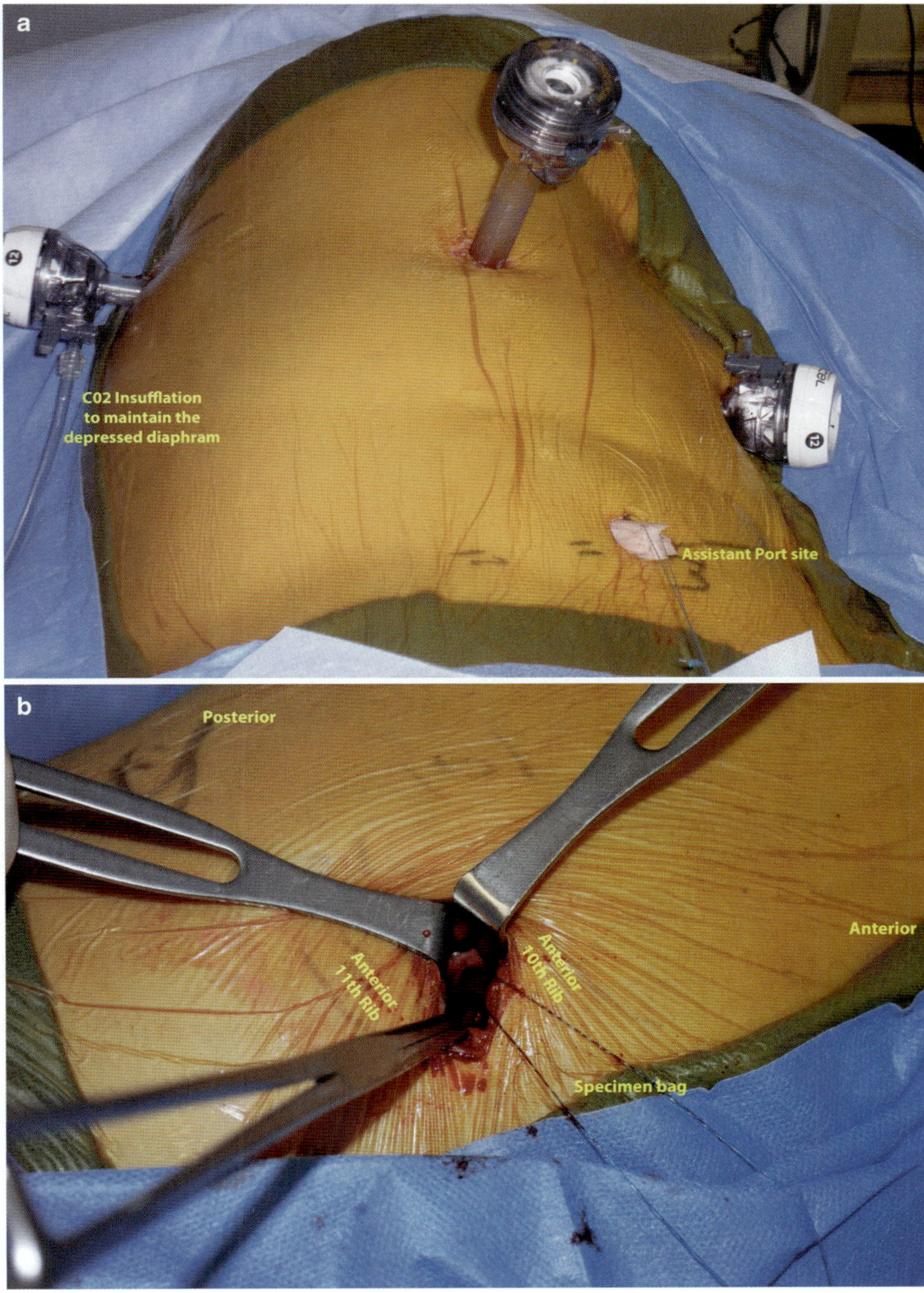

Fig. 7.2 (**a**) Retrieval of specimen bag through assistant port. (**b**) Opening of the assistant port site for specimen removal. (**c**) Exposure of specimen removal site for repair of diaphragm

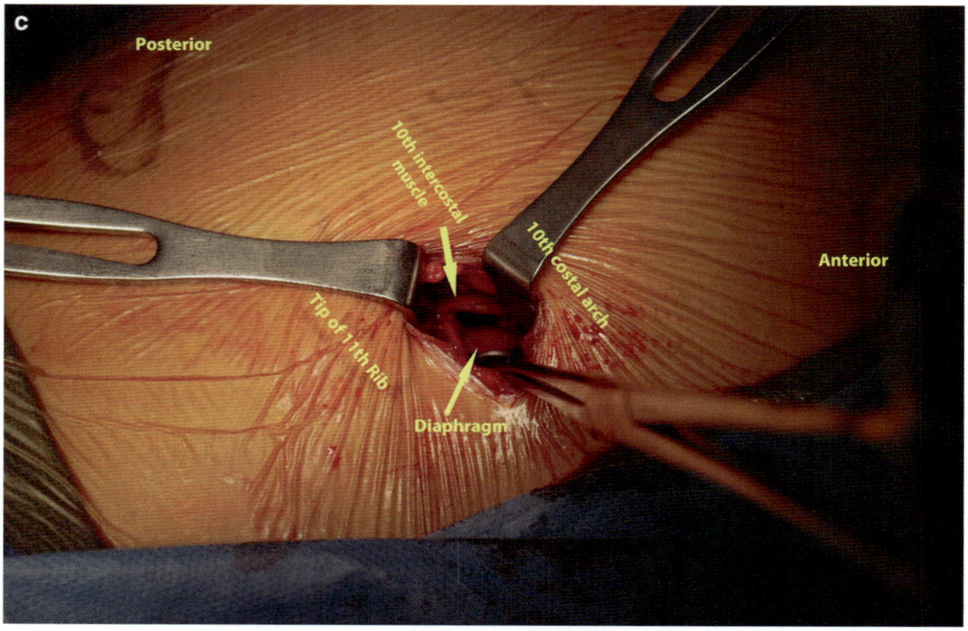

Fig. 7.2 (continued)

Table 7.1 Patient characteristics ($n=200$)

Male/female	90/110
Median age (years)	68.0 (20–92)
Median tumor diameter (cm)	2.0 (0.5–8.5)
Tumor location	
RUL	52
RML	18
RLL	27
RML and RLL	4
LUL	36
LLL	21
Histology	
NSCLC	125
Small cell carcinoma	1
Carcinoid	18
Benign	26
Metastatic	29
Lymphoma	1
Pathological stage (NSCLC $n=26$)	
Stage IA/IB	106
Stage IIA/IIB	22
Stage IIIA	16
Stage IV (T3N0M1)	2
Type of anatomical resection	
Lobectomy	154
Bilobectomy/pneumonectomy	4/1
Segmentectomy	35
Enbloc/sleeve lobectomy	3/3

Table 7.2 Results

Mean/median operative time (min)	100/90 (30–279)
Mean/median total operating room time (min)	180/175 (82–370)
Median docking time (min)	12 (6–20)
Median chest tube duration (days)	1.5 (1–35)
Median length of ICU stays (days)	0 (0–15)
Median length of hospital stay (days)	3 (1–44)
Median chest tube drainage (cc)	300 (90–2,000)
Median lymph nodes stations removed	5 (4–8)
Median operative blood loss (cc)	70 (25–500)

by which we gauge the success of a newly adopted operative procedure. Additional measures, including procedural blood loss and perioperative complications are equally important and need to be evaluated as part of the metrics. Our analysis of the learning curve has shown that certain components of the curve differ greatly between groups of surgeons as defined by their training level. Not only does the surgeon's level of training impact the implementation of robotic surgery into a surgeon's practice, but also careful patient selection should minimize surgeon frustration while learning how to operate a robotic

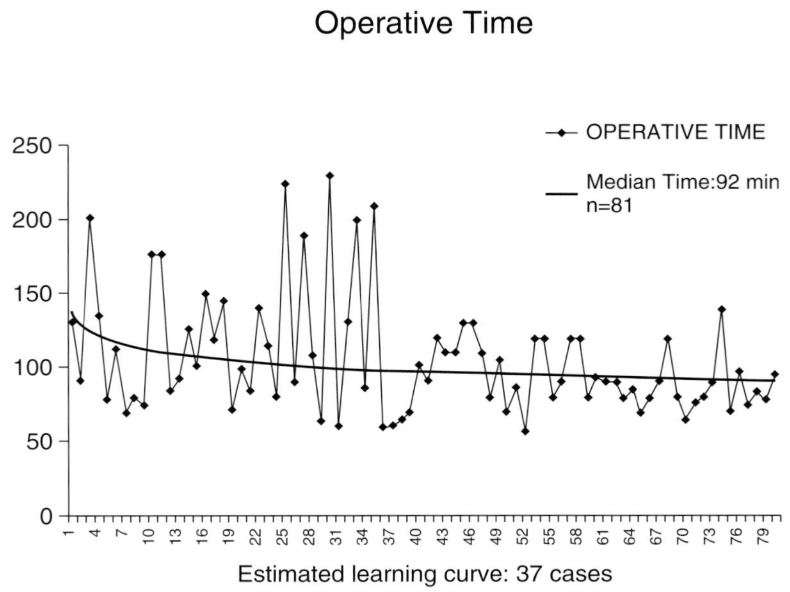

Fig. 7.3 Learning curve for robotic-assisted lobectomy

surgical instrument. Attention to matching surgeon experience, surgeon robotic preparation, and patient/case selection provides a successful path to optimize the safety of the robotic procedure, minimizing perioperative risk and establishing the development of a robotic skill set which will preserve equivalent oncological outcomes to VATS or open. Robotic technology allows surgeons to replicate their preferred technique now using a minimally invasive approach. Advancements achieved in medical simulation should shorten the learning curve and increase the use of minimally invasive techniques. Taking into account the morbidity, mortality, and short-term outcome measures for our series, the number of cases require to reach the learning-curve plateau was approximately 34 cases (Fig. 7.3).

Abbas and colleagues in an unpublished series of 103 patients undergoing robotic lobectomy for NSCLC have also demonstrated a shortened learning curve with overall complication and major morbidity of 21 % and 6 %, respectively, and a mortality of 0 %. Oncological outcomes have also remained a concern with the introduction of robotic-assisted lobectomy for NSCLC. However, a recent study has reported robust long-term follow-up data on survival or outcome measure for robotic-assisted pulmonary resection. Park and colleagues reported on a multi-institutional review of the long-term oncological results following robotic lobectomy, utilizing CALGB consensus technique, on 325 patients. The authors concluded that "long-term stage-specific survival is acceptable and consistent with prior results for VATS and thoracotomy" [18].

Complications

A systematic review of the conventional video-assisted thoracoscopic surgery versus thoracotomy performed by Whitson and associates [19] reported the overall complications in numerous series of VATS lobectomy from 1995 to 2006 ranged from 6 to 34.2 %. The two largest series reported by McKenna and associates [20] and Onaitis and associates [21] reviewed the full spectrum of complications occurring in patients undergoing conventional video-assisted lobectomy.

Table 7.3 Perioperative complications ($n=52$)

60-day mortality	3 (1.5 %)
Supraventricular arrhythmia	6 (3.0 %)
Myocardial infarction/CVA	2 (1.0 %)
Pneumonia	8 (4.0 %)
Effusion requiring drainage	17 (8.5 %)
Prolonged air leak (greater than 6 days)	15 (7.5 %)
Mural thrombus	1 (0.5 %)
Bleeding requiring transfusion	2 (1.0 %)
Splenectomy	1 (0.5 %)
Conversion for difficulty	2 (1.0 %)
Conversion for bleeding	1 (0.5 %)
Return to OR for bleeding	1 (0.5 %)
Transfusion for bleeding	2 (1.0 %)
Postoperative pneumothorax	3 (1.5 %)

In these series, the 30-day morbidity rates were 15.3 % and 23.8 %, respectively. The most common complications included air leak ≥7 days, atrial fibrillation, pleural drainage ≥7 days, and pneumonia. The 60-day mortality and overall complication rate for our study cohort was 1.5 % and 26 %, respectively (Table 7.3).

In our series, the majority of complications occurred in patients who underwent a lobectomy (90 %). Four patients who underwent a segmental resection suffered a complication. Forty-seven patients following a lobectomy suffered complications. The majority of complications were grades 2 or 3 [22]. The most common complications occurring following a complete port-access robotic-assisted segmentectomy or lobectomy were similar to complications observed after conventional VATS lobectomy and included pneumonia, symptomatic postoperative effusion, and air leak for more than 6 days. A summary of the literature regarding the perioperative outcomes of robotic lobectomy and systematic review and meta-analysis on pulmonary resection by robotic video-assisted thoracic surgery confirms the safety of robotic pulmonary lobectomy, with reported results similar to that of VATS lobectomy [23, 24]. However, several procedural-related complications are specific to complete port-access robotic-assisted pulmonary resection. These include complications related to the insertion of the para-diaphragmatic assistant port and specimen retrieval from this location. Potential injury to the ipsilateral diaphragm and abdominal viscera exists. In our experience, entrance into the abdomen through the diaphragm can occur on rare occasions. The risk of trans-diaphragmatic placement of a port and secondary injury of abdominal organs may be increased in patients with previous intra-abdominal or thoracic surgery, pleural adhesions, paralysis of the ipsilateral diaphragm, hepatosplenomegaly, or obesity. In patients with any of these potential risk factors, reverse Trendelenburg, the use of continuous CO_2 insufflation, placement of the assistant port under direct visualization and within the anterior 9th intercostal space, facilitate post placement and ensure entrance of the chest cavity well above the diaphragm. With these basic maneuvers, safe placement of the para-diaphragmatic port can be accomplished.

As an added advantage, extraction of the specimen bag is accomplished at the site of the para-diaphragmatic port located at the confluence of the anterior 10th intercostal muscle and adjacent diaphragm. In our series, few complications have been realized as a result of this technique of specimen retrieval. There are several inherent benefits to utilizing this para-diaphragmatic technique for extraction of the lung specimen. Due to the anterior and posterior fixation of the upper rib cage and the limited elasticity of the rib cage and intercostal muscle, removal of large specimens or tumors greater than 3 cm requires creation of a utility thoracotomy ranging from 3 to 8 cm. Theoretically, chronic post-thoracotomy pain is secondary to injury to the intercostal nerve, localized rib trauma, or disruption of the costovertebral and costosternal joints. Various differences exist among the described VATS lobectomy techniques, and a complete port-access video-assisted lobectomy may be technically feasible. However, there is an inherent need for specimen retrieval via a utility incision. Even without active rib retraction, the intercostal nerve can be inadvertently injured, and the sternocostal and costovertebral joints can be disrupted by excessive traction. By utilizing the para-diaphragmatic specimen retrieval, we believe there is no risk to rib injury, costosternal or costovertebral separation. The specimen is retrieved through the soft tissues of the upper abdomen and diaphragm that are inherently more forgiving than the rib cage. In addition, the main trunks of the intercostal nerves do not traverse the confluence of the abdominal and chest wall cavity in this location, thus, limiting the risk of nerve injury.

Excessive bleeding from a major vascular injury from a pulmonary artery or vein during a minimally invasive video-assisted pulmonary resection can be troublesome and dangerous because of limited access. Historically, catastrophic bleeding event during VATS lobectomy have been rare. The largest series of VATS lobectomies by McKenna and coworker [20] reported only 6 (0.5 %) patients in their series required conversion to thoracotomy for bleeding. In our series of 200 complete port-access robotic-assisted pulmonary resections, there was one (0.5 %) patient (number 46) who sustained an injury to the superior segmental branch while undergoing an attempted right lower lobe superior segmentectomy. The injury resulted in the need to convert to a conventional VATS approach with a utility incision in order to place a clip on the small vessel. Eventually the patient required a right lower lobectomy to achieve an R0 resection.

Tips and Pitfalls

Vascular Isolation

In our experience, the robotic dissection of critical structures is precise, and the added three-dimensional high-definition imaging makes the procedure inherently more accurate than with conventional instruments performed through a utility incision. Reduced tactile feedback has been recognized as a weakness of the robotic technique. However, the advanced imaging and accuracy of dissection achieved with the robotic technique offsets this minor limitation. Theoretically, the etiology of major vascular injury during a minimally invasive pulmonary resection occurs as a result of aggressive traction, direct puncture, or electrocautery injury. In our experience, the injury that is most likely to occur during robotic-assisted dissection of the pulmonary vessels is a small tear in a side branch of the pulmonary vein or lobar arteries. This type of injury is different than injuries that occur most frequently in conventional VATS lobectomy. During a VATS lobectomy, maximal traction is placed on the lobe in order to expose and dissect around the respective vessel. This predisposes the origin of the vessel to an avulsion injury. Once this type of injury occurs, it often requires conversion to a traditional thoracotomy to achieve exposure and vascular control. Our techniques model the traditional open lobectomy technique, where the major arterial inflow to the lobe is divided by dissection through the major pulmonary fissure. During dissection of the pulmonary arterial branches with robotic instrument, the lung is lying in the natural position and requires minimal to no retraction during these maneuvers. Although opponents of total endoscopic anatomical resection have strongly emphasized safety as a major obstacle to adoption of endoscopic techniques, an inadvertent traction or avulsion injury is unlikely to occur. *In an effort to avoid a major fatality during a vascular injury, we recommend that gauze fashioned into a tightly rolled "cigar" be placed within the chest cavity at all times.* This gauze can be utilized for general hemostasis as well as for applying pressure in the event of major bleeding, thus allowing time for conversion thoracotomy. The gauze can be grasped with the anterior robotic instrument to hold pressure on the site of bleeding. Meanwhile, the posterior and midaxillary ports can be removed, and a standard thoracotomy can be performed unhindered.

Camera Selection

Our technique utilizes a 0° camera for two reasons. During the conduct of the operation, a 0° camera will be operating at a 60–90° angle with respect to the chest wall. When using a 30° camera, the camera will operate at a 20–40° angle with respect to the chest wall. As a result of this difference, the 30° camera impedes the ability of the bedside assistant to access the assistant port. In addition, the 30° camera causes excessive torque on the rib above and below the port site, thus risking rib fracture or intercostal nerve injury. Proper positioning of the camera port is critical to achieving visualization of all intended structures. *In order to optimize visual exposure, we recommend placing the camera port one interspace below the oblique fissure in the midaxillary line and make the initial port incision directly over the middle of the rib. In the case of malpositioning, the port can be moved above or below the respective rib without changing the incision site*. In the event that there is poor exposure to the inferior most aspect of the inferior pulmonary ligament, or adhesions prevent mobilization of the lower lobe, the camera can be briefly docked to the para-diaphragm access port to divide these attachments. Additional maneuvers include releasing CO_2 from the thorax, which will allow the diaphragm to move cephalad, bringing the ligament into view or temporarily utilizing a 30° scope in the down-to position to visualize the ligament for safe division.

Haptics Feedback and Retraction

One of the most recognized differences between the robotic technique as compared to the VATS technique is that it requires the surgeon to operate through a console some distance from the patient's bedside. As a result, the surgeon cannot take advantage of tactile feedback as in traditional surgery. During the conduct of the operation, manipulation and retraction of the lung parenchyma is necessary. With loss of tactile feedback, the surgeon may have difficulty determining the extent of traction placed on the visceral pleura or hilar structures. Several technical maneuvers can be utilized to avoid iatrogenic injury that may lead to prolonged air leaks or excessive bleeding. During a robotic-assisted hilar lymph node dissection, exposure is necessary to perform a systematic lymph node dissection. In an effort to reduce iatrogenic injuries to the lung parenchyma, we recommend utilizing "passive" retraction rather than "active" retraction to manipulate the lung around the chest cavity as previously described. By avoiding excessive traction on the lung parenchyma being left behind, limited iatrogenic injury will be created.

Lymph Node Dissection

Unnecessary bleeding during the lymph node dissection will obscure the surgical field requiring the bedside assistant to clear the field with suction. During dissection of the mediastinal and hilar lymph node stations, the use of two maneuvers will minimize bleeding and expedite the dissection. The lymph node dissection should be conducted along the perivascular Layer, stripping all this fatty lymph node tissue en bloc away from the mediastinal structures. The surgeon should avoid "active" traction on the lymph nodes to avoid capsule disruption that will lead to bleeding that is difficult to control. With the use of a bipolar dissector, the collection of lymph nodes can be precisely dissected away from the adjacent mediastinal structures until the majority of the nodes are free of attachments. Then the entire collection of nodes can then be gently lifted out of its respective bed, and the remaining attached tissue can be transected. Exposure of the deep subcarinal and paratracheal nodes is achieved by countertraction on adjacent structures rather than grasping and pulling on the nodal packet.

Discussion

Anatomical lobectomy with systematic mediastinal lymphadenectomy performed through a posterolateral thoracotomy remains the "gold standard" for treatment of early-stage non-small cell lung cancer [1]. Even with advancements in thoracoscopic minimally invasive instruments, conventional lobectomy remains the preferred method. Opponents have argued that VATS lobectomy has not been shown to be the superior approach when compared to muscle-sparing thoracotomy and potentially exposes the patient to the risk of major complications during pulmonary resection in a closed chest [25]. In order to offset the restrictions imposed by a complete endoscopic VATS platform, a "utility" thoracotomy (ranging from 2 cm to 8 cm with varying degrees of rib spreading for extraction of the specimen and/or facilitating the anatomical dissection [9, 10]) has become an integral element of the VATS lobectomy technique. With access through a utility thoracotomy, surgeons are able to make use of conventional surgical instruments to conduct vascular isolation and mediastinal lymph node dissection. The use of conventional instruments in this manner provides sufficient flexibility and increased degrees of freedom in order to perform an effective anatomical lung resection. The utility thoracotomy has also provided safe and reliable access to hilar structures in the event of major vascular injury. VATS lobectomy with a utility thoracotomy has made this procedure more acceptable to thoracic surgeons who would otherwise be uneasy with performing a technically challenging procedure through port access with conventional endoscopic instruments. Consequently, few authors perform totally endoscopic major pulmonary resection [26, 27].

Despite the maturation of minimally invasive surgery, VATS lobectomy is generally reserved for a small population of patients who present with a peripheral early-stage I NSCLC. The technical limitations of the VATS platform, when faced with potential hilar (N1) lymph node involvement, central, or T3 lesions, management of these patients with VATS technique may make it difficult to achieve a complete resection of mediastinal and hilar disease. Other techniques have included limitations on the extent of hilar dissection and the use of simultaneous ligation of the hilar structures [28]. *Because of the non-anatomical dissection, these techniques have largely been discouraged.* When compared with lobectomy performed by conventional thoracotomy, the various methods of VATS lobectomy have been shown to be associated with numerous advantages, but the techniques remain elusive to the majority of practicing thoracic surgeons [6, 7].

The introduction of robotic technology combined with improved three-dimensional video platforms and wristed instrumentation has accelerated the acceptance of this technology into the thoracic surgeons practice. The da Vinci surgical system represents the most advanced robotic tool in order to perform individual isolation and ligation of the pulmonary vasculature, bronchus, and complete systematic lymph node dissection. By incorporating the da Vinci surgical system into a minimally invasive platform for pulmonary resection, surgeons can accomplish a safe and reliable video-assisted anatomical thoracoscopic lung resection without the need for a utility thoracotomy. In our experience, complete port-access robotic-assisted lung resection can be performed with individual isolation of the pulmonary artery and division of its branches. During this phase of the operation, a thorough removal of the hilar (N1) and mediastinal (N2) lymph nodes can be performed. One of the main benefits of robotic-assisted techniques is the meticulous dissection that can be conducted in a nearly bloodless field. With the use of a robotic platform, precise dissections, lymphadenectomy, and vascular isolation can be performed with safety and reliability.

Robotic video-assisted thoracoscopic pulmonary resection is contraindicated in most patients with unresectable clinical stage IIIA or IIIB non-small cell lung cancer and in central lesions involving proximal bronchus, carina, or pulmonary artery that may require sleeve pneumonectomy or major vascular reconstruction, similar to contraindications to conventional VATS pulmonary resection. However, large lesions greater than 5 cm and more advanced clinically operable NSCLC are not felt to be a contraindication to robotic-assisted pulmonary resection. In our experience, patients with clinically resectable NSCLC who undergo a complete port-access robotic video-assisted thoracoscopic lung resection experience low mortality and morbidity rates that compare favorably to conventional open and VATS lobectomy.

In conclusion, the technique of complete port-access robotic video-assisted thoracoscopic pulmonary resection continues to be an evolving technique and will require further refinements. The technique described was specifically designed to limit the need for unnecessary chest wall trauma and to provide reliable endoscopic access to the chest cavity in order to perform complex intrathoracic surgical procedures, a technique that would improve upon conventional VATS pulmonary resection while having the potential for reducing mortality and morbidity.

References

1. Ginsburg RJ, Rubinstein LV. Randomized trial of lobectomy versus limited resection for T1N0 non-small cell lung cancer. Ann Thorac Surg. 1995;60:615–23.
2. Walker WS, Carnochan FM, Pugh GC. Thoracoscopic pulmonary lobectomy. J Thorac Cardiovasc Surg. 1993;106:1111–7.
3. Kirby TJ, Rice TW. Thoracoscopic lobectomy. Ann Thorac Surg. 1993;56:784–6.
4. Lewis RJ. The role of video-assisted thoracic surgery for cancer of the lung: wedge to lobectomy by simultaneous stapling. Ann Thorac Surg. 1993;56:762–8.
5. Swanson SJ, Herndon J, D'Amico TA, et al. Results of CALGB 39802 feasibility of VATS lobectomy for lung cancer. Proc Am Soc Clin Oncol. 2002;21:290a.
6. Daniels LJ, Balderson SS, Onaitis MW, D' Amico TA. Thoracoscopic lobectomy: a safe and effective strategy for patients with stage I lung cancer. Ann Thorac Surg. 2002;74:860–4.
7. Whitson BA, Andrade RS, et al. Video-assisted thoracoscopic surgery is a more favorable than thoracotomy for resection of clinical stage I non-small cell lung cancer. Ann Thorac Surg. 2007;83:1965–70.
8. Mack MJ, Scruggs GR, Kelly KM, Shennib H, Landreneau RJ. Video-assisted thoracic surgery: has technology found it place? Ann Thorac Surg. 1997;64:211–5.
9. Iwasaki M, Kaga K, Nishiumi N, et al. Experience with the two-windows method for mediastinal lymph node dissection in lung cancer. Ann Thorac Surg. 1998;65:800–82.
10. Kirby TJ, Mack MJ, Landreneau RJ, Rice TW. Initial experience with video-assisted thoracoscopic lobectomy. Ann Thorac Surg. 1993;56:1248–53.
11. Melfi FM, Menconi GF, Marianin AM, et al. Early experience with robotic technology for thoracoscopic surgery. Eur J Cardiothorac Surg. 2002;21:864–8.
12. Park JB, Flores RM, Rusch VW. Robotic assistance for video-assisted thoracic surgical lobectomy: technique and initial results. J Thorac Cardiovasc Surg. 2006;131:54–9.
13. Gharagozloo F, Margolis M, Tempesta B. Robot-assisted thoracoscopic lobectomy for early-stage lung cancer. Ann Thorac Surg. 2008;85:1880–6.
14. Dylewski MD, Ohaeto AC, Pereira JF. Pulmonary resection using a total endoscopic robotic-assisted approach. Semin Thorac Cardiovasc Surg. 2011;23(1):36–42.
15. Gharagozloo F, Margolis M, Tempesta B, et al. Robotic-assisted lobectomy for early-stage lung cancer: report of 100 consecutive cases. Ann Thorac Surg. 2009;88:330–84.
16. Park BJ, Flores RM. Cost comparison of robotic, video-assisted thoracic surgery and thoracotomy approaches to pulmonary lobectomy. Thorac Surg Clin. 2008;18(3):297–300. vii.
17. Veronesi G, Galetta D, Maisonneuve P, Melfi DF, Schmid RA, Borri A, Vannucci F, Spaggiari L. Four-arm robotic lobectomy for the treatment of early-stage lung cancer. J Thorac Cardiovasc Surg. 2010;140:19–25.
18. Park BJ, Melfi F, Mussi A, Maisonneuve P, Spaggiari L, Da Silva RK, Veronesi G. Robotic lobectomy for non-small cell lung cancer (NSCLC): long-term oncologic results. J Thorac Cardiovasc Surg. 2012;143(2):383–9.
19. Whitson BA, Groth SS, Duval SJ, Swanson SJ, Maddaus MA. Surgery for early-stage non-small cell lung cancer: a systematic review of the video-assisted thoracoscopic surgery versus thoracotomy approaches to lobectomy. Ann Thorac Surg. 2008;86:2008–18.
20. McKenna RJ, Houck W, Fuller CB. Video-assisted thoracic surgery lobectomy: experience with 1100 cases. Ann Thorac Surg. 2006;81:421–6.
21. Onaitis MW, Petersen RP, Balderson SS, et al. Thoracoscopic lobectomy is a safe and versatile procedure. Ann Surg. 2006;244(3):420–5.
22. Cancer Therapy Evaluation Program, Common Terminology Criteria for Adverse Events, Version 3.0, DCTD, NCI, NIH, DHHS. Published date August 9, 2006. Accessed 31 Mar 2003
23. Takagi H, et al. Perioperative results of robotic lung lobectomy: summary of the literature. Surg Endosc. 2012;26(12):3697–9.
24. Cao C, Manganas C, Ang SC, Yan TD. A systematic review and meta-analysis on pulmonary resections by robotic video-assisted thoracic surgery. Ann Cardiothorac Surg. 2012;1(1):3–10.
25. Kirby TJ, Mack MJ, Landreneau RJ, Rice TW. Lobectomy—video-assisted thoracic surgery verses muscle-sparing thoracotomy. A randomized trial. J Thoracic Cardiovasc Surg. 1995;109(5):997–1001.
26. Shiraishi T, Shirakusa T, Miyoshi T, Hiratsuka M, Yamamoto S, Iwasaki A. A completely thoracoscopic lobectomy/segmentectomy for primary lung cancer: technique, feasibility and advantages. Thorac cardiovasc Surg. 2006;54:202–7.
27. Gossot D. Technical tricks to facilitate totally endoscopic major pulmonary resection. Ann Thorac Surg. 2008;86:323–32.
28. Lewis RJ, Caccavale RJ, Sisler GE, Bocage JP, Mackenzie JW. VATS simultaneously stapled lobectomy. Ann Thorac Surg. 1997;64:1869–71.

8 Robotic Pulmonary Resection Using a Completely Portal Four-Arm Technique

Robert James Cerfolio and Ayesha S. Bryant

The principle investigator of this study (Robert Cerfolio) has lectured for Intuitive (Sunnyvale, CA).

Introduction

Over the past several years, minimally invasive surgery (MIS) such as robotic surgery has become the standard of care in urology and gynecology; it has also steadily gained a place as standard of care in thoracic surgery. One of the factors that have prompted the shift towards robotic surgery is the limitation of video-assisted thoracoscopic surgery (VATS). VATS is limited by a two-dimensional view, ergonomic discomfort, and counterintuitive movement and non-wristed instruments. The robot, on the other hand, provides a magnified three-dimensional view, small 5 and 8 mm wristed instruments, and the ability for the surgeon to drive his own camera and provide his own retraction. However, robotic surgery requires a longer setup time, higher initial capital costs, in-depth training of the entire team, a lack of haptic feedback, and the need for more specialized and costly equipment compared to VATS. Despite these issues that slow robotic adoption, most thoracic surgeons who have used both the robot and VATS for mediastinal and esophageal operations believe the robotic approach affords distinct advantages. However, the role of the robot for pulmonary resection remains controversial.

R.J. Cerfolio, M.D., F.A.C.S., F.C.C.P. (✉)
A.S. Bryant, M.D., M.S.P.H.
Division of Cardiothoracic Surgery, University of Alabama at Birmingham, 703 19th Street S, ZRB 739, Birmingham, AL 35294, USA
e-mail: rcerfolio@uab.edu

Definitions and Nomenclature of Robotic Thoracic Surgery

Robotic pulmonary resection is performed using several different techniques. A standardized nomenclature system has been proposed by an international robotic committee (publication pending). A completely portal technique (no access incisions are used) has been championed by Dylewski and by us at the University of Alabama at Birmingham (UAB). We favor using four arms and thus have coined the term "*completely portal robotic lobectomy* (*CPRL*)" *technique that uses either three or four arms.* A "completely portal operation" is defined as an operation where only ports are used (e.g., incisions that are only as large as the size of the trocars placed in them), the air in the pleural space or chest cavity does not communicate with the ambient air in the operating room, carbon dioxide is insufflated in the chest, and the portal incision(s) is/are not enlarged at any time during the operation to be larger than the trocars placed through them except for the removal of a specimen that is contained in a bag [1]. The number of robotic arms implemented during the operation is also included in the nomenclature and will be separated by a hyphen after the type of operation is specified. Thus we prefer a CPRL-4 and Dylewski has used a CPLR-3 approach for several years with outstanding results.

Robotic operations that make a utility incision are being defined as robotic-assisted procedures (RA). A utility incision is defined as an incision

K.C. Kim (ed.), *Robotics in General Surgery*, DOI 10.1007/978-1-4614-8739-5_8,

in the chest that may or may not have trocars or robotic arms placed through it; the incision allows communication between the ambient air in the operating room and the pleural space, is less than 5 cm in size, does not spread the ribs, and CO_2 insufflation is utilized selectively. Each has its advantages and disadvantages.

Procedure Overview

Patient Positioning

The patient is placed in a standard lateral decubitus positioning. We have devised a technique, as shown in the following Fig. 8.1, that avoids arm boards and bean bags and places the patients' arms on the operating room table with blankets in between them.

We do not routinely use arterial lines, central lines, Foley catheters, or epidurals. The avoidance of the commonly used devices above quickens the operative setup and reduces unnecessary delays prior to surgery.

Robotic Positioning and Docking

Because we use a four-arm technique, the robot must be driven in over the patient head on a 15–30° angle as shown in Fig. 8.2. This allows the third arm and the robotic arm next to it (for right-sided operation it is arm 2, for left-sided operation it is arm 1) ample room to prevent collisions between the robotic arms.

Operative Technique and Trocar Placement of CPRL-4

We prefer the CPRL-4 method [2]. As shown in Fig. 8.1, the pleural space is entered over the top of the eighth rib using a 5 mm port in the proposed camera port first. We have continued to evolve our technique to improve it, and recently we have started to place the camera port first instead of the most anterior port first. This avoids accidental entry into the abdomen. In order to do this, one must first carefully plan the most posterior port for robotic arm 3. Measurements using a

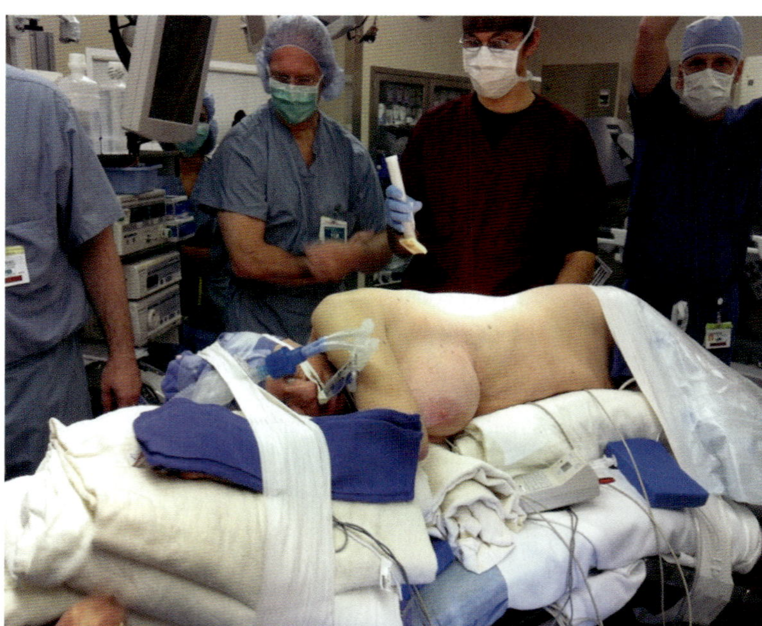

Fig. 8.1 Patient positioning

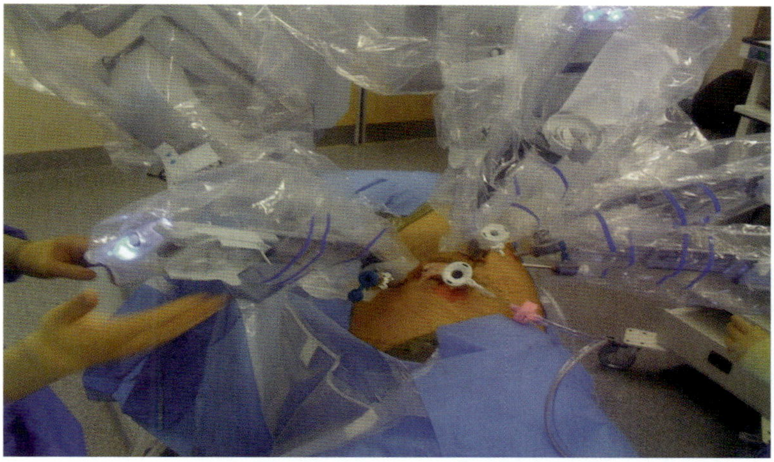

Fig. 8.2 Robot being driven in over the patient

ruler should be marked on the patient's skin prior to any incisions. Once the marks are made, the camera incision is made first. A 5 mm VATS camera is used to ensure entry into the pleural space and warmed CO_2 is insufflated to drive the diaphragm inferiorly. The incisions are all carefully marked out with a pen and measured to ensure that there is at least 9 cm between it and the more posterior robotic arm and then 10 cm between it and robotic arm 3, which always serves as the most posterior robotic arm as shown in Fig. 8.3.

Robotic arm 3 is a 5 mm port, which is placed a few cm anterior to the spinous processes of the vertebral bodies. A paravertebral block is performed posteriorly using a local anesthetic and a 21 gauge needle from ribs 3 to 11. The needle is used to help select the ideal location for the second incision, the most posterior incision. The location chosen is two ribs below the major fissure and as far posterior in the chest as possible, just anterior to the spinal processes of the vertebral body. A small 5 mm incision is made and a 5 mm reusable metal da Vinci trocar is placed. This will be the position for robotic arm 3. The next few incisions are carefully planned and once again marked or remarked or changed on the skin prior to making them. Ten centimeters anteriorly to the most posterior incision and along the same rib (most commonly rib 8), a third incision is planned. It is an incision for an 8 mm port and its trocar is an 8 mm metal reusable da Vinci trocar that will be docked with robotic arm 2. A 12 mm plastic disposable port is used for the 12 mm camera and if the 8 mm camera is used, an 8 mm metal reusable trocar is placed. Prior to making these two incisions, a small 21 gauge needle is used to identify the most anteriorly inferior aspect of the chest that is just above the diaphragmatic fibers. This incision will have a 15 mm port and serve as the access port. A plastic disposable trocar is used. No robotic arms are attached to the trocar that is placed in this incision. This incision is carefully planned. It is made just above the diaphragm as anterior and inferior as possible and, importantly, in order to be in between the ports used for robotic arm 1 and the camera. The access port can be alternatively placed more posterior if anatomy dictates between the camera and robotic arm 2. It should be two or three ribs lower than these two ports. This affords room for the bedside assistant to work. Once these incisions are carefully planned and their location is confirmed, they are made and the appropriate trocars are placed. Finally, the initial 5 mm anterior port that was made first and used to introduce the VATS camera to identify the internal landmarks is then dilated to a 12 mm double cannulated port for robotic arm 1. The robot is driven over the patient's shoulder on a 15° angle and attached to the four ports. In general, only four robotic instruments were used for all of these operations—the Cadiere grasper, a 5 mm bowel grasper (used

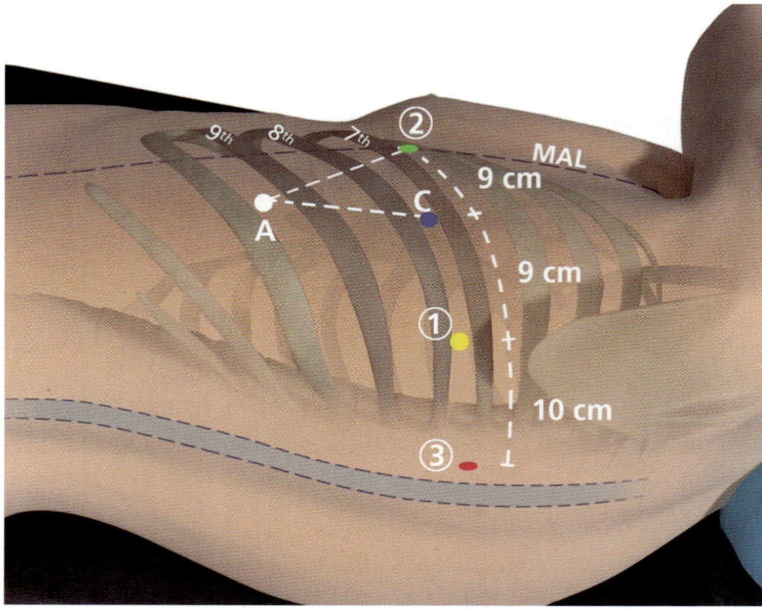

Fig. 8.3 CPRL-4 technique features entering the pleural space using a 5 mm port anteriorly in the midaxillary line (MAL) over the top of the seventh rib and then using a 5 mm VATS camera to make all other incisions based on internal anatomy. The *circled numbers* in the figure represent the robotic arms used. (C) is for the camera port, (A) is for the 15 mm access port (which can also be placed between the camera and robotic arm 2 is space is not adequate more anteriorly). Note that robotic arm 3 is a 5 mm port, robotic arm two is an 8 mm port, the camera can be an 8 or 12 mm port depending on the camera used, and robotic arm 1 is a 12 mm port. The area with the *dashed lines* is the area where no incisions are made and is the most posterior third of the area between the mid-spine and the post edge of the scapula

exclusively through the most posterior port that is attached to robotic arm 3 which serves as a retractor of the lung), the Maryland forceps, and a cautery spatula.

Once the arms are in the chest under direct vision, we use a zero-degree camera to reduce pain and rubbing on the intercostal nerve and use it the entire operation usually.

Step-by-Step Operative Technique of a Robotic Right Upper Lobectomy

First the pleural space is inspected and explored to ensure there are no metastatic lesions on the diaphragm or the parietal or visceral pleura. Dissection is started at the N2 mediastinal lymph nodes. If the lung deflates well, the nodes #9, #8, and #7 can be can be completely removed. If the lung does not deflate sufficiently, it is best to start at the #7 station and then move cephalad towards the trachea and remove #10R and separate the azygos vein off of the trachea. Removal of the lymph nodes first opens up the anatomy and affords visual inspection of the N2 nodes.LN# 9

The dissection is carried down between the hilar structures and the phrenic nerve. The phrenic nerve is gently swept down to remove the #10R lymph node avoiding the small phrenic vein that goes to the large #10R lymph node that is routinely found in this area. Develop the bifurcation between middle and upper lobe veins by bluntly dissecting it off of the underlying pulmonary artery. It can be encircled with the Cadiere forceps or curved bipolar dissector and a vessel loop. The #10R lymph node between the anterior–apical pulmonary artery branch and the superior pulmonary vein should be removed or swept up towards the lung. This exposes the anterior apical pulmonary artery branch. The dissection is continuing of the hilar tissue to cleanly expose the main pulmonary artery. Encircle the superior pulmonary vein with an 8 cm vessel loop and retract it off the pulmonary artery behind it. Using the vessel loop as a guide, the linear stapling device is passed across the right superior pulmonary vein and fired. Next the anterior apical trunk pulmonary artery branch is encircled with a vessel loop and transected with a linear stapler in the same fashion as the vein. In both cases the stapler is brought in from the assistant non-robotic port. Exposure might be improved by using the left-hand *EndoWrist* instrument to deflect the trachea downward and enable the tip of the stapler device to go above the trachea. The operation is now changed to a posterior approach in contrast to continue this anteriorly as done commonly via VATS lobectomy. The RUL bronchus' anatomy is exposed. Its upper aspect is seen coming off the trachea. The dissection is continued inferiorly to expose the inferior edge of the RUL bronchus and free it from the bronchus intermedius. Once the anatomy is identified, a Cadiere forceps can be placed under the RUL bronchus to confirm complete dissection of it. Further lymph node dissection (10R and 11R, hilar and interlobar) is continued along the right main bronchus and the bifurcation between the bronchus intermedius with the upper lobe bronchus identified. Encircle the right upper lobe bronchus with a vessel loop and transect with a linear stapler (gold, green, or purple load). Care must be taken to apply only minimal retraction on the specimen to avoid tearing of any small remaining anterior PA branches.

Next, the posterior segment of the pulmonary artery is exposed. The surrounding N1 nodes can be removed and the posterior artery can be encircled with a vessel loop and taken with a vascular stapler. A vessel-sealing device or titanium clips applied by the *EndoWrist* Small Clip Applier could be used if the vessel is less than 6 mm in size. The only step left is the completion of the fissure between the upper and middle lobes, which can be difficult. The anterior aspect of the pulmonary artery is carefully inspected to ensure there are no PA branches remaining. If so these are usually quite small and can be easily torn and must be carefully ligated. The fissure between the right upper lobe and the right middle lobe is now taken with a gold or purple stapler. Usually this is done anterior to posterior; however, if the space between the middle lobe pulmonary artery and the right middle lobe vein is already developed, it can be done in the reverse direction, from posterior to anterior; this allows the stapler to be directed away from the PA. If the stapler is brought in anteriorly, then as the fissure is completed, the main pulmonary artery should be seen and the stapler should be placed just above it and again ensuring that all small PA branches to the RUL have been taken. The right middle lobe PA branch can be easily seen and should be preserved. The RUL must be lifted up to ensure the specimen bronchus is included in the resected specimen. The lobe, now free of any attachments, is placed remotely anteriorly and the remaining LN dissection of station 2R and 4R should be performed. The specimen is then bagged and removed. With completion of the lymph node dissection and the lobe completely resected, an "Anchor" bag is inserted into the chest from the assistant port. The lobe is held freely up in the dome of the chest by the thoracic grasper. This is to utilize gravity to facilitate bagging of the lobe.

The Anchor bag is placed below the freely hanging lobe. The lobe is then dropped and pushed into the bag. Visualize that the complete specimen is contained in the bag while the assistant slowly closes the "Anchor" bag. The strings of the bag are brought out through the 15 mm access port. A small 20 Fr chest tube is placed apically and posteriorly via the most anterior port and guided into position by the *EndoWrist* instrument in the arm. Once completed, CO_2 is turned off and the right thorax vented. The incisions are carefully inspected from inside via the camera to make sure there is no venous bleeding that was tamponaded by the CO_2.

Robotic-Assisted Compared to Completely Portal

Other series which used a robotic-assisted lobectomy (RAL) technique have come from Melfi (Italy) and Parks (United States). Recently the two have combined their series and reported long-term follow-up in 2012. In this report,

Park et al. [4] evaluated 325 patients who underwent robotic lobectomy for early stage NSCLC who also showed minimal morbidity and mortality. Veronesi and Melfi in 2010 recently reported the safety of a four-arm robotic-assisted (RAL-4) lobectomy (using a 3–4 cm access incision as employed by VATS surgeons) in 54 patients. However, Melfi now uses a completely portal technique. Dylewski and Ninan in 2010 reported the effectiveness of a completely portal robotic lobectomy using three arms (CPRL-3) in 74 patients [3, 4]. Survival rates were similar to those for similar-staged patients who underwent lobectomy by VATS or thoracotomy.

Outcomes Review

The largest series of a completely portal robotic lobectomy using four arms was our series published in 2011. It had 168 patients that underwent robotic pulmonary resection of which 104 had a lobectomy. In that paper on patients with NSCLC, we matched (3–1) to patients who had a pulmonary resection via nerve- and rib-sparing thoracotomy. In that study 16 patient had a CPRS-4 (segmentectomy) as well. The results of our study are summarized in Table 8.1. The technical changes made were the following: adding the fourth robotic arm posterior and using a 5 mm port so the surgeon can retract the lung for himself; placing a vessel loop around the artery, vein, bronchus, and fissures to help guide the stapler; the removal of the tumor above the diaphragm; and using CO_2 insufflation. Results of CPRL-4 after technical modifications show a trend in reduction of median operative times and reduction in conversion rates.

Discussion

Minimally invasive techniques are the future of thoracic surgery and most all-surgical specialties. The robot currently represents the ultimate MIS tool. One of the reasons to perform MIS includes immunologic benefits that may lead to improved survival for patients with non-small cell lung cancer [5–8]. The adoption of the robot for pulmonary resection will depend on several factors: the availability of the robotic platform to the thoracic surgeon, the true cost of the operation, the measured and perceived benefit to the patient, hospital, and surgeon, and the time it takes to perform the operation. Most importantly is the surgeon's current enthusiasm for the VATS lobectomy that he or she performs. If a team is already adroit with VATS lobectomy and they believe that the lymph node dissection is adequate, the desire to adopt robotic pulmonary resection into their practice will be low. However, if their lymph node dissection during VATS lobectomy was, as in our experience, suboptimal and difficult to teach, then it will probably be high.

In conclusion, the current literature shows that robotic surgery is safe and efficient and has similar survival rates compared to the open and VATS approaches for patients with NSCLC. The surgeon can provide an R0 resection in patients with cancer, even those with large tumors (up to 10 cm). In addition, an outstanding mediastinal and hilar lymph node resection is achievable. Technical modifications have led to decreased operative times and may improve teachability, as well as decrease patient morbidity and surgeon

Table 8.1 Summary of results from the CPRL-4 paper

	Robotic group	Matched group (thoracotomy)	P-value
Blood loss (ml)	35	90	0.03
Chest tube duration (days)	1.5	3.0	<0.001
Morbidity	27 %	38 %	0.05
Pain score at 3 weeks postoperatively	2.5/10	4.4/10	0.04
Mortality	0 %	3.1 %	0.11
Median hospital length of stay (days)	2.0	4.0	0.02

From Cerfolio RJ, Bryant AS, Skylizard L, Minnich DJ. Initial consecutive experience of completely portal robotic pulmonary resection with 4 arms. J Thorac Cardiovasc Surg. 2011; 142(4): 740–6 with permission frustration during the learning curve. Even though hospitals are acquiring more robots for other specialties besides thoracic surgery, the capital cost, service contract costs, and equipment costs have to be carefully considered and studied. Patient selection is critical, especially during the learning curve. Surgeon's teams that are earlier in their learning should start their robotic experience with wedge resections and/or mediastinal tumor resections. When the team is ready for a lobectomy, small T1 or T2 lesions should be chosen in patients without enlarged or calcified mediastinal or hilar lymph nodes. The preoperative CT scan should be carefully examined and complete fissures improve attractiveness of early case selection. Finally we believe that lower lobes are a better place to start than upper lobes.

References

1. Cerfolio RJ, Dylewski M, Parks Bernard, Veronesi G, Kernstine K, Melfi F. International consensus paper for definitions and nomenclature for robotic thoracic and pulmonary resection. Ann Thorac Surg; 2012.
2. Cerfolio RJ, Bryant AS, Skylizard L, Minnich DJ. Initial consecutive experience of completely portal robotic pulmonary resection with 4 arms. J Thorac Cardiovasc Surg. 2011;142(4):740–6.
3. Ninan M, Dylewski MR. Total port-access robot assisted pulmonary lobectomy without utility thoracotomy. Eur J Cardiothorac Surg. 2010;38:231–2.
4. Park BJ, Melfi F, Mussi A, Maisonneuve P, Spaggiari L, Da Silva RK, Veronesi G. Robotic lobectomy for non-small cell lung cancer (NSCLC): long-term oncologic results. J Thorac Cardiovasc Surg. 2012;143:383–9.
5. Mahtabifard A, DeArmond DT, Fuller CB, McKenna Jr RJ. Video-assisted thoracoscopic surgery for stage 1 non-small cell lung cancer. Thorac Surg Clin. 2007;17:223–31.
6. Whitson BA, Groth SS, Duval SS, Swanson SJ, Maddaus MA. Surgery for Early Stage Non-small cell lung cancer: a systematic review of the video-assisted thoracoscopic surgery versus thoracotomy approach to lobectomy. Ann Thorac Surg. 2008;86:2008–18.
7. Yan TD, Black D, Bannon PG, McCaughan M. Systematic review and meta-analysis of randomized and non-randomized trials on safety and efficacy of video-assisted thoracic surgery lobectomy for early stage non-small cell lung cancer. J Clin Oncol. 2009;27:2553–62.
8. Flores RM, Ihekweasu UN, Rizk N, Dycoco BA, Bains MS, Downey RJ. Patterns of recurrence and incidence of second primary tumors after lobectomy by means of video-assisted thoracoscopic surgery (VATS) versus thoracotomy for lung cancer. J Thorac Cardiovasc Surg. 2011;141:59–64.

Part IV

Surgical Techniques: *Stomach*

9 Gastric Cancer: Partial, Subtotal, and Total Gastrectomies/Lymph Node Dissection for Gastric Malignancies

Woo Jin Hyung and Yanghee Woo

Introduction

The management of gastric cancer patients requires a multidisciplinary approach with surgery, the mainstay of curative treatment. Radical gastric resection and appropriate lymphadenectomy is the standard of care. Operative procedures for gastric cancer can be technically challenging especially as minimally invasive approaches. Many gastric cancer surgeons have adopted robotic technology to assist them in the technically challenging procedure of gastrectomy with - lymphadenectomy [1–4]. With additional robotic surgery training, experienced laparoscopic gastric cancer surgeons can safely provide the advantages of minimally invasive surgery to their patients. Adherence to the oncologic principles of gastric cancer treatment can assure the patients that the long-term survival benefits of surgery will not be compromised.

W.J. Hyung, M.D., Ph.D. (✉)
Department of Surgery, Yonsei University College of Medicine, 50 Yonsei-ro Seodaemun-gu, Seoul 120-752, Republic of Korea
e-mail: wjhyung@yuhs.ac

Y. Woo, M.D.
Division of GI/Endocrine Surgery, Center for Excellence in Gastric Cancer Care, Columbia University Medical Center, New York, NY, USA

Department of Surgery, Columbia University College of Physicians and Surgeons, New York, NY, USA

Department of Surgery, New York Presbyterian Hospital, New York, NY, USA
e-mail: yw2263@columbia.edu

Indications

Robotic surgery can be applied to those gastric cancer operations where conventional laparoscopic approach is indicated [5–10]. Currently, minimally invasive surgery is most commonly performed for early gastric cancer patients without perigastric lymph node (LN) involvement, and these patients are good candidates for robotic gastrectomy with limited lymphadenectomy. This is based on the recommendations of the Japanese gastric cancer treatment guidelines and classification [11, 12]. However, robotic technology may be most ideal for patients with locally advanced gastric cancer without evidence of distant metastases that require gastrectomy and D2 lymphadenectomy since robotic surgery provides the advantages of increase dexterity of movement for more precise dissection along the vessels during retrieval of perivascular soft tissues containing N2 lymph nodes [5].

Indications for robotic gastrectomy with limited lymphadenectomy:

- Stage IA ($cT_1N_0M_0$) by 7th AJCC TNM classification
- Mucosal and submucosal tumors not eligible for endoscopic resection
- Failed endoscopic mucosal resection or endoscopic submucosal dissection

Indications for robotic gastrectomy requiring D2 lymphadenectomy:

- Stage IB ($cT_1N_1M_0$; $cT_2N_0M_0$)
- Stage IIA ($cT_2N_1M_0$)

K.C. Kim (ed.), *Robotics in General Surgery*, DOI 10.1007/978-1-4614-8739-5_9,

At this time, no evidence is available to support robotic surgery for serosa-positive tumors (T4a) or tumors which have invaded adjacent organs (T4b) nor for palliative procedures.

Preoperative Work-Up

A comprehensive and thorough preoperative work-up of patients undergoing robotic surgery for gastric cancer is essential to guide each step of surgeon's operation. Preoperative planning for robotic gastric cancer surgery begins with pathologic confirmation of the diagnosis, which should be done by endoscopic biopsy. The operative planning requires complete evaluation of the patient's clinical status, the identification of the location of the tumor, and the local extent of disease. Therefore, we recommend that all patients scheduled for robotic gastric cancer operations have at least the following preoperative work-up:

- Upper endoscopy with biopsy (to confirm diagnosis and identify the location of the tumor)
- Endoscopic ultrasound (to evaluate for invasion depth and nodal status)
- CT Scan of the abdomen and pelvis (to evaluate for invasion depth, nodal status, and distant metastasis)

Operative Strategy

Pertinent Anatomy

Robotic gastrectomy and lymphadenectomy requires an intimate knowledge of the gastric anatomy, especially the gastric vessels and the accompanying nodal stations as defined by the Japanese Gastric Cancer Association [11, 12]. The robotic procedural steps are described in relation to the dissection of the lymph node stations required for D2 lymphadenectomy and should not deviate from the standard of care operations, which are performed both by open or laparoscopic approaches.

Operating Room Configuration

The configuration of the operating room should provide a safe and convenient environment for the patient and the entire team of surgeons, anesthesiologists, scrub technologists, and circulating nurses. The optimal configuration of the robot, the surgeon console, the surgical cart, the anesthesia cart, the bedside assistant position, and the monitors during a robotic gastrectomy is described relative to the patient on the operating table as the center of the room. Specific characteristics of robotic surgical system and operating room configuration have been previously described in detail [4, 8–10, 13–17]:

- The robot system is placed directly cephalad to the patient with the center of the robotic cart aligned with the patient's head.
- The anesthesia cart and the anesthesiologist are positioned to the left side of the patient's head for easy access to the patient's airway.
- The patient-side assistant stands to the lower left side of the patient with the scrub nurse, scrub table, and the main assistant monitor on the opposite side.
- The vision cart can be placed at the foot of the operating table or if space does not allow for this configuration, the vision cart can be placed to the patient's upper right.
- The surgeon console is positioned in the left lower edge of the operating room to provide the surgeon with a view of the patient and the overall access to the operating room.

Patient Positioning, Port Placement, Robot Docking, and Preparation of the Operative Field

Under general anesthesia the patient is positioned in supine with arms tucked at both sides. Sequential compression stockings and urinary catheter are placed. The entire abdomen from the nipple line to the suprapubic region is prepared and draped in the standard sterile fashion. Five ports, two non-robotic 12 mm trocars and three 8 mm robotic trocars, are used for robotic gastrectomy (Fig. 9.1).

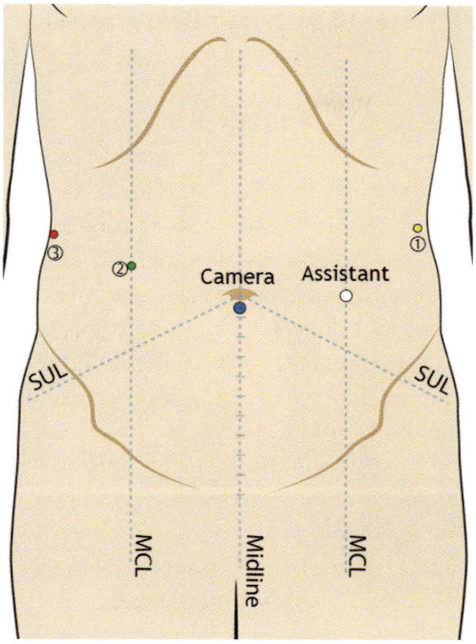

Fig. 9.1 Ports used for robotic gastrectomy

The proper placement of the ports are essential to ease of the robotic arm use during operation, and therefore, care should be taken to ensure that the port placement is accurate and adjusted for patient's abdominal wall girth as well as the intra-abdominal anatomy. Once the ports have been correctly inserted, the patient is placed in 15° reverse Trendelenburg position and the surgical cart is aligned and brought straight in to the head of the patient. The robot arms are ready to be docked as described below. Instruments should be inserted into the abdominal cavity under direct visualization as in any laparoscopic operation:

- The camera arm: the infraumbilical port (C)
- The 1st arm: curved bipolar Maryland forceps [1]
- The 2nd and the 3rd arms: the ultrasonic shears or a monopolar device and the Cadiere forceps, interchangeably

Three key maneuvers to optimize exposure and facilitate accurate resection during the main operation are recommended before proceeding with the main operative procedure.

Gastric Decompression

Gastric decompression should be performed to manipulate the stomach and to make the uncluttered view of the upper abdomen. This can be done with either the insertion of an orogastric/nasogastric tube or with a percutaneously placed needle (e.g., long 18–20 gauge spinal needle) [18].

Liver Retraction

To maximize the full use of the three robotic arms during robotic gastrectomy, a self-sustaining retraction of the left lobe of the liver is required. Proper liver retraction is necessary for adequate exposure of the hepatoduodenal and hepatogastric ligaments for complete dissection of the suprapancreatic lymph nodes and clearance of the soft tissues along the lesser curve of the stomach. Before beginning the dissection for the gastrectomy, any of the several described techniques may be used to retract the liver including the suture-gauze liver suspension method [19–21].

Intraoperative Determination of the Resection Extent

To determine the extent of resection, intraoperative tumor localization is required. Most lesions cannot be readily visualized due to the lack of serosal involvement or palpated during a robotic operation. Several methods of intraoperative tumor localization have been employed. These include preoperative endoscopic tattooing of the tumor, intraoperative endoscopy [8], or laparoscopic ultrasound [9, 22]. The authors prefer using preoperatively placed endoclips and an intraoperative abdominal x-ray, which has been found to be very successful [23].

Procedure of Robotic Distal Subtotal Gastrectomy and D2 LN Dissection

Five Major Steps and Associated Vascular Landmarks

1. Left side dissection: left gastroepiploic vessels
2. Right side dissection and duodenal transection: anterior superior pancreaticoduodenal vein and the right gastroepiploic vessels
3. Hepatoduodenal ligament and suprapancreatic dissection: right gastric artery, proper hepatic artery, portal vein, and celiac axis

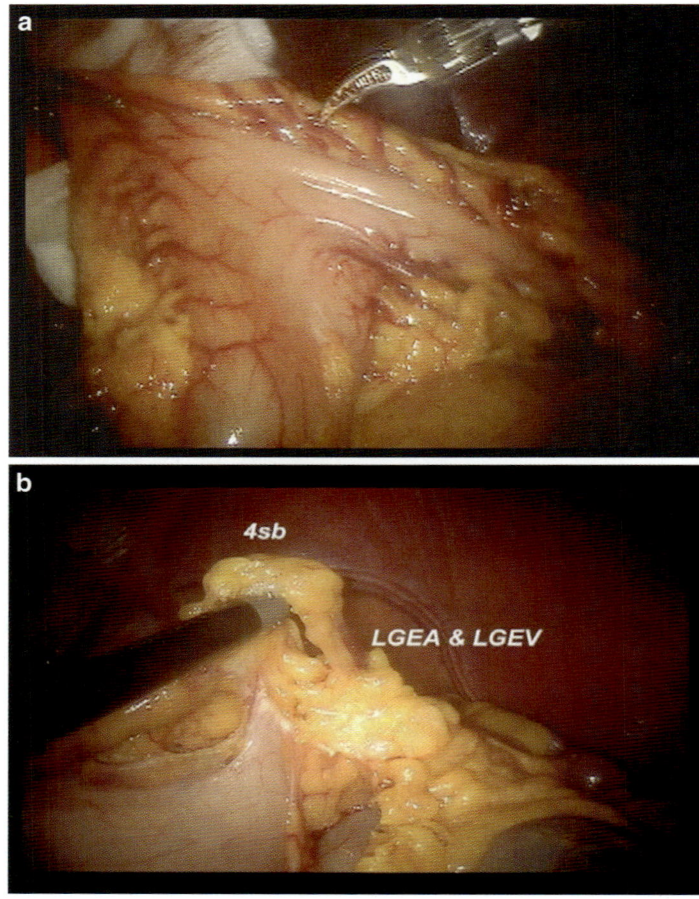

Fig. 9.2 (**a**) Greater curve of the stomach is retracted cephalad and toward the anterior abdominal wall creating a fanning effect to facilitate the greater curve dissection of the #4 lymph node station. (**b**) Division of the gastrocolic ligament proximally allows for the identification of the root of the LGEA and LGEV and retrieval of the 4sb

4. Approach to the left gastric vessels and the splenic vessels
5. Lesser curvature dissection and proximal gastric resection

Left Side Dissection

The left side dissection begins with a partial omentectomy from mid-abdomen toward the left gastroepiploic vessels along the greater curvature of the body the stomach. The necessary exposure of the omentum is achieved by grasping the soft tissues on the edge of the greater curvature of the stomach using the robot arm #3 (Cadiere) and pulling superiorly and anteriorly to create a draping of the greater omentum. This allows for safe division and efficient retrieval of LN stations 4sb and 4d (Fig. 9.2a):

- Begin 4–5 cm from the greater curvature of the stomach near the mid-transverse colon and enter the lesser sac and divide the greater omentum toward the lower pole of the spleen.
- Near the lower pole of the spleen, identify, ligate, and divide the left gastroepiploic vessels at their roots (Fig. 9.2b).
- Identify the first short gastric vessel and clear the greater curvature of the stomach toward the proximal resection margin.

Right Side Dissection and Duodenal Transection

The second major step moves the focus of the operation to the patient's right side. Right side dissection begins with mobilization of the distal stomach from the head of the pancreas and dissection of the soft tissues containing LN station #6. The borders of LN station #6 is defined by right gastroepiploic vein (RGEV), anterior superior pancreaticoduodenal

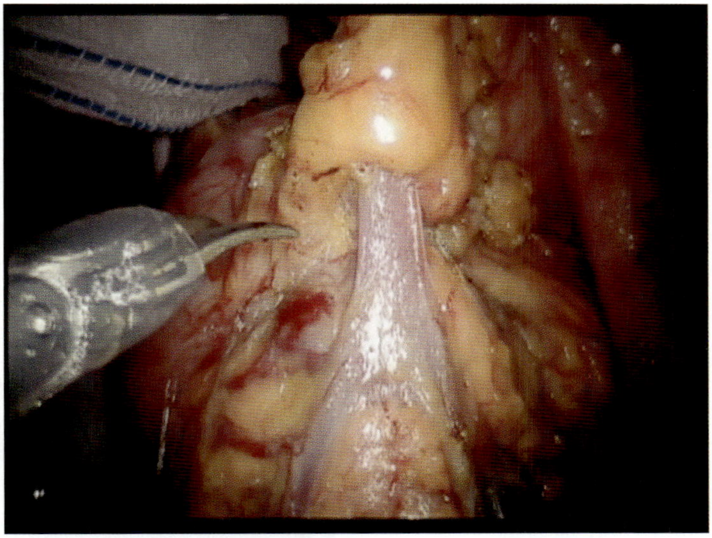

Fig. 9.3 The soft tissue containing lymph node station #6 has been cleared above the ASPDV to identify the root of RGEV on the head of the pancreas before ligation and division

vein (ASPDV), and the middle colic vein (MCV) (Fig. 9.3):

- Release the posterior stomach attachments to the anterior surface of the pancreas and the first portion of the duodenum from the colon.
- Dissect the soft tissues on the head of the pancreas until the RGEV and ASPDV are identified.
- Isolate, ligate, and divide the RGEV as it joins the ASPDV.
- Retrieve the soft tissues anterior to and superior to the ASPDV and superior to the MCV on both sides of the RGEV.
- Identify the right gastroepiploic artery which is usually located behind the RGEV ligate and divide it as it branches from the gastroduodenal artery (GDA).
- Release the attachments anterior to the GDA until the common hepatic artery (CHA). Free the immediate supraduodenal area using caution to avoid injury to the GDA and PHA (4″×4″ gauze placed anterior to the GDA may provide a visual mark to identify the area of dissection). The duodenum approximately 2 cm distal to the pylorus has been cleared, transect using an Endo-linear stapler.

Hepatoduodenal Ligament and Suprapancreatic Dissection

- Proper en bloc retrieval of soft tissues in the hepatoduodenal ligament and the suprapancreatic region is one of the most challenging steps of the D2 lymphadenectomy. After identification and ligation of the right gastric artery, a meticulous and precise dissection along the proper hepatic artery (PHA), the portal vein (PV), and the CHA is essential to success. Identify and dissect along the PHA to the origin of the RGA. Ligate and divide the RGA and retrieve the associated soft tissue of LN station #5 (Fig. 9.4).
- Carefully lift and dissect to free the soft tissues containing LN station #12a, which is anterior and medial to the PHA and medial to the PV (Fig. 9.5a).
- Additional exposure with the third arm by upper lifting of the liver and gentle downward retraction of the CHA by the assistant maybe necessary during this portion of the procedure.
- Continue dissection inferiorly along the PHA to clear the soft tissues superior to the CHA, which contain LN station #8a.
- Identify and ligate left gastric vein, which will become visible during the clearance of the soft tissues in the suprapancreatic area as it drains into the portal vein (*Caution*: *In some cases, the left gastric vein drains into the splenic vein and can be found running anterior to the splenic artery*).

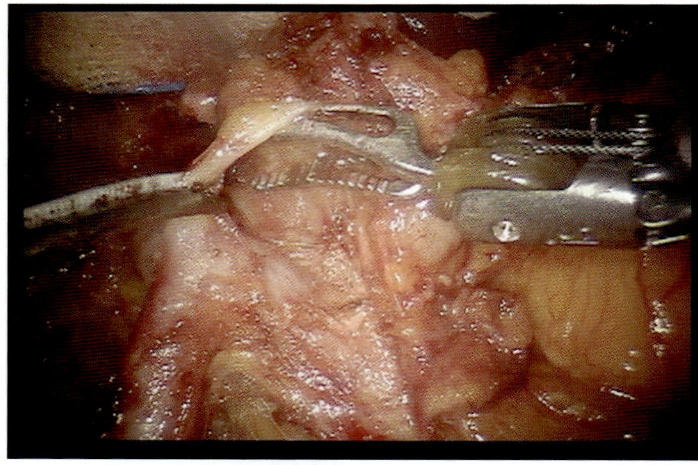

Fig. 9.4 Isolation of the right gastric artery is being performing using the Maryland dissector in arm #1 (*right*) with the harmonic in arm #2 (*left*)

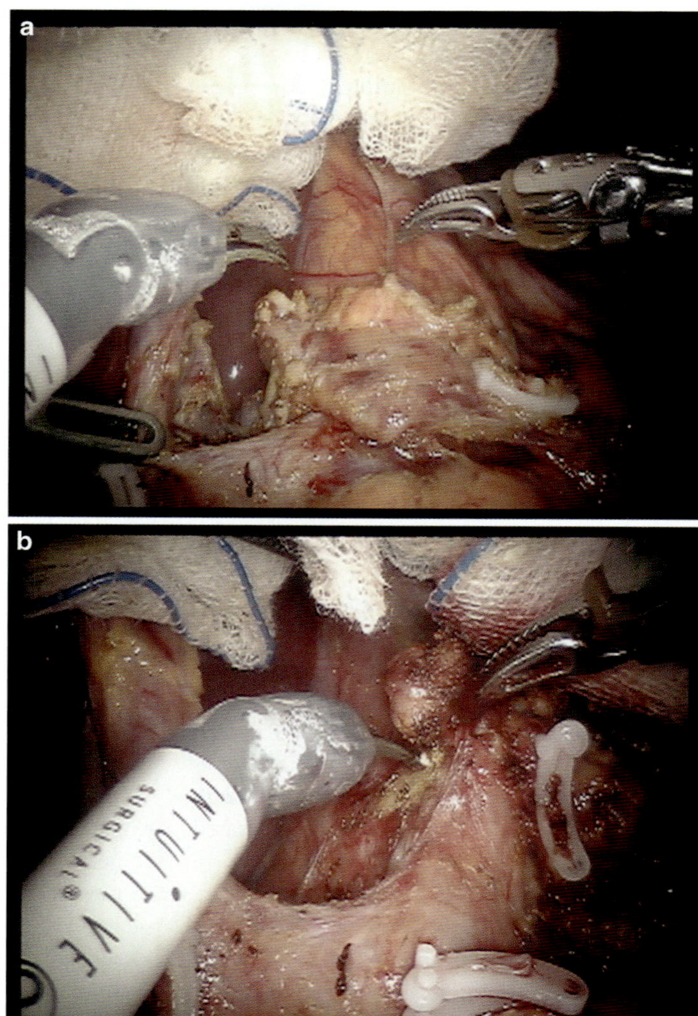

Fig. 9.5 (**a**) The portal vein is exposed in the hepatoduodenal ligament after on block lymphadenectomy has been performed to retrieve lymph node stations 12a and 8. (**b**) Dissection is being carried out along the celiac axis after division of the left gastric artery to retrieve the #9 lymph nodes

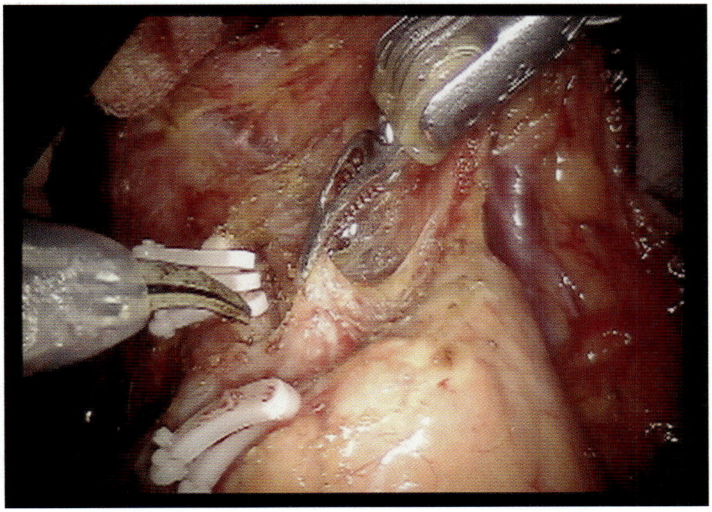

Fig. 9.6 The soft tissues along the left gastric artery (LGA) and splenic vessels are retrieved as LN station #7 and #11p, respectively

- Skeletonize the CHA toward the celiac axis to retrieve the soft tissues around the celiac artery, which contain LN station #9 (Fig. 9.5b).

Approach to the Left Gastric Artery and the Splenic Vessels

The soft tissues along the left gastric artery (LGA) and splenic vessels are retrieved as LN station #7 and #11p, respectively (Fig. 9.6):

- To improve access to the origin of the LGA as it branches from the celiac axis, divide the retroperitoneal attachments along the lesser curvature of the stomach.
- Using the Cadiere grasper (the robot arm #3), grasp the soft tissues containing the distal portion of the LGA by the stomach and lift the pedicle superiorly and anteriorly to tent up the LGA.
- Clear the soft tissues surrounding the root of the LGA for more complete exposure and identification then securely ligate and divide the LGA at its root.

After placing the stomach in the left upper quadrant, dissect the soft tissues off of the anterior surface of the splenic artery and continue to skeletonize the artery until the splenic vein is exposed. Retrieve lymph node station #11p along the splenic vessels until halfway point is reached.

Lesser Curvature Dissection and Proximal Resection

- At this point in the operation, the proximal stomach is freely retracted to the patient's left to improve exposure of the remaining attachments of the lesser curvature of the stomach to the retroperitoneum and the diaphragmatic crus. The soft tissues along the intra-abdominal esophagus, the right cardia, and the lesser curvature of the stomach containing LN stations #1 and #3 are cleared until the proximal resection margin. Perform the truncal vagotomy at this time by dividing the anterior and posterior branches of the vagus nerve.
- Be sure to fully mobilize the stomach from its posterior attachments to prepare for proximal gastric resection. Confirm the proximal resection line from the greater curvature to the lesser curvature with sufficient margin and divide the stomach using a 60 mm blue load Endo-linear stapler ensuring sufficient proximal margin (Reloads are usually required).

This completes the procedure of robotic D2 lymphadenectomy for distal subtotal gastrectomy.

Procedure of D2 Lymphadenectomy During Total Gastrectomy

The recommended procedure for advanced gastric adenocarcinoma located in the upper body of the stomach is a total gastrectomy with D2 lymphadenectomy. D2 lymphadenectomy for a proximal gastric adenocarcinoma requires the retrieval of LN #11d (along the distal splenic vessels)

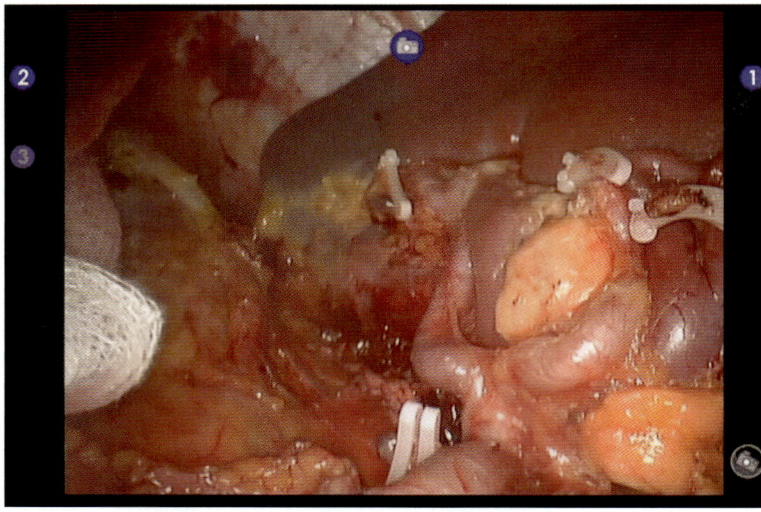

Fig. 9.7 Spleen-preserving total gastrectomy

and LN #10 (in the splenic hilum). The procedure can be performed using two different methods: spleen-preserving total gastrectomy or total gastrectomy with splenectomy.

Complete dissection of the splenic hilum to preserve the spleen during LN #10 retrieval is challenging and complex procedure which may lead to unexpected bleeding and prolonged operative time. While splenectomy-related postoperative complications, such as subphrenic abscesses and post-splenectomy syndrome, are well known [7], spleen preservation might be recommended for experienced surgeons.

Spleen-Preserving Total Gastrectomy (Fig. 9.7)

Robotic spleen-preserving total gastrectomy requires three of the following additional steps:

- After the division of the left gastroepiploic vessels, the dissection continues along the greater curvature of the stomach to ligate and divide the short gastric vessels. The esophagophrenic ligament is released to completely free the left side of the stomach. This portion of the procedure is facilitated by retracting the stomach to the right side of the patient to expose the left diaphragmatic crus.
- Approach to the splenic hilum by first identifying the distal splenic vessels dorsal to the distal pancreas and carefully skeletonizing the vessels toward the spleen.
- To ensure retrieval of the LN #10, completely removal the soft tissues encasing the splenic hilum must be achieved.
- Then, return to the proximal splenic vessels to retrieve the remaining soft tissues along the distal splenic artery and vein for the LN #11p and 11d dissection.

Reconstruction

After robotic gastric resection and complete lymph node dissection, several methods for creation of an intracorporeal or extracorporeal gastrointestinal anastomosis have been described. The advantages and disadvantages to each approach exist. The surgical extent and surgeon's preference dictate the selection of the gastrointestinal reconstruction after robotic gastric cancer surgery. In general, stapled anastomoses are preferred as it is less time consuming, but sutured anastomosis using robot assistance is another option [8]. Reconstruction using the stapling device requires the patient-side assistant and can be an opportunity for a hybrid operation. Therefore, many methods used during laparoscopic gastroduodenostomy, gastrojejunostomy, and esophagojejunostomy can be applied after robotic gastric resections [3, 4, 9–11]:

- Gastroduodenostomy, gastrojejunostomy, or Roux-en-Y gastrojejunostomy
- Intracorporeal or extracorporeal
- Linear or circular staplers including transoral anvil placement

Postoperative Management

Postoperative management of patients who have undergone robotic gastrectomy is identical to those patients who have undergone a laparoscopic gastrectomy for gastric cancer. The patients are monitored for ability for oral intake while given appropriate fluid maintenance, pain control, deep vein thrombosis prophylaxis, and blood tests:

- Gastrointestinal function is expected to return approximately in 3 days after operation in patients without complications.
- Oral intake is resumed on postoperative day (POD) 2 and advanced as tolerated usually to liquid diet (POD3), soft diet (POD4), and regular diet (POD5).
- Median length of hospital stay is usually 5 days without complications.

Complications

The reported complication rates for robotic gastrectomy vary. The largest series evaluating the short-term outcomes of robotic and laparoscopic gastric cancer surgery report wound-related issues, intraluminal bleeding, and anastomotic leakage to be the most common complications encountered after robotic gastrectomies [1]. These complications are not directly related to robot assistance since the ports placements and anastomoses are not performed using the robot.

In general the morbidity and mortality associated with radical gastrectomies depend on the extent of resection, LN dissection, experience of the surgeon, and the experience of the institution where the surgery is being performed [12–14]. Many of the complications are related to the extent of LN dissection and expectedly are higher with D2 lymphadenectomy than for D1 lymphadenectomy. Improved surgical outcomes have been reported with spleen-preserving total gastrectomies when compared to total gastrectomy with splenectomy. No differences in complication rates have been found between laparoscopic and robotic gastric cancer surgeries.

Other possible complications are:

- Intra-abdominal fluid collections/abscesses
- Intraluminal and intra-abdominal bleeding
- Pancreatitis/pancreatic leak/pancreatic fistula
- Anastomotic leak/stricture
- Gastroparesis or ileus
- Obstruction

Benefits for the Patient

- Less pain
- Shorter length of hospital stay
- Decreased blood loss
- Faster gastrointestinal recovery
- Faster physical recovery
- Better quality of life after surgery
- Better cosmesis

Benefits for the Surgeon

The robotic surgery system facilitates the process of performing laparoscopic surgery and provides the surgeon with ergonomics, 3D view, control of 4 arms, and accuracy of dissection, shorter learning curve that is provided by the inherent functions of the robotic system. This computer-enhanced surgical system thus allows surgeons to overcome various difficulties of laparoscopic surgery [4, 8]. The benefits specific to robotic gastric cancer operation is realized during the most difficult portions of the procedure including the dissection of the splenic vessels, isolation of the esophageal crux, and the suprapancreatic lymphadenectomy.

Dissection of Splenic Vessels

The small branches of the splenic vessels are easily identified and preserved allowing a pancreas–spleen-preserving D2 lymph node dissection, thanks to image magnification, tremor filtering, and fine circumferential robotic arm movements. This approach allows surgeons to drive the vascular dissection around and to completely clear the lymphatic tissue without any vascular injury with minimal intraoperative bleeding [13, 14].

Isolation of Diaphragmatic Crura

It is a fundamental step to an en bloc dissection of cardia lymph nodes and is greatly facilitated by wristed instruments that allow complete encircling of the distal esophagus [13, 15]. Moreover, the four-arm robotic surgery system will facilitate the insertion of the anvil head into the esophageal stump that could be not so easy to do in conventional laparoscopy [15], and esophagojejunostomy, which is usually performed in the deep and narrow space of the abdominal cavity, is feasible to execute by the robot-sewing technique [24].

Lymphadenectomy Include LN #14v, #8a, #9, #11p, #11d, and #12a

Relatively difficult areas to access during laparoscopic lymphadenectomy include LN #14v, #8a, #9, and #11. Moreover, the infrapyloric area and the superior mesenteric vein, including LN stations #6 and #14v, are the most frequent sources of intraoperative bleeding, while the suprapancreatic area including stations #7, #8a, and #9 is the second most frequent source [13, 25]. If the dissection along these vessels is easily conducted, the risk of bleeding can be reduced and lymphadenectomy can be better performed. The EndoWrist, tremor filtration, stable operative platform, and three-dimensional vision offered by the robotic surgical system aid the surgeon to perform a more accurate lymph nodes and vessels dissection [25].

Some authors have recently reported a new integrated robotic approach for suprapancreatic D2 nodal dissection that appears to be safe and feasible, even though the number of patients in the study was small [26]. Actually, the role of LN #14v lymphadenectomy in distal gastric cancer is controversial. Dissection of LN #14v had been a part of D2 gastrectomy defined by the 2nd edition of the Japanese classification, but it has been excluded from the latest edition [11]. However, D2 (+ No. 14v) may be beneficial in tumors with apparent metastasis to the LN # 6.

Disadvantages

- Longer operative time
- Initial cost of robot for hospital
- Financial burden to patient
- Limited training opportunities

Results

Robotic surgery for gastric cancer treatment is a relative novel, but experience in the field is growing. While many studies have studied laparoscopic versus open gastric cancer surgery and demonstrated many benefits of minimally invasive surgery without the loss of oncologic standards, the evaluation of the robotic approach to treatment of gastric cancer patients is in its infant stages. Phase III clinical trials support the safety and effectiveness of LG with lymph node dissection for the treatment of patients with EGC [6]. Laparoscopic gastric cancer surgery has been shown to produce better early postoperative outcome than conventional open surgery with comparative long-term survival. Robotic system is a new technology that holds significant promises for facilitating laparoscopic treatment of gastric cancer, although scientific evidence is still lacking.

Outcomes Review

The currently available studies are summarized. Ten case series evaluating robotic gastric cancer surgery with a total of 299 patients have been published between 2007 and 2012 (Table 9.1) [9, 13, 15–17, 26–30]. The two largest studies were by Song et al. [9] in 2009 in which they summarized their initial 100 cases of robot-assisted gastrectomy with lymph node dissection followed by another one [17] in 2011 with 61 patients. In general, these case series supported the safety and

Table 9.1 Casa series of RG for gastric cancer

Author/year	No. of patients	Type of surgery (STG/TG)	D2 LN dissection	Mean OT (min)	Mean EBL (ml)	No. of resected LN	LOS (days)	Morbidity %
Anderson et al. [16]	7	7/0	–	420	300	24 (17–30)	4 (3–9)	14.3
Patriti et al. [15]	13	9/4	13	286.0	103.0	28.1 ± 8.3	11.2 ± 4.3	46.2
Song et al. [9]	100	67/33	42	231.3	128.2	36.7 ± 13.3 (11–83)	7.8 (5–175)	14
Hur et al. [24]	7	5/2	0	205	–	36	9	14
Liu et al. [27]	9	2/5 (1WG + 1PG)	–	150–440	10–100	19–24 (D1) 28–38 (D2)	–	11
Isogaki et al. [17]	61	46/14 (1PG)	39	388 (STG) 520 (TG)	61.8 (STG) 150 (TG)	43 ± 14 (TG) 42 ± 18 (STG)	13.3 (8–43)	4
D'Annibale et al. [13]	24	13/11	24	267.5	30	28 (23–34)	6 (5–8)	8
Lee et al. [28]	12	12/0	0	253	135	46 (21–115)	6.6 ± 1.6	8
Yu et al. [29]	41	29/12	–	225 (STG) 285 (TG)	150 ± 127 (STG) 180 ± 157 (TG)	34.2 ± 18.5	–	5
Uyama et al. [26]	25	25/0	18	361	51.8 ± 38.2 (4–123)	44.3 ± 18.4 (26–95)	12.1 ± 3.2	11.2

TG total gastrectomy, *STG* subtotal gastrectomy, *WG* wedge resection, *PG* proximal gastrectomy, *OT* operative time, *LOS* length of hospital stay, *EBL* estimated blood loss

Table 9.2 NRCT robotic versus open gastrectomy for gastric cancer

Author/year	Pernazza et al. [33]		Caruso et al. [31]	
Approach (R/O)	R	O	R	O
No. of patients	45	45	29	120
Resection type (STG/TG)	21/24	–	17/12	83/37
D2 LND	45	–	29	120
No. LN examined	34	–	28	32
EBL (ml)	–	–	198 ± 202	386 ± 96
LOS (days)	–	–	9.6 ± 2.8	13.4 ± 8.5
Morbidity (%)	24.5	13.3	41.4	42.5
Mortality (30 days, %)	4.4	8.9	0	3.3
Median follow-up (months)	26	26	25	44

R robotic, *O* open, *TG* total gastrectomy, *STG* subtotal gastrectomy, *OT* operative time

feasibility of robotic gastric cancer operations. Robotic gastrectomy with D2-lymphadenectomy demonstrated adequate lymph node harvest and optimal R0-resection rates with low postoperative morbidity and short hospital stays [13, 16, 28]. Several retrospective studies from Europe and Asia have compared the use of robotic gastrectomy with laparoscopic or open approaches. Again, these studies concluded that D2 lymph node dissection is technically feasible [31] and had the benefit of less operative blood loss and shorter postoperative hospital stay than laparoscopic and open gastrectomy groups [32]. Most common robotic disadvantages were found to be longer operative time, higher costs, loss of tactile sensation, and the lack of oncologic results and long-term outcomes.

Subsequently, two studies compared robotic gastrectomy and open gastrectomy for gastric cancer (Table 9.2). For the first time, Pernazza et al. compared survival between the two groups with a mean follow-up of 26 months and found no difference [33]. The second study conducted using a strictly matched-case-controlled method demonstrated no significant difference between the number of lymph nodes obtained during the laparoscopic and open procedures [31]. In addition, all resected margins in this study were free of tumor in the robotic group, whereas tumor involvement was present in the margin of two specimens in the open group. The conclusion of this trial is that robot-assisted gastric with D2 lymph node dissection is safe, technically feasible, and oncologically effective compared to open surgery.

Investigations comparing robotic gastrectomy versus laparoscopic gastrectomy (Table 9.3) and robotic gastrectomy versus laparoscopic gastrectomy versus open gastrectomy (Table 9.4) have resulted in several publications most of which were conducted in early gastric cancer with the exception of one study which included advanced gastric cancer patients.

All reports included patient characteristics, intraoperative factors, postoperative complications, and oncologic parameters. Kim et al. [25] was the first to compare robotic technique with both the open and laparoscopic ones in a small group of patients. According to the authors, robotic gastrectomy offers better short-term surgical outcomes than the open and laparoscopic methods in terms of blood loss and hospital stay. The largest of the studies involving 236 robotic gastrectomies and 591 laparoscopic gastrectomies, while not randomized, supported outcomes of several of the smaller studies, which found less blood loss and shorter hospital stay in the robotic gastrectomy group. Moreover, a study by Woo et al. demonstrated that robotic approach permits the experienced surgeon to follow oncologic parameters [36]. All resection margins in the robotic gastrectomy group were negative for cancer involvement and the number of lymph nodes retrieved per extent of robotic dissection was sufficient and did not differ from the laparoscopic gastrectomy group. While these studies show promising results for robotic gastric cancer operations, the studies reveal a much longer operative time using the robotic approach and still long-term oncologic outcomes results.

Table 9.3 NRCT Robotic versus laparoscopic gastrectomy for gastric cancer [34]

Author/year	Type of approach	No of patients	Type of surgery (STG/TG/)	D2 LN dissection (/)	No. of resected LN	OT (min)	Blood loss (ml)	Hospital stay (days)	Morbidity %
Pugliese et al. [34]	R	18	18	18	25 ± 4.5 (18–40)	344 ± 62 (240–460)	90 ± 48 (50–200)	10 ± 3 (10–13)	6
	L	52	0/52	52	31 ± 8 (20–45)	235 ± 23 (145–360)	148 ± 53 (45–250)	10 ± 2.6 (7–24)	12.5
Eom et al. [35]	R	30	0/30	20	30.2 (13–60)	229.1 (165–307)	152.8 (10–500)	7.9 (7–20)	13
	L	62	0/62	34	33.4 (10–67)	189.4 (125–272)	88.3 (10–400)	7.8 (5–17)	6
Woo et al. [36]	R	236	62/172	105	39.0	219.5	91.6	7.7	11
	L	591	108/481	279	37.4	170.7	147.9	7.0	13.7
Yoon et al. [30]	R	36	36/0	–	42.8 ± 12.7	305.8 ± 115.8	–	8.8 ± 3.3	16.7
	L	65	65/0	–	39.4 ± 13.4	210.2 ± 57.7	–	10.3 ± 10.8	15.4

R robotic, *L* laparoscopic, *TG* total gastrectomy, *STG* subtotal gastrectomy, *OT* operative time

Table 9.4 NRCT robotic versus laparoscopic versus open gastrectomy for gastric cancer

Author/year	Kim et al. [25]			Huang et al. [35]		
Approach (R/O)	R	L	O	R	L	O
No. of patients	16	11	12	39	64	586
Resection type (STG/TG)	16/0	11/0	12/0	32/7	34/5	407/179
Extent of LND (D1 + α or β/D2)	2/14	3/8	0/12	5/34		120
OT (min)	259	204	127	430	350	320
No. LN examined	41.1 ± 10.9	37.4 ± 10.0	43.3 ± 10.4	32.0 + 13.7	26.0 + 12.4	34.0 + 14.8
EBL (ml)	30	45	45	50	100	400
LOS (days)	5	7	7	7	11	12
Morbidity (%)	0	9	16	15	16	15

R robotic, *L* laparoscopic, *O* open, *TG* total gastrectomy, *STG* subtotal gastrectomy, *OT* operative time

Future Aspects

Operative Time and Costs

A major concern regarding robotic gastric cancer surgery as with other operations is the significantly longer operating time and higher costs associated with robotic surgery when compared to the open and laparoscopic approaches. As studies have demonstrated, it is expected that once the surgeon and the robotic surgical team overcome the initial learning curve the operation time will be improved.

The cost remains a major issue. A detailed analysis of the actual overall cost of undergoing a robotic gastrectomy is still lacking and maybe difficult to determine, especially since healthcare prices vary to widely among the many countries where robotic gastric cancer operations are currently being performed. Currently, prospective multicenter studies comparing the cost-effectiveness of open versus laparoscopic gastrectomy [3] and robotic versus laparoscopic gastrectomy for gastric cancer are planned as secondary outcomes of more comprehensive study designs (ClinicalTrials.gov. Identifier NCT01309256).

Oncologic Outcomes

Multicenter, randomized, controlled trials are undoubtedly needed to establish the oncologic adequacy of most new drugs. However, it is unlikely that such a trial comparing robotic versus laparoscopic surgery for gastric cancer will be necessary. As robotic surgical systems are advancements in technology, an improved tool to perform more precise and accurate laparoscopic surgery, surgeons and patients may not wait for the results of such potential studies.

Moreover, it is expected that the rapid development of surgical technology will provide more useful diagnostic and therapeutic tools to benefit both the patients as well as the surgeons in the near future. In the meantime, the surgeons are pushing the frontier of robotic surgical systems application and in the treatment of gastric cancer it will be in its role in the treatment of advanced gastric cancers. In the near future, new approaches to gastric cancer management will provide novel opportunities of treatment, including improved chemotherapeutic agents, more effective combinations, immunochemotherapy, and molecular-targeted therapies. In this context, minimally invasive surgery could play a key role in improving postoperative course and accelerating times to adjuvant treatments [15], and especially robotic surgery might be a correct alternative to laparoscopic approach or the first choice for selected cases.

Conclusions

Robotic surgery for gastric cancer is a safe and feasible operation. The short-term benefits of robotic gastrectomy parallel that of laparoscopy. Surgical oncologists who treat gastric cancer patients can readily adhere to the oncologic principles of gastric cancer treatment including no touch technique, negative margins, and adequate LN dissection. The adoption of robotic surgery for the treatment of gastric cancer patients may improve the quality of surgery for the patient and offer a shorter learning curve for the surgeon.

References

1. Kitano S, Shiraishi N, Uyama I, Sugihara K, Tanigawa N, Japanese Laparoscopic Surgery Study Group. A multicenter study on oncologic outcome of laparoscopic gastrectomy for early cancer in Japan. Ann Surg. 2007;245(1):68–72.
2. Huscher CG, Mingoli A, Sgarzini G, Sansonetti A, Di Paola M, Recher A, et al. Laparoscopic versus open subtotal gastrectomy for distal gastric cancer: five-year results of a randomized prospective trial. Ann Surg. 2005;241(2):232–7.
3. Kim HH, Hyung WJ, Cho GS, Kim MC, Han SU, Kim W, et al. Morbidity and mortality of laparoscopic gastrectomy versus open gastrectomy for gastric cancer: an interim report–a phase III multicenter, prospective, randomized Trial (KLASS Trial). Ann Surg. 2010;251(3):417–20.
4. Giulianotti PC, Coratti A, Angelini M, Sbrana F, Cecconi S, Balestracci T, et al. Robotics in general surgery: personal experience in a large community hospital. Arch Surg. 2003;138:777–84.
5. Hyung WJ. Robotic surgery in gastrointestinal surgery. Korean J Gastroenterol. 2007;50:256–9.
6. Baek SJ, Lee DW, Park SS, Kim SH. Current status of robot-assisted gastric surgery. World J Gastrointest Oncol. 2011;3(10):137–43.
7. Buchs NC, Bucher P, Pugin F, Morel P. Robot-assisted gastrectomy for cancer. Minerva Gastroenterol Dietol. 2011;57(1):33–42.
8. Hashizume M, Sugimachi K. Robot-assisted gastric surgery. Surg Clin North Am. 2003;83:1429–44.
9. Song J, Oh SJ, Kang WH, Hyung WJ, Choi SH, Noh SH. Robot-assisted gastrectomy with lymph node dissection for gastric cancer: lessons learned from an initial 100 consecutive procedures. Ann Surg. 2009;249:927–32.
10. Hyung WJ, Woo Y, Noh SH. Robotic surgery for gastric cancer: a technical review. J Robot Surg. 2011;5(4):241–9.
11. Japanese Gastric Cancer Association. Japanese classification of gastric carcinoma: 3rd English edition. Gastric Cancer. 2011;14:101–12.
12. Japanese Gastric Cancer Association. Japanese gastric cancer treatment guidelines (ver. 3). Gastric Cancer. 2011;14:113–23.
13. D'Annibale A, Pende V, Pernazza G, Monsellato I, Mazzocchi P, Lucandri G, et al. Full robotic gastrectomy with extended (D2) lymphadenectomy for gastric cancer: surgical technique and preliminary results. J Surg Res. 2011;166(2):e113–20.
14. Song J, Kang WH, Oh SJ, Hyung WJ, Choi SH, Noh SH. Role of robotic gastrectomy using Da Vinci system compared with laparoscopic gastrectomy: initial experience of 20 consecutive cases. Surg Endosc. 2009;23:1204–11.
15. Patriti A, Ceccarelli G, Bellochi R, Bartoli A, Spaziani A, Di Zitti L, et al. Robot-assisted laparoscopic total and partial gastric resection with D2 lymph node dissection for adenocarcinoma. Surg Endosc. 2008;22:2753–60.
16. Anderson C, Ellenhorn J, Hellan M, Pigazzi A. Pilot series of robot-assisted laparoscopic subtotal gastrectomy with extended lymphadenectomy for gastric cancer. Surg Endosc. 2007;21:1662–6.
17. Isogaki J, Haruta S, Man-I M, Suda K, Kawamura Y, Yoshimura F, et al. Robot-assisted surgery for gastric cancer: experience at our institute. Pathobiology. 2001;78(6):328–33.
18. Hyung WJ, Song C, Cheong JH, Choi SH, Noh SH. Percutaneous needle decompression during laparoscopic gastric surgery: a simple alternative to nasogastric decompression. Yonsei Med J. 2005;46(5):648–51.
19. Woo Y, Hyung WJ, Kim HI, Obama K, Son T, Noh SH. Minimizing hepatic trauma with a novel liver retraction method: a simple liver suspension using gauze suture. Surg Endosc. 2011;25(12):3939–45.
20. Shinohara T, Kanaya S, Yoshimura F, Hiramatsu Y, Haruta S, Kawamura Y, et al. A protective technique for retraction of the liver during laparoscopic gastrectomy for gastric adenocarcinoma: using a Penrose drain. J Gastrointest Surg. 2001;15(6):1043–8.
21. Shabbir A, Lee JH, Lee MS, Park do J, Kim HH. Combined suture retraction of the falciform ligament and the left lobe of the liver during laparoscopic total gastrectomy. Surg Endosc. 2010;24:3237–40.
22. Hyung WJ, Lim JS, Cheong JH, Kim J, Choi SH, Song SY, et al. Intraoperative tumor localization using laparoscopic ultrasonography in laparoscopic–assisted gastrectomy. Surg Endosc. 2005;19(10):1353–7.
23. Kim HI, Hyung WJ, Lee CR, Lim JS, An JY, Cheong JH, et al. Intraoperative portable abdominal radiograph for tumor localization: a simple and accurate method for laparoscopic gastrectomy. Surg Endosc. 2011;25(3):958–63.
24. Hur H, Kim JY, Cho YK, Han SU. Technical feasibility of robot-sewn anastomosis in robotic surgery for gastric cancer. J Laparoendosc Adv Surg Tech A. 2010;20:693–7.
25. Kim MC, Heo GU, Jung GJ. Robotic gastrectomy for gastric cancer: surgical techniques and clinical merits. Surg Endosc. 2010;24:610–5.
26. Uyama I, Kanaya S, Ishida Y, Inaba K, Suda K, Satoh S. Novel integrated robotic approach for suprapancreatic D2 nodal dissection for treating gastric cancer: technique and initial experience. World J Surg. 2012;36(2):331–7.

27. Liu FL, Lv CT, Qin J, Shen KT, Chen WD, Shen ZB, et al. Da Vinci robot-assisted gastrectomy with lymph node dissection for gastric cancer: a case series of 9 patients. Zhonghua Wei Chang Wai Ke Za Zhi. 2010;13(5):327–9.
28. Lee HH, Hur H, Jung H, Jeon HM, Park CH, Song KY. Robot-assisted distal gastrectomy for gastric cancer: initial experience. Am J Surg. 2011;201(6):841–5.
29. Yu PW, Tang B, Zeng DZ, Zhao YL, Shi Y, Hao YX, et al. Robotic-assisted radical gastrectomy using Da Vinci robotic system: a report of 41 cases. Zhonghua Wei Chang Wai Ke Za Zhi. 2012;15(2):121–4.
30. Yoon HM, Kim YW, Lee JH, Ryu KW, Eom BW, Park JY, et al. Robot-assisted total gastrectomy is comparable with laparoscopically assisted total gastrectomy for early gastric cancer. Surg Endosc. 2012;26:1377–81.
31. Caruso S, Patriti A, Marrelli D, Ceccarelli G, Ceribelli C, Roviello F, et al. Open vs. robot-assisted laparoscopic gastric resection with D2 lymph node dissection for adenocarcinoma: a case–control study. Int J Med Robot. 2011;7(4):452–8.
32. Glantzounis G, Ziogas D, Baltogiannis G. Open versus laparoscopic versus robotic gastrectomy for cancer: need for comparative-effectiveness quality. Surg Endosc. 2010;24:1510–2.
33. Pernazza G, Gentile E, Felicioni L, Tumbiolo S, Giulianotti PC. Improved early survival after robotic gastrectomy in advanced gastric cancer. Surg Laparosc Endosc Percutan Tech. 2006;16(8):286.
34. Pugliese R, Maggioni D, Sansonna F, Costanzi A, Ferrari GC, Di Lernia S, et al. Subtotal gastrectomy with D2 dissection by minimally invasive surgery for distal adenocarcinoma of the stomach: results and 5-year survival. Surg Endosc. 2010;24:2594–602.
35. Huang KH, Lan YT, Fang WL, Chen JH, Lo SS, Hsieh MC, et al. Initial experience of robotic gastrectomy and comparison with open and laparoscopic gastrectomy for gastric cancer. J Gastrointest Surg. 2012;16(7):1303–10.
36. Woo Y, Hyung WJ, Pak KH, Inaba K, Obama K, Choi SH, et al. Robotic gastrectomy as an oncologically sound alternative to laparoscopic resections for the treatment of early-stage gastric cancers. Arch Surg. 2011;146:1086–92.

Suggested Reading

Eom BW, Yoon HM, Ryu KW, Lee JH, Cho SJ, Lee JY, et al. Comparison of surgical performance and short-term clinical outcomes between laparoscopic and robotic surgery in distal gastric cancer. Eur J Surg Oncol. 2012;38(1):57–63.

Heemskerk J, Van Gemert WG, De Vries J, Greve J, Bouvy ND. Learning curves of robot-assisted laparoscopic surgery compared with conventional laparoscopic surgery: an experimental study evaluating skill acquisition of robot-assisted laparoscopic tasks compared with conventional laparoscopic tasks in inexperienced users. Surg Laparosc Endosc Percutan Tech. 2007;17:171–4.

Jayaraman S, Quan D, Al-Ghamdi I, El-Deen F, Schlachta CM. Does robotic assistance improve efficiency in performing complex minimally invasive surgical procedures? Surg Endosc. 2010;24(3):584–8.

Pugliese R, Maggioni D, Sansonna F, Ferrari GC, Forgione A, Costanzi A, et al. Outcomes and survival after laparoscopic gastrectomy for adenocarcinoma. Analysis on 65 patients operated on by conventional or robot-assisted minimal access procedures. Eur J Surg Oncol. 2009;35:281–8.

Part V

Surgical Techniques: *Bariatric*

Robotic Roux-en-Y Gastric Bypass

10

Erik B. Wilson, Hossein Bagshahi, and Vicky D. Woodruff

Overview

The gastric bypass procedure was initially developed in the 1960s by Drs. Mason and Ito [1] and based on the weight loss observed after ulcer treatment in which patients had part of the stomach removed. Over the ensuing decades the procedure has been modified into the current form using a Roux-en-Y limb of intestine to produce the Roux-en-Y gastric bypass (RYGBP), sometimes referred to as proximal gastric bypass. The Roux-en-Y connects a limb of the intestine to a much smaller stomach pouch which prevents the bile from entering the upper part of the stomach and esophagus, thereby effectively bypassing the remaining stomach and first segment of the small intestine. In 1994 Drs. Wittgrove and Clark performed the first laparoscopic Roux-en-Y which enabled precise manipulation of tissue and enhanced the visual field [2]. Unfortunately, it also introduced significant postural stresses on the surgeon due to the body habitus of the patient. The advent of robotic-assisted Roux-en-Y gastric bypass in 2001 eliminated the stresses on the surgeon and introduced several additional enhancements [3]. Minimally invasive surgeons who adopted robotic digital platforms early on have developed refinement of techniques and protocols that lead to safe and effective applications for Roux-en-Y gastric bypass with very low reported morbidity and mortality [4].

This chapter provides a procedure overview and explores our experience with (1) patient positioning, (2) trocar placement, (3) a step-by-step account of the full robotic-assisted procedure, and (4) advantages and limitations of robotic-assisted RYGBP.

Procedure Overview

Roux-en-Y gastric bypass for morbid obesity is ranked in the top three most challenging advanced minimally invasive procedures in modern general surgery [4]. As such, technique variations have developed and a robust discussion has revolved around creating the gastric pouch, gastrojejunal anastomosis, and jejunojejunal anastomosis. This chapter discusses a full robotic-assisted approach

E.B. Wilson, M.D. (✉)
Department of Surgery, University of Texas Health Science Center/Memorial Hermann Hospital, 6431 Fannin Street, MSB4.162, Houston, TX 77030, USA
e-mail: erik.b.wilson@uth.tmc.edu

H. Bagshahi, M.D.
Department of Surgery, Harris Methodist Hospital, 800 Fifth Avenue, Suite 404, Fort Worth, TX 76104, USA

Reshape Bariatric and General Surgery of Fort Worth, 800 Fifth Avenue, Suite 404, Fort Worth, TX 76104, USA
e-mail: hbagshahi@gmail.com

V.D. Woodruff, Ph.D.
Department of Surgery, University of Texas Health Science Center, 6431 Fannin Street, Suite 4.294, Houston, TX 77030, USA
e-mail: vicky.woodruff@uth.tmc.edu

K.C. Kim (ed.), *Robotics in General Surgery*, DOI 10.1007/978-1-4614-8739-5_10,

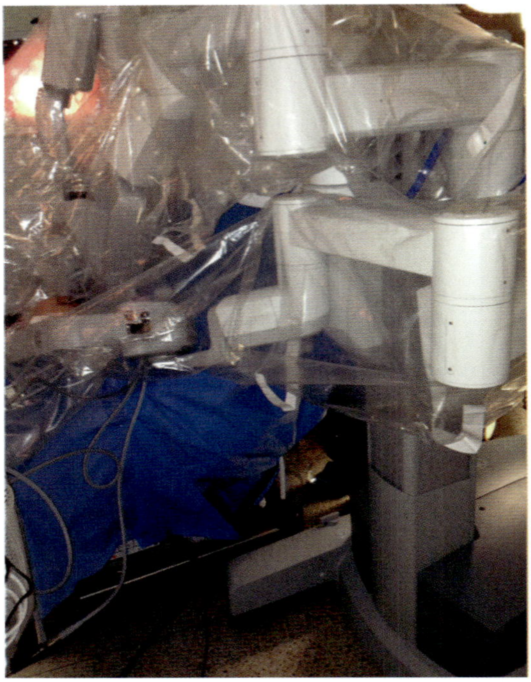

Fig. 10.1 Parallel docking view showing foot of patient

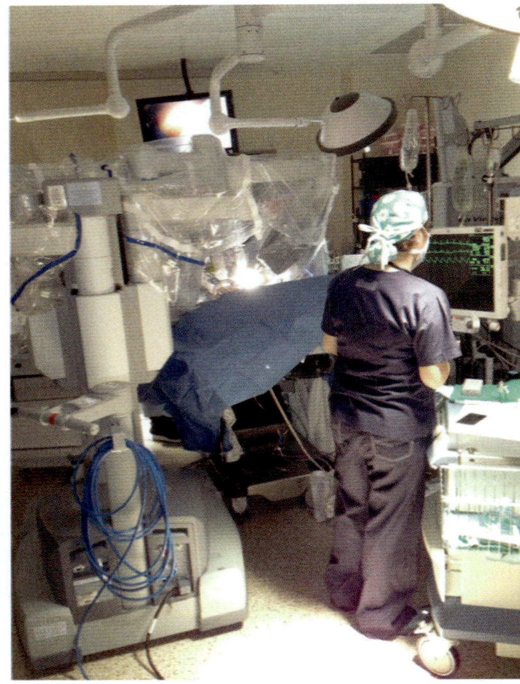

Fig. 10.2 Parallel docking view showing position of anesthesiologist with head of patient accessible

to dissect and create the gastric pouch, to create a two-layered hand-sewn gastrojejunal anastomosis, and to perform a jejunojejunal anastomosis with a 60 mm linear stapler. Robotic assistance then hand-sews the common enterotomy defect and closure of the mesenteric defects. The details of the procedure are explored in this chapter.

Patient Positioning

Early in our experience we adopted a modification to the traditional cart position (over the patient's head with both arms extended outward). The "parallel-docking" (Figs. 10.1 and 10.2) position with the patient's right arm extended allows better access for anesthesia while leaving the head access open for intraoperative endoscopy and a leak test, performed at the end of the procedure. Prior to docking the robotic arms, a footboard is positioned and 20° reverse Trendelenburg is used. Finally, a gastric lavage tube is placed preoperatively to facilitate pouch creation and to stent the gastrojejunal anastomosis while sewing.

Trocar Placement

A total of five or six trocar ports are placed for robotic-assisted RYGBP. The order of placement is shown in Figs. 10.3 and 10.4 and is as follows (1) a peritoneal entry with a zero degree scope on a 5 mm optical viewing in the right upper quadrant just to the right of the midclavicular line, one finger width below the costal margin—this port is subsequently changed to the robotic "number two arm" after all other ports have been placed, (2) a 12 mm umbilical port for the robotic camera, (3) a 5 mm left upper quadrant port placed at the level of the umbilicus at the anterior axillary line with the "number three robotic arm" docked, (4) the area between the umbilical port and left anterior axillary line port is bisected and an 8 mm robotic port is placed with the "number one robotic arm" docked, (5) a 12 mm right mid-abdominal assistant port is placed halfway between the umbilical port and the RUQ port, and (6) if the liver is small, we prefer to use a 3 mm retractor or an internal liver retractor fashioned out of a Penrose drain and sutures (Fig. 10.5), reducing the need for an epigastric incision. A sixth port is created if the liver is large, in which case an epigastric incision is made to facilitate a Nathanson liver retractor (Fig. 10.5) in order to elevate the left lateral lobe. When completed, the patient cart is ready to be docked. This trocar placement allows for the Roux-en-Y gastric bypass procedure to be accomplished without the reported challenge of moving the robot from one quadrant to another. Both upper and lower quadrants are easily visible and manageable for work without re-placing trocars and extending surgical and anesthesia time.

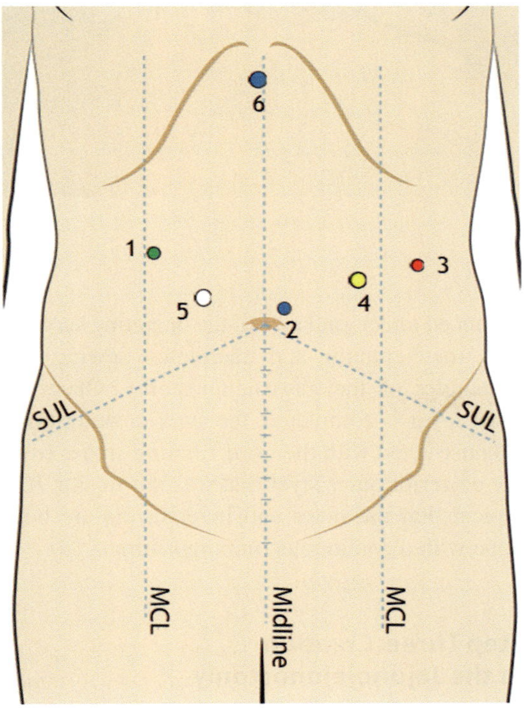

Fig. 10.3 Diagram of port placement

Three-Step Procedure

Step 1: Creation of the Gastric Pouch

The angle of His is identified with the fundus retracted laterally. The peritoneum, over the angle of His, is dissected with ultrasonic shears or scissors and carried posterior to identify the path for a linear stapler and the left crus of the diaphragm. Next, the pars flaccida is identified and opened. At this point it is important to identify the left gastric artery and its branches onto the lesser curve for preservation, as this will be the main blood supply to the gastric pouch and the gastrojejunal anastomosis. The mesentery to the lesser curve of the stomach is divided by a vascular load linear stapler. A retrogastric plane in the lesser curve is then created and the dissection is carried up to the angle of His. Once accomplished, two serial applications of a 60 mm linear stapler are used to create a 20 mL gastric pouch.

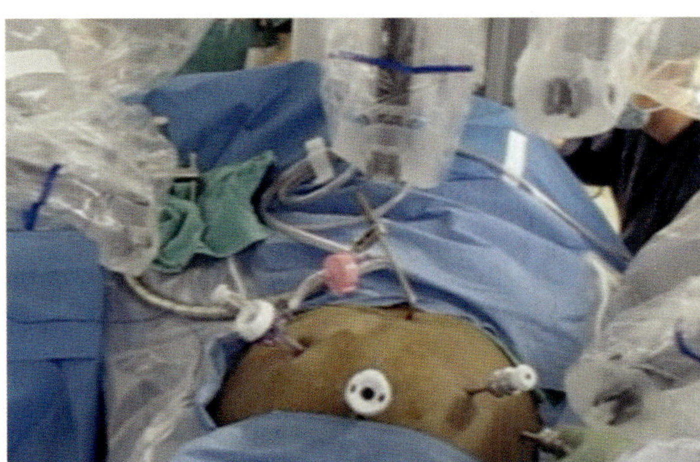

Fig. 10.4 Nathanson liver retractor

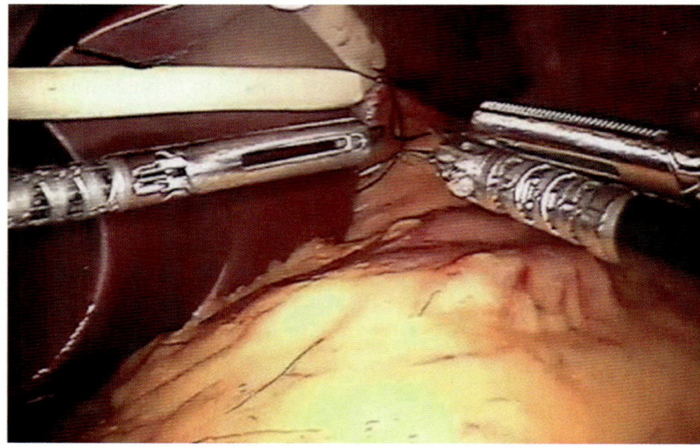

Fig. 10.5 Internal liver retractor

Step 2: Creation of the Gastrojejunal Anastomosis

The greater omentum is divided with an ultrasonic scalpel, to the level of the transverse colon. The proximal jejunum is identified at the ligament of Treitz and extended into the upper abdomen. It is critical to ensure that an adequate length of jejunum is measured to avoid tension on the anastomosis (approximately 50–70 cm is suggested). It is equally important to properly orient the jejunum so that proximal and distal ends are not misidentified during the creation of the gastrojejunal anastomosis.

Once the area to be anastomosed has been identified, the number three robotic arm is used to maintain and properly orient the jejunum in the upper abdomen. The outer posterior layer of the anastomosis is created first using a long 2-0 Vicryl suture. After the posterior outer layer is completed, the suture and needle are left in situ and attention is focused on constructing the inner layer of the gastrojejunal anastomosis. Using the number two robotic arm, the gastrotomy and enterotomy are performed with 8 mm robotic scissors while monopolar cautery is activated. The inner layer of the anastomosis is also performed with a running 2-0 Vicryl suture. Once the bowel has been opened, the posterior inner row is created. After this step has been performed, the gastric tube placed preoperatively is advanced under guidance of the operating surgeon into the jejunum and facilitates sewing the remainder of the gastrojejunostomy. Once the inner layer is completed, the anterior outer layer is constructed with the same running suture from the posterior outer layer that was left in situ. It is typical that the outer and inner layers are both done with a continuous running suture.

Step Three: Creation of the Jejunojejunostomy

We prefer to create an approximate 150 cm Roux limb. The Roux limb is measured out and draped into the RUQ. The number three robotic arm is utilized to place a stay suture at the estimated distal staple line and line up the bowel with the direction of the linear stapler. A harmonic scalpel is then used to make the enterotomies, followed by a 60 mm linear stapler to create the anastomosis. The common enterotomy that remains is closed with a single running layer of 2-0 Vicryl.

After the creation of the jejunojejunostomy, a silk suture is used to close the mesenteric defect between the Roux limb and the biliary limb of the small bowel. At this point, an intraoperative endoscopy is performed to evaluate a gastrojejunostomy. This ensures passage of the gastroscope into the Roux limb and ensures passage is airtight. The robot is then undocked.

Advantages to Robotic-Assisted Roux-en-Y Gastric Bypass (RARYGB)

A comparison of complication rates against standard laparoscopic techniques shows lower morbidity and mortality rates for robotic procedures [5]. A study by Yu et al. reviewed the first 100 robotic gastric bypasses during surgeons' learning curves and found no anastomotic leaks and no mortality [6]. Standard laparoscopic gastrointestinal leak rates are commonly reported up to 6.3 % and mortality up to 2 % [7, 8]. A series of studies between 2002 and 2008 presented data on operative times and complications after robotically assisted Roux-en-Y gastric bypass [3, 6, 8–11]. A total of 603 patients received either totally robotic (129 patients) or a hybrid robotic procedure (474 patients). An average operative time of 201 min was long; however, the leak rate was significantly low at 0.3 % (2 fistulas or leaks). This was remarkable since the current-day literature reported fistula and leak rates at 6.7 % [8]. The safety of the robotic operation was supported with a 0 % 30 day mortality. At the time, the hybrid procedure, consisting of robotic gastrojejunostomy and laparoscopy for the remainder of the case, was more popular. However, Wilson reported, "Since 2008, the totally robotic approach has become more common with improved instruments and techniques where the robot is docked at the beginning of the case and the console surgeon performs the entire procedure with the help of a bedside assistant to deploy any staplers needed for creations of the gastric pouch and intestinal reconstruction (described earlier)" [4]. Additionally, the advent of the FDA's approval of the robotic stapler has created the potential for a completely robotic one-surgeon operation, reducing the need for skilled bedside assistance.

Reduced operative times are another advantage, once the learning curve is overcome. Sanchez et al. recounted a randomized trial of RARYGB versus LRYGB with significantly shorter operative times for the robotic approach. The RARYGB took 130.8 min versus 149.4 min for the LRYGB ($p=0.02$). The largest difference was in patients with a BMI >43 kg/m^2, for whom the difference in procedure time was 29.6 min faster for RARYGB ($p=0.009$) [12].

Snyder et al. reported a nonrandomized cohort study of 356 LRYGB cases against 249 RARYGB which directly compared laparoscopic hand-sewn versus robotic hand-sewn gastrojejunostomies. Demographics showed no difference between the two patient populations, mortality was nonexistent in both groups, and major complication rates were similar between the two groups. Conversely, the gastrointestinal leak rate was 1.7 % for LRYGB and 0 % for RARYGB, which was significantly lower in the robotic group ($p=0.04$), emphasizing a clinical benefit from the precision of robotics [6].

The advantages that directly benefit the surgeon include a relief from painful ergonomic positioning and postures that affect the neck, shoulders, and back. The superior upper abdominal visualization allows for robotic preciseness and eliminates shying away from the challenges that come from patients with prior surgery in the abdominal area. In the morbidly obese patient, the surgeon enjoys a notable advantage from robotics regarding improved mechanical efficiency against large thick abdominal walls and large livers, due to fatty infiltration. In these cases, robotics allows for more precise reconstruction of the anatomy and effectively working in small spaces where laparoscopy struggles.

Limitations to Robotic Roux-en-Y Gastric Bypass

Literature repeats limitations associated with the steep learning curve for manipulating the robot between 12 and 15 cases to normalize outcomes, extended time to dock the robot, difficulty moving between quadrants, and lack of tactile sense [6, 11]. Certainly, learning new technology and skills can take time; however, surveys of robotic general surgeons show the learning curve is related primarily to the setup and docking of the system and this improves with training. Performing Roux-en-Y gastric bypass at a console requires the surgeon to follow the same principles and knowledge based on open and laparoscopic surgery.

It is the suggestion of our practice that surgeons new to robotics first pay close attention to proper patient selection, initially screening out patients with BMIs ≥40 until a proficient skill level is achieved. Additionally, we suggest a hybrid approach to perform different steps of a gastric bypass until adequate skills are developed to perform the bypass totally robotically [13–15]. The hybrid approach docks the robot for a smaller portion of the case and as more experience is added, the robot is utilized for a greater portion of the procedure until total robotic bypass is achieved. A parallel approach suggests that early on, many surgeons are best suited to dock only 3 arms of the system until the potential trocar and arm interference issues are understood and managed. The forth arm may be added after the procedure has been tried and analyzed. In the end, robotic surgeons need to evolve their procedures because a standard robotic approach does not usually exist [4].

While it is generally accepted that RARYGB has a reported learning curve phase, few studies have published length of operative times during this ramp-up period. To provide to address this oversight, we first reviewed our initial learning curve cases to find operative times ranged from 148 to 437 min, with a mean of 254 min [16]. These times reflect a hybrid laparoscopic and robotic approach due to early learning and account for the extended times. There were no leaks or deaths. Four patients had one complication each, comprised of reoperation, incisional hernia, pulmonary embolus, and recurrent umbilical hernia. We contend these results demonstrate the feasibility and safety during the learning curve phase of RARYGB. With 800 additional cases performed, our mean operating time is 90 min and continuing to move downward.

A common argument, however, is that cases are not reproducible to other surgeons and practices. Tieu et al. looked at outcomes from 1,100 consecutive RARYGB cases at 2 high-volume centers that routinely perform RARYGB located in the Houston Texas Medical Center and a private practice in Maine [17]. The mean operative time was 155 min. There were no conversions. The mean body mass index was 39.8 kg/m^2 at 3 months postoperatively (70 % follow-up). Complications were few and included 1 case of gastrojejunal anastomotic leak (0.09 %) and 4 strictures (0.36 %). The mortality rate was zero. More recently, we reported outcomes of 1,695 cases of RARYGB from 3 high-volume centers in Texas, Maine, and Florida. Mortality for the series was zero at 30 days with 2 leaks (0.12 %) and 3 abscesses (0.18 %) [13, 17]. If leaks and abscesses were combined (5 total), the 0.29 % remains an exceptionally low infection rate after gastric bypass, which is favorable against any leak rates reported in the literature. Stricture requiring dilation was also low at 0.29 %. These data support the RARYGB is translatable and reproducible in other practices and hospitals with continued outstanding results.

Lastly, a common perception is that because the surgeon cannot tactically feel the tissue directly, or indirectly as with laparoscopic instruments, the robot is dangerous. Actually, there are some crude haptics that occur if the instruments bump or hit each other, transmitting a tactile sensation back to the surgeon's console. Otherwise, the concern is valid to the point that the surgeon must maintain visual contact through the monitor to guide the instrumentation and ensure appropriate and safe manipulation is preserved. Even so, it has been our experience that as time working with the robot is logged, the visual cues become so strong a faux tactile sensation can be realized. Until then, the trade-off is better control over the surgical instruments and a better view of the surgical site.

Conclusion

The future is fast approaching with the advent of single incision or natural orifice approaches as well as new integrated fluorescence imaging capability that provides real-time, image-guided identification of key anatomical landmarks using near-infrared technology. Interactive digital platforms between the robot, digital medical records, and digital imaging are already being designed.

This capability may allow access to preoperative CAT scans or MRIs at the push of a button that will direct the surgeon away from potential danger or navigate through visceral fat, safely behind organs and anatomic structures to the point of interest. The bottom line is that robotic-assisted surgery extends the capabilities of minimally invasive surgeons with the added benefit of stable 3D visualization and increased dexterity. RARYGB is safe and effective and reduces the learning curve of gastric bypass. Although the operative time might be increased initially, the complication rates, most notably of anastomotic leak, are extremely low.

There remain concerns about costs, but as more industry investments continue and more competition develops in this area, robotics will become the primary mechanism for surgical interaction with a patient, because a digital platform will allow for infinite opportunities to make surgery safer, better, faster, and ultimately cheaper.

References

1. Mason EE, Ito C. Gastric bypass in obesity. Surg Clin North Am. 1967;47:1345–51.
2. Wittgrove AC, Clark GW, Tremblay LJ. Laparoscopic gastric bypass. Roux-en-Y: preliminary report of five cases. Obes Surg. 1994;4:353–7.
3. Hubens G, Balliu L, Ruppert M, Gypen B, Van Tu T, Vaneerdeweg W. Roux-en-Y gastric bypass procedure performed with the da Vinci robot system: is it worth it? Surg Endosc. 2008;22(7):1690–6.
4. Wilson EB. The evolution of robotic general surgery. Scand J Surg. 2009;98(2):125–9.
5. Wilson, EB, Snyder B, Yu S, et al. Robotic bariatric surgery outcomes with laparoscopic biliopancreatic diversion and gastric bypass. Presentation in American Society of Metabolic and Bariatric Surgery; 2008 June; Washington, DC.
6. Yu SC, Clapp BL, Lee MJ, et al. Robotic assistance provides excellent outcomes during the learning curve for laparoscopic Roux-en-Y bypass: result from 100 robotic assisted gastric bypasses. Am J Surg. 2006; 192(6):746–9.
7. Flum DR, Salem L, Elrod JA, et al. Early mortality among medicare beneficiaries undergoing bariatric surgical procedures. JAMA. 2005;294(15):1903–8.
8. Blachar A, Federle MP, Pealer KM, et al. Gastrointestinal complications of laparoscopic Roux-en-Y gastric bypass surgery. Radiology. 2002;223(3): 625–32.
9. Mohr CJ, Nadzam GS, Alami RS, Sanchez BR, Curet MJ. Totally robotic laparoscopic Roux-en-Y Gastric bypass: results from 75 patients. Obes Surg. 2006; 16(6):690–6.
10. Hagen ME, Inan I, Pugen F, Morel P. The da Vinci surgical system in digestive surgery. Rev Med Suisse. 2007;3(117):1622–6.
11. Buchs NC, Pugin F, Bucher P, Hagen ME, Chassot G, Koutny-Gong P, Morel P. Learning curve for robot-assisted Roux-en-Y gastric bypass. Surg Endosc. 2012;26(4):1116–21.
12. Parini U, Fabozzi M, Contul RB, Millo P, Loffredo A, Allieta R, Nardi Jr M, Lale-Murix E. Laparoscopic gastric bypass performed with the Da Vinci intuitive robotic system: preliminary experience. Surg Endosc. 2006;20(4):279–83.
13. Snyder BE, Wilson T, Scarborough T, et al. Lowering gastrointestinal leak rates: a comparative analysis of robotic and laparoscopic gastric bypass. J Robot Surg. 2008;2:159–63.
14. Sanchez BR, Mohr CJ, Morton JM, et al. Comparison of totally robotic laparoscopic Roux-en-Y bypass and traditional laparoscopic Roux-en-Y gastric bypass. Surg Obes Relat Dis. 2005;1(6):549–54.
15. Wilson E. Robotic gastric bypass. Presentation in American Society of Metabolic and Bariatric Surgery Annual Conference, Atlanta, GA; 2012 June.
16. Snyder B, Wilson T, Woodruff V, Wilson E. Robotically assisted revision of bariatric surgeries is safe and effective to achieve further weight loss. World J Surg; March 2013 [EPub Ahead of Print].
17. Tieu K, Allison N, Snyder B, Wilson T, Toder M, Wilson E. Robotic-assisted Roux-en-Y gastric bypass update from 2 high-volume centers. Surg Obes Relat Dis. 2012;9(2):284–8.

Robotic Sleeve Gastrectomy

11

Jorge Rabaza and Anthony M. Gonzalez

General Overview

The ever-increasing global epidemic of obesity is a cause for worldwide concern. It is estimated that if the trend continues, nearly half of all Americans will be obese by 2030 [1]. Comorbidities such as type II diabetes, hypertension, increased triglycerides and hypercholesterolemia, and sleep apnea contribute to obesity as one of the United States' leading causes of death [2]. The field of bariatric surgery has proven to be most effective and safe in the treatment of this disease.

The three most common procedures performed for weight loss in the United States and universally are the laparoscopic Roux-en-Y gastric bypass (LRYGB), the laparoscopic adjustable gastric band procedure (LAGB), and the sleeve gastrectomy (SG). The sleeve gastrectomy (SG) is a restrictive bariatric surgical procedure best described as a partial left gastrectomy of the fundus and body of the stomach so as to create a long tubular "sleeve" along the lesser curvature (Fig. 11.1). The weight loss and resolution of comorbidities are attributed not only to the restrictive nature of the procedure but also to restriction by the pylorus, decreased ghrelin, increased satiety, increased gastric emptying, and faster small bowel transit times with a component of malabsorption [3–6] (Table 11.1).

Historically, the SG evolved over time from other procedures. In 1988, Doug Hess performed the first sleeve gastrectomy as part the duodenal switch [7]. Anthone in 1997, while performing a duodenal switch in a young patient with common bile duct stones, limited the procedure to only a sleeve gastrectomy due to the complexity of the procedure. In this specific patient, he observed excellent weight loss results with the sleeve alone. Subsequently, between 1997 and 2001, he completed 21 sleeve gastrectomies with similar results [8]. Gagner [9] is credited with performing the first laparoscopic sleeve gastrectomy (LSG) in very high-BMI patients as a first stage with subsequent laparoscopic gastric bypass Roux-en-Y (LGBYP).

Recently, the American Society for Metabolic and Bariatric Surgery (ASMBS) updated their position statement on sleeve gastrectomy as a bariatric procedure [10]. Based on several prospective randomized controlled trials and matched cohort studies, the ASMBS recognizes the SG as an acceptable primary bariatric procedure and as a first stage for a Roux-en-Y gastric bypass (RYGB) or a duodenal switch (DS). Furthermore, the SG has been found to have a risk/benefit profile somewhere between that of the laparoscopic adjustable band (LAGB) and the RYGB [11–13]. The sleeve gastrectomy has several advantages

J. Rabaza, M.D. (✉)
South Miami Hospital, Baptist Health Medical Group, 7800 SW 87 Avenue, Suite B-210, Miami, FL 33173, USA
e-mail: jorgera@baptisthealth.net

A.M. Gonzalez, M.D.
Bariatric Surgery, Baptist Health Medical Group, 7800 SW 87 Avenue, Suite B-210, Miami, FL 33173, USA
e-mail: anthonygonzalezmd@me.com

K.C. Kim (ed.), *Robotics in General Surgery*, DOI 10.1007/978-1-4614-8739-5_11,

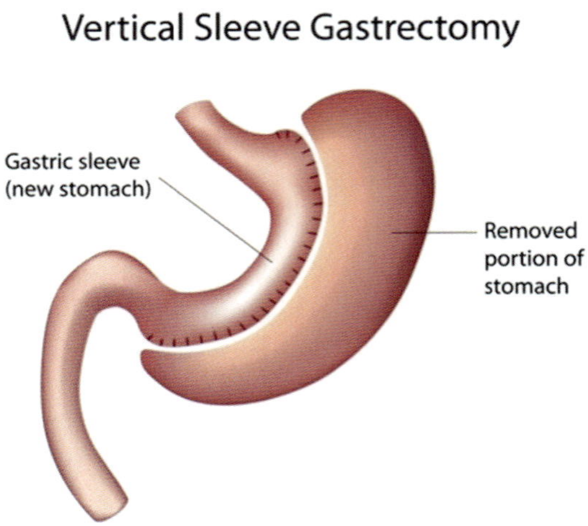

Fig. 11.1 Sleeve gastrectomy diagram

Table 11.1 Mechanism of the sleeve gastrectomy

• Decreased gastric volume
• Restriction by the pylorus
• Decreased ghrelin
• Increased gastric emptying
• Decreased small bowel transit time with malabsorption
• Increased glucagon-like peptide 1 and YY

Table 11.2 Considerations for the sleeve gastrectomy

Advantages	Limitations
• Relatively simple and quick procedure • Short learning curve • Access to stomach maintained • Good early results • Extremely low morbidity and mortality • Can use for failed LAGB • Can convert to RYGB for severe reflux • Can convert to duodenal switch (DS) or RYGB for insufficient weight loss	• No long-term results • Infrequent complications are difficult to treat • Irreversible • Early and late GERD

and few limitations (Table 11.2). Although long-term results are not available as they are for the LAGB and the RYGB, Sarela et al. [14] published very favorable results at 8–9 years with 69 % excess weight loss.

Although complications are rare, they can be very problematic to treat. Gastric leaks following a sleeve gastrectomy can be a very difficult and complex management problem. The average reported leak rate is approximately 2.7 % [15]. For revisional surgery, it can be greater than 10 % [16]. The most common area for leak occurrence is at the gastroesophageal junction. Leaks are caused by local tissue ischemia combined with increased intraluminal pressure of the sleeve. A tight sleeve is a risk factor for a leak, and it is thought that the size of the bougie used is inversely proportional to the rate of leakage [17]. Patients with a distal stricture or a functional obstruction caused by a spiraling staple line are also at a greater risk. Leaks can be repaired surgically, however, usually requiring a multidisciplinary approach, which includes percutaneous drainage, endoscopic stenting and clipping by the gastroenterologist, and maximization of nutrition to enhance healing.

Stricture or stenosis is most common at the incisura angularis. Proper creation of the sleeve with lateral traction and appropriate bougie size when stapling at incisura is key in preventing strictures. Treatment options for stricture can be endoscopic dilatation, seromyotomy, or conversion to a RYGB.

One of the most recent advances in the field of bariatric surgery has been the introduction of the da Vinci robotic platform (Intuitive Surgical, Sunnyvale, CA). Although the role of the robot in bariatric surgery has been found to be advantageous in the RYGB [18, 19], its role in the SG is less clear. Ayloo et al. [20] presented their initial experience with robotic-assisted sleeve gastrectomy (RASG), concluding the RASG can be performed safely with excellent outcomes. Diamantis et al. [21] reported their limited series also with similar results.

Our group originally adopted the use of the da Vinci system with the intent of reducing the high complication rates for revisional bariatric surgery in patients with previous RYGB or vertical banded gastroplasties (VBG). The Michigan Bariatric Surgery Collaborative, in a large multivariate analysis, found that the LSG had less risk for serious complications when compared with RYGB (OR 2.46 versus 3.58, respectively). Although the rate of staple-line dehiscence is low in laparoscopic sleeve gastrectomies, these complications are feared and extremely problematic. Having taken care of some of these troublesome complications, it was our thought that the current limitations of laparoscopic surgery (such as limited range of motion, poor ergonomics, lack of depth perception, and surgeon fatigue) could be risk factors for these rare but serious complications. Thus, we also adopted the da Vinci system for the sleeve gastrectomy.

Patient Positioning

The patient is placed in the supine position with the arms extended. The robot is docked straight over the head of the patient, and anesthesia is positioned on the patient's right side (Fig. 11.2). The bedside assistant stands on the patient's right side and the robotic monitor is placed across from the assistant on the patient's left. Because the anesthesia's positioning to the right of the patient, a peripheral IV should ideally be placed in the right upper extremity. After induction of anesthesia, a Foley catheter is placed, a footboard is properly secured, and straps are placed at the level of the upper thighs. An upper body-warming blanket is placed. The abdomen is then prepped from the nipple line to the suprapubic area. An orogastric tube is then placed to decompress the stomach. Lastly, the patient is draped without the traditional anesthetic barrier in order to allow the robot to be docked over the head. It is important always to ensure that the anesthesiologist has instant and unobstructed access to the head of the patient. Prior to docking the robot, the patient is placed in the reverse Trendelenburg position at approximately 15–20°.

Trocar Placement

A three-arm technique plus an assistant trocar is utilized. The camera trocar, which is a 12 mm long trocar, is positioned above the umbilicus via a transverse or vertical incision. The two robotic working arms, which can be 5 or 8 mm robotic trocars, are positioned at the anterior axillary line on both sides and just above the level of the camera port (Figs. 11.3 and 11.4). A 12 mm nonrobotic port is then placed approximately halfway between a line from the umbilical port to the right robotic port and slightly inferior. The liver is retracted with a Nathanson Hook Liver

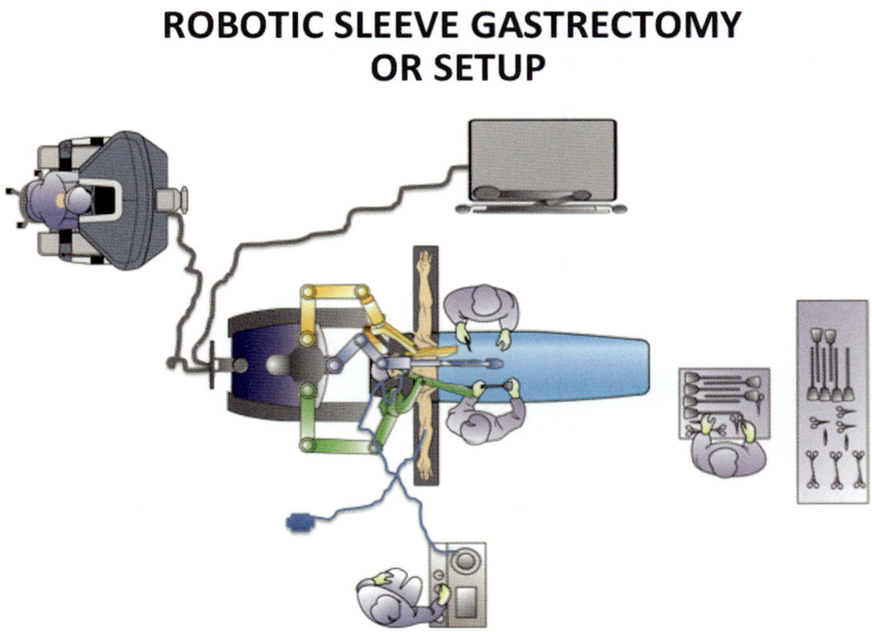

Fig. 11.2 Operating room layout

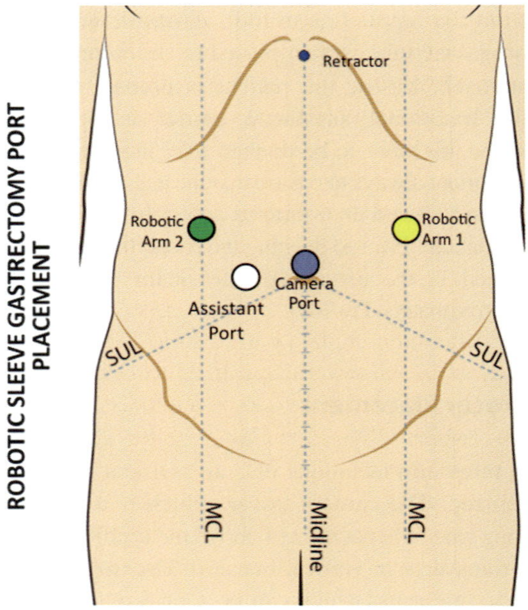

Fig. 11.3 Robotic sleeve gastrectomy port placement

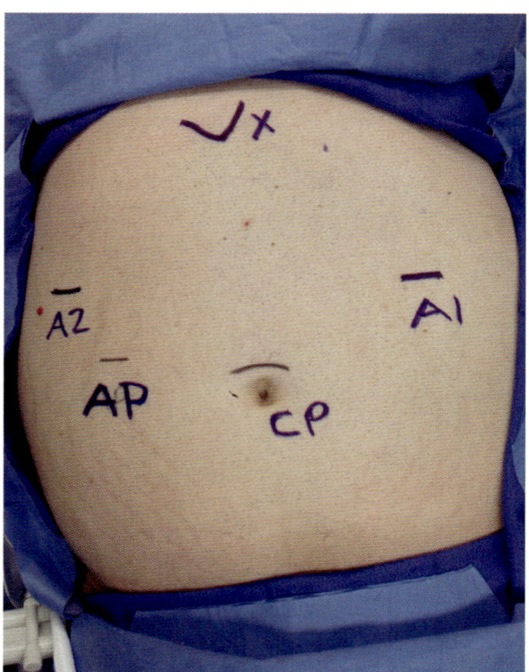

Fig. 11.4 Robotic sleeve gastrectomy port placement

Retractor (Mediflex Surgical Products), which is placed just below the xiphoid and held in place with a retractor that is mounted to the bed over

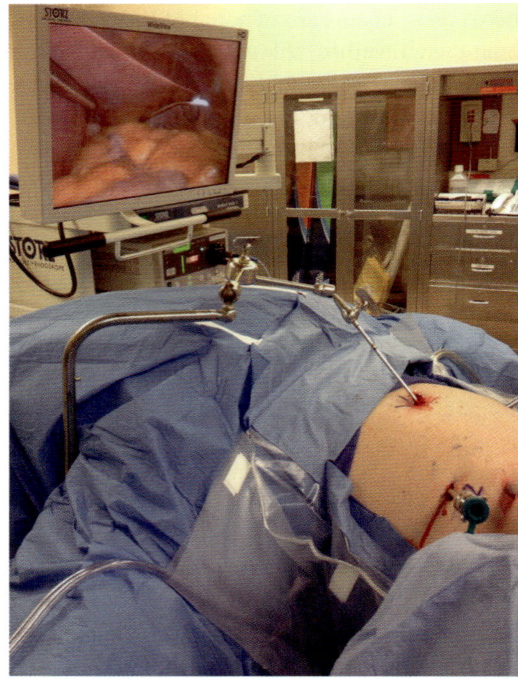

Fig. 11.5 Nathanson retractor position

the patient's right shoulder (Fig. 11.5). Finally the robot is docked directly above the patient's head (Fig. 11.6).

Step-by-Step Review of the Critical Elements of the Robotic Sleeve Gastrectomy

The first step of the robotic sleeve gastrectomy (RSG) is identification of the pylorus (Fig. 11.7). Approximately 4–6 cm proximal to the pylorus, the vascular attachment of the gastrocolic ligament is divided with the use of an energy source such as the Harmonic scalpel or the EndoWrist vessel sealer. This is typically started a little distal to the midpoint of the greater curvature where it is easier to enter the lesser sac than it is closer to the pylorus.

Once the target area to begin the dissection is decided, the console surgeon grasps the stomach with a double fenestrated bowel grasper and gently elevates it while the assistant provides countertraction of the gastrocolic ligament. We typically use the harmonic scalpel as the energy source (Fig. 11.8). It is important to stay close to the stomach wall in order to avoid injury to the underlying colon. Once the lesser sac is entered, the dexterity of the console surgeon's left grasper allows easier orientation of the Harmonic scalpel along the greater curvature. Another technique involves tucking the left grasper under the stomach and elevating it for further exposure.

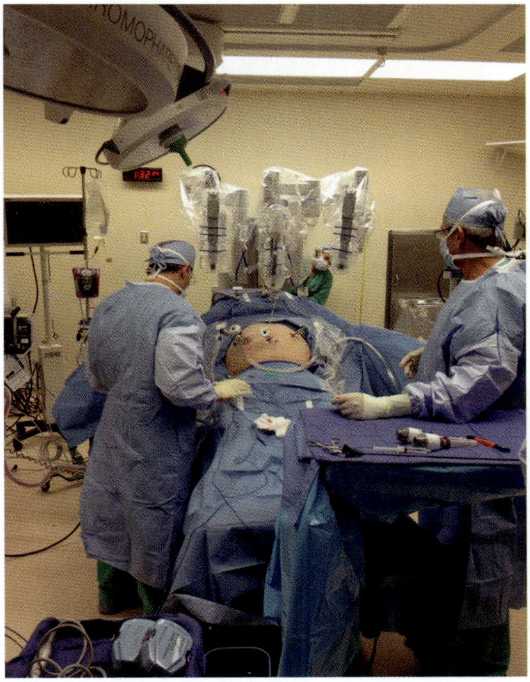

Fig. 11.6 Robot docked overhead

The dissection continues cephalad toward the angle of His and the short gastric vessels. Once the short gastric vessels are located, care must be taken to avoid troublesome bleeding. This is aided by the superior high-definition, three-dimensional view that the robot provides. Alternatively, the short gastric vessels can be divided after completing the gastric stapling portion, which allows the specimen to be retracted laterally and the vessels to be approached medially, which often provides a better and safer exposure for dividing the gastrosplenic attachments and the short gastric vessels. After the short gastric vessels are divided at the upper pole of the spleen (Fig. 11.9), the attachments between the fundus and left crus must be divided (Fig. 11.10) for two reasons: first, to avoid a large fundus at the superior portion of the stomach (neofundus) (Fig. 11.11) and, second, to clearly identify the gastroesophageal junction and to avoid stapling close to this area.

Once this is completed, it is imperative to aggressively dissect in the area of the phreno-esophageal ligament in search of an occult hiatal hernia. If a hernia is identified, it should be repaired in order to avoid disabling GERD later

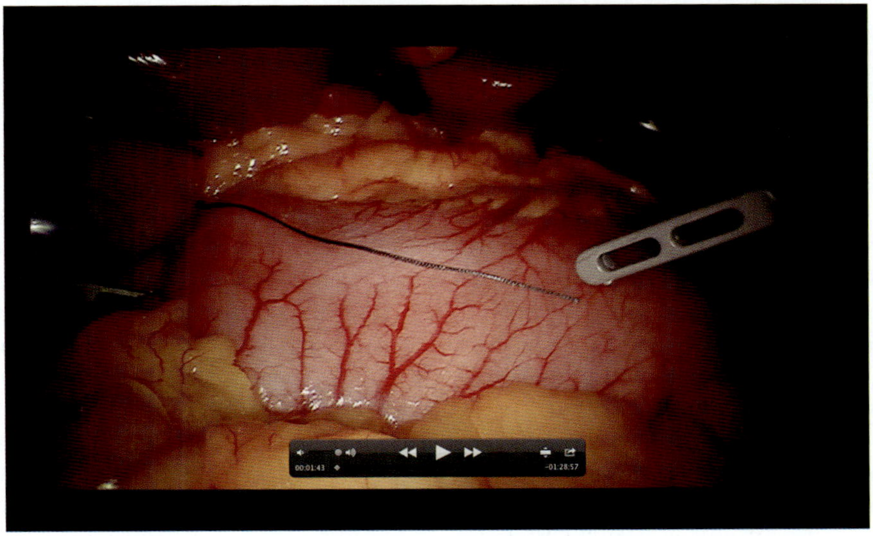

Fig. 11.7 Locating the pylorus

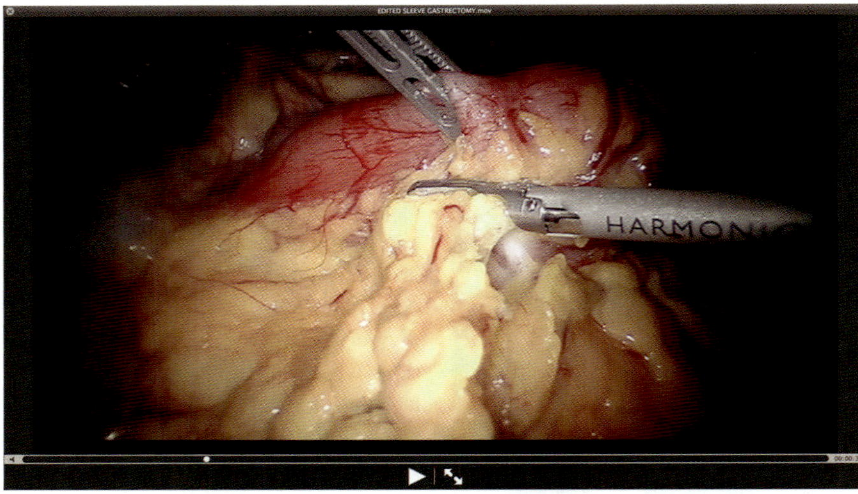

Fig. 11.8 Begin division of gastrocolic ligament

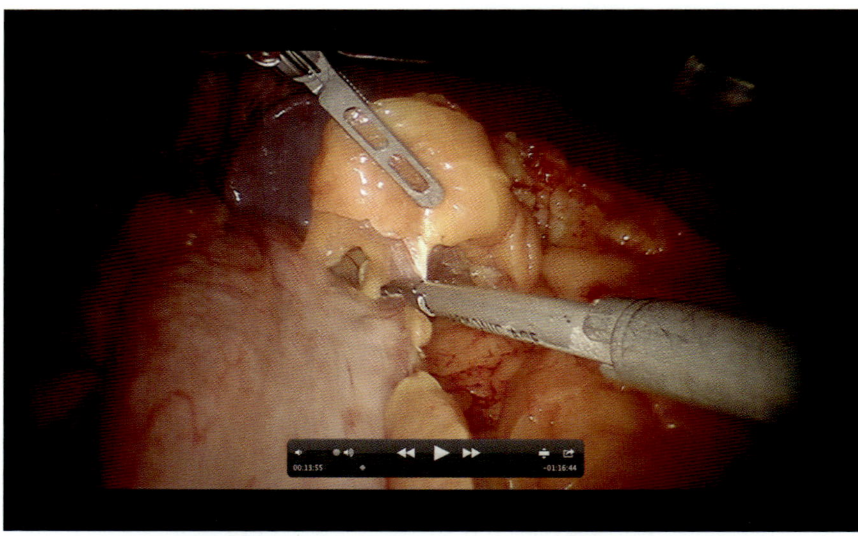

Fig. 11.9 Takedown of short gastric vessels

on. We prefer to perform the repair after creation of the gastric sleeve. Next, the distal portion the gastrocolic ligament can then be divided to approximately 4–6 cm proximal to the pylorus. Once this is completed, the usually flimsy posterior adhesions of the stomach to the underlying pancreas are divided in order to fully mobilize the stomach (Fig. 11.12). It is our opinion that mobilization is not complete until the lesser curvature vessels are identified from the posterior aspect of the stomach. This will obviate a larger than intended sleeve construction.

Once the vessels are divided and the stomach is well mobilized, the creation of the gastric sleeve is started. First the anesthesiologist is instructed to remove the temperature probe and the orogastric tube and a 32–36 Fr bougie is carefully passed orally. The bougie is used to calibrate the gastric pouch. The bedside assistant surgeon provides lateral traction of the stomach, while the

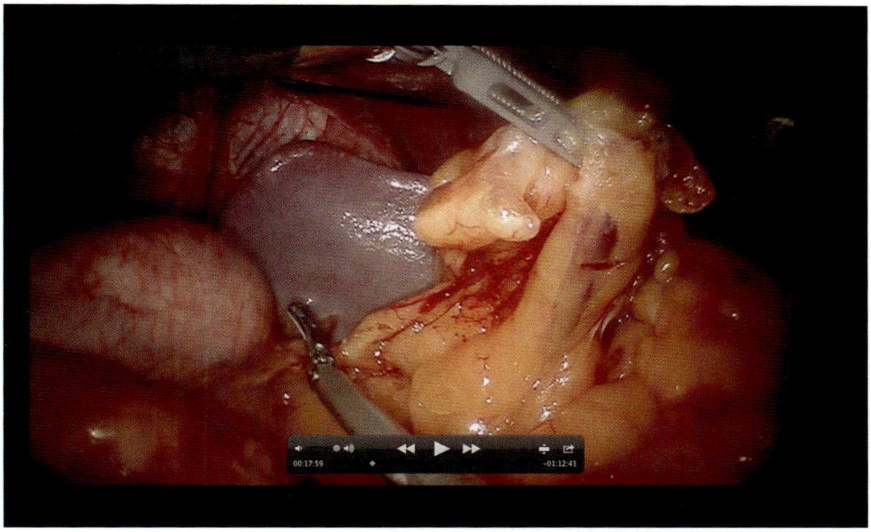

Fig. 11.10 Division of attachments between the fundus and the left crus

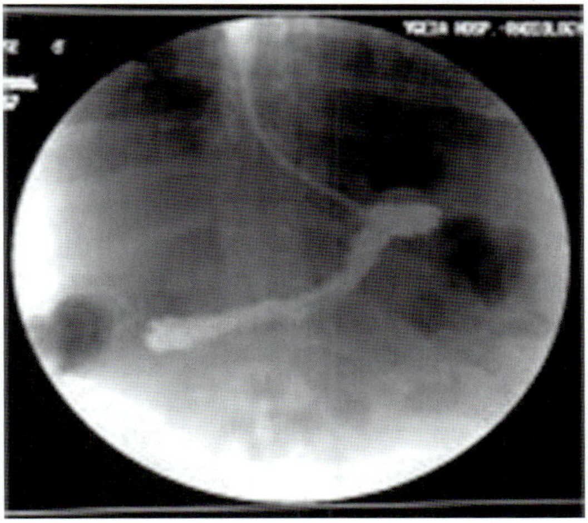

Fig. 11.11 Upper GI of neofundus

console surgeon, with the aid of the articulating bowel grasper, gently guides the bougie into the proximal duodenum (Fig. 11.13).

Once the calibration tube/bougie is in place, the transection begins. This is a critical first step, and careful attention should be paid to the angle of the stapler and its proximity to the incisura angularis. Because of the thickness of the tissue in this area, the first firing is performed with a green cartridge of the Echelon 60 mm stapler (2.0 mm). The console surgeon again gently retracts the tip of the bougie medially toward the duodenum with the articulating left-hand grasper and lateral retraction of the greater curvature with the right hand. The assistant bedside surgeon then introduces the stapler. The stapler is placed across the antrum in a more horizontal than vertical orientation, paying close attention to the incisura at all times (Figs. 11.14 and 11.15). This technique allows a "wide turn" at the area of the incisura, obviating a stricture or spiraling.

The transection is then continued proximally along the lateral edge of the bougie while maintaining lateral symmetrical traction. This technique is greatly facilitated by the dexterity and maneuverability of the robotic wristed instruments. This portion of the transection is performed with nothing less than a blue cartridge. As the staple line progresses proximally, it is important not to allow the staple line to spiral either anteriorly or posteriorly because this can lead to a functional obstruction (Fig. 11.16). The final critical step of the RSG is the completion of the transection at the angle of His. Most bariatric surgeons generally stay away from the gastroesophageal junction during the last staple firing in order to avoid a leak. However, leaving too large a fundus can lead to insufficient weight loss

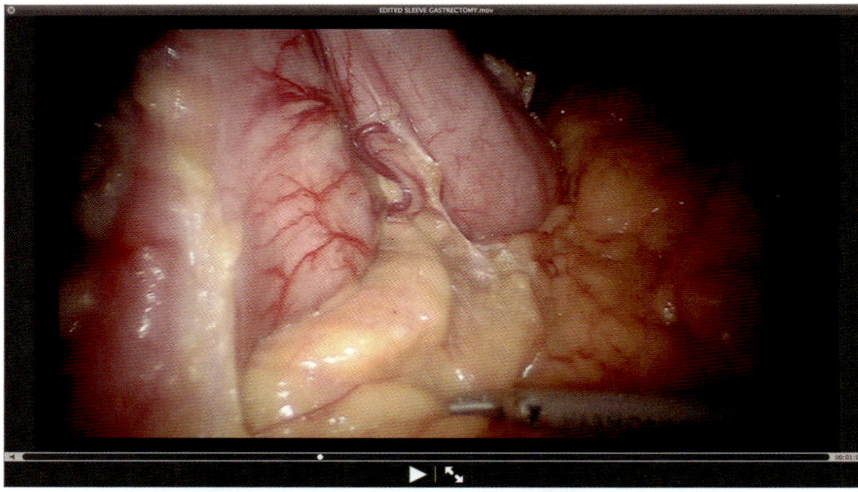

Fig. 11.12 Posterior dissection and complete gastric mobilization

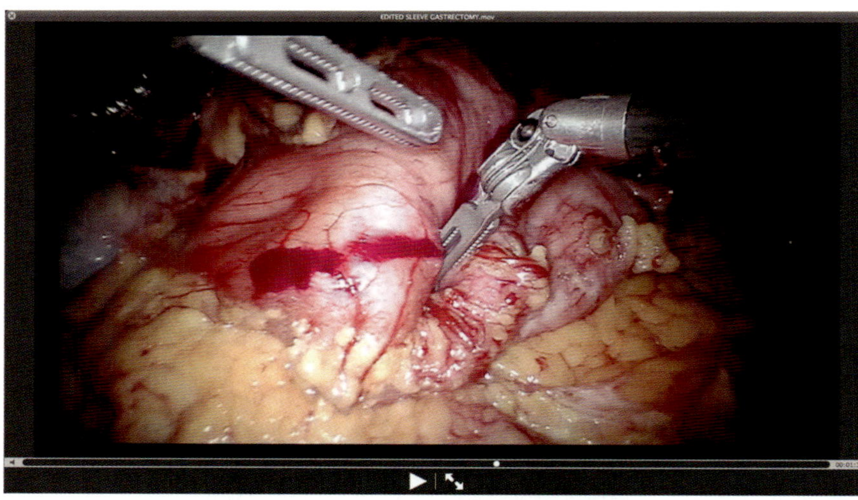

Fig. 11.13 Placement of bougie

or incapacitating gastroesophageal reflux. During the last firing, it is important that the console surgeon visualize 1–2 cm of gastric serosa just medial (left) to the stapler (Fig. 11.17). The early "aggressive" dissection of the hiatus at the beginning of the case, in search of a hiatal hernia, will also help in identifying the GE junction.

The consensus among most bariatric surgeons is that reinforcing the staple line will decrease bleeding. One of the authors of this chapter uses buttress material to reinforce the staple line, while the other reinforces the staple line by oversewing (Fig. 11.18). If an imbricating suture is used to reinforce the staple line, then it should be done with the bougie in place. Once the procedure is completed, the staple line is carefully examined for bleeding. The staple line is also examined for spiraling. If spiraling is found, the previous divided gastrocolic fat is sutured to the staple line to prevent kinking or further spiraling.

After the procedure is completed, we prefer intraoperative endoscopy, not only to ensure an

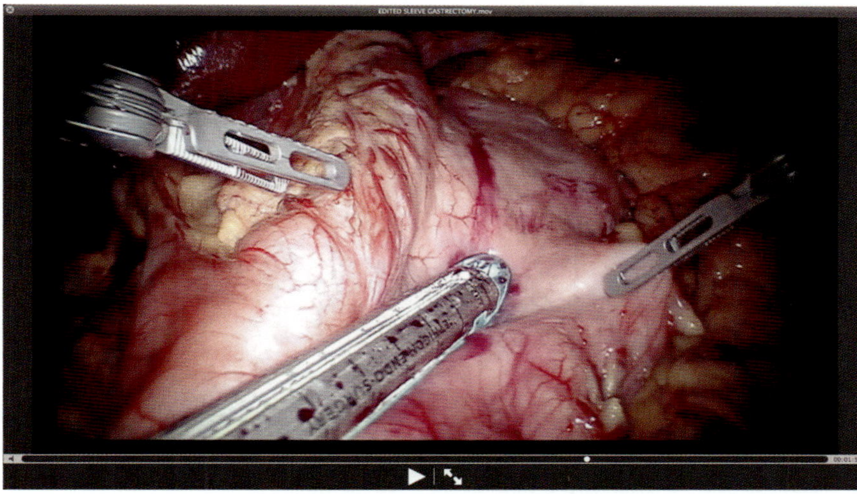

Fig. 11.14 Critical first firing of *staple line*

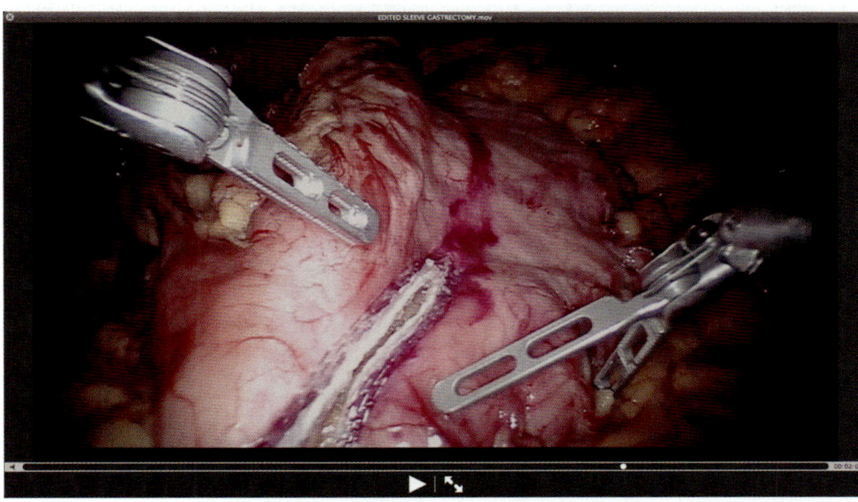

Fig. 11.15 Critical first firing of *staple line*

intact staple line with air leak test but also to ensure a uniform unobstructed lumen. Generally, a drain is not necessary with most cases, but should be considered in difficult or revisional cases. Fibrin glue is occasionally applied over the staple line when indicated. The resected stomach is removed via the assistant port site or the umbilical site. Closure of this fascial site is important to prevent an immediate postoperative incarcerated incisional hernia.

All patients undergo an upper gastrointestinal series the following day with water-soluble contrast. If the study shows no leak or stricture, the patient is started on a clear liquid diet and discharged home the next day. They are advanced to full liquid diet for 2 weeks and then a solid soft diet for 2 more weeks. Follow-up is at 1 week; 6 weeks; 4, 8, and 12 months; and then every 6 months thereafter.

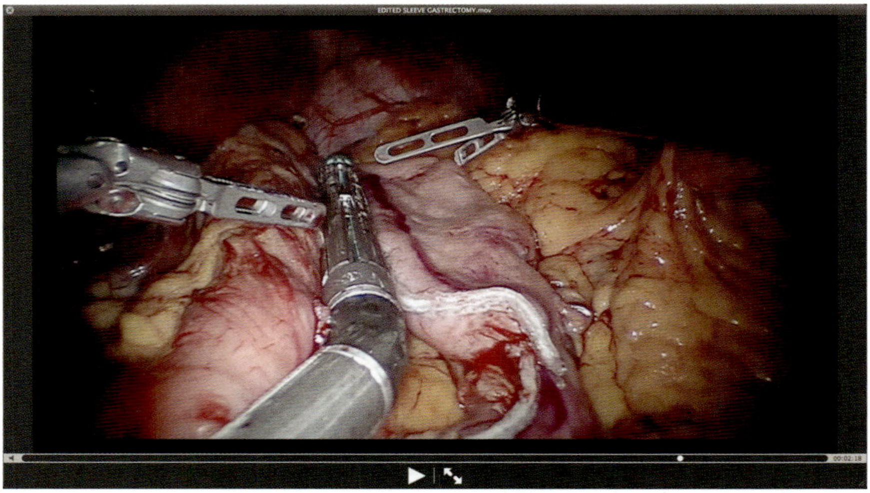

Fig. 11.16 Second firing beyond incisura

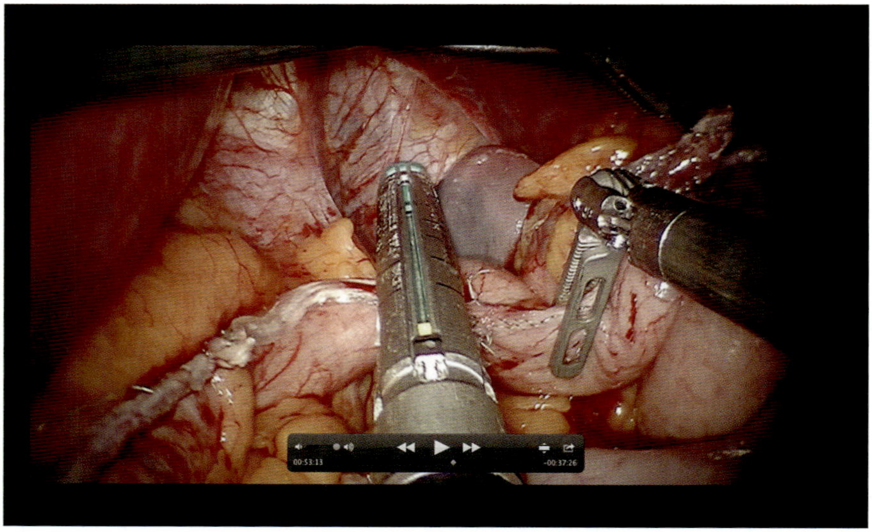

Fig. 11.17 Proximal portion of sleeve gastrectomy

Review of Literature

Robotic surgery has emerged in different surgical specialties (as gynecology, urology) with obvious benefits demonstrated in these areas. The use of the robot in bariatric surgery has been restricted only to those surgeries that are considered complex, such as revisions or bypass surgery; there are only a few papers that report the use of the robot for sleeve gastrectomies (Table 11.3).

We presented our preliminary experience in patients who underwent an RSG as treatment for morbid obesity and made a comparison with a meta-analysis of the standard laparoscopic approach in order to have a better understanding of both platforms. A total of 3,148 LSG patients from 22 studies were analyzed and compared with 134 RSG patients. This series represents one

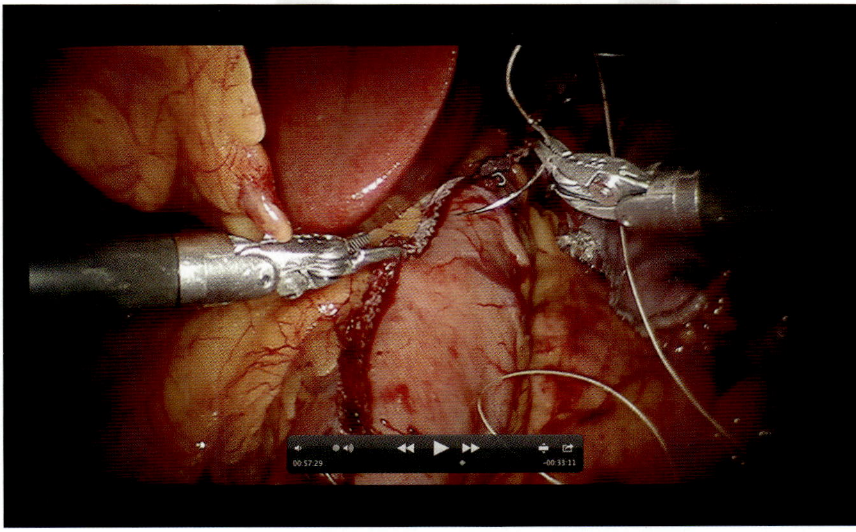

Fig. 11.18 Oversewing of *staple line*

Table 11.3 Review of literature

	Diamantis et al. [21]	Ayloo et al. [20]	Abdalla et al. [22]	Elli et al. [23]	Vilallonga et al. [24]	Gonzalez et al. [25]
Year	2011	2011	2012	2012	2012	2012
Number of patients	19	30	5	1	32	134
Leaks	0	0	0	0	0	0
Strictures	0	1 (3.3 %)	0	0	0	0
Bleeding	0	0	1 (20 %)	0	0	1 (0.7 %)
Mortality	0	0	0	0	0	0
Conversions	0	0	NP	0	0	0
Surgical time	95.5 ± 11.5	135 ± 28	NP	158	77.5 (56–130)	106.6 ± 48.8
Hospital length of stay	4	NP	NP	4	NP	2.2 ± 0.6

of the few published RSG experiences and the largest one to date. Comparison of three of the most common major complications after an LSG (leak, bleeding, and stricture) as well as the surgical time and hospital length of stay was reviewed, since these variables may have a direct relation with surgical technique.

Our conclusions were that both laparoscopic and robotic techniques are safe and feasible, showing good results in every measured parameter. However, surgical time was faster during the laparoscopic approach, and hospital length of stay was shorter with the robotic approach. The leak rate was slightly lower in the robotic platform (1.97 % vs. 0 %, $p=0.101$); however, there were no differences in strictures, bleeding, and mortality.

Conclusion

As obesity rates continue to rise in the United States, more bariatric procedures are needed to battle this growing problem. The sleeve gastrectomy has proven to be an excellent procedure for resolution of morbid obesity and its comorbid medical issues. The use of the robot in sleeve gastrectomy has been reported sparingly, but our experience, the largest reported to date, demonstrates that the robotic approach has similar results to its laparoscopic counterpart. Although the enhanced dexterity of the robot greatly facilitates reinforcing the staple line by suturing, until recently, the use of the robot in sleeve gastrectomies has been limited by the lack of a robotic stapler, which essentially assigns the stapling portion of the procedure, arguably the most critical portion of the procedure, to the bedside surgeon. The recent FDA approval of the robotic stapler, however, will now allow the entire procedure to be completed by the console surgeon. Further experience with larger numbers and randomization is necessary to determine its clear benefit in sleeve gastrectomies.

References

1. Wang Y, Beydoun MA, Liang L, Caballero B, Kumanyika S, Shiriki K. Will all Americans become overweight or obese? Estimating the progression and cost of the US obesity epidemic. Obesity. 2008;16: 2323–30.
2. Mokdad AH, Marks JS, Stroup DF, Gerberding JL. Actual causes of death in the United States, 2000. JAMA. 2004;291:1238–45.
3. Braghetto I, Davazo C, Korn O, et al. Scintigraphic evaluation of gastric emptying in obese patients submitted to sleeve gastrectomy compared to normal subjects. Obes Surg. 2009;19:1515–21.
4. Karamanakis SN, Vagenas K, Kalfarentzos F, Alexandrides TK. Weight loss, appetite suppression, and changes in fasting and postprandial ghrelin and peptide-YY levels after Roux-en-Y gastric bypass and sleeve gastrectomy: a prospective, double blind study. Ann Surg. 2008;247:408–10.
5. Shah S, Shah P, Todkar J, Gagner M, Sonar S, Solav S. Prospective controlled study of effect of laparoscopic sleeve gastrectomy on small bowel transit time and gastric emptying half time in morbidly obese patients with type 2 diabetes mellitus. Surg Obes Relat Dis. 2010;6:152–7.
6. Tymitz K, Engel A, McDonough S, Hendy MP, Kerlakian G. Changes in ghrelin levels following bariatric surgery: review of the literature. Obes Surg. 2011;21:125–30.
7. Hess DS, Hess DW. Biliopancreatic diversion with a duodenal switch. Obes Surg. 1998;8:267–82.
8. Hamoui H, Anthone GJ, Kaufman HS, Crookes PF. Sleeve gastrectomy in the high-risk patient. Obes Surg. 2006;16:1445–9.
9. Regan JP, Inabnet WB, Gagner M. Early experience with two-stage laparoscopic roux-en-Y gastric bypass as an alternative in the super-super obese patient. Obes Surg. 2003;13:861–4.
10. ASMBS Clinical Issues Committee. Updated position statement on sleeve gastrectomy as a bariatric procedure. Surg Obes Relat Dis. 2012;8:21–6.
11. Abbatini F, Rizzello M, Casella G, et al. Long-term effects of laparoscopic sleeve gastrectomy, gastric bypass, and adjustable gastric banding on type 2 diabetes. Surg Endosc. 2010;24:1005–10.
12. Bohdjalian A, Langer FB, Shakeri-Leidenmühler S, et al. Sleeve gastrectomy as sole and definitive bariatric procedure: 5-year results for weight loss and ghrelin. Obes Surg. 2010;20:535–40.
13. Jacobs M, Biscand W, Greg E. Laparoscopic sleeve gastrectomy: a retrospective review of 1- and 2-year results. Surg Endosc. 2010;24:781–5.
14. Sarela AI, Dexter SPL, O'Kane M, Menon A, McMahon MJ. Long-term follow-up after laparoscopic sleeve gastrectomy: 8–9-year results. Surg Obes Relat Dis. 2012;8(6):679–84. doi:10.1016/j.soard.2011.06.020. ISSN 1550–7289.
15. Brethauer SA, Hammel JP, Schauer PR. Systematic review of sleeve gastrectomy as staging and primary bariatric procedure. Surg Obes Relat Dis. 2009;5(4): 469–75.
16. Ramalingam G, Anton CK. Our 1-year experience in laparoscopic sleeve gastrectomy. Obes Surg. 2011; 21(12):1828–33.
17. Gagner M. Leaks after sleeve gastrectomy are associated with smaller bougies: prevention and treatment strategies. Surg Laparosc Endosc Percutan Tech. 2010;20:166–9.
18. Snyder BE, Wilson T, Leong BY, Klein C, Wilson EB. Robotic-assisted Roux-en-Y gastric bypass: minimizing morbidity and mortality. Obes Surg. 2010;20: 265–70.
19. Deng JY, Lourié DJ. 100 Robotic-assisted laparoscopic gastric bypasses at a community hospital. Am Surg. 2008;74:1022–5.
20. Ayloo S, Buchs NC, Addeo P, Bianco FM, Giulianotti PC. Robot-assisted sleeve gastrectomy for supermorbidly obese patients. J Laparoendosc Adv Surg Tech A. 2011;21:295–9.
21. Diamantis T, Alexandrou A, Nikiteas N, Giannopoulos A, Papalambros E. Initial experience with robotic sleeve gastrectomy for morbid obesity. Obes Surg. 2011;21:1172–9.
22. Abdalla RZ, Garcia RB, Luca CR, Costa RI, Cozer CO. Brazilian experience in obesity surgery robot-assisted. Arq Bras Cir Dig. 2012;25(1):33–5. English, Portuguese: PMID: 22569976.
23. Elli EF, Masrur MA, Giulianotti PC. Robotic sleeve gastrectomy after liver transplantation. Surg Obes Relat Dis. 2013;9(1):e20–2. PMID: 22365186.
24. Vilallonga R, Fort JM, Gonzalez O, Caubet E, Boleko A, Neff KJ, Armengol M. The initial learning curve for robot-assisted sleeve gastrectomy: a surgeon's experience while introducing the robotic technology in a bariatric surgery department. Minim Invasive Surg. 2012;2012:347131. doi:10.1155/2012/347131. PMID: 23029610.
25. Gonzalez AM, et al. Robotic sleeve gastrectomy: experience of 134 cases and comparison with a systematic review of the laparoscopic approach. Obes Surg. 2013.

Robotic Biliopancreatic Diversion: Robot-Assisted (Hybrid) Biliopancreatic Diversion with Duodenal Switch

12

Ranjan Sudan and Sean Lee

General Overview of Current Applications

The first robot-assisted biliopancreatic diversion with duodenal switch operation (BPD/DS) was performed in October 2000, only months after the Food and Drug Administration approved the da Vinci surgical system for use in general surgery in July 2000 [1]. Subsequently, Roux-en-Y gastric bypass, laparoscopic adjustable band operations, and sleeve gastrectomy have all been performed using the da Vinci platform [2, 3]. However, the focus of this chapter will be the hybrid BPD/DS. The BPD/DS is a malabsorptive bariatric procedure that has been performed by laparotomy for over 20 years. It was first described by Marceau et al. [4] and by Hess and Hess [5]. The laparoscopic BPD/DS was first described by Ren et al. in 2000 [6], but complication rates were high for patients with BMI >60 kg/m^2 [7]. The BPD/DS is a technically challenging operation and the vast majorities were still being performed by laparotomy in 2010 [8].

R. Sudan, M.D. (✉)
Department of Surgery, Duke University Medical Center, Trent Drive, Durham, NC 27710, USA
e-mail: ranjan.sundan@duke.edu

S. Lee, M.D.
Division of Metabolic and Weight Loss Surgery, Duke University Medical Center, Box 2834, Durham, NC 27710, USA
e-mail: seanmleemd@gmail.com

Our group adopted the da Vinci platform with the hope of reducing both the technical challenges faced in laparoscopic approaches to this operation and the resulting high complication rates. Initially we performed the operation totally robotically, but the first-generation robot had limited mobility, only two working arms, and shorter instrument lengths that significantly limited our ability to access the three abdominal quadrants involved in this procedure, the right lower quadrant for the ileoileostomy, the left upper quadrant for the sleeve, and the right upper quadrant for the duodenoileostomy. Thus, the totally robotic approach initially required multiple docking positions. We first performed the ileoileostomy with the patient cart docked toward the foot end with the patient in lithotomy position. After completion of this part of the operation, we disconnected the anesthetic lines, rotated the patient bed 180°, reconnected the anesthetic lines and tubes, docked the da Vinci from the head end, and performed the rest of the procedure in the right upper and left upper abdominal quadrants.

Although we had no complications related to these maneuvers, the process had potential for errors and was also quite time consuming. Therefore, in the interest of patient safety and time conservation, we adopted a hybrid technique in which conventional laparoscopy was used to perform the ileoileostomy and the sleeve gastrectomy, while the robot was used for a sutured duodenoileostomy. The duodenoileostomy is considered the most crucial portion of the BPD/DS, and laparoscopic techniques using a

K.C. Kim (ed.), *Robotics in General Surgery*, DOI 10.1007/978-1-4614-8739-5_12,

circular stapler, a linear cutting stapler, or hand suturing have been described for this anastomosis. Since the robot allows for precise suturing, we have found that the robot-sutured anastomosis is reliable, widely patent, and not prone to strictures. It also preserves the maximum possible length of the first part of the duodenum. In fact, in the last 12 years of our experience, no patient has suffered from a stricture in this location.

The newest generation robot (Si) has three instrument arms and has an extended reach allowing for greater flexibility in working in different quadrants. We have therefore started performing the ileoileostomy and sleeve gastrectomy portions robotically with a single docking. However, the procedures in the strictest sense are still not totally robotic because robotic staplers are not available for general use. Once these are available we will be able to develop a totally robotic BPD/DS procedure. Although we look forward to continuing advancement in the field of surgical robotics, for the purposes of this chapter, we will focus on our hybrid technique with which we have 11 years of experience. This method is also less challenging for those users who are early in their learning curve with the da Vinci system and thus recommend this technique as a starting point.

Patient Positioning

The patient is positioned supine. After induction of anesthesia, a Foley catheter is placed. Arterial or central venous catheters are not routinely placed. The patient is secured to the bed with belts, a footboard is placed to facilitate extreme bed positioning as required, and pressure points are protected adequately to prevent against a neuropathy because of the long duration of these procedures. The arms are placed on adjustable arm boards and are secured with bandages so they do not slip off when the patient is tilted in either the Trendelenburg or reverse-Trendelenburg positions. A lower-body warming blanket is used to keep the upper body free of obstructions so that it does not interfere with robot docking. Adequate slack in the anesthetic lines and tubes is ensured and is kept low profile so that the robot can be positioned over the patient's right shoulder without interference from the anesthetic cart. The abdomen is prepped and draped to expose the upper body from the umbilicus to the xiphoid and from the right anterior axillary line to the left anterior axillary line. A large bore stomach-sizing tube (Allergan®) is used to decompress the stomach. It is subsequently used for sizing the sleeve and instilling dye into the stomach for a duodenoileostomy leak test. The drapes are dropped over the head and cover the patient's face. The traditional barrier between the surgical field and the anesthesiologist is deliberately avoided so that the surgeon may stand above the patient's shoulders and operate in the lower abdomen with laparoscopic instruments so that the robot can dock without interference.

Trocar Placement

The abdomen is entered with a Veress needle in the left upper quadrant. A 0°, 10 mm laparoscope is then placed through a 12 mm optical trocar, and the abdominal cavity is entered under direct visualization in the midline about 15 cm below the xiphoid. After confirming the absence of injury related to Veress needle and the trocar insertions, additional ports are placed. An 8 mm robot trocar is placed in the right anterior axillary line at the edge of the right lobe of the liver and a second robotic trocar is placed just lateral to the left midclavicular line. Accessory 12 mm ports are placed in the left anterior axillary line and the right midclavicular line at about the horizontal level as the camera port. These port positions are individualized to a certain extent based on the patient's body habitus and the size of the liver (Fig. 12.1). All port sites are preinjected with a long-acting local anesthetic prior to incision.

Key Steps

The patient is positioned in the Trendelenburg position and tilted slightly to the left. A 30°, 10 mm conventional laparoscopic camera is used in the umbilical port site. Previously, we began the operation by performing an appendectomy because most open surgeons routinely did so to prevent confounding the anatomy if an appendectomy was needed later. Although performing an appendectomy did not add to our complication rate or duration of the procedure, we have stopped performing a routine appendectomy because of our experience with laparoscopic gastric bypass patients who rarely need an appendectomy after bariatric surgery. The diagnosis of appendicitis using computerized tomography is quite accurate, and since robotic duodenal switch results in minimal right lower quadrant adhesions in most patients, subsequent appendectomy should be straightforward.

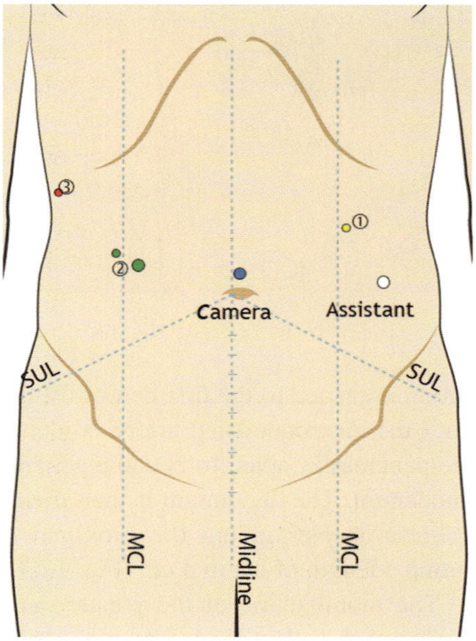

Fig. 12.1 Port positions

We now begin by identifying the ileocecal junction and marking the ileum at 100 cm and 250 cm proximal to it with sutures. The bowel is then divided at the 250 cm mark using a linear cutter stapler and the mesentery is divided toward its root using the harmonic scalpel to mobilize the bowel. The bowel proximal to the 250 cm mark becomes the biliary limb and the bowel distal to it will become the alimentary limb. The biliary limb is then anastomosed to the ileum at the 100 cm mark using a 60 mm long conventional laparoscopic linear stapler. The enterotomies for the stapler are created using an ultrasonic shear and are closed using a single-layer running 2-zero suture using conventional intracorporeal laparoscopic suturing (Fig. 12.2).

The mesenteric defect between the biliary limb and the common channel is closed with running nonabsorbable sutures.

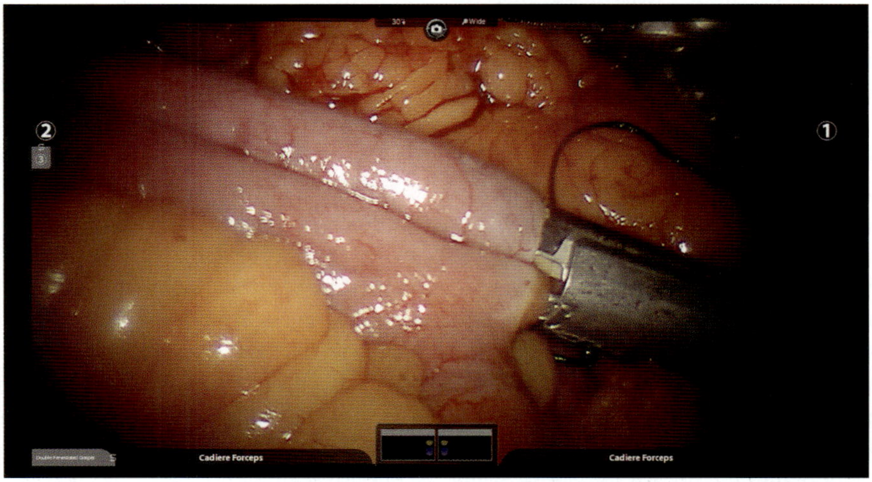

Fig. 12.2 Side-to-side ileoileostomy

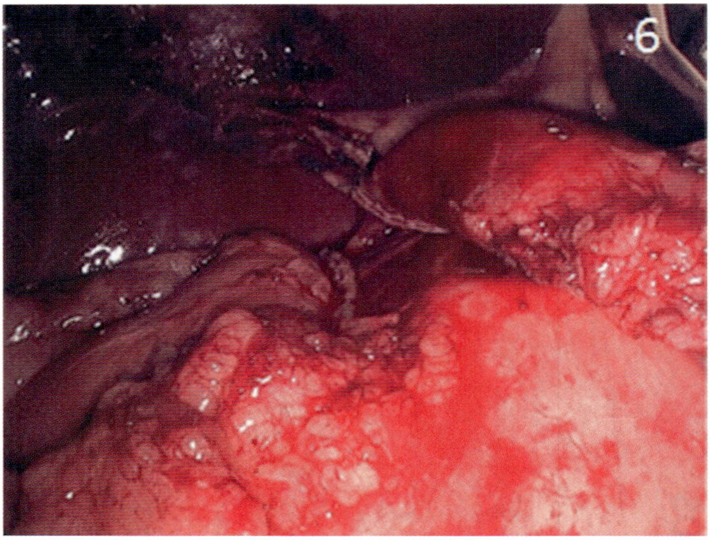

Fig. 12.3 Division of duodenum

The patient is then placed in a reverse Trendelenburg position. A Nathanson liver retractor is placed through a stab incision near the xiphoid and used to elevate the left lobe of the liver. If the falciform ligament obscures visualization, it may need to be excised or we will sometimes attach it to the anterior abdominal wall.

Open surgeons have performed routine cholecystectomy in the past, and we continue to perform routine cholecystectomy for several reasons. The risk of gallstone formation is likely even higher than in gastric bypass patients due to the wasting of bile salts. There is no remnant stomach after BPD/DS, and the alimentary and biliopancreatic limbs are very long, making purely endoscopic techniques to retrieve common bile duct stones and ERCP essentially impossible. In addition, performing a cholecystectomy in the presence of scarring after a duodenoileostomy that lies immediately adjacent to the gallbladder is likely to be more difficult than after a RYGB where the anastomosis is in the left upper quadrant. The cholecystectomy is performed using standard laparoscopic techniques, although admittedly the procedure is made somewhat cumbersome by the port placement for the BPD/ DS.

The preparation for a sleeve gastrectomy begins by mobilizing the greater curvature of the stomach using an ultrasonic device. The mobilization is carried to the first part of the duodenum until the gastroduodenal artery is identified and the pancreas is noted to become adherent to the duodenum. The duodenum is then divided using a linear stapler giving the proximal duodenal stump a length of about 4 cm (Fig. 12.3).

The mobilization of the greater curvature of the stomach is then carried proximally inside the gastroepiploic arcade until the highest short gastric vessels are divided and the angle of His is exposed (Fig. 12.4). It is beneficial to detach any of the filmy adhesion between the posterior wall of the stomach and the pancreas to allow the stomach to be freely mobilized. Using the 34 French sizing tube as a guide, a sleeve gastrectomy is performed to create a stomach tube with a capacity of 150 ml s (Fig. 12.5).

The distal stomach is stapled with at least 4.8 mm leg length staplers (green loads), and as the stomach becomes less thick, the loads can be switched to a leg length of 3.5 mm. The use of staple-line reinforcements is optional. Our preference is to use robotic suturing with absorbable suture to oversew the distal stomach where it is thickest, and staples may not approximate the edges of the stomach. Particular care is taken to not narrow the stomach near the incisura. The central diaphragm is carefully inspected and any hiatal hernia identified is repaired.

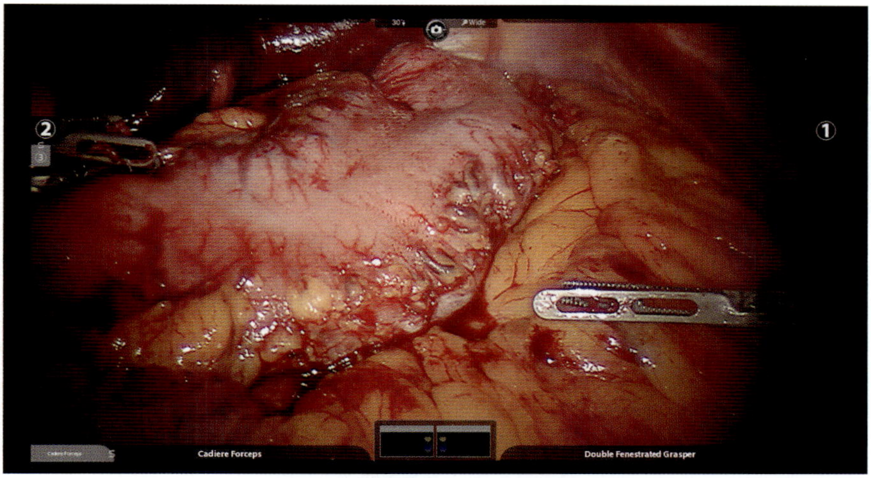

Fig. 12.4 Mobilization of greater curvature

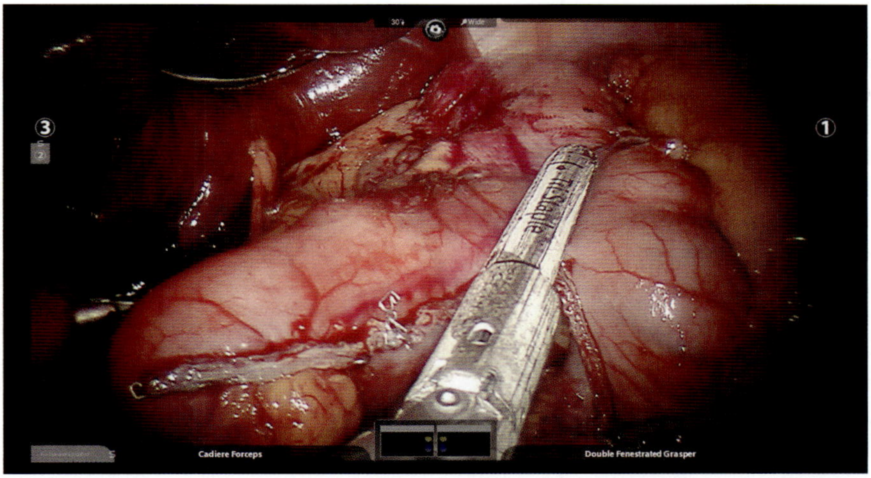

Fig. 12.5 Sleeve gastrectomy

The alimentary limb is then taken retrocolic to the right of the middle colic vessels and delivered close to the first part of the duodenum. The robot is then docked over the right shoulder (Fig. 12.6).

The camera is inserted through the umbilical port and a needle driver inserted through the left midclavicular port (arm 1). The second robotic arm is placed using a port-in-port technique through the right midclavicular port (arm 2), and the accessory arm is used through the right anterior axillary port (arm 3). The instruments on the right side are usually Cadiere graspers as this allows handling of the bowel and retraction on the suture. Arms 1 and 2 are used for suturing, whereas arm 3 is used for retraction of a stay suture that helps align the orientation of the enterotomies for suturing. The posterior seromuscular running layer is first started using running 2-zero nonabsorbable suture. An enterotomy is then made in the duodenum and in the ileum using the robotic hook cautery. A full-thickness running layer of 2-zero absorbable

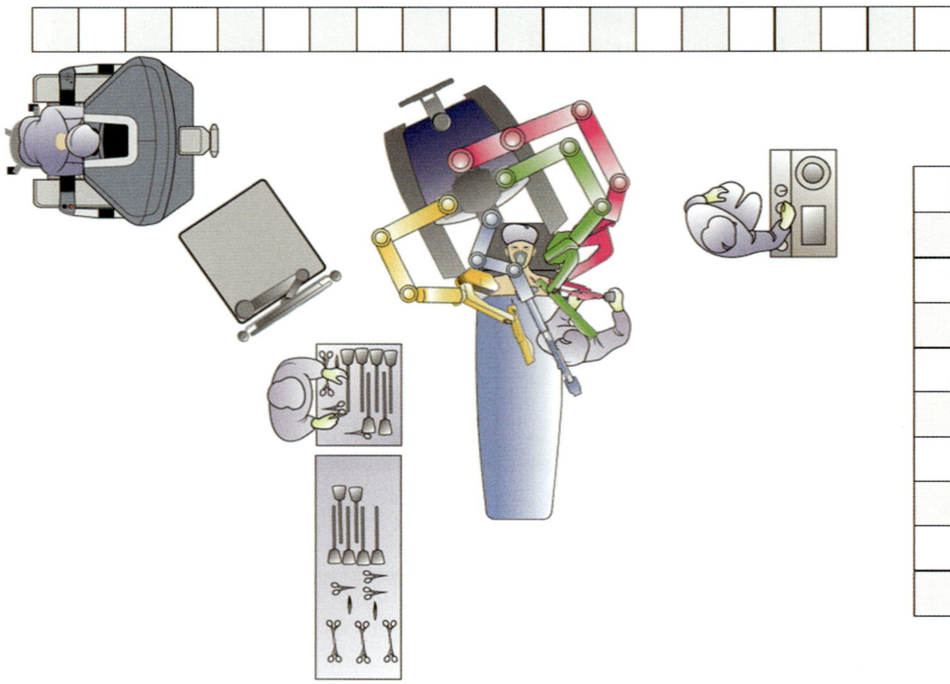

Fig. 12.6 Operating room layout

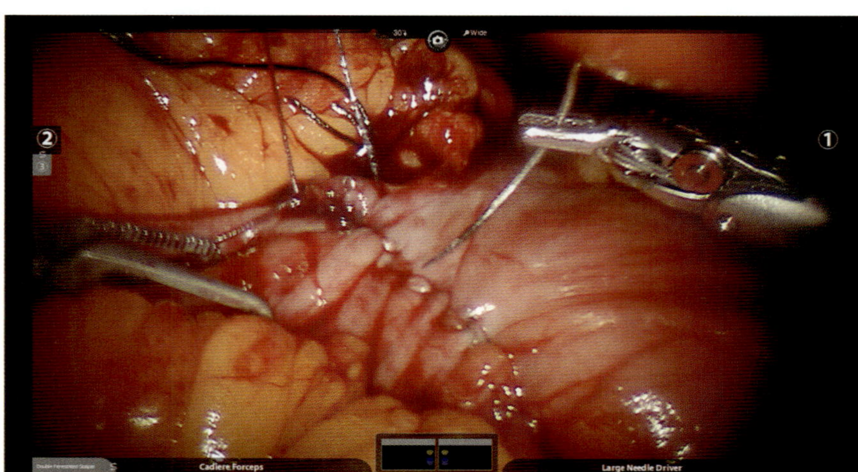

Fig. 12.7 Proximal alimentary limb anastomosis

suture is started posteriorly and completed anteriorly. The anterior seromuscular layer of nonabsorbable suture completes the two-layer hand-sewn anastomosis (Fig. 12.7).

At this stage methylene blue is instilled in the stomach using the orogastric tube. The mesenteric defect between the mesentery of the alimentary limb and the retroperitoneum (Petersen's defect) is closed using running nonabsorbable suture. After confirming the absence of leaks and ensuring hemostasis, an endoscopic leak check is optional. We tend to perform endoscopy to rule out leaks, evaluate for luminal staple-line bleeding, and to ensure patency of the lumen. Once endoscopy is completed, the robot is undocked, the ports are removed under direct visualization, and the resected specimens (gallbladder and greater curvature of stomach) are removed. We place a suture on one end of the stomach specimen and use it as a handle to remove the stomach through the midline port site. Using this technique we rarely have to enlarge the fascial defect to extract the specimen. Skin is closed with absorbable subcuticular suture.

Discussion of Advantages, Limitations, and Relative Contraindications

The indications for a BPD/DS are the same as for any bariatric operation: a BMI >35 kg/m^2 with significant medical comorbidities or a BMI >40 kg/m^2. In practical terms, the operation is very good for patients with severe diabetes and hypercholesterolemia, but not so good for patients with severe gastroesophageal reflux disease. Patients should not have this operation if there is a specific reason why they should avoid malabsorption, such as in those with Crohn's disease or severe osteoporosis.

The learning curve of the robotic BPD/DS for a novice in laparoscopic and robotic techniques is about 50 cases. Age and male gender have been considered risk factors for bariatric surgery, but our own analysis of patient outcomes has not borne this out. Patient-related factors such as enlarged livers, excessive abdominal wall torque, and significant intraabdominal adiposity did increase the risk for complications. The need for adhesiolysis from prior abdominal operations such as open cholecystectomy increased the duration, but not the risk of complications from a robotic BPD/DS. We found very enlarged livers greatly increased the degree of difficulty of a case initially [9]. However, with increasing experience we have developed greater skill using the accessory arm for retraction purposes and we are able to perform operations on patients with difficult anatomy with greater ease. This likely also translates into greater safety for the patient. Based on these findings we recommend performing a robotic BPD/DS on patients whose anatomy is likely to be difficult only after a surgeon has mastered the technique in simpler patients.

Laparoscopic BPD/DS in patients with a BMI >60 has been reported to have a high mortality [7]. However, in the last 12 years, we have not experienced any short- or long-term mortality in our patients, and other authors have also reported no increase in mortality for high-BMI patients [10]. Leak rates in our early experience were similar to those seen in the learning curve of the laparoscopic Roux-en-Y gastric bypass, and these rates have improved considerably since our first 50 cases. Patients seeking BPD/DS tend to be heavier as certain insurance companies will not approve the procedure for patients with a BMI <50 kg/m^2. This can increase the degree of difficulty of a case, and novice surgeons are cautioned about taking on more difficult cases such as those with high BMI early in their experience.

One limitation of the da Vinci surgical system is that it is not able to operate easily in multiple quadrants. In order to access widely separated areas of the abdomen, or when changing the position of the bed to enhance the intraabdominal view, redocking of the robot is required. This is time-consuming and could pose added risk to the patient. We have overcome this limitation by using a hybrid laparoscopic/robotic technique. Another limitation is the loss of haptic sensation, which is especially problematic when grasping bowel as this can lead to bowel injuries. This was responsible for a leak and conversion to open surgery in a patient early in our experience. Since then, double fenestrated instruments have been developed that are more suitable for grasping bowel and are now in use. A third limitation is the lack of articulation in the robotic harmonic and its short length. This can limit the reach in patients with long torsos. Although this can often be overcome by inserting the trocars deeper, it may necessitate the repositioning of trocars to an extent that makes the operation awkward. A new energy device (ERBE) is now available, but we do not yet have experience with it. As robotic technology advances, so our technique continues to evolve. We have recently begun to utilize a totally robotic technique that we hope to introduce in the near future.

Review of Outcomes

In our series of over 180 BPD/DS, we have had no mortality. Our leak rate for primary operations is the same as that for a laparoscopic Roux-en-Y gastric bypass, at around 2 %. However, this number includes our entire experience including the learning curve. Our conversion rate is also very low. After three conversions within our first 17 cases, we have not had to convert anyone to open surgery. We now use the robotic platform exclusively to perform all our BPD/DS operations including revisions (such as conversion of adjustable gastric banding or vertical banded gastroplasty to BPD/DS).

Large retrospective reviews as well as smaller comparative studies have shown that excess body weight loss and resolution of comorbid conditions (such as hypertension and type II diabetes mellitus) are superior for BPD/DS compared to gastric bypass [11–13]. Mortality and postoperative complication rates are slightly higher for the BPD/DS in these studies, but there is significant variability in these rates amongst reports in the literature. Our data is in line with this literature, and we have reported a leak rate of 5.8 % and a conversion to open surgery in 2.2 %, with improvement in these rates over time in our first 47 patients [1].

Operative times and hospital length of stay is generally longer for the BPD/DS than gastric bypass as well. One prospective comparative study showed mean operative times of 206 min for BDP/DS and 91 min for LRYGB [14], and another reported times of 239 and 135 min, respectively, for conversion of failed gastric banding to BPD/DS or gastric bypass [15]. Our experience with the hybrid robotic procedure has been that it does require longer operative times [1]. On an average, a robotic case including a cholecystectomy and training time for fellows is approximately 5 h.

Length of stay is also significantly longer for the BPD/DS compared to gastric bypass. This ranges between 4 and 5 days for BPD/DS and between 2 and 4 days for Roux-en-Y gastric bypass [13, 14]. Our experience aligns with these data also and reflects a difference in the approach to postoperative management between the BPD/DS and gastric bypass patient groups. Whereas we advance gastric bypass patients to a liquid diet on the first postoperative day irrespective of bowel function, BPD/DS patients are kept NPO until first flatus. This usually takes 3–5 days and thus our length of stay averages around 4 days after BPD/DS.

Conclusions

We have described a technique to perform a BPD/DS using a hybrid laparoscopic/robotic approach that is safe and time efficient and that yields efficacy commensurate with reports of other BPD/DS techniques.

References

1. Sudan R, Puri V, Sudan D. Robotically assisted biliary pancreatic diversion with a duodenal switch: a new technique. Surg Endosc. 2007;21(5):729–33.
2. Jacobsen G, Berger R, Horgan S. The role of robotic surgery in morbid obesity. J Laparoendosc Adv Surg Tech A. 2003;13(4):279–83.
3. Ayloo S, et al. Robot-assisted sleeve gastrectomy for super-morbidly obese patients. J Laparoendosc Adv Surg Tech A. 2011;21(4):295–9.
4. Marceau P, et al. Biliopancreatic diversion with a new type of gastrectomy. Obes Surg. 1993;3(1):29–35.
5. Hess DS, Hess DW. Biliopancreatic diversion with a duodenal switch. Obes Surg. 1998;8(3):267–82.
6. Ren CJ, Patterson E, Gagner M. Early results of laparoscopic biliopancreatic diversion with duodenal switch: a case series of 40 consecutive patients. Obes Surg. 2000;10(6):514–23. discussion 524.
7. Kim WW, et al. Laparoscopic vs. open biliopancreatic diversion with duodenal switch: a comparative study. J Gastrointest Surg. 2003;7(4):552–7.
8. DeMaria EJ, et al. Baseline data from American society for metabolic and bariatric surgery-designated bariatric surgery centers of excellence using the bariatric outcomes longitudinal database. Surg Obes Relat Dis. 2010;6(4):347–55.

9. Sudan R, et al. Multifactorial analysis of the learning curve for robot-assisted laparoscopic biliopancreatic diversion with duodenal switch. Ann Surg. 2012; 255(5):940–5.
10. Buchwald H, et al. Duodenal switch operative mortality and morbidity are not impacted by body mass index. Ann Surg. 2008;248(4):541–8.
11. Buchwald H, et al. Bariatric surgery: a systematic review and meta-analysis. JAMA. 2004;292(14): 1724–37.
12. Buchwald H, Oien DM. Metabolic/bariatric surgery Worldwide 2008. Obes Surg. 2009;19(12):1605–11.
13. Prachand VN, Davee RT, Alverdy JC. Duodenal switch provides superior weight loss in the superobese (BMI >or=50 kg/m^2) compared with gastric bypass. Ann Surg. 2006;244(4):611–9.
14. Sovik TT, et al. Randomized clinical trial of laparoscopic gastric bypass versus laparoscopic duodenal switch for superobesity. Br J Surg. 2010;97(2):160–6.
15. Topart P, Becouarn G, Ritz P. Biliopancreatic diversion with duodenal switch or gastric bypass for failed gastric banding: retrospective study from two institutions with preliminary results. Surg Obes Relat Dis. 2007;3(5):521–5.

Part VI

Surgical Techniques: *Hepatobiliary/ Pancreas*

Robotic Pancreaticoduodenectomy (Whipple Procedure)

13

Martin J. Dib, Tara Kent, and A. James Moser

Introduction

The major technical aspects of pancreatoduodenectomy (PD) to resect tumors of the periampullary region have not changed significantly since it was first established in the early twentieth century. Allen O. Whipple published the first case series of a single-stage PD in 1945, and Traverso and Longmire described the addition of pylorus preservation in 1978 [1, 2]. The high postoperative mortality rates prevented the widespread use of PD for several decades, but advancements in critical care, anesthesia, and attention to surgical detail led to significant outcome improvements [3, 4]. The most recent refinements have focused on minimally invasive adaptations, taking the advantages of technological innovations in complex resections and anastomotic reconstructions.

The first laparoscopic PD was published by Gagner and Pomp in 1994 [5]. Reports of totally laparoscopic PDs have been published by Palanivelu et al. [6] and Kendrick and Cusatti [7], although less than 200 reports of laparoscopic PDs are found in the English literature since Garner's first description. The slow adoption of laparoscopic PDs is a result of the technical burdens and complexity of this procedure [8].

Robotic-assisted surgery, with magnified stereoscopic visualization and computer-enhanced 540° movement of the surgical instruments, has the potential to overcome the technical impediments to recreating time-tested techniques for open pancreatic surgery in a minimal access technique. Variations of robotic-assisted PD and its preliminary outcomes have been published by groups led by Giulianotti, Melvin, and Moser and Zeh [9–15].

Selection Criteria

Selection criteria for attempting minimally invasive resection for pancreatic cancer are of equal importance to the technical aspects and must address potential oncological hazards including the likelihood of residual tumor at the surgical margin and adequacy of lymph node sampling. We select patients for robotic-assisted PD (RAPD) using a validated predictive model to maximize the likelihood of R0 surgical resection among patients with pancreatic cancer [16]. Three factors are evaluated: evidence for any vascular involvement on preoperative CT scan, abnormal lymph nodes on endoscopic ultrasound (EUS), and tumor

M.J. Dib, M.D. • T. Kent, M.D., F.A.C.S.
Department of Surgery, Beth Israel Deaconess Medical Center, 330 Brookline Avenue, Stoneman 9th Floor, Boston, MA 02215, USA
e-mail: mdib@bidmc.harvard.edu; dibmartin@gmail.com; tkent@bidmc.harvard.edu

A.J. Moser, M.D., F.A.C.S. (✉)
Institute for Hepatobiliary and Pancreatic Cancer, Beth Israel Deaconess Medical Center, 330 Brookline Avenue, Boston, MA 02215, USA
e-mail: jmoser1@bidmc.harvard.edu

K.C. Kim (ed.), *Robotics in General Surgery*, DOI 10.1007/978-1-4614-8739-5_13,

diameter greater than 2.6 cm on EUS. RAPD is offered only to patients at low-predicted risk of a non-R0 outcome: (a) EUS stage 1A; (b) absence of vascular involvement on CT and EUS stage less than or equal to 2A; and (c) absence of vascular involvement on CT and EUS stage 2B, but largest tumor diameter <2.6 cm.

Position, Equipment, and Trocar Placement

The patient is positioned supine on a split-leg table with the right arm tucked and the left arm extended, and the robot is docked from straight over the patient's head. Seven laparoscopic ports are required (Fig. 13.1a, b). A 5-mm optical separator is used to access the peritoneal cavity in the left subcostal region. The camera port is placed 2–3 cm superior and to the right of the umbilicus to improve exposure of the portal vein. Two 5-mm ports are placed in the right upper quadrant and later converted to 8-mm robotic trocars. A 5-mm port for the laparoscopic liver retractor is inserted in the anterior axillary line. Two assistant ports are placed in the lower quadrants. Once resectability is ensured, a 5-cm extraction incision is created and sealed with a GelPoint® access device, through which a 10-mm port is inserted for the passage of needles, staplers, and extraction bags.

Step 1: Mobilization of the Right Colon and Pancreatic Head

Following laparoscopic staging, the right colon is mobilized and rotated medially to expose the root of the mesentery. A flexible liver retractor is used to retract segment 4 cranially. An extended Kocher maneuver is performed to release the proximal jejunum from the ligament of Treitz. The jejunum is transected with a 3.5-mm linear cutting stapler 10 cm distal to the former ligament of Treitz and marked with an Endo Stitch 50–60 cm downstream to mark the intended location of the duodenojejunostomy.

Step 2: Division of the Gastrocolic Omentum, Proximal Duodenum, and Jejunum

The gastrocolic omentum is divided with LigaSure. The groove between the gastroepiploic vascular pedicle and the duodenum is opened

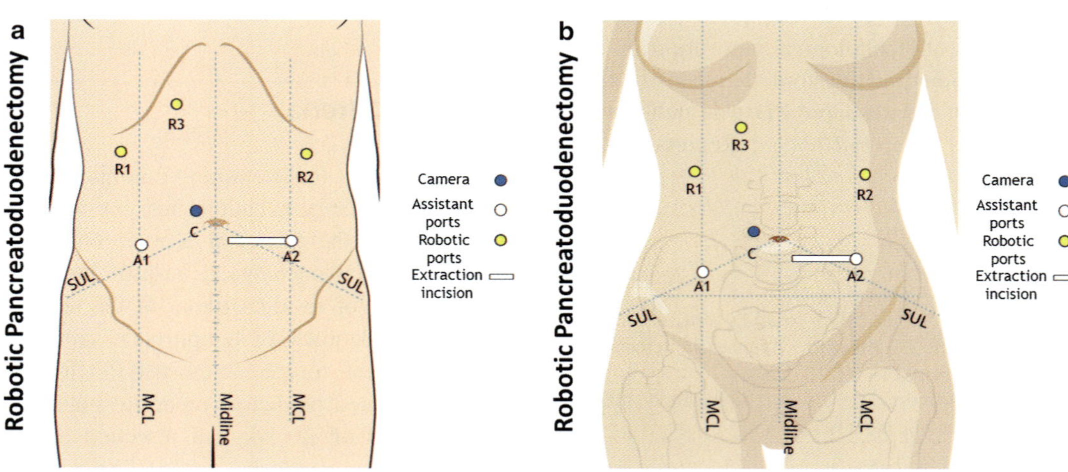

Fig. 13.1 Position of the ports during a robotic-assisted pancreatoduodenectomy in male (**a**) and female (**b**). The camera port (C) is placed to the right of the umbilicus. Robotic ports (R1, R2, R3) are placed along the subcostal margin as shown. Assistant ports (A1, A2) are placed at the midclavicular line slightly inferior to the umbilicus and the extraction incision as an extension of A2 medially

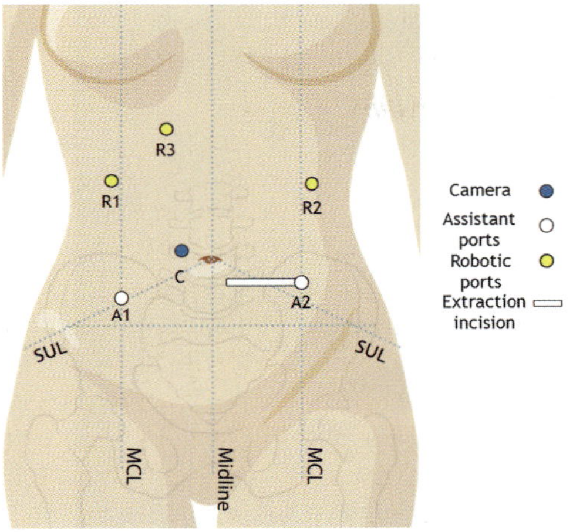

Fig. 13.2 Room setup. The patient is positioned supine on a split-leg table, and the robot is docked from straight over the patient's head. The robotic surgeon operates the console while the laparoscopic surgeon sits between the patient's legs. A *triangle* of safety is created between the robotic surgeon, the laparoscopic surgeon, and the scrub nurse, ensuring direct visualization among them

with the LigaSure. The right gastric artery is mobilized from the hepatic artery and divided to free the proximal duodenum. The duodenum is divided with a linear cutting stapler, after which the gastroepiploic pedicle is divided with a vascular stapler.

Step 3: Docking the Robot

The robot is brought over the patient's head with arms 2 and 3 on the patient's right and the patient positioned right side up in steep reverse Trendelenburg (Fig. 13.2). The robotic surgeon operates the console while the laparoscopic surgeon sits between the patient's legs.

Step 4: Portal Dissection and Division of the Bile Duct

The common hepatic artery (CHA) lymph node is resected and retrieved. The CHA is followed into the porta hepatis. The gastroduodenal artery (GDA) is temporarily occluded to confirm continued flow within the CHA and then ligated and divided with a vascular stapler. The PV is exposed and dissected into the hepatic hilum. The portal lymph nodes are swept into the specimen, searching for an aberrant right hepatic artery. The bile duct is divided with a stapler whenever possible to minimize contamination of the peritoneum with bile. The distal bile margin is resected and sent to pathology.

Step 5: Mobilization of the Portal Vein and Division of the Pancreatic Neck

The origin of the right gastroepiploic vein is identified as it enters the SMV and divided. The SMV is dissected free from the pancreatic neck, and an articulated laparoscopic grasper is used to pass an umbilical tape beneath the pancreas. 2-0 silk sutures are placed to occlude the transverse pancreatic arteries at the inferior and superior borders of the pancreas. The gland is divided with cautery scissors in an attempt to identify and sharply transect the pancreatic duct.

Step 6: Division of the Retroperitoneal Margin

The pancreas is elevated from the retroperitoneum using the third robotic arm. Venous tributaries on the lateral margin of the SMV-PV, superior pancreaticoduodenal vein, and tributaries from the first jejunal vein to the uncinate process are ligated with 3-0 silk ties and divided sharply. Arterial branches from the SMA are either divided with the LigaSure or controlled proximally with a silk tie and clip and transected distally with the LigaSure. The specimen is retrieved in a specimen bag and examined by frozen section. Gold fiducials are placed in cases of suspected malignancy. Lastly, antegrade cholecystectomy is performed.

Step 7: Reconstruction

A duct-to-mucosa pancreaticojejunostomy is performed using a modified Blumgart technique. Interrupted 5-0 Vicryl sutures are placed around the pancreatic duct to facilitate visualization. 2-0

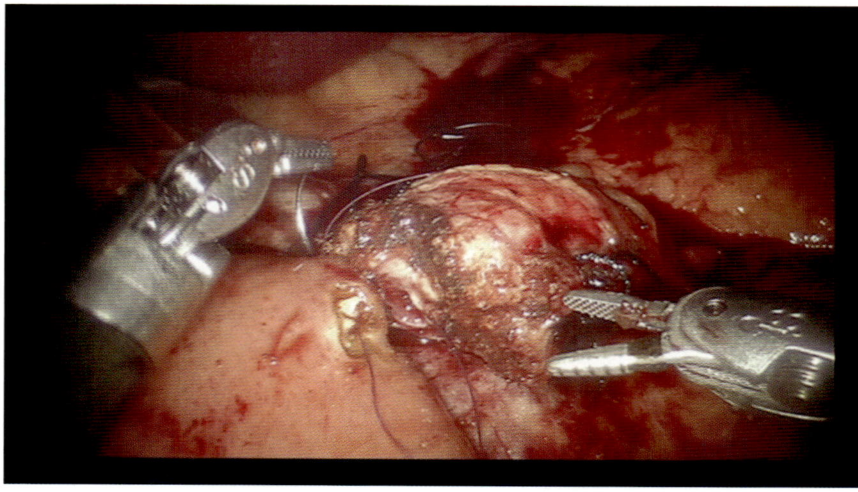

Fig. 13.3 Pancreaticojejunostomy. Picture demonstrates the corner stitch of the duct-to-mucosa anastomosis performed using a modified Blumgart technique with interrupted 5-0 Vicryl sutures and 2-0 silk horizontal mattress sutures to anchor the seromuscular layer of the jejunum

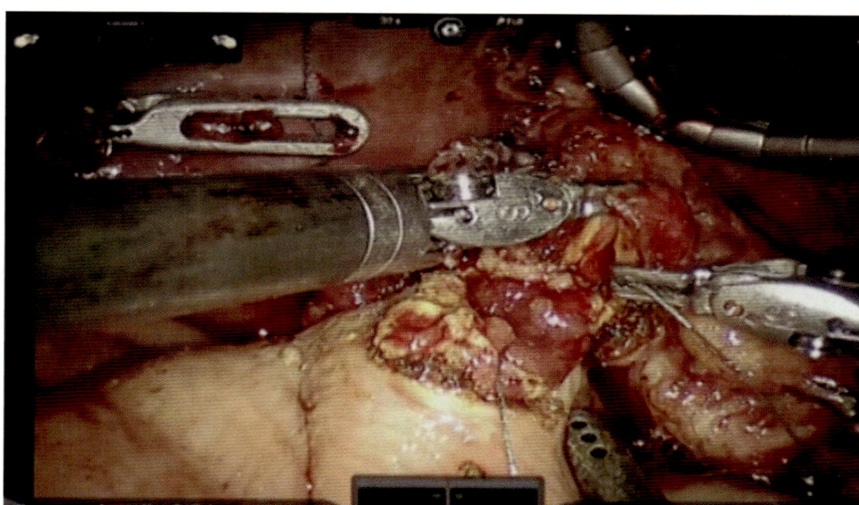

Fig. 13.4 Hepaticojejunostomy. Picture demonstrates the back row of the single-layer end-to-side anastomosis created with interrupted 5-0 Vicryl

silk horizontal mattress sutures are passed through the pancreas to anchor the seromuscular layer of the jejunum. A small enterotomy is made in the jejunum with robotic scissors, and an interrupted duct-to-mucosa anastomosis is completed (Fig. 13.3). The anastomosis is completed with an anterior layer of 2-0 silk sutures. A single-layer end-to-side hepaticojejunostomy is created with interrupted 5-0 Vicryl (Fig. 13.4). A running technique is used for ducts >5 mm in diameter when visualization is optimal. Finally, an antecolic, two-layer duodenojejunostomy is performed (Fig. 13.5). A posterior layer of interrupted seromuscular 2-0 silk sutures is placed,

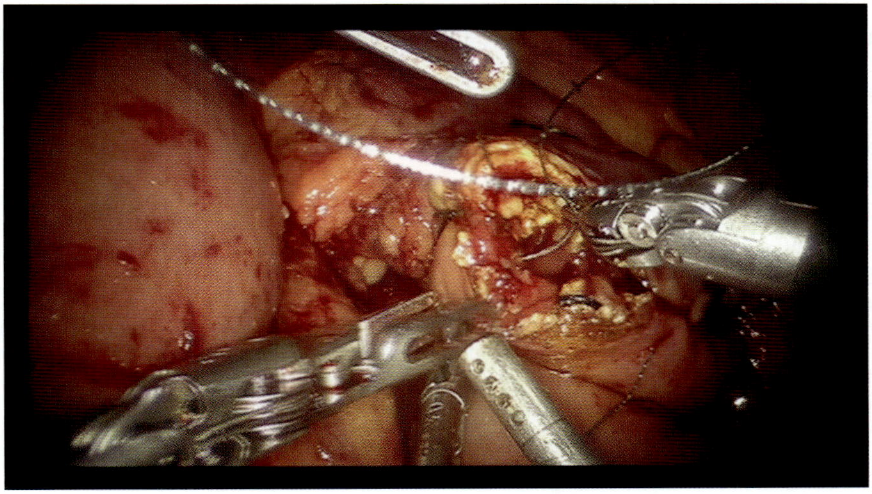

Fig. 13.5 Duodenojejunostomy. Picture demonstrates the anterior corner stitch of the antecolic, two-layer anastomosis, with interrupted seromuscular 2-0 silk sutures posteriorly, followed by a full-thickness running 3-0 Vicryl after the duodenum and jejunum are opened

followed by full-thickness running 3-0 Vicryl after the duodenum and jejunum are opened. Two round 19 F surgical drains are placed: one anterior and one posterior to the biliary and pancreatic anastomoses. The robot is undocked, and the right lower quadrant incision and camera port are closed. The skin is closed with a monofilament subcuticular closure.

Outcomes

Analysis of outcomes in our first 50 patients undergoing attempted RAPD demonstrated a median age of 72 years (range 27–85). The predominant indications for surgery were pancreatic ductal carcinoma (14, 28 %), neuroendocrine tumor (10, 20 %), ampullary adenocarcinoma (9, 18 %), and intraductal papillary mucinous neoplasm (9, 18 %). The median duration of attempted RAPD was 568 min (IQR 536–629) including the time to undock and convert to an open procedure in eight patients (16 %). Median blood loss was 350 mL (IQR 150–625), and 11 patients (22 %) required transfusion during their index hospital stay. Conversion to open procedure was required in eight patients (16 %), and the reasons for conversion were failure to progress ($n=4$), unsuspected abutment of the PV by tumor ($n=2$), and unsuspected microscopic tumor at the pancreatic neck margin ($n=2$) by frozen section. At intention-to-treat analysis, pancreatic fistula as defined by the International Study Group of Pancreatic Surgery occurred in ten patients (20 %). The margin-negative resection rate was 89 %, and the median number of lymph nodes collected was 18 [12, 14, 15].

Conclusion

Robotic-assisted pancreatoduodenectomy (RAPD) allows the recreation of time-tested techniques for open pancreatic surgery through a minimally invasive approach. The robotic platform is able to overcome the current limitations of laparoscopic surgery, including limited range of motion, poor surgeon ergonomics, and lack of 3D view. Early outcomes of robotic-assisted major pancreatic resection are comparable to laparoscopic and open approaches. Technological innovations and increased surgeon familiarity with this approach will lead to greater adoption and acceptance. Next-generation robots may expedite these efforts, hopefully at lower cost.

References

1. Whipple AO. Pancreaticoduodenectomy for Islet carcinoma: a five-year follow-up. Ann Surg. 1945;121(6): 847–52.
2. Traverso LW, Longmire Jr WP. Preservation of the pylorus in pancreaticoduodenectomy. Surg Gynecol Obstet. 1978;146(6):959–62.
3. Howard JM. Pancreatico-duodenectomy: forty-one consecutive Whipple resections without an operative mortality. Ann Surg. 1968;168(4):629–40.
4. Crist DW, Sitzmann JV, Cameron JL. Improved hospital morbidity, mortality, and survival after the Whipple procedure. Ann Surg. 1987;206(3):358–65.
5. Gagner M, Pomp A. Laparoscopic pylorus-preserving pancreatoduodenectomy. Surg Endosc. 1994;8(5): 408–10.
6. Palanivelu C, Rajan PS, Rangarajan M, Vaithiswaran V, Senthilnathan P, Parthasarathi R, Praveen RP. Evolution in techniques of laparoscopic pancreaticoduodenectomy: a decade long experience from a tertiary center. J Hepatobiliary Pancreat Surg. 2009; 16(6):731–40.
7. Kendrick ML, Cusati D. Total laparoscopic pancreaticoduodenectomy: feasibility and outcome in an early experience. Arch Surg. 2010;145(1):19–23.
8. Gagner M, Palermo M. Laparoscopic Whipple procedure: review of the literature. J Hepatobiliary Pancreat Surg. 2009;16(6):726–30.
9. Giulianotti PC, Sbrana F, Bianco FM, Elli EF, Shah G, Addeo P, Caravaglios G, Coratti A. Robot-assisted laparoscopic pancreatic surgery: single- surgeon experience. Surg Endosc. 2010;24(7):1646–57.
10. Narula VK, Mikami DJ, Melvin WS. Robotic and laparoscopic pancreaticoduodenectomy: a hybrid approach. Pancreas. 2010;39(2):160–4.
11. Moser AJ, Zeh HJ. Robotic pancreaticoduodenectomy. In: Fischer JE, Jones DB, Pomposelli FB, Upchurch Jr GR, editors. Fischer's mastery of surgery, vol. 133A. 6th ed. Philadelphia, PA: Lippincott Williams & Wilkins; 2011. p. 92–9.
12. Zureikat AH, Nguyen KT, Bartlett DL, Zeh HJ, Moser AJ. Robotic-assisted major pancreatic resection and reconstruction. Arch Surg. 2011;146(3):256–61.
13. Nguyen KT, Zureikat AH, Chalikonda S, Bartlett DL, Moser AJ, Zeh HJ. Technical aspects of robotic-assisted pancreaticoduodenectomy (RAPD). J Gastrointest Surg. 2011;15(5):870–5.
14. Zeh III HJ, Bartlett DL, Moser AJ. Robotic-assisted major pancreatic resection. Adv Surg. 2011;45:323–40.
15. Zeh HJ, Zureikat AH, Secrest A, Dauoudi M, Bartlett D, Moser AJ. Outcomes after robot-assisted pancreaticoduodenectomy for periampullary lesions. Ann Surg Oncol. 2012;19(3):864–70.
16. Bao P, Potter D, Eisenberg DP, Lenzner D, Zeh HJ, Lee Iii KK, Hughes SJ, Sanders MK, Young JL, Moser AJ. Validation of a prediction rule to maximize curative (R0) resection of early-stage pancreatic adenocarcinoma. HPB (Oxford). 2009;11(7):606–11.

Robotic Distal Pancreatectomy

14

Anusak Yiengpruksawan

Introduction

Similar to cholecystectomy and adrenalectomy, the surgical approach to distal pancreatectomy is evolving from an open to a minimally invasive procedure [1–3]. The safety and feasibility of minimally invasive distal pancreatectomy (DP) has been shown to be equal, if not superior, to its open counterpart [3–9]. Unlike laparoscopic cholecystectomy, which is technically straightforward and commonly performed by most general surgeons, laparoscopic distal pancreatectomy is a much more complex and a less common procedure. In addition, certain technical disadvantages associated with laparoscopy and the steep learning curve required to master the technique have limited the global adoption of the laparoscopic DP approach and remain limited to a few pancreatic surgeons and centers.

Compared to laparoscopic surgery, the robotic approach has several advantages. The greatest advantage is that robotic surgery brings the open-surgery "feeling" or "experience" to the minimally invasive environment by providing the surgeon with intuitive hand-eye coordination, three-dimensional vision, and dexterity enhancement. The endowrist technology enables the surgeon to perform meticulous, delicate, and complex tasks such as knot tying, suturing, and vascular or lymph node dissection. For robotic distal pancreatectomy, these advantages are especially of significance when splenic vessels are to be preserved or extended lymphadenectomy is required in cancer cases. The main drawback of robotic surgery is the lack of tactile feedback, which forces the surgeon to rely on visual guidance. With the advent of da Vinci robotic technology, surgeons with experience in open pancreatic procedures, but with limited laparoscopic skills, can achieve proficiency in minimally invasive pancreatectomy in an efficient and safe manner.

Application of the robotic platform to pancreatic resection has evolved in a similar fashion as laparoscopic pancreatectomy, with the left-sided (distal) pancreas as an initial procedure. A standard distal pancreatectomy requires only extirpation compared to that of the right-sided (proximal) pancreas (i.e., Whipple procedure), which mandates complex vascular dissection in addition to gastrointestinal reconstruction. Technical details of robotic distal pancreatectomy were initially described by Giulianotti and later by others [10–14]. This chapter describes the technical approach to robotic DP, including technical tips, culminating from the author's 10-year experience in robotic pancreatic surgery.

A. Yiengpruksawan, M.D., F.A.C.S. (✉)
Department of Surgery, The Valley Minimally Invasive and Robotic Surgery Center, The Valley Hospital, North van Dien Avenue, Ridgewood, NJ 07450, USA
e-mail: yienga@mac.com

K.C. Kim (ed.), *Robotics in General Surgery*, DOI 10.1007/978-1-4614-8739-5_14,

Procedure Overview (Fig. 14.1)

The standard position for DP begins by placing the patient in an oblique 30° right lateral position (left side up) supported by a pillow or a roll of linen sheet behind the left mid-back, with both arms tucked along the body and protected by foam protectors. Next, "fine tuning" of the initial positioning prior to docking the robot should be performed and will depend on the tumor location. For more proximal pancreatic lesions (pancreatic neck), the patient is placed in a less-oblique angle (almost supine) with the table placed in a reverse Trendelenburg position to allow for adequate exposure of the portal-SMV junction if necessary. For true pancreatic tail lesions, additional obliquing of the patient to 45° allows the stomach to fall to the right, which improves exposure as well as facilitates the splenectomy portion of the procedure.

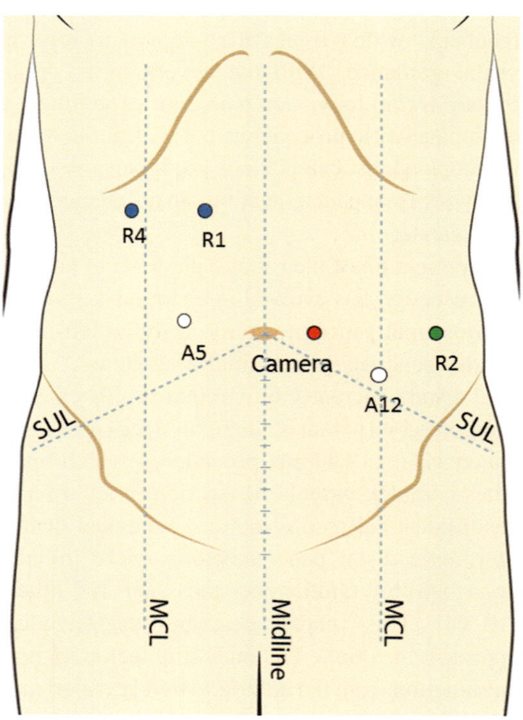

Fig. 14.1 Patient and port positioning

Pneumoperitoneum Technique

To achieve initial pneumoperitoneum, the left subcostal approach using a Veress needle technique is preferred. The insufflation tubing is connected to the needle, and the insertion is done under continuous CO_2 flow. The entry into the peritoneal cavity is confirmed by a drop in CO_2 pressure to near zero. [*TIP*: *The needle insertion under pressure-monitoring technique is especially helpful in an obese patient. The ideal puncture site is just right below the costal margin between the midclavicular and anterior axillary lines. Lifting the abdomen up prior to needle insertion can help separate the omentum from the anterior abdominal wall. Gastric decompression prior to the procedure is mandatory to prevent inadvertent puncture of the distended stomach. This technique is contraindicated in patients with splenomegaly, portal hypertension, or bowel distention.*] However, in a patient with previous left upper abdominal surgery, an open (Hassan's) technique is used with the camera port. The camera port (12 mm) is placed 3–4 cm to the left of the umbilicus or at the umbilicus if the lesion is near the pancreatic neck.

Trocar Placement

As in patient positioning, choosing locations for trocar placement should be based on patient's body habitus, location of the lesion, and the extent of dissection and/or resection. After placement of the camera port as described above, three robotic trocars (8 mm) and a 12 mm accessory ports are placed. The 12 mm accessory port and one robot port are placed on the patient's left, while two robotic ports and, occasionally, an additional 5 mm accessory port may be needed on the patient's right, and all are placed under direct vision. Robotic trocars are usually placed first. [*TIP*: *Choosing the placement sites for the fourth arm and accessory ports after the docking of the surgical cart to the camera, right and left instrument ports, allows the surgeon to assess the possibility of robotic arm collision and whether the accessory ports are accessible before making incisions*.] The left robotic port (R2) is placed along the left anterior axillary line at the level of the umbilicus. The right robotic port (R1) is then placed on the right upper abdomen along the pararectal (for distal lesion) or midclavicular (for more midline lesion) line, 3–4 cm above the umbilicus, while the fourth robotic port (R4) is placed along the right midclavicular (for distal lesion) or anterior axillary line (for more midline lesion) at the same level as the right robotic port. A 12 mm accessory port is then placed between the camera port and the left robot port and 4–5 cm inferiorly. The 5 mm accessory port, if needed, is positioned on the right abdomen in a mirror image to the 12 mm accessory port.

Once the trocars are placed and patient positioning confirmed, docking of the robot is then performed. The surgical cart is brought in superiorly, approximately 20° to the left of the patient's longitudinal axis. It is important to place the robot's fourth arm on the patient's right side (surgeon's left) prior to docking. Once docked, robotic instruments are placed through the robotic trocars. The R1 port holds the bipolar forceps, the R2 port uses a monopolar cautery hook, and the R4 holds the grasper forceps.

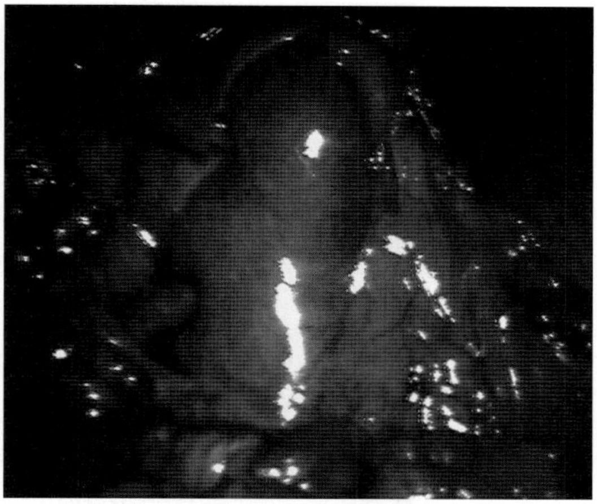

Fig. 14.2 Firefly fluorescence imaging showing illuminating spleen

Technique

Step 1: Exposure of the Pancreatic Neck, Body, and Tail

Using the grasper forceps (R4), the anterior wall of the mid-gastric body is grasped close to the greater curvature and lifted cranially to open the lesser sac space. The gastrocolic attachments are divided below and along the gastroepiploic arcade from the prepyloric antrum to the fundus using the electrocautery hook and the bipolar coagulator. With lesions located close to the pancreatic neck, the right-sided dissection of the omentum should be carried out until the right gastroepiploic vessels and the duodenum are fully exposed. This step will help in localizing and exposing the superior mesenteric vein as it courses underneath the pancreatic neck. Short gastric vessels may be divided at this stage if splenectomy is planned. However, they should be left intact if a surgeon intends to preserve the spleen using Warshaw's technique (en bloc resection of splenic vessels). [*TIP*: *Viability of spleen can be assessed more definitively by injecting ICG dye and shining infrared light on the spleen ("firefly" fluorescence imaging). If there is blood flow into the spleen, it will illuminate fluorescence green (Fig. 14.2). If majority of the spleen does not illuminate, splenectomy should then be performed.*]

Once the greater curve of the stomach is adequately mobilized, complete mobilization of splenic flexure of the colon is generally accomplished prior to pancreatic mobilization. This can be performed by continuing the dissection from a medial to lateral approach or a lateral to medial approach, depending on patient anatomy, tumor size, and location.

The pancreatogastric fold (ligament) is next divided to fully expose the pancreatic body. Care is taken not to injure the left gastric vein unless subtotal pancreatectomy is to be performed. The mobilized stomach is retracted superiorly and held cranially either by the fourth arm or a retractor via an accessory port. [*TIP*: *Suturing the stomach to the falciform ligament and diaphragm frees up the fourth arm, which would otherwise be used to hold up the stomach. In addition, having the stomach fixed in position helps to create a*

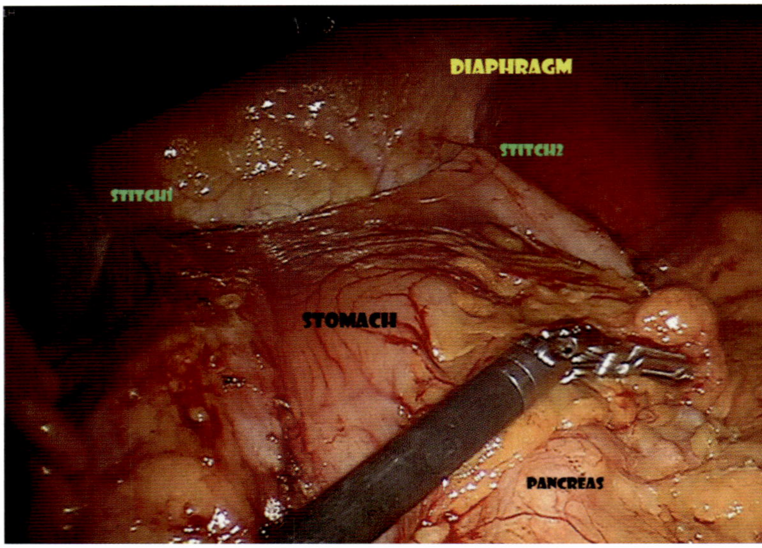

Fig. 14.3 Tagging of stomach to the anterior abdominal wall

stable operative field (Fig. 14.3).] Intraoperative ultrasound of the pancreas, using a laparoscopic 8 MHz probe, can be performed if the lesion is small and in the proximal pancreas. Ultrasound images can be displayed in the surgeon console using the TilePro system.

Step 2: Mobilization of the Pancreas and Spleen and Identification of the Proximal Splenic Vessels

Once the greater curve of the stomach and splenic flexure of the colon are mobilized, and the lesion is identified, the transverse mesocolon is retracted inferiorly to define the inferior border of the pancreas. The peritoneum overlying the inferior border of the pancreatic body is incised using the cautery hook and the loose areolar tissue posterior to the pancreas. Dissection is carried out toward the patient's left along this plane. For pancreaticosplenectomy, mobilization of the spleen together with the distal pancreas in continuity is preferred. This approach is more efficient and less time consuming and involves less bleeding, since dissection is along the same plane leading to the splenorenal and splenophrenic ligaments, both of which are quite avascular. The fourth arm (R4) retracts the spleen medially, providing exposure of the splenorenal and splenophrenic attachments. Retraction is facilitated by leaving a small "tag" of splenorenal peritoneum connected to the spleen to be used as a handle for grasping and to prevent splenic bleeding secondary to retraction injury.

As the dissection continues to the left, the pancreas is gently lifted and rotated upward and held by the fourth arm grasper forceps. As the posterior border of the dissection proceeds, the splenic vein is identified about halfway to two-thirds superiorly from the lower border of the pancreas (Fig. 14.4). In some patients, the tortuous part of the splenic artery may be found immediately after identifying the splenic vein, indicating that the dissection has reached the superior edge of the pancreas. The lesser sac bursa is then entered by continuing the dissection between the artery and lymphatic tissue until the bursa cavity is visualized. Sometimes it is much easier to come around the upper edge of the pancreas near the upper pole of the spleen since there is less fatty lymphatic tissue and the peritoneum is much better defined. A vessel loop or an umbilical tape can then be passed behind the pancreas and looped around it to help in further

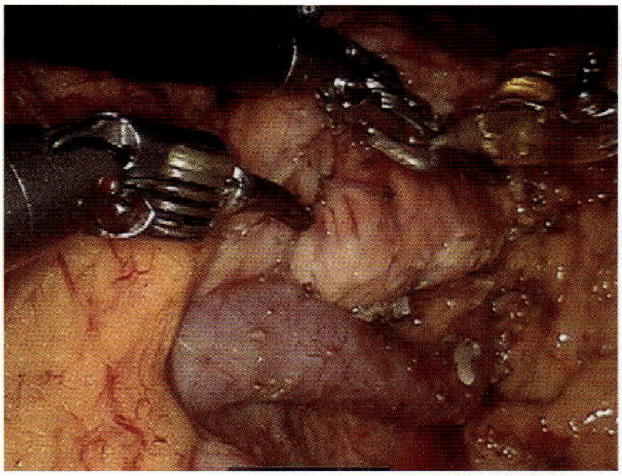

Fig. 14.4 Splenic vein

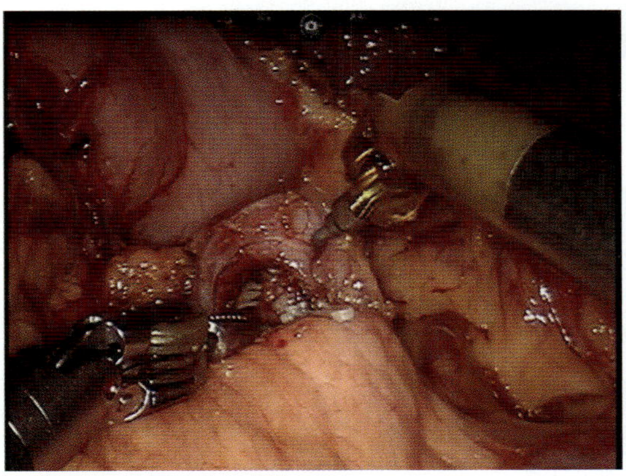

Fig. 14.5 Splenic artery

pancreatic mobilization ("hanging" technique). Control of splenic artery at this location is sufficient if the margin of the proximal pancreatic resection is distal to it. For subtotal pancreatosplenectomy, it is essential to isolate and control the artery near its origin from the celiac trunk. This dissection requires an anterior approach to reach the superior aspect of the pancreas (Fig. 14.5) [*TIP*: *To locate the origin of the splenic artery, often it is easier to start from the common hepatic artery (since it is readily recognized) and then trace back toward the celiac trunk. Lymph node dissection can also be simultaneously performed. The left gastric vein may have to be divided for better exposure. Nuisance bleeding from lymphatic tissue around the celiac region can be controlled with bipolar energy or with just pressure gauze. To avoid inadvertent ligation of celiac trunk or common hepatic artery, the splenic artery should be exposed well into the pancreas or ligated distal to the left gastric artery. The latter artery may form a common trunk with the splenic artery or arises separately from the celiac trunk.*]

Step 3: Pancreatic and Vascular Transection

Transection of pancreas for en bloc splenectomy can be performed together with splenic vessels or separately, depending on ease of dissection. The pancreas is mobilized proximally up to the portosplenic junction (Fig. 14.6), and the splenic artery and vein are identified.

If the vessels can be isolated, it is preferable to divide the splenic artery first and then the vein to avoid splenic congestion, but it is not essential. The vessel can be divided using a vascular stapler or clips (Hem-o-loks®). If the lesion is found adherent to splenic vein close to the portal vein trunk, partial resection (Figs. 14.7 and 14.8) or resection of the portal vein with reconstruction may be necessary.

Once the vessels have been controlled, the pancreas is subsequently divided with an endo-GIA stapler (Fig. 14.9). Bioabsorbable staple line reinforcement strips placed on the stapler cartridge (Seamguard®) can be used to reinforce the stump to prevent pancreatic leak. Closure of stapler jaws should be slow and gradual to allow for smooth tissue approximation.

If the vessels cannot be safely dissected from the pancreatic parenchyma, or the pancreas is too thick for the stapler, the pancreas is divided in a stepwise fashion using a combination of cutting, cauterization, and suture ligation (Fig. 14.10). Care must be taken during this approach that the vessels, which are partially exposed, can be protected at all times. The proximal stump of the pancreas is then closed using running 3-0 Prolene suture, and fibrin glue may be applied to decrease pancreatic leak. If the pancreatic duct is visible, it is first transfixed with the same suture.

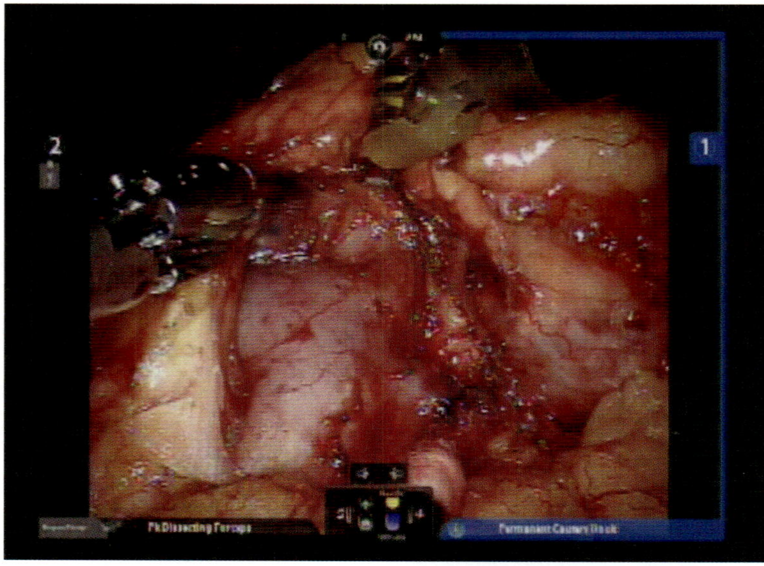

Fig. 14.6 Portomesenteric-splenic junction

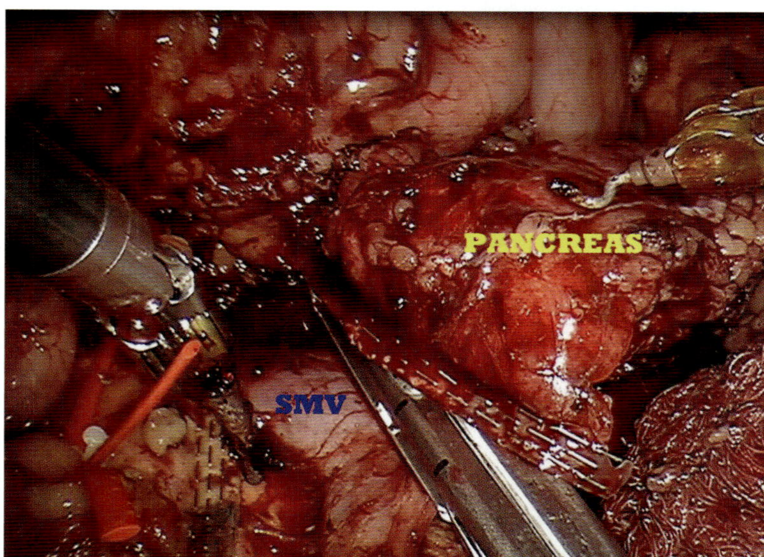

Fig. 14.7 Partial resection of SMV

Step 4: Splenic-Preserving Distal Pancreatectomy

Splenic preservation may be attempted for certain histologies and anatomy. There are two approaches for splenic preservation, which are dictated by location of the lesion. For far distal tumors, a lateral to medial approach may be used. For body lesions, it is often safer to approach splenic preservation from a medial to lateral approach. [*TIP*: *Knowledge of the relationship between the pancreatic tail and spleen from*

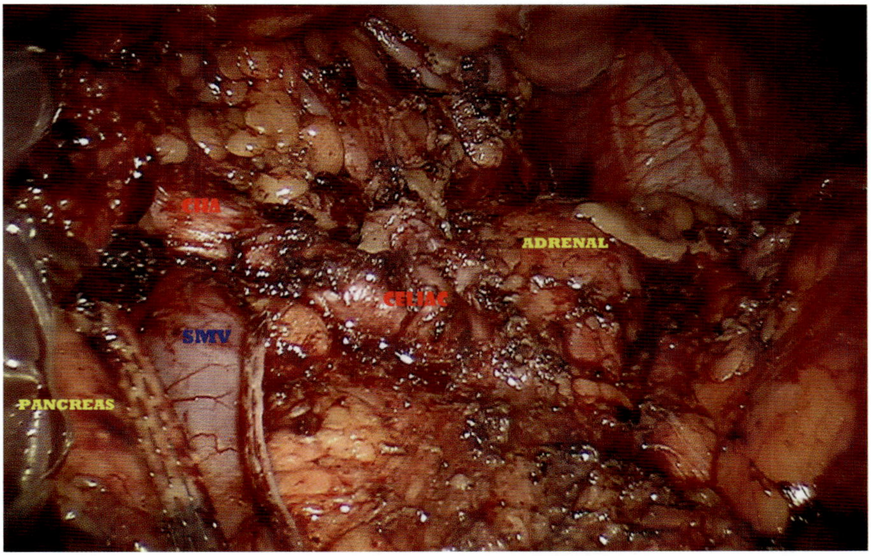

Fig. 14.8 Celiac trunk after wedge resection of SMV

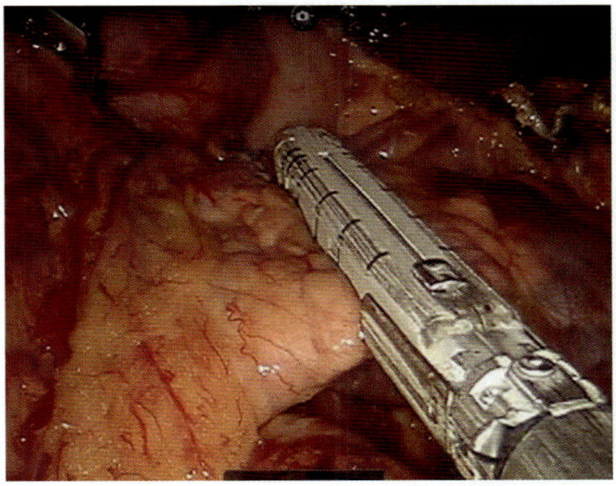

Fig. 14.9 Pancreatic transection with staplers

preoperative imaging study facilitates the distal dissection. In some patients, a short pancreatic tail or lack of one creates a wide gap; in others the tail may lie snugly near the splenic hilum. For the latter, the splenic flexure may have to be completely detached from the spleen in order to safely free the tail from the hilum.]

Medial to Lateral Approach

Similar to pancreaticosplenectomy, the pancreas is mobilized proximally up to the portosplenic junction (Fig. 14.6), and the splenic artery and vein are identified. A plane is developed between the pancreas and the splenic vein, and pancreas parenchyma is transected proximal to the lesion.

After the pancreas is transected, the distal stump is grasped and carefully retracted laterally toward the left while it is dissected away from the vessels (Figs. 14.11 and 14.12). There are 3–4 short perforating vessels into the pancreatic body that require meticulous dissection to achieve adequate length before they can be ligated with fine sutures and divided. Stay sutures may be placed on the stump to allow for easy manipulation of the pancreas. Using the fourth arm (R4) to hold and stabilize the pancreas during the dissection makes the process much more efficient and safer. During the dissection and mobilization, there are two areas requiring particular attention. The first area is at the looping portion of the splenic artery. Here, it is important to dissect along the curvature of the artery while paying careful attention to the medially located splenic vein (Fig. 14.11). In some instances, the splenic artery may form a smooth curve and appear to run parallel to the vein (Fig. 14.12). It is, therefore, important to study preoperative images and know the topographic anatomy, including the vascular pattern before the

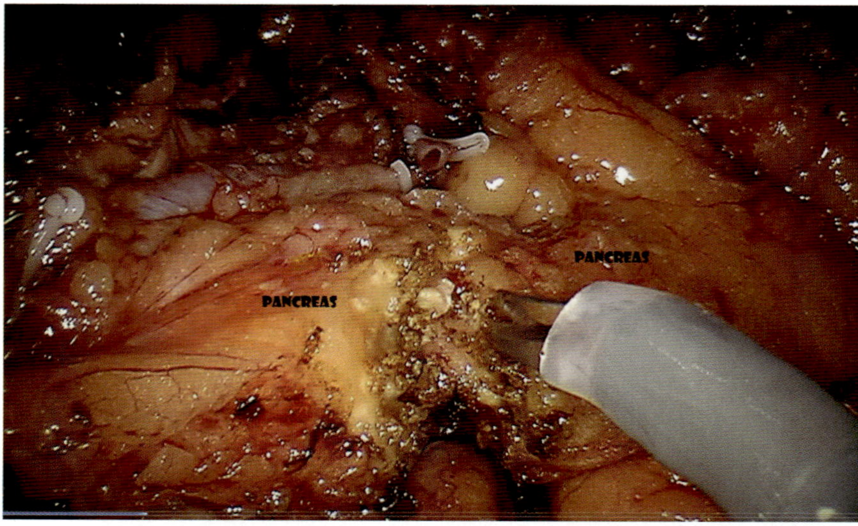

Fig. 14.10 Manual transection of pancreas

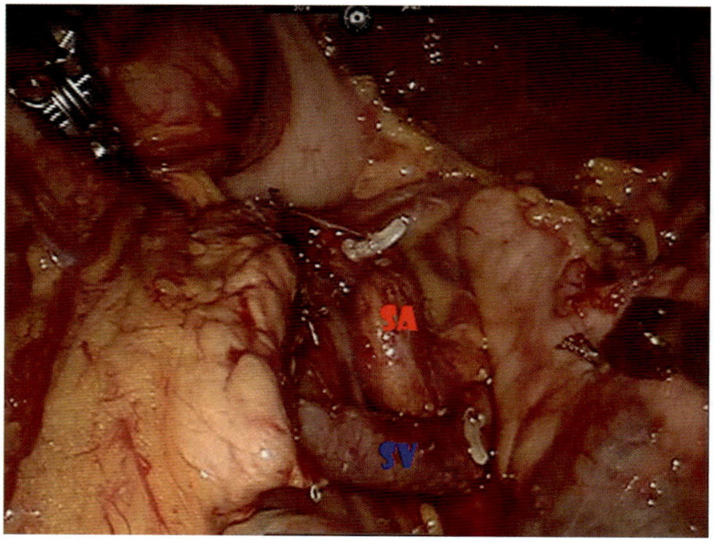

Fig. 14.11 Tortuous splenic artery (SA)

surgery. The second area is around the tail of the pancreas where several vessels may be found clustered together and can be easily injured.

Lateral to Medial Approach

Lateral to medial approach is often used when the lesion is in the distal tail. As described above, preoperative evaluation of the CT scan with particular attention to the relationship of the tail of the pancreas and spleen should be noted. For this approach, complete mobilization of the splenic flexure of the colon should be done initially. Once the tail of the pancreas and spleen are fully exposed, the tail of the pancreas is retracted medially and downward. Small perforating vessels are controlled with the bipolar electrocautery or clips. The pancreas can be divided once a margin of at least 2 cm proximal to the lesion is achieved.

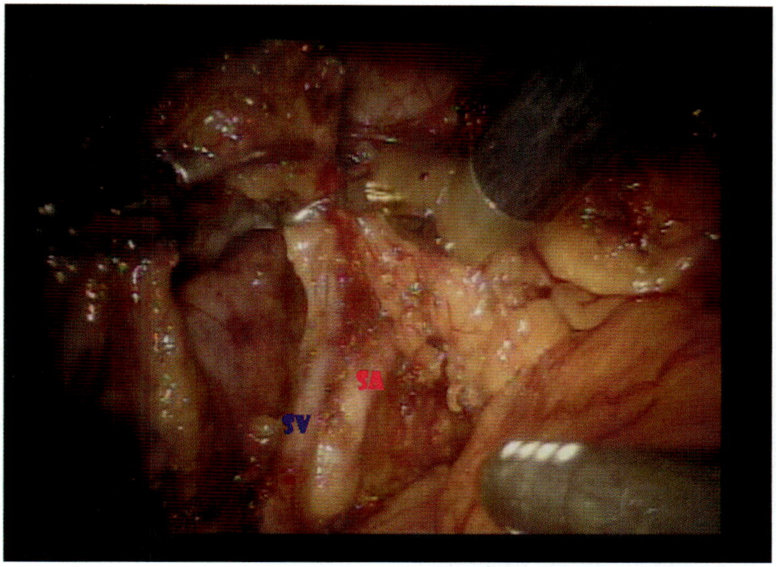

Fig. 14.12 Straight splenic artery

Step 5: Specimen Extraction

The resected specimen is placed in the endobag placed through the 12 mm accessory port. The specimen is brought out either through the enlarged 12 mm accessory port incision (for a small specimen) or a Pfannenstiel incision (for a larger specimen). [*TIP*: *When a Pfannenstiel incision is made, it is better to keep pneumoperitoneum for easy access into the peritoneal cavity. This is especially helpful in an obese patient with thick preperitoneal fat. Care should be taken to prevent splashing of blood when the peritoneum is open.*] After adequate hemostasis is confirmed, a closed-suction drain may be placed in the pancreatic bed and brought out through the left instrument port incision.

Discussion

Indications to proceed with the robotic approach to distal pancreatectomy should be determined by surgeon's experience with pancreatic surgery and robotic surgery. While it is quite possible to resect most pancreatic lesions through a robotic approach, it is recommended that early on in the learning curve, the surgeon begin with a simple distal pancreatosplenectomy for benign lesions. However, before attempting one's first robotic DP, the surgeon should familiarize himself/herself with robotic surgery in general and observe a similar procedure performed by other experienced robotic surgeons. In terms of institutional credentialing, most institutions require that for the initial experience, robotic surgery should be done under the supervision of an expert surgeon. Ideally, this is performed using a dual console system, which allows the experienced surgeon to assist directly. It must be emphasized that a low threshold for conversion and the use of common sense should always be considered in the early learning stage.

Published Outcome Studies to Date

Since 2003, there have been several published articles on robotic DP. However, most were case reports describing technical aspects of robotic

DP. The first report with outcome analysis was from Giulianotti et al. [11] who studied their series of 46 robotic DPs over 10 years span. Their robotic-to-open conversion rate was 6.5 % with a postoperative pancreatic fistula rate of 20.9 %. These results compared favorably with those from laparoscopic studies. The other published series by Waters et al. [12] described 17 robotic DP and compared them to open DP and laparoscopic DP. Their conversion rate was 6 % but with a reduced amount of blood loss in robotic DP group. However, the operative time was higher in robotic DP group in comparison to open DP and laparoscopic. Both studies observed a better trend toward successfully preserving splenic vessels when compared to laparoscopic and open groups. Our own (unpublished) series of 84 robotic distal pancreatectomy patients performed between January 2002 and December 2011 also showed outcomes similar to above reports. During the first 5-year period, our robotic-to-open conversion rate was as high as 18.4 % but has decreased significantly since. There was no conversion in the last 2 years. Our overall pancreatic fistula rate was 20 %, out of which 5 % was of ISGPF grade B and/or C pancreatic fistulas. There was no perioperative mortality, and the median length of stay was 5 days.

As for robotic DP for pancreatic ductal carcinoma, although perioperative outcomes such as tumor margins and number of harvested lymph nodes were similar to [11–13] both laparoscopic and open groups, long-term survival outcomes have not yet been adequately analyzed. Therefore, a randomized multi-institutional controlled study is needed to evaluate its efficacy and cost-effectiveness before it can be recommended for routine use.

Acknowledgments Lawrence Harrison, M.D., a new addition to the Valley Robotic Program, for his critiques, comments, and corrections of this chapter.

Nino Carnevale, M.D. for his consistent support and assistance during the development of the Valley Robotic Program.

References

1. Fernandez-Cruz L, Marinez I, Gilabert R, Cesar-Borges G, Astudillo E, Navarro S. Laparoscopic distal pancreatectomy combined with preservation of the spleen for cystic neoplasm of the pancreas. J Gastrointest Surg. 2004;8:439–501.
2. Pietrabissa A, Moretto C, Boggi U, Di Candio G, Mosca F. Laparoscopic distal pancreatectomy: are we ready for a standardized technique? Semin Laparosc Surg. 2004;11:179–83.
3. Uranues S, Alimoglu O, Todoric B, Toprak N, Auer T, Rondon L, Sauseng G, Pfeifer J. Laparoscopic resection of the pancreatic tail with splenic preservation. Am J Surg. 2006;192:257–61.
4. Papanivelu C, Shetty R, Jani K, Sendhikumar K, Rajan PS, Maheshkumar GS. Laparoscopic distal pancreatectomy: results of a prospective non-randomized study from a tertiary center. Surg Endosc. 2007;21:373–7.
5. Pryor A, Means JR, Pappas TN. Laparoscopic distal pancreatectomy with splenic preservation. Surg Endosc. 2007;21:2326–30.
6. Honore C, Honore P, Meurisse M. Laparoscopic spleen-preserving distal pancreatectomy: description of an original posterior approach. J Laparoendosc Adv Surg Tech A. 2007;17:686–9.
7. Bruzoni M, Sasson AR. Open and laparoscopic spleen preserving, splenic vessel-preserving distal pancreatectomy: indications and outcomes. J Gastrointest Surg. 2008;12:1202–6.
8. Nau P, Melvin WS, Narula VK, Bloomston PM, Ellison EC, Muscarella P. Laparoscopic distal pancreatectomy with splenic conservation: an operation without increased morbidity. Gastroenterol Res Pract. 2009;2009:846340.
9. Xie K, Zhi YP, Xu XW, Chen K, Yan JF, Mou YP. Laparoscopic distal pancreatectomy is as safe and feasible as open procedure: a meta-analysis. World J Gastroenterol. 2012;18:1959–67.
10. Melvin W, Needleman B, Krause K, Ellison E. Robotic resection of a pancreatic neuroendocrine tumor. J Laparoendosc Adv Surg Tech A. 2003;13:33–6.
11. Giulianotti P, Sbrana F, Bianco F, Elli E, Shah G, Addeo P, et al. Robot-assisted laparoscopic pancreatic surgery: single-surgeon experience. Surg Endosc. 2010;24:1646–57.
12. Waters J, Canal D, Wiebke E, Dumas R, Beane J, Aguilar-Saavedra J, et al. Robotic distal pancreatectomy: cost effective? Surgery. 2010;148:814–23.
13. Yiengpruksawan A. Technique for laparobotic distal pancreatectomy with preservation of spleen. J Robot Surg. 2011;5:11–5.
14. Buchs NC, Volonte F, Pugin F, Bucher P, Jung M, Morel P. Robotic pancreatic resection: how far can we go? Minerva Chir. 2011;66:603–14.

15 Robotic Hepatic Resections: Segmentectomy, Lobectomy, Parenchymal Sparing

M. Shirin Sabbaghian, David L. Bartlett, and Allan Tsung

Introduction and History

Since Langenbuch first described a planned hepatic resection in 1888 [1], the practice of liver resection has evolved tremendously. Improved understanding of hepatic anatomy [2–5], monumental advances in surgical and anesthesia technique [6–11], greater use of intraoperative ultrasound [12, 13], improved preoperative imaging techniques, and eventually the incorporation of vascular stapling devices [14] as well as energy-induced hemostasis [15–17] have all contributed to improved outcomes from liver surgery [18–20]. With these improved outcomes realized, indications for hepatic resection have been broadened to include patients with benign disease as well as select patients with abnormal liver function.

As comfort with liver surgery has grown, minimally invasive techniques have been applied with the intent to take advantage of the benefit they can bring, including less postoperative pain, decreased time of ileus, decreased length of stay, fewer postoperative complications, and improved cosmesis [21–23]. Most recently, robotic technology has been applied for use in liver surgery. Since the introduction of robotic technology to the operating room in 1985 [24], telepresence has emerged with its development inspired mostly by military intent [25]. Advances with this technology have taken such great strides that robotic techniques are able to surpass limitations of laparoscopic surgery. For example, robotic technology enables instrument movement with seven degrees of freedom (comparable to the human wrist) instead of just four degrees with laparoscopic equipment; robotic optics are three dimensional, not two; surgeon tremor is eliminated; the robot does not tire during long and sometimes repetitive procedures, and robotic surgery offers the surgeon an opportunity to operate in an optimal and comfortable position. These advantages enable an improved ability to finely dissect (particularly along the hilum of the liver), reconstruct, and maintain vascular control even in more challenging locations [26]. This theoretically makes robotic-assisted liver resection a safer minimally invasive approach, allowing for the completion of more complex procedures. The first reported robot-assisted liver resection took place in the Czech Republic in 2006 [27]. Since then, multiple centers have used robot-assistance for liver resection, and success has been reported with

M.S. Sabbaghian, M.D. • D.L. Bartlett, M.D.
Division of Surgical Oncology, Department of Surgery, University of Pittsburgh Medical Center, 5150 Centre Avenue, Pittsburgh, PA 15232, USA
e-mail: sabbaghianms@upmc.edu

A. Tsung, M.D. (✉)
Division of Hepatobiliary and Pancreatic Surgery, Department of Surgery, University of Pittsburgh Medical Center, Liver Cancer Center, Montefiore Hospital, 3459 Fifth Avenue, 7 South, Pittsburgh, PA 15213, USA
e-mail: tsunga@upmc.edu

K.C. Kim (ed.), *Robotics in General Surgery*, DOI 10.1007/978-1-4614-8739-5_15,

outcomes comparable to the laparoscopic approach, including similar short-term oncologic outcomes [28].

As success as well as investigation of the robotic-assisted liver resection continues, it is anticipated that more groups will adopt this technique. This chapter describes our methods of commonly performed liver resections—right hepatectomy, left hepatectomy, left lateral sectionectomy, and nonanatomic resection—using robotic assistance.

Indications for Robotic-Assisted Hepatectomy

As robotic assistance is a more recently applied technology, appropriate patient selection has not been explicitly defined. Currently, we recommend using the Louisville Statement [29] as a guide. This summary of the consensus conference for applications of laparoscopic liver surgery recommends surgery with minimally invasive technique for patients with a single lesion of 5 cm or less located in segments 2–6. It suggests that major liver resection can be performed with minimally invasive technique but only by those experienced both with liver surgery as well as minimally invasive liver resection. Importantly, the consensus conference suggests that the surgeon should be facile with minimally invasive technique, including the skill of intracorporeal suturing should bleeding become an issue.

Technique of Robotic-Assisted Hepatectomy

The technique of robotic-assisted hepatectomy is, as intended, the same as for open surgery except minimally invasive equipment is used. Smooth teamwork between two experienced surgeons (one at the console and one assisting) familiar with liver anatomy is imperative for these robotic-assisted procedures. This enables proper exposure, identification, and control of major structures as they are/should be encountered.

Patient Positioning, Room Setup

The patient is positioned supine with the arms tucked and legs split. The robot sits undocked at the patient's head. While we oblige what the room allows, anesthesia usually works at the patient's left shoulder and the scrub nurse at the patient's right side. One surgeon stands at the patient's right, one between the legs, and an additional surgeon or assistant on the patient's left (Fig. 15.1).

The patient will be in 30° reverse Trendelenburg position for the duration of the case after ports are placed.

Right Hepatectomy

Access is gained to the abdominal cavity via a 5 mm port ideally in the left upper quadrant (LUQ), and pneumoperitoneum of 12 mmHg is created. Additional ports are placed using a 5 mm, 30° scope for visualization (Fig. 15.2). Additional port sites include the 12 mm camera port to the right of the umbilicus, a robotic port at the right mid-abdomen on the anterior axillary line and another robotic port to the left of the umbilicus. A 12 mm assist port is place 8–10 cm inferolaterally to the camera port (this port will be used for larger instruments, such as the ultrasound and the stapler), and a 5 mm assist port is placed 8–10 cm inferolaterally to the left abdominal robotic port. The scope is changed to a 10 mm, 30° scope and placed in the camera port. Lastly, the LUQ port is changed to a robotic port.

Step 1

The round and falciform ligaments are divided using hook cautery (Fig. 15.3), exposing the anterior surface of the hepatic veins.

Step 2

The ligamentous attachments of the right liver are dissected. With the patient's right side up, the gallbladder fundus is retracted superiorly via a grasper in the LUQ port, and the right lobe of the liver is retracted anteriorly using a closed grasper in the right mid-abdominal port.

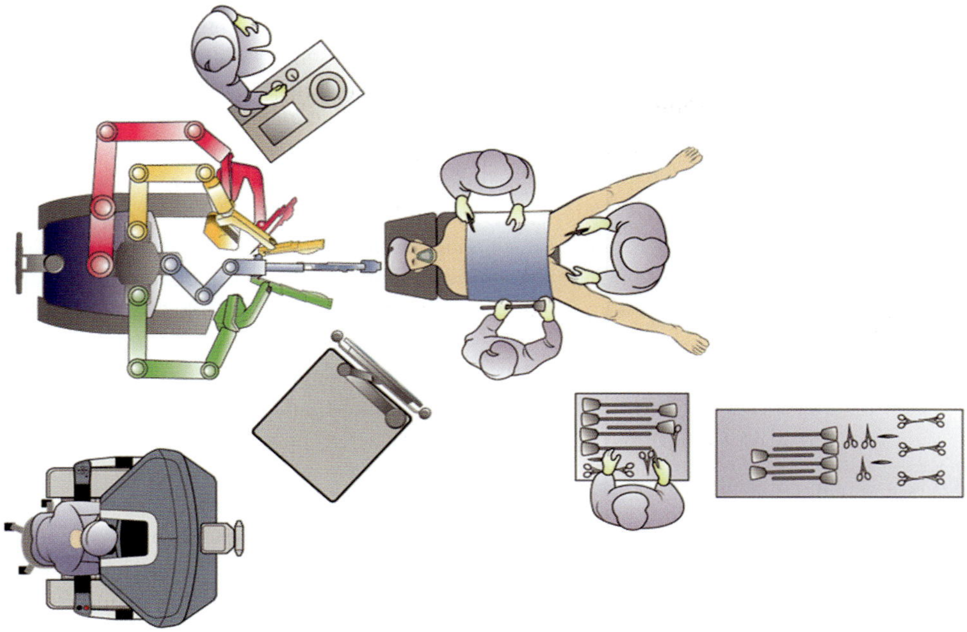

Fig. 15.1 Suggested room setup

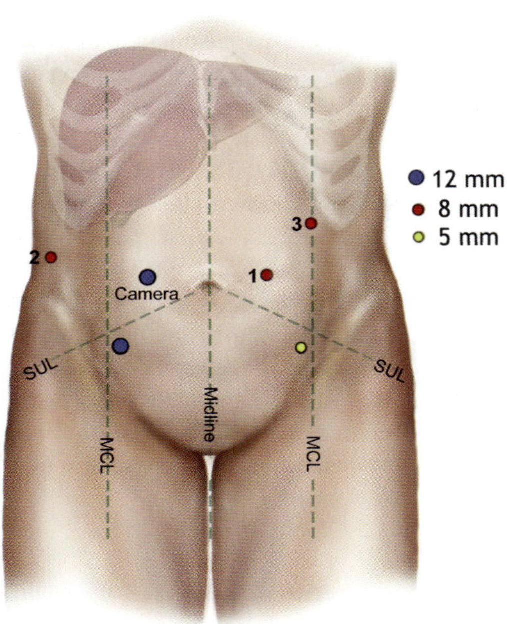

Fig. 15.2 Port placement, right hepatectomy (Used with kind permission from Randal S. McKenzie/McKenzie Illustrations)

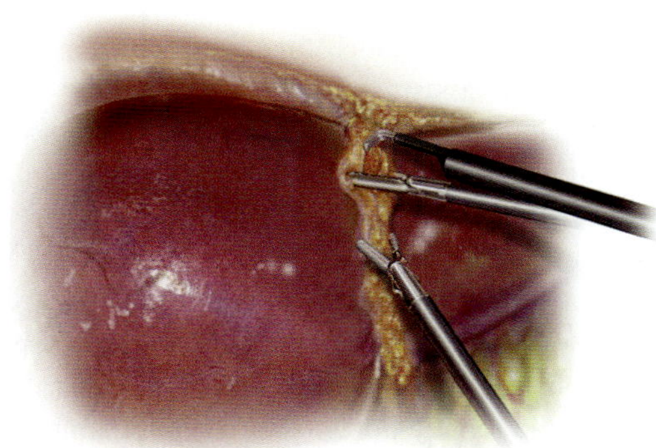

Fig. 15.3 Laparoscopic dissection of the falciform ligament (Used with kind permission from Randal S. McKenzie/McKenzie Illustrations)

The hepatic flexure is dissected and the colon is reflected inferiorly. Attachments to the duodenum are also dissected from the liver as necessary. Gerota's fascia, once exposed, is pushed posteriorly using another closed grasper. A cautery device is used to divide the right triangular

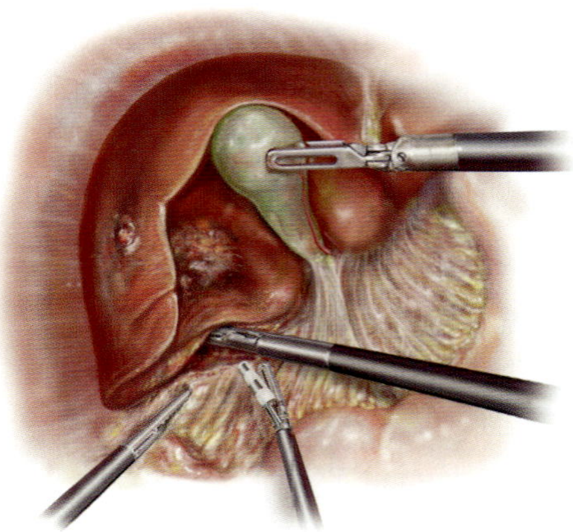

Fig. 15.4 Laparoscopic dissection of the right triangular ligament. A grasper is used to retract the gallbladder superiorly. A closed grasper is used to lift the right liver up while another instrument pushes Gerota's fascia posteriorly, exposing the right triangular ligament (Used with kind permission from Randal S. McKenzie/McKenzie Illustrations)

and coronary ligaments up to the right hepatic vein/inferior vena cava (IVC) (Fig. 15.4).

Step 3

Laparoscopic ultrasound of the liver is performed via the 12 mm assist port to confirm anatomy and ensure that the procedure will include the pathology that is anticipated.

Step 4

The robot is docked. The camera arm should be aligned with the patient's head, and the camera is docked in the camera port (Fig. 15.2). Arm 1 docks in the robotic port to the left of the umbilicus, Arm 2 docks in the right robotic port, and Arm 3 docks in the LUQ port.

Step 5

Cholecystectomy and portal dissection. With a grasper in the robotic Arm 3 retracting the fundus of the gallbladder superiorly, a bipolar grasper in robotic Arm 2 holds lateral retraction on the infundibulum while a robotic hook in Arm 1 dissects around the cystic artery and duct. After identifying the critical view, the cystic artery and duct are clipped and transected (as with a laparoscopic cholecystectomy) via the 12 mm assist port. The gallbladder should stay in situ until the portal dissection is completed. It *should be noted that this is different from the open technique…in the open technique, the gallbladder is separated from the gallbladder fossa, but the cystic duct remains intact to allow for a cholangiogram to be performed after hepatic parenchymal transection*. While maintaining superior retraction of the gallbladder, portal tissue is retracted laterally via the bipolar grasper in robotic Arm 2. The hepatoduodenal ligament is dissected using hook cautery in robotic Arm 1. The right hepatic artery (HA) is identified and defined (Fig. 15.5). If space allows, this is stapled using a vascular load, roticulating stapler through the 12 mm assist port. Otherwise, this can be tied robotically, clipped with the robotic clip applier via robotic Arm 1, and then transected. Next, the right portal vein (PV) is identified and defined. A silk tie is placed around it (this is not tied), and robotic Arm 2 retracts this tie superolaterally to expose the full length of the vein (Fig. 15.6). A vascular load, roticulating stapler is used through the 12 mm assist port to ligate and transect the right portal vein. The right hepatic duct (HD) is identified and defined. A dissecting forceps may be more beneficial than the hook if the duct is deep within adjacent tissue. The right HD is tied distally and then transected proximally (Fig. 15.7). It is important to identify bile coming from the proximal duct. Once bile is identified, the proximal duct can be clipped to maintain a clean field. The free, distal end of the right HD is doubly clipped to prevent leak. Note that during this time, the two assist ports are used to help expose as necessary. Once the portal dissection is completed, the gallbladder is dissected from the gallbladder fossa, placed in a laparoscopic bag, and removed from the abdominal cavity.

Step 6

The IVC is dissected. For exposure, the gallbladder fossa is gently pushed superiorly using a surgical sponge sponge within a grasper via robotic Arm 3 (Fig. 15.8). Suction is used in the 12 mm assist port to push the right kidney posteriorly. The IVC is exposed. The liver is mobilized from the

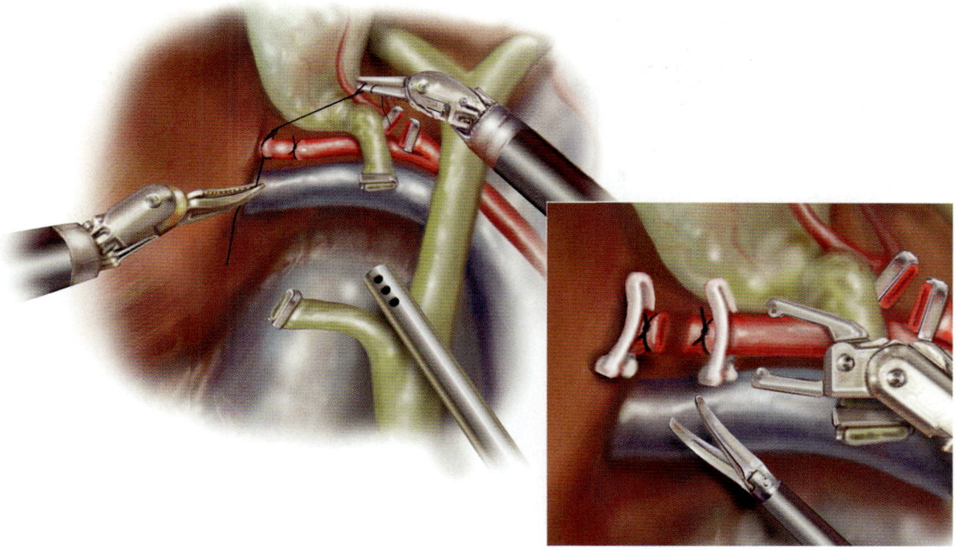

Fig. 15.5 Right hepatic artery dissection and ligation. If unable to use a stapling device, the artery is tied, clipped, and ligated. Note that exposure is achieved by using a grasper in robotic Arm 3 to grasp the gallbladder fundus and retract it superiorly (Used with kind permission from Randal S. McKenzie/McKenzie Illustrations)

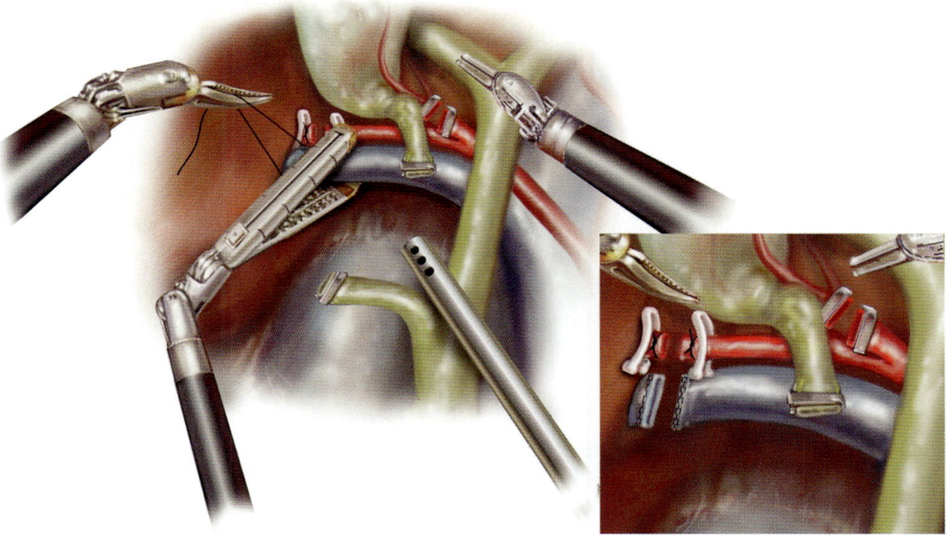

Fig. 15.6 Right portal vein ligation. A silk tie is used to retract the vein and expose its full length, allowing the roticulating stapler to fit with ease (Used with kind permission from Randal S. McKenzie/McKenzie Illustrations)

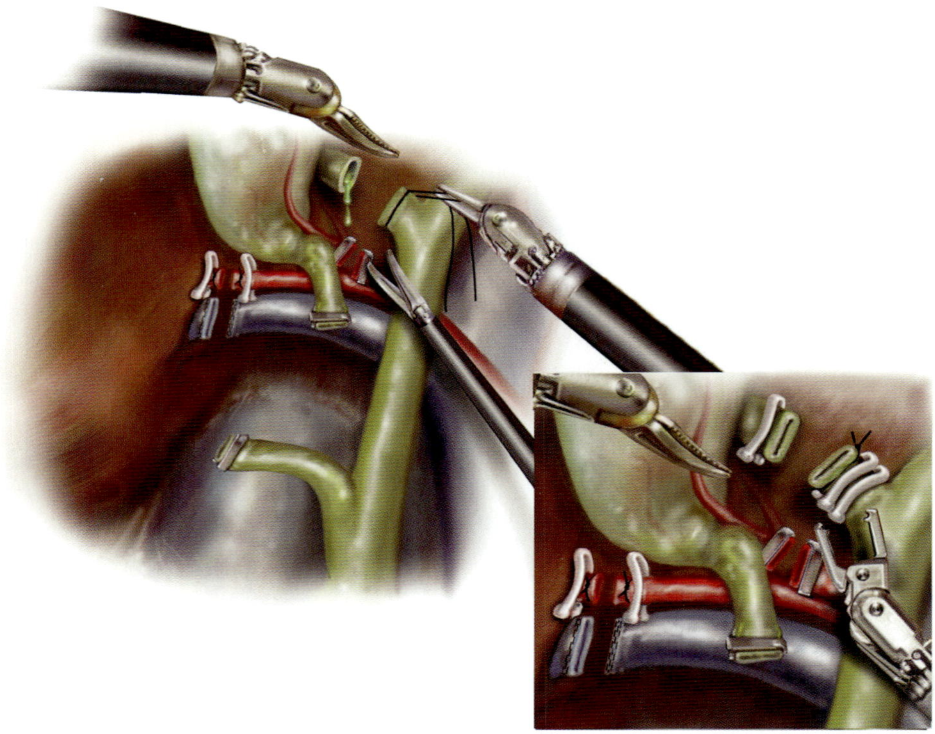

Fig. 15.7 Right hepatic duct division. It is important to identify bile coming from the proximal duct after transection. Both ends are ligated with robotic clips (Used with kind permission from Randal S. McKenzie/McKenzie Illustrations)

inferior vena cava by identifying and ligating short hepatic veins. Using a dissector in robotic Arm 2 and cautery in robotic Arm 1, the short hepatic veins are ligated with clips and silk ties, as appropriate. To clip, a robotic clip applier is passed through robotic Arm 1. To tie, a needle driver in robotic Arm 1 is used with a robotic dissector in Arm 2. This is done up to the right hepatic vein.

Step 7

The parenchyma is transected. All retracting instruments are removed, allowing the liver to drop. The line of transection is defined using hook cautery, following the line of demarcation on the liver's anterior surface. Ultrasonography is repeated to ensure again that the pathology will be included in the point of transection. Figure-of-eight stitches using 0-size absorbable suture are placed on either side of the line of transection, and these are retracted to either side using robotic ports (Fig. 15.9). The parenchyma is coagulated, placing clips when appropriate. Progress is made along the line of transection until the right hepatic vein is encountered. Using a vascular load, roticulating stapler through the 12 mm assist port, the right hepatic vein is stapled intraparenchymally. The remaining parenchyma is divided as necessary.

Step 8

The specimen is collected using a laparoscopic bag. Hemostasis on the resection bed of the liver is ensured. The proximal falciform ligament is tacked to the diaphragm with a single figure of eight stitch. The robot is undocked, and the specimen is removed from the abdominal cavity. Fascia is incised at the extraction point as necessary.

Step 9

The abdomen is closed. Laparoscopic equipment is used to remove ports under direct visualization

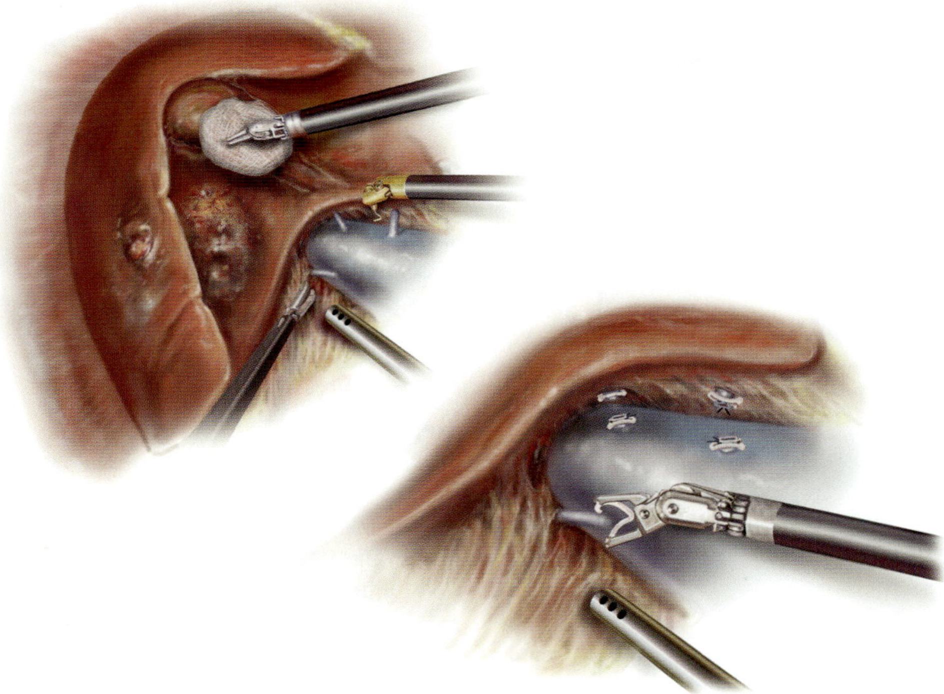

Fig. 15.8 IVC dissection. For exposure, the gallbladder fossa is gently pushed superiorly using a surgical sponge within a grasper via robotic Arm 3 (Used with kind permission from Randal S. McKenzie/McKenzie Illustrations)

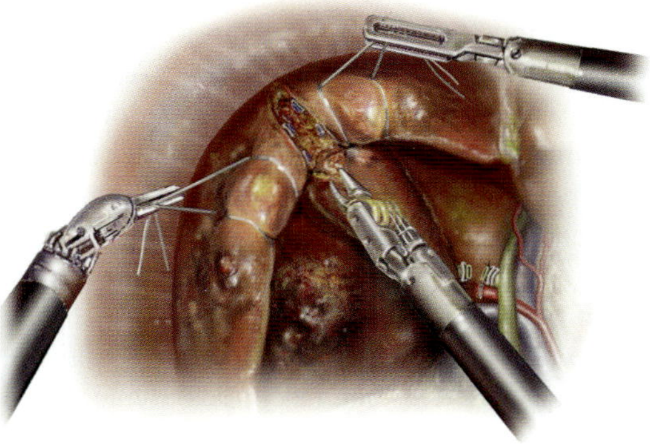

Fig. 15.9 Figure-of-eight stitches are placed on either side of the line of transection, and these are retracted to either side using robotic instruments. The parenchyma is coagulated, placing clips when appropriate. Progress is made along the line of transection until the right hepatic vein is encountered, and this is stapled intrahepatically. The remaining parenchyma is divided as necessary (Used with kind permission from Randal S. McKenzie/McKenzie Illustrations)

and close fascia. Fascia at the extraction site may need to be closed from the outside in standard manner. The skin is closed.

Left Hepatectomy

Access is gained to the abdominal cavity via a 5 mm port ideally in the LUQ, and pneumoperitoneum of 12 mmHg is created (Fig. 15.10).

A 5 mm, 30° scope is used to visualize additional port placement, including a supraumbilical, 12 mm port for the camera; a right, subcostal robotic port at the midclavicular line; a left, robotic port at the anterior axillary line; a 12 mm assist port 8–10 cm inferolateral and to the right of the camera port; and a 5 mm assist port 8–10 cm inferolateral and to the left of the camera.

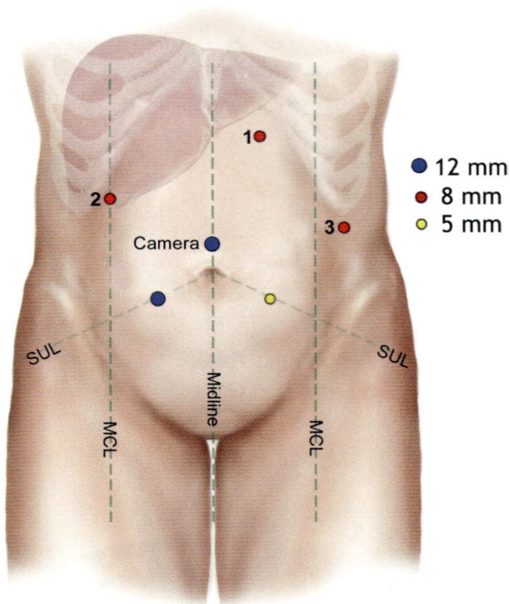

Fig. 15.10 Port placement for left hepatectomy and left lateral sectionectomy (Used with kind permission from Randal S. McKenzie/McKenzie Illustrations)

The scope is changed to a 10 mm, 30° scope for use in the camera port, and the LUQ port is changed to a robotic port.

Step 1

The round and falciform ligaments are divided using hook cautery, exposing the anterior surface of the hepatic veins.

Step 2

With the patient's left side slightly turned up, the ligamentous attachments of the left liver are dissected with a cautery device. This includes the left triangular and coronary ligaments up to the left hepatic vein. The left liver is then pushed anteriorly with a closed grasper in the right, subcostal port, allowing for exposure of the undersurface of the left liver. The gastrohepatic ligament is divided close to the left lateral segments and caudate lobe using cautery in one of the left-sided ports while a grasper in the 12 mm assist port retracts. A replaced left hepatic artery is isolated and divided at this time, if present.

Step 3

Laparoscopic ultrasound of the liver is performed through the 12 mm assist port to confirm anatomy and ensure that the procedure will include the pathology that is anticipated.

Step 4

The robot is docked. The camera arm should be aligned with the patient's head, and the camera is docked in the camera port. Arm 1 is docked in the left subcostal port; Arm 2 is docked in the right robotic port, and Arm 3 in the left port at the anterior axillary line.

Step 5

Portal dissection. With a closed grasper in robotic Arm 2, the left liver is retracted anteriorly. Hook cautery is used in robotic Arm 1 to dissect the left portal structures while a suction tip or grasper is used in the 12 mm assist port to retract. The left HA is identified and dissected, then tied robotically, clipped with the robotic clip applier via robotic Arm 1, and transected. Next, the left PV is identified. A grasper in robotic Arm 3 grasps the ligamentum teres to retract the liver anteriorly, allowing a grasping instrument in Arm 2 to retract portal tissue. After the left PV is further defined, a silk tie is placed around it (this is not tied), and robotic Arm 1 retracts this tie superiorly and to the left to expose the full length of the vein. A vascular load, roticulating stapler is used through the 12 mm assist port to ligate and transect the left PV. The left HD is identified and defined, using a dissecting forceps in robotic Arm 1 and a grasper in robotic Arm 2 for lateral retraction of adjacent portal tissue. The duct is tied distally and then transected proximally. Bile is identified from the proximal duct. This can be clipped to maintain a clean field. The free, distal end of the left HD is doubly clipped to prevent leak.

Step 7

The parenchyma is transected, and the left hepatic vein is controlled intraparenchymally. All retracting instruments are removed, allowing the liver to drop. The line of transection is defined using hook cautery, following the line of demarcation on the liver's anterior surface. Ultrasonography is repeated to ensure again that the pathology will be included in the point of transection. Figure-of-eight stitches using 0-size absorbable suture are placed on either side of the line of transection, and these are retracted to either side using robotic ports. The parenchyma is coagulated and divided, placing clips when appropriate. Progress is made up to the left hepatic vein, which is then ligated and transected using a vascular load, roticulating stapler through the 12 mm assist port.

Steps 8 and 9

Same as for right hepatectomy, although the falciform does not need to be stitched to the diaphraghm.

Left Lateral Sectionectomy

Port placement and steps 1–4 are similar to left hepatectomy.

Step 5

Parenchymal transection. The line of transection is defined just lateral to the falciform ligament. Ultrasound is repeated to ensure that the pathology is included within the specimen. Figure-of-eight stitches using 0-size absorbable suture are placed on either side of the line of transection, and these are retracted to either side using robotic ports. The parenchyma is coagulated and divided, placing clips when appropriate. A roticulating, vascular load stapler can be used via the 12 mm assist port as defined pedicles for segments II and III are encountered. The specimen is collected, and the abdomen is closed as with right and left hepatectomies.

Nonanatomic Resection

Note that guidelines from the Louisville Statement are important to consider for this type of liver resection. Optimal port placement varies dependent on where the lesion is. Ligamentous attachments are taken down as necessary. Laparoscopic ultrasound is performed prior to resecting the lesion to ensure that the specimen can be removed in its entirety by wedge resection. The robot is docked. The circumference of resection is defined with hook cautery according to what is appropriate by surgical or oncologic guidelines. Ultrasound is repeated. If possible, figure-of-eight stitches using 0-Polysorb™ are placed on either side of the line of transection, and these are retracted to either side using robotic ports. The parenchyma is coagulated and divided, placing clips when appropriate. Otherwise, the parenchyma is coagulated along the resection line using appropriate retraction, delivering the lesion out of the liver bed. The specimen is placed in a laparoscopic specimen bag, hemostasis is ensured, and the specimen is removed. The robot is undocked. Laparoscopic equipment is used to close fascia and remove ports under direct visualization. The skin is closed.

Current Experience

Review of the world literature reveals 9 case reports/series containing unique groups of patients undergoing robotic liver resection for a total of 144 cases [26, 30–38]. A majority (70 %) of these cases have been performed for malignancy—39 % hepatocellular carcinoma, 29 % colorectal cancer metastases, 11 % other primary hepatobiliary malignancy, 11 % other metastases, and 10 % not documented. Benign lesions have included hemangioma (34 %), focal nodular hyperplasia (21 %), adenoma (17 %), pyogenic abscess (10 %), hepatolithiasis (3 %), and not documented (14 %). The most common procedures reported have been left lateral sectionectomy in 37 patients (26 %), segmentectomy in 34 (24 %), and right hepatectomy in 28 (19 %). Other procedures performed include left hepatectomy in 16 (11 %), wedge resection in 15 (10 %), bisegmentectomy in 10 (7 %), extended right hepatectomy in 3 (2 %), and extended left hepatectomy in 1 (1 %).

Operative outcomes of these patients have been evaluated. Morbidity experienced from robotic-assisted liver resection was 14.6 %, and this seems comparable to the 10.5 % (between 0 and 50 %) reported in the laparoscopic literature [23]. Reported liver-related morbidity for the robotic group included bile leak in 6 (4 %), transient liver failure in 2 (1.4 %), and ascites in 1 (0.7 %). Surgical-related morbidity consisted of pleural effusion in 3 (2 %), wound infection in 1 (0.7 %), ileus in 1, and bladder injury in 1. General postoperative morbidity included transient ischemic attack in 2 (1.4 %) and deep vein thrombosis in 2. Perioperative mortality was zero for the robotic-assisted cases, and this is comparable to 0.3 % in laparoscopic cases [23]. For other outcomes, including operative time, estimated blood loss (EBL), and length of stay (LOS), conclusions are difficult to ascertain. It is suspected that case complexity as well as the learning curve of the surgeon/robotic surgery team are relevant to this, as demonstrated for other types of surgical procedures and techniques [39–42]. Estimated blood loss has been reported between 5 mL and 2 L in 8 studies. Giulianotti et al suggest that major resections were associated with higher EBL compared to minor resections and that cirrhotic patients experienced greater blood loss when compared to non-cirrhotic patients [32]. Length of stay has been reported between 3 and 26 days. It is difficult to draw a conclusion from this as some suggest a cultural difference between nations for this variable. Regarding oncologic outcomes, all but one study evaluating margins of resection demonstrated that R0 resections were achieved using this technique. Long-term outcomes are not available given the recent application of this technology among few patients.

Ultimately, current experience with robotic-assisted liver resection supports that this form of surgery is safe and effective in appropriate hands. Additional study and comparison of this technique to open and laparoscopic surgery should be pursued.

Summary

Robotic assistance can safely be applied to liver surgery in the appropriate setting. It has many theoretical advantages that are potentially useful for the field, and the technology is only improving as engineers, scientists, and surgeons collaborate. For example, the Raven device is now being tested for use as a more compact, lighter, less expensive surgical tool with open-source software [43]. Additional efforts are also being made to develop systems that can respond to touch and communicate this with the operating surgeon as well as systems that can function autonomously to assist the surgeon. Altogether, robotic-assisted surgery's overall use, particularly in liver surgery, will likely expand in the future. Further investigation into its appropriate role is necessary.

Acknowledgments The authors would like to acknowledge Randal McKenzie/McKenzie Illustrations for figures 2–10.

References

1. Langenbuch D. Ein fall von resektion eines linksseitigen schnurlappens der leber. Heilung Berl Klin Wochenschr. 1888;25:37–8.
2. Couinaud C, editor. Etudes anatomiques et chirurgicales. Paris: Masson; 1957.
3. Cantlie J. On a new arrangement of the right and left lobes of the liver. J Anat Physiol. 1897;32:4–9.
4. Hjortsjo CH. The topography of the intrahepatic duct systems. Acta Anat (Basel). 1951;11(4):599–615.
5. McIndoe AH, Counsellor V. The bilaterality of the liver. Arch Surg. 1927;15:589–612.
6. Fortner JG, Shiu MH, Kinne DW, Kim DK, Castro EB, Watson RC, et al. Major hepatic resection using vascular isolation and hypothermic perfusion. Ann Surg. 1974;180(4):644–52.
7. Huguet C, Nordlinger B, Bloch P, Conard J. Tolerance of the human liver to prolonged normothermic ischemia. A biological study of 20 patients submitted to extensive hepatectomy. Arch Surg. 1978;113(12):1448–51.
8. Huguet C, Nordlinger B, Galopin JJ, Bloch P, Gallot D. Normothermic hepatic vascular exclusion for extensive hepatectomy. Surg Gynecol Obstet. 1978;147(5):689–93.
9. Kousnetzoff M, Pensky J. Sur la resection partielle du foie. Rev Chir. 1896;16:954–92.
10. Melendez JA, Arslan V, Fischer ME, Wuest D, Jarnagin WR, Fong Y, et al. Perioperative outcomes of major hepatic resections under low central venous pressure anesthesia: blood loss, blood transfusion, and the risk of postoperative renal dysfunction. J Am Coll Surg. 1998;187(6):620–5.
11. Pringle JH. V. Notes on the arrest of hepatic hemorrhage due to trauma. Ann Surg. 1908;48(4):541–9.
12. Bismuth H, Castaing D, Garden OJ. The use of operative ultrasound in surgery of primary liver tumors. World J Surg. 1987;11(5):610–4.

13. Castaing D, Kunstlinger F, Habib N, Bismuth H. Intraoperative ultrasonographic study of the liver. Methods and anatomic results. Am J Surg. 1985;149(5):676–82.
14. Fong Y, Blumgart LH. Useful stapling techniques in liver surgery. J Am Coll Surg. 1997;185(1): 93–100.
15. Geller DA, Tsung A, Maheshwari V, Rutstein LA, Fung JJ, Marsh JW. Hepatic resection in 170 patients using saline-cooled radiofrequency coagulation. HPB (Oxford). 2005;7(3):208–13.
16. Saiura A, Yamamoto J, Koga R, Sakamoto Y, Kokudo N, Seki M, et al. Usefulness of LigaSure for liver resection: analysis by randomized clinical trial. Am J Surg. 2006;192(1):41–5.
17. Weber JC, Navarra G, Jiao LR, Nicholls JP, Jensen SL, Habib NA. New technique for liver resection using heat coagulative necrosis. Ann Surg. 2002; 236(5):560–3.
18. Belghiti J, Hiramatsu K, Benoist S, Massault P, Sauvanet A, Farges O. Seven hundred forty-seven hepatectomies in the 1990s: an update to evaluate the actual risk of liver resection. J Am Coll Surg. 2000;191(1):38–46.
19. Dimick JB, Pronovost PJ, Cowan Jr JA, Lipsett PA. Postoperative complication rates after hepatic resection in Maryland hospitals. Arch Surg. 2003; 138(1):41–6.
20. Jarnagin WR, Gonen M, Fong Y, DeMatteo RP, Ben-Porat L, Little S, et al. Improvement in perioperative outcome after hepatic resection: analysis of 1,803 consecutive cases over the past decade. Ann Surg. 2002;236(4):397–406. discussion –7.
21. Cai XJ, Yang J, Yu H, Liang X, Wang YF, Zhu ZY, et al. Clinical study of laparoscopic versus open hepatectomy for malignant liver tumors. Surg Endosc. 2008;22(11):2350–6.
22. Koffron AJ, Auffenberg G, Kung R, Abecassis M. Evaluation of 300 minimally invasive liver resections at a single institution: less is more. Ann Surg. 2007;246(3):385–92. discussion 92–4.
23. Nguyen KT, Gamblin TC, Geller DA. World review of laparoscopic liver resection-2,804 patients. Ann Surg. 2009;250(5):831–41.
24. Kwoh YS, Hou J, Jonckheere EA, Hayati S. A robot with improved absolute positioning accuracy for CT guided stereotactic brain surgery. IEEE Trans Biomed Eng. 1988;35(2):153–60.
25. Satava RM. Robotic surgery: from past to future–a personal journey. Surg Clin North Am. 2003;83(6): 1491–500. xii.
26. Chan OC, Tang CN, Lai EC, Yang GP, Li MK. Robotic hepatobiliary and pancreatic surgery: a cohort study. J Hepatobiliary Pancreat Sci. 2011;18(4): 471–80.
27. Ryska M, Fronek J, Rudis J, Jurenka B, Langer D, Pudil J. Manual and robotic laparoscopic liver resection. Two case-reviews. Rozhl Chir. 2006;85(10): 511–6.
28. Kitisin K, Packiam V, Bartlett DL, Tsung A. A current update on the evolution of robotic liver surgery. Minerva Chir. 2011;66(4):281–93.
29. Buell JF, Cherqui D, Geller DA, O'Rourke N, Iannitti D, Dagher I, et al. The international position on laparoscopic liver surgery: the Louisville Statement, 2008. Ann Surg. 2009;250(5):825–30.
30. Abood GJ, Tsung A. Robotic-assisted surgery: improved tool for major liver resections? J Hepatobiliary Pancreat Sci. 2013;20(2):151–6.
31. Berber E, Akyildiz HY, Aucejo F, Gunasekaran G, Chalikonda S, Fung J. Robotic versus laparoscopic resection of liver tumours. HPB (Oxford). 2010;12(8):583–6.
32. Giulianotti PC, Coratti A, Sbrana F, Addeo P, Bianco FM, Buchs NC, et al. Robotic liver surgery: results for 70 resections. Surgery. 2011;149(1):29–39.
33. Giulianotti PC, Sbrana F, Bianco FM, Addeo P. Robot-assisted laparoscopic extended right hepatectomy with biliary reconstruction. J Laparoendosc Adv Surg Tech A. 2010;20(2):159–63.
34. Ji WB, Wang HG, Zhao ZM, Duan WD, Lu F, Dong JH. Robotic-assisted laparoscopic anatomic hepatectomy in China: initial experience. Ann Surg. 2011;253(2):342–8.
35. Lai EC, Yang GP, Tang CN. Robot-assisted laparoscopic pancreaticoduodenectomy versus open pancreaticoduodenectomy - A comparative study. Int J Surg. 2012;10(9):475–9.
36. Tomulescu V, Stanciulea O, Balescu I, Vasile S, Tudor S, Gheorghe C, et al. First year experience of robotic-assisted laparoscopic surgery with 153 cases in a general surgery department: indications, technique and results. Chirurgia (Bucur). 2009;104(2): 141–50.
37. Wakabayashi G, Sasaki A, Nishizuka S, Furukawa T, Kitajima M. Our initial experience with robotic hepato-biliary-pancreatic surgery. J Hepatobiliary Pancreat Sci. 2011;18(4):481–7.
38. Choi SB, Park JS, Kim JK, Hyung WJ, Kim KS, Yoon DS, et al. Early experiences of robotic-assisted laparoscopic liver resection. Yonsei Med J. 2008;49(4): 632–8.
39. Gill J, Booth MI, Stratford J, Dehn TC. The extended learning curve for laparoscopic fundoplication: a cohort analysis of 400 consecutive cases. J Gastrointest Surg. 2007;11(4):487–92.
40. Hardacre JM. Is there a learning curve for pancreaticoduodenectomy after fellowship training? HPB Surg. 2010;2010:230287.
41. Tekkis PP, Senagore AJ, Delaney CP, Fazio VW. Evaluation of the learning curve in laparoscopic colorectal surgery: comparison of right-sided and left-sided resections. Ann Surg. 2005;242(1):83–91.
42. Tseng JF, Pisters PW, Lee JE, Wang H, Gomez HF, Sun CC, et al. The learning curve in pancreatic surgery. Surgery. 2007;141(5):694–701.
43. An open-source robo-surgeon. The Economist. Technology Quarterly 2012 Mar 3; Q1.

Part VII

Surgical Techniques: *Colon and Rectum*

Robotic Right Colectomy: Four-Arm Technique

16

Gyu Seog Choi

Introduction

Colorectal cancer is the second leading cause of cancer-related deaths in the USA. There were 102,900 cases of colon cancer and 39,670 cases of rectal cancer in 2010 [1]. The overall prevalence of colorectal cancer was 1,139,710 in 2009 [2]. Minimally invasive techniques have been used to perform colon cancer surgery for more than 20 years, and the use of laparoscopic colectomy has proven beneficial to patients during convalescence. Several randomized trials have shown that laparoscopic colectomy is associated with similar oncological outcomes to open surgery [3–6]. After the Food and Drug Administration approved the da Vinci® surgical robot system (Intuitive Surgical, Sunnyvale, CA, USA) for intra-abdominal surgery in 2000, robotic approaches have been used for minimally invasive colon cancer surgery. This introduction of surgical robot systems in colon cancer treatment has been shown to be safe and effective, particularly when dealing with complex procedures.

This chapter will cover the indications for robotic right colectomy, techniques from port placement to specimen extraction including intracorporeal anastomosis and natural orifice specimen extraction (NOSE), and treatment outcomes. Both medial-to-lateral and lateral-to-medial approaches can be used to perform robot-assisted right colectomy for colon cancers. The techniques described here are based on the lateral-to-medial approach.

Indications and Contraindications

The same criteria for laparoscopic colectomy are applied to robotic right colectomy. According to the National Comprehensive Cancer Network Guidelines (version 3, 2012), laparoscopic colectomy can be considered based upon the following criteria [7].

- Surgeon with experience performing laparoscopically assisted colorectal operations.
- No disease in rectum or prohibitive abdominal adhesions.
- No locally advanced disease.
- Not indicated for acute bowel obstruction or perforation from cancer.
- Thorough abdominal exploration is required.
- Consider preoperative marking of small lesions.

Patients with contraindications for creating a pneumoperitoneum, with a tumor greater than 8 cm in diameter, or with an advanced tumor with adjacent organ invasion are also contraindicated for robotic colectomy.

G.S. Choi, M.D., Ph.D. (✉)
Colorectal Cancer Center, Kyungpook National University Medical Center, 807, Hogukro, Buk-gu, Daegu, 702-210, South Korea
e-mail: kyuschoi@mail.knu.ac.kr

K.C. Kim (ed.), *Robotics in General Surgery*, DOI 10.1007/978-1-4614-8739-5_16,

Preoperative Assessment and Patient Preparation

For accurate preoperative staging of colon cancers, assessments consist of a physical examination, colonoscopy, biopsy, measurement of carcinoembryonic antigen, and abdominopelvic computed tomography (CT) scan. A positron emission tomography (PET)-CT scan is not routinely indicated, but can be used to obtain additional information.

After the patient has been admitted for robot-assisted right colectomy, preoperative mechanical bowel preparation is dependent on the surgeon's preference and is identical to that of open or laparoscopic surgery.

The intraoperative preparation includes shaving the patient from the costal margin to the pubic bone. The abdomen and pelvic area are prepared and draped in the usual sterile fashion. Thromboembolic stockings and sequential compression devices are placed to prevent deep vein thromboses. A Foley catheter is inserted. Intravenous antibiotics are administered immediately before the skin incision. Placement of a nasogastric or orogastric tube is optional.

Position, Port Placement, and Docking

Patient Position

The patient is placed supine or in the lithotomy position (necessary to perform transvaginal specimen extraction in female patients). Both arms are alongside the body to prevent any possibility of shoulder injury and to gain space for the patient cart and surgical assistants. After the patient has been draped and the placement of ports has been completed, the table is placed in a 10–15° Trendelenburg position and rolled to the left 10–15°. This positioning allows the small bowel to move aside under gravity and expose the right mesocolon.

Port Placement

For optimal port placement in robotic surgery, the unique concept of "camera cone" is important. This is an imaginary conical area that the

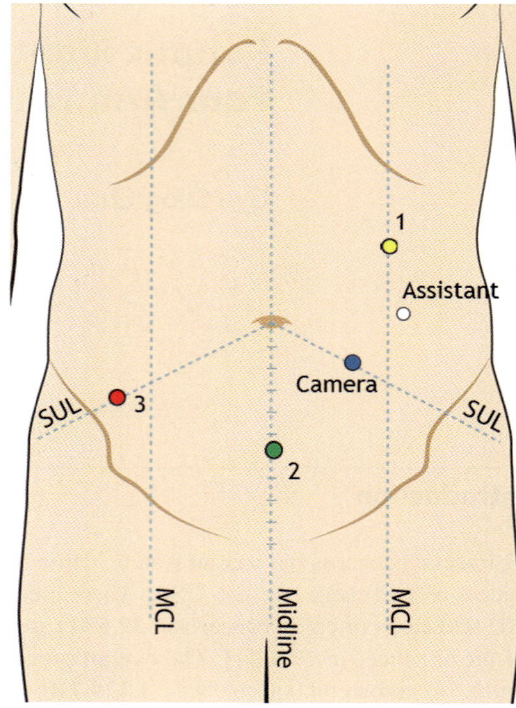

Fig. 16.1 Port placement

da Vinci system can cover in a single docking. Ideally, the surgical target should be placed within this camera cone; the camera port should be at the tip, and all other ports should be placed outside it. With this principle, we use five ports including one robot camera port, three robot arm ports, and one port for an assistant. At first, abdominal insufflation is established using a Veress needle or with open trocar placement by the Hasson technique at the level of the anticipated camera port. A 12-mm camera port is placed 5 cm to the left of and 2.5 cm below the umbilicus. Three 8-mm ports for the robot arms are placed along an imaginary curvilinear line across the left upper quadrant to the right lower quadrant and out of the camera cone, as shown in Fig. 16.1.

- The da Vinci camera port (12 mm) is placed 5 cm to the left of and 2.5 cm below the umbilicus. The distance to the symphysis pubis should be ~16–18 cm.
- The da Vinci arm port ① (8 mm) is placed 7–8 cm below the left costal margin and on the left midclavicular line.

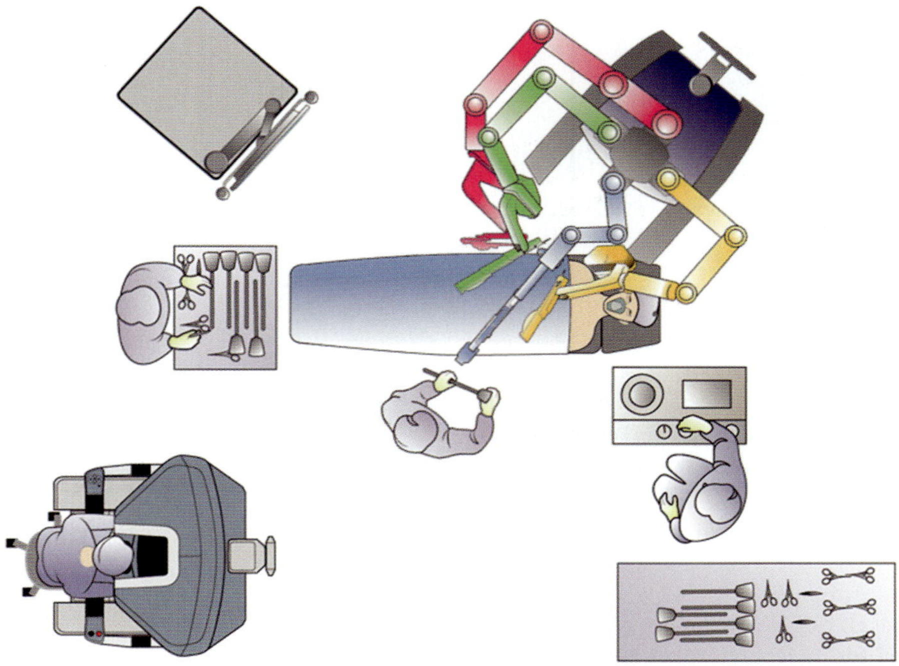

Fig. 16.2 Configuration of the operating room after docking the patient cart

- The da Vinci arm port ② (8 mm) is placed on the midline and 4 cm above the symphysis pubis.
- The da Vinci arm port ③ (8 mm) is placed 2–3 cm lateral to the midclavicular line and 2–3 cm above the anterior superior iliac spine.
- The assistant's port (5 mm) is placed 8–10 cm caudal and 1–2 cm lateral to the da Vinci arm port ①. This port is used for suction/irrigation, ligation, and additional retraction.
- The distance between all ports should be at least 8 cm.

The location of the camera port should be consistent. The instrument arm ports need to be adjusted based on the tumor's location (cecum to transverse colon) and the patient's height.

Patient Cart Docking

The patient is placed in a Trendelenburg position and tilted to the left before introduction of the patient cart. This is positioned obliquely at the right upper quadrant of the abdomen. It is angled 45° from the perpendicular relative to the patient. The robot arms are docked to the trocars.

Figure 16.2 shows an overhead view of the recommended operating room setup for robotic right colectomy after introducing the patient cart. There should be a clear view of the patient from the surgeon's console, a tension-free cable connection to the equipment, and clear pathways for the operating team to move freely.

- The patient-side assistant is on the patient's left side.
- The scrub nurse is at the patient's feet but can stand at the right side of an assistant surgeon according to the arrangement of the operating room.
- The main assistant monitor is located at the right of the patient toward the feet.
- An anesthesiologist is positioned at the head of the patient. Alternatively, an anesthesiologist can be positioned at the patient's feet by fixing the lines of the ventilator along the operation table.

Surgical Techniques

A 0° endoscope, monopolar curved scissors (arm ①); bipolar Cadiere forceps (arm ②); and double-fenestrated grasper (arm ③) are used. Robot arm

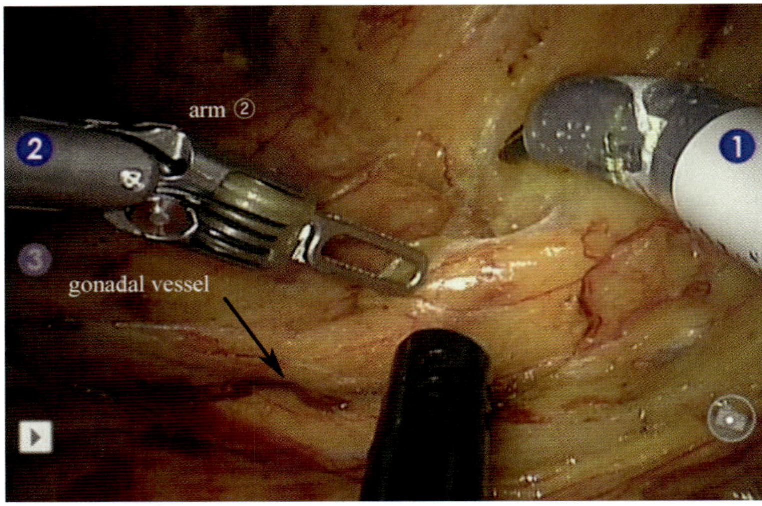

Fig. 16.3 Exposure of the peritoneal attachment by retracting the appendix and terminal ileum with the grasper in the robotic arm

① is used for dissection, robot arm ② for major retraction or countertraction, and robot arm ③ for minor retraction.

Mobilization of Ascending Colon and Terminal Ileum

The small intestine is placed toward the left upper abdominal quadrant, and the inferior dissection starts at the retrocecal recess. This work is continued over the duodenum to the head of the pancreas. At the same time, the lateral attachments of the ascending colon are taken down starting at the right paracolic gutter and moving cranially to the hepatic flexure until the ascending colon is mobilized completely.

1. Lifting and retracting the appendix and terminal ileum caudally and superiorly with the grasper in arm ③ provides major retraction to expose the peritoneal attachment along the right iliac vessels (Fig. 16.3).
2. Additional exposure can be gained by retraction of the grasper in arm ② and by the assistant using a laparoscopic port.
3. Dissection through the avascular plane between the ileocecum and the retroperitoneal layer is done with the monopolar scissors in arm ①. The right gonadal vessels and the ureter should be identified and preserved retroperitoneally.
4. Lifting the mesentery of the terminal ileum exposes the avascular plane over the duodenum and the head of the pancreas (Fig. 16.4).

Vascular Control and Lymphadenectomy

When the colonic mobilization is completed, vascular control is initiated by placing the bowels in the normal anatomical position. The extent of any necessary vascular control depends on the tumor location, planned anastomosis location, and the patient's anatomy. All lymph nodes and adipose tissue at the right side of the superior mesentery artery are removed sequentially from the ileocolic artery to the middle colic artery. The right colonic branches of the superior mesentery artery and vein are ligated with a Hem-o-Lok clip™ or sealing device (e.g., EndoWrist One Vessel Sealer™ or LigaSure™ or EnSeal™). Our recommendation for lymphadenectomy in this area is to maintain tension in the right mesocolon by elevating the ileocolic vessels using a grasper through arm ③ and in the middle colic vessels with a grasper through the assistant port while this procedure is being finished.

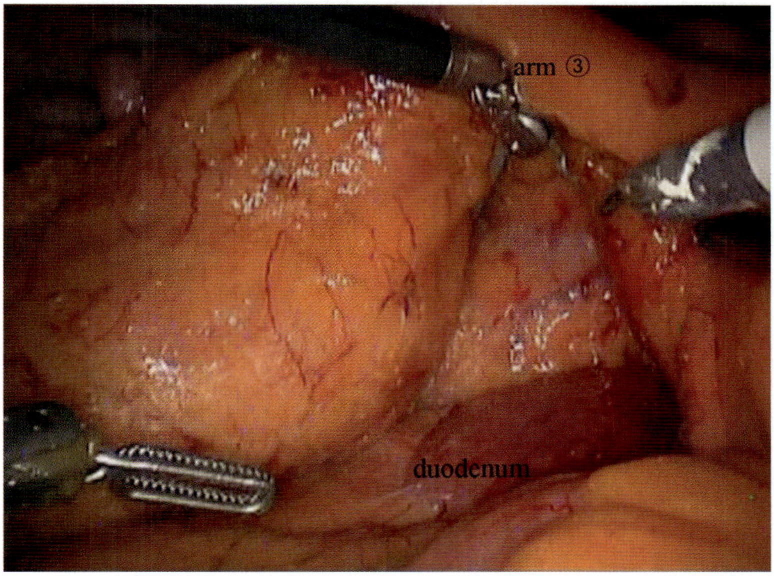

Fig. 16.4 Lifting the mesentery of the terminal ileum to expose the avascular plane over the duodenum and the head of the pancreas

1. For ileocolic vessel division, arm ③ is used to lift up the ileocolic pedicle (Fig. 16.5).
2. The ileocolic vessels are skeletonized up 1–2 cm above the root and ligated at 1–1.5 cm from the root (Fig. 16.6).
3. Once the ileocolic vessels have been divided, lymphadenectomy is continued along the superior mesenteric artery to the root of right colic and middle colic arteries. Ligation of the right colic and middle colic vessels depends on the tumor location (Fig. 16.7).
4. The assistant's port can be used to introduce hemostatic instruments (e.g., clips, *LigaSure*™, or *EnSeal*™) for ligating vessels. The assistant can use a laparoscopic bowel grasper to push the middle colic pedicle superiorly for additional exposure to the superior mesenteric axis during lymphadenectomy.

Final Mobilization

After all vessels have been securely divided and lymphadenectomy is completed, the transverse mesocolon is opened just above the head of the pancreas to enter the lesser sac. The transverse mesocolon is divided from its root to the colon. The marginal artery and vein are controlled with clips or a sealing device. Colon mobilization is completed with partial omentectomy along the colon up to the resection site.

Ileocolic Anastomosis and Specimen Extraction

Two approaches can be used to create the anastomosis: extracorporeal and intracorporeal anastomosis. In an extracorporeal anastomosis, the mobilized right colon and terminal ileum are extracted through a 5–7 cm minilaparotomy. The skin incision is covered using a wound protector. Side-to-side anastomosis is created using a standard linear stapler. However, as generally used in a laparoscopic approach, extension of the camera port (normally a transumbilical incision) for extraction of specimens and creating an anastomosis is not indicated in the robotic approach because the camera port is far lateral to the umbilicus. This is why most surgeons prefer an intracorporeal anastomosis to the cosmetically inferior extracorporeal one.

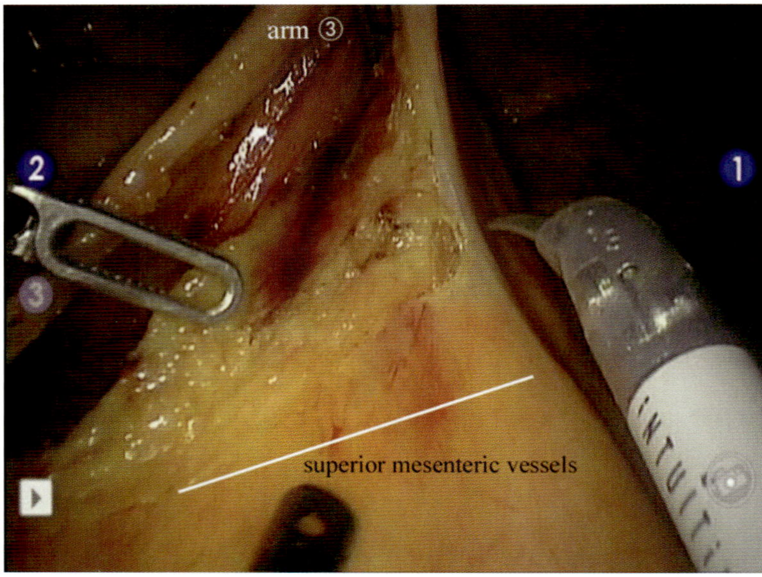

Fig. 16.5 Robot arm ③ is used to lift up the ileocolic pedicle and perform a lymphadenectomy around the ileocolic vessels

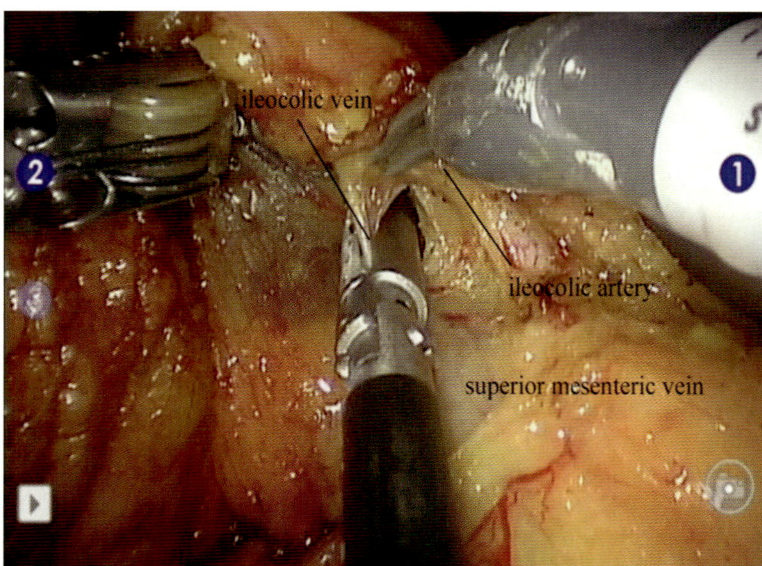

Fig. 16.6 Division of the ileocolic vein

Intracorporeal Anastomosis

1. For this, the mesentery of the ileum and transverse colon is divided at the selected anastomosis location. A sealing device is used for dividing the mesentery to control bleeding. The ileum is then skeletonized in preparation for anastomosis in a well-vascularized area.
2. The monopolar curved scissors in arm ① are replaced with a needle driver. The transverse colon and ileum are approximated with double stay sutures placed near the planned

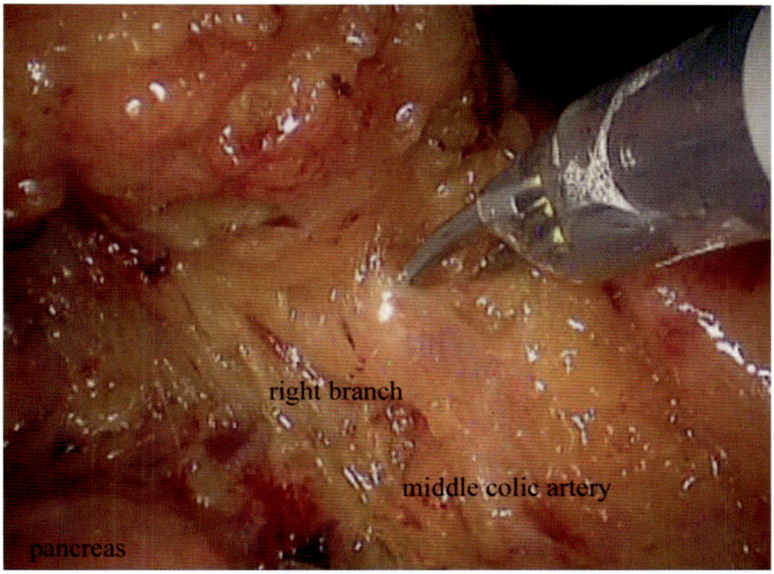

Fig. 16.7 Lymphadenectomy around the right branch of the middle colic artery

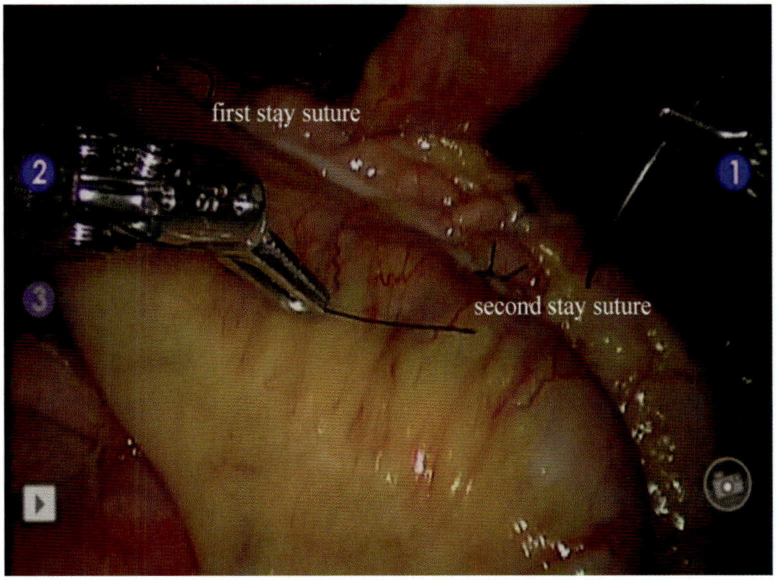

Fig. 16.8 Stay sutures for approximating the free taenia of the transverse colon to the antimesenteric border of the ileum

enterotomy site. Additional single stay sutures are placed about 7–8 cm distal to the initial double stay sutures, approximating the free taenia of the transverse colon to the antimesenteric border of the ileum (Fig. 16.8). Monopolar curved scissors in arm ① are used to create enterotomies.

3. A port for robotic arm ② is temporarily undocked and replaced by 12-mm laparoscopic port. A linear stapler is introduced

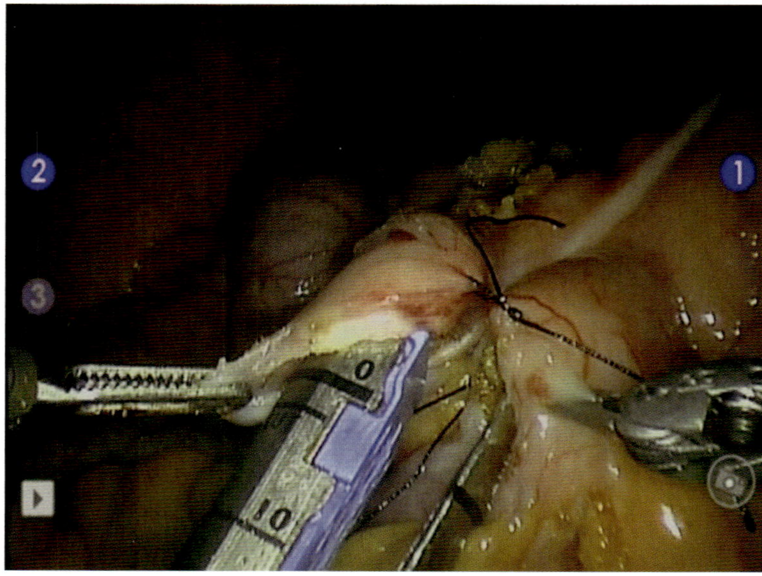

Fig. 16.9 Insertion of a linear stapler in the enterotomies

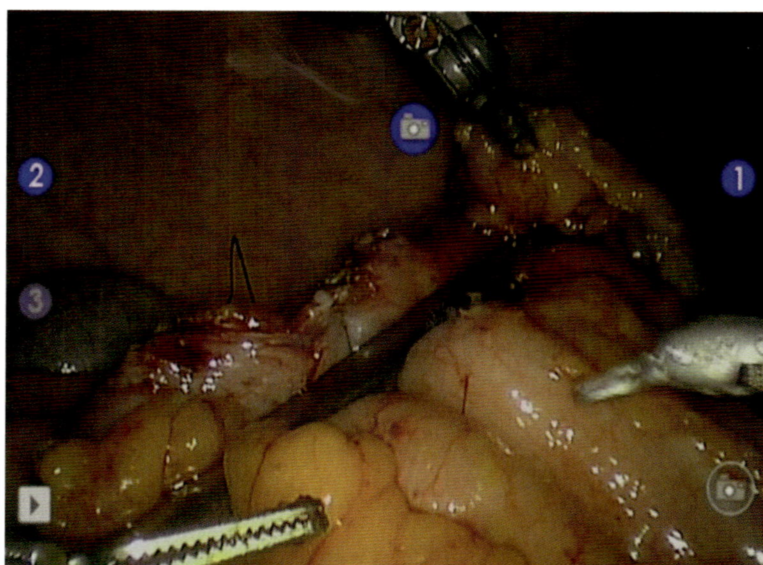

Fig. 16.10 Final closure of the anastomosis using a linear stapler

through the port and inserted in the enterotomies (Fig. 16.9). The grasper in arm ③ is used to lift the stay sutures upward to prevent inadequate stapling. Placing another liner stapler across the colon and ileum distal to the enterotomies completes the anastomosis (Fig. 16.10). The enterotomies can also be closed using robotically placed sutures.

4. A plastic bag and a wound protector are used to protect contamination during specimen extraction. After placing the specimen into the bag, the ileal end of the specimen is separated

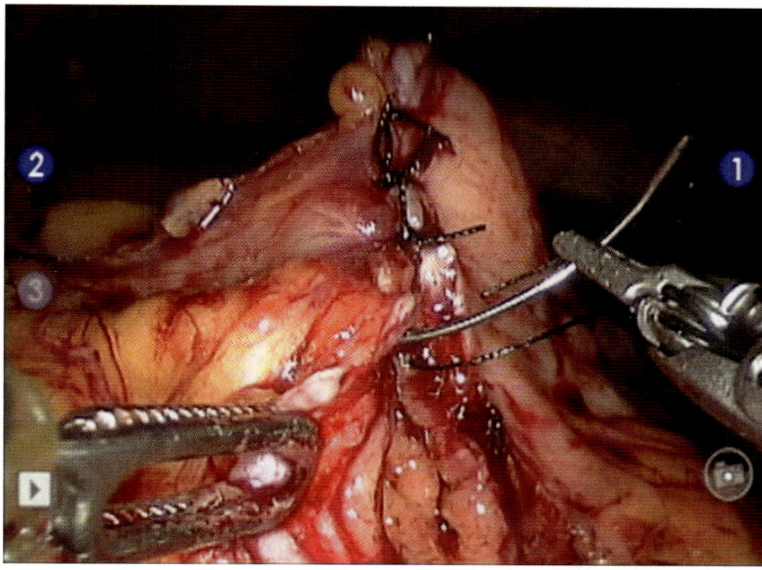

Fig. 16.11 Hand-sewn colocolic anastomosis

from the transverse colon to avoid the specimen folding during extraction.

5. The specimen is extracted through an extension of the trocar incision or via Pfannenstiel incision.

There are other options for performing intracorporeal ileocolic anastomosis. Iso- or antiperistaltic side-to-side anastomoses using a linear stapler with robotic hand-sewn closure of the enterotomies are the most commonly practiced manner. A fully hand-sewn anastomosis is somewhat time-consuming but can be attempted for selective cases, especially for colocolic anastomosis after a transverse colectomy (Fig. 16.11).

The advantages of intracorporeal anastomosis are minimal colonic mobilization, little chance of rotation of the bowels, and reduced size of the incision needed for extracting specimens. In addition, the surgeon is able to choose the best site of incision according to the patient's history of abdominal surgery, for example, previous Caesarean section or appendectomy incisions.

NOSE Procedure

1. In female patients, the NOSE technique can be applied selectively using a transvaginal incision.
2. Patients with a large tumor (>5 cm in its smaller diameter), severe pelvic adhesions, pelvic inflammatory diseases, or of childbearing age are contraindications for this procedure.
3. A 12-mm laparoscopic trocar is placed transvaginally through the posterior fornix vaginally (Fig. 16.12). Linear stapling devices are introduced through the trocar to perform anastomosis as described above.
4. The specimen is wrapped in a sterile bag and removed though an extension of the transvaginal trocar incision.
5. The colpotomy is closed intra-abdominally or transvaginally using a running suture.

Exploration and Wound Closure

Once the specimen is removed, the minilaparotomy incision is covered with a glove or other means, and insufflations are reestablished. Conventional laparoscopy is used to check the operation field and trocar sites.

- Any bleeding should be checked.
- The orientation of the anastomosed bowel should be checked.
- The small bowel and omentum should be reoriented necessarily.
- The trocar sites should be checked for bleeding.

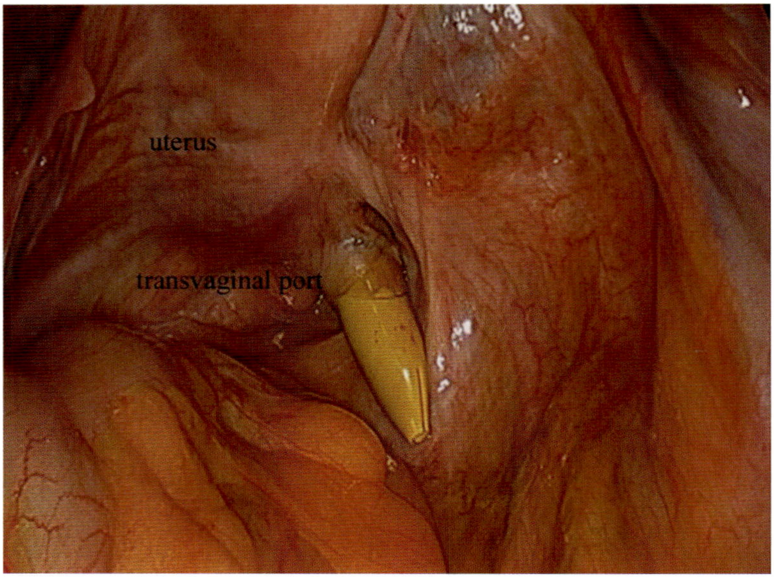

Fig. 16.12 A 12-mm transvaginal trocar

- All trocar sites greater than 8 mm in diameter should be closed with 2-0 absorbable sutures at the fascial level.

Postoperative Treatment

The patient's postoperative management is no different from those of conventional open and laparoscopic colectomy approaches. The in-hospital course depends on the surgeon's experience and preference. If necessary, the patient can be transferred to an intensive care unit until all vital signs are stable.

- Stable patients can be transferred to the recovery room and to the regular nursing floor.
- The patient is encouraged to be ambulatory the day after surgery.
- The clinical recovery process can follow the individual center's policy including any early recovery protocol.
- The patient can be discharged from the hospital 3–5 days postoperatively if stable and if there is no sign of bleeding or adverse events.

Results

The surgical outcomes of robot-assisted right colectomy of colon cancer are summarized in Table 16.1. According to these retrospective and prospective studies, robot-assisted right colectomy for patients with colon cancers is technically safe and feasible [8–10]. Robotic right colectomy showed good convalescence outcomes similar but not superior to those of minimally invasive surgery. Patients had short mean hospital stays of 4.3–7.9 days. The overall postoperative complication rate has been reported as up to 24 % and includes ischemia, colitis, anastomosis leakage, and ileus (Table 16.1). Two reports concluded that effective lymphadenectomy along the superior mesenteric vessels and easier intracorporeal anastomosis could be the potential benefit of robotic surgery [11, 15]. Experience with robotic right colectomy demonstrated considerably low conversion rates (~2.5 %) compared with laparoscopic colon resection with reported conversion rates of 11–29 % [3–6]. However, these impressions have

Table 16.1 Results of robot-assisted right colectomies for patients with colon cancer

Authors	Year	Design	No. of cases (cancer)	OP time (min)	Blood loss (mL)	Conversions (*n*)	LOS (days)	Intraoperative complications (*n*)	Postoperative complications (*n*)	No. of harvested LNs
Delaney et al. [8]	2003	NR	1	267	100	–	5	–	1	NR
Rawlings et al. [9][a]	2006	Prosp	17	218	66	0	5.2	NA	NA	NR
Spinoglio et al. [10]	2008	NR	18	NA	NA	0	NA	NA	NA	NA
D'Annibale et al. [11]	2010	Prosp	50	224	20	0	7	0	2	18.7
deSouza et al. [12][a]	2010	NR	40	158	50	1	5	0	8	16
Luca et al. [13]	2011	Prosp	33	191	6.1	0	5	0	24	26.6
Park et al. [14]	2012	Prosp	35	195	36	0	7.9	0	17	29.9
Trastulli et al. [15]	2012	Prosp	20	328	55	0	4.5	0	5	17.6
Deutsch et al. [16][a]	2012	Retro	18	219	76	NA	4.3	2	NA	21.1

LNs lymph nodes, *LOS* length of hospital stay, *NA* not applicable, *NR* not reported, *OP* operation, *Prosp* prospective, *Retro* retrospective

[a]Studies include both benign and malignant cases

not yet been translated into objective clinical outcomes. Recently, we conducted a randomized comparative study of robotic versus laparoscopic right hemicolectomy and concluded that robotic approach for this particular procedure was feasible and effective but not recommended for routine use because of its high cost and long operation time [14]. Other comparative studies including long-term oncological outcomes have not been reported.

Conclusions

Robot-assisted right colectomy for patients with colon cancers is technically safe and feasible. The improved surgical technique arises from the inherent properties of the robotic system such as the elimination of tumor, a three-dimensional view, and ambidextrous capability. These potential advantages can lessen the technical difficulties of vascular control and lymphadenectomy during right colon cancer surgery. However, objective evidence of its efficacy is insufficient at present. Further studies comparing short-term outcomes, long-term oncological outcomes, and cost-related benefits of robotic, laparoscopic, and open techniques are needed to determine the utility and efficacy of this technology in the field of colon cancer surgery.

References

1. Jemal A, et al. Cancer statistics. CA Cancer J Clin. 2010;60:277–300.
2. Howlader N et al. SEER cancer statistics review, 1975–2009 (Vintage 2009 Populations), National Cancer Institute, Bethesda, MD. http://seer.cancer.gov/csr/1975_2009_pops09/, based on November 2011 SEER data submission, posted to the SEER web site, April 2012. Accessed 10 Dec 2012.
3. Lacy AM, et al. Laparoscopy-assisted colectomy versus open colectomy for treatment of non-metastatic colon cancer: a randomized trial. Lancet. 2002;359: 2224–9.
4. Veldkamp R, et al. Laparoscopic surgery versus open surgery for colon cancer: short term outcomes of a randomised trial. Lancet Oncol. 2005;6:477–84.
5. Guillou PJ, et al. Short-term endpoints of conventional versus laparoscopic-assisted surgery in patients with colorectal cancer (MRC CLASICC trial): multicentre, randomised controlled trial. Lancet. 2005;365:1718–26.
6. Fleshman J, et al. Laparoscopic colectomy for cancer is not inferior to open surgery based on 5-year data from the COST Study Group trial. Ann Surg. 2007;246:655–62. discussion 662–664.
7. NCCN clinical practice guidelines in oncology: colon cancer (v.3.2013). The National Comprehensive Cancer Network. http://www.nccn.org. Accessed 10 Dec 2012.
8. Delaney CP, et al. Comparison of robotically performed and traditional laparoscopic colorectal surgery. Dis Colon Rectum. 2003;46:1633–9.
9. Rawlings AL, et al. Telerobotic surgery for right and sigmoid colectomies: 30 consecutive cases. Surg Endosc. 2006;20:1713–8.
10. Spinoglio G, et al. Robotic colorectal surgery: first 50 cases experience. Dis Colon Rectum. 2008;51: 1627–32.
11. D'Annibale A, et al. Robotic right colon resection: evaluation of first 50 consecutive cases for malignant disease. Ann Surg Oncol. 2010;17:2856–62.
12. deSouza AL, et al. Robotic assistance in right hemicolectomy: is there a role? Dis Colon Rectum. 2010; 53:1000–6.
13. Luca F, et al. Surgical and pathological outcomes after right hemicolectomy: case-matched study comparing robotic and open surgery. Int J Med Robot. 2011; 7:298–303.
14. Park JS, et al. Randomized clinical trial of robot-assisted *versus* standard laparoscopic right colectomy. Br J Surg. 2012;99:1219–26.
15. Trastulli S, et al. Robotic right colectomy for cancer with intracorporeal anastomosis: short-term outcomes from a single institution. Int J Colorectal Dis. 2013;28:807–14. Accessed 10 Dec 2012.
16. Deutsch GB, et al. Robotic vs. laparoscopic colorectal surgery: an institutional experience. Surg Endosc. 2012;26:956–63.

Robotic Right Colectomy: Three-Arm Technique

17

Henry J. Lujan and Gustavo Plasencia

Since 2000, robotic-assisted surgery has been increasing in popularity, especially for cardiac, gynecologic, and urologic procedures [1]. Recently, increased interest in robotic techniques for colon resection has emerged. The first robotic colectomies were reported by Weber et al. in 2002 and included one right colectomy [2]. Since then, the da Vinci® surgical robot (Intuitive Surgical, Sunnyvale, CA) has been shown to be safe and effective for colorectal procedures by other authors [1, 3–6]. Nevertheless, the role of robotic surgery has not yet been established for colorectal surgery.

Laparoscopic colectomy has been shown to have significant advantages over open colectomy [7–9]. Laparoscopic colectomy is even considered the gold standard by some authors [10, 11]. Robotic colorectal surgery today may be in the same position that laparoscopic surgery was 20 years ago [12, 13]. Despite first being described by Jacobs et al. in 1991, laparoscopic colectomy has been slow to be adopted as the preferred approach to colon and rectal diseases. Estimates for the percentage of laparoscopic colectomies performed in the USA range from 20 to 40 % and for laparoscopic rectal resection range from 10 to 15 % [14, 15].

H.J. Lujan, M.D., F.A.C.S., F.A.S.C.R.S. (✉)
G. Plasencia, M.D., F.A.C.S., F.A.S.C.R.S.
Department of Surgery, Jackson South Community Hospital, Miami, FL 33157, USA
e-mail: hlujan15@me.com; guspmd@aol.com

Initially, laparoscopic colectomy took longer and was more expensive than conventional open colectomy. However, with time, it proved to offer significant advantages to the patient, including quicker return of bowel function, less postoperative pain, shorter hospital stay, and lower postoperative morbidity and mortality [9]. Robotic surgery purportedly offers advantages to overcome the limitations of laparoscopic surgery [6]. Some surgeons believe this could lead to wider use of minimally invasive surgery for colorectal resections.

Robotics for colorectal surgery has been shown to be safe and feasible, and perioperative and pathologic outcomes appear to be equivalent to laparoscopic surgery. However, most authors believe that the robot will have the greatest impact on rectal resection [1, 6, 16]. It seems ideally suited for pelvic dissection, where the superior visualization and articulating instruments facilitate exposure, retraction, and difficult dissection. It is hypothesized that these advantages will result in lower conversion rates and higher rates of adoption. Furthermore, possible advantages of better mesorectal excision, better preservation of nerves, and easier operation in the obese are all areas of ongoing investigation. But, for partial colectomy, the benefits are more difficult to foresee. In the literature, modest advantages in visualization and possibly decreased blood loss seem to be offset by longer operative times and higher costs thus far [1, 6, 16–20].

If nothing else, robotic right colectomy is an ideal case for a surgeon's initial experience with

K.C. Kim (ed.), *Robotics in General Surgery*, DOI 10.1007/978-1-4614-8739-5_17,

robotic techniques [19]. It is a familiar procedure to general and colorectal surgeons alike and is technically easier than other colon procedures with relatively short operative times. It is commonly used as learning and/or teaching tool. It is a procedure that is easily converted to either laparoscopic or open colectomy with relatively little clinical consequence.

The indications and setting for right colectomy are well described and include benign and malignant conditions, elective, urgent, and emergent operations. Benign conditions include inflammatory bowel disease, volvulus, diverticular disease, arteriovenous malformations, ischemic colitis, and polyps not amenable to endoscopic removal. Adenocarcinoma, carcinoid tumor, and appendiceal tumors account for most malignant diseases. Surgery for the right colon is usually elective. However, urgent indications include nearly obstructing lesions, ischemic colitis, and hemorrhage. There are only a few emergent indications, with perforation, complete obstruction, and refractory hemorrhage the most common [21].

Technique

Our three-arm technique for robotic right colectomy with intracorporeal anastomosis is described below. We modified this technique from the description by Rawlings et al. [17]. The patient is under general anesthesia in the supine position. Room setup is shown in Fig. 17.1a, b. Pneumoperitoneum can be achieved with a Veress needle.

As an alternative, open laparoscopic entry (Hasson technique) or visual entry systems (Optiview/Visiport) can be used per surgeon's preference. A total of four ports (three robotic ports and one assistant port) are placed as shown in Figs. 17.2 and 17.3.

An extra long 12 or 8.5 mm periumbilical port for the camera is placed. Usually 2 cm below and 2 cm lateral to the umbilicus (depending on the patient's body habitus). A left upper quadrant and suprapubic 8 mm robotic trocars are placed for arms 1 (R1) and 2 (R2). Five mm robotic trocars and arms can be used, but this limits the instrument options and degrees of articulation with today's available instrumentation, and, therefore, we prefer 8 mm ports at this time. In cases of polyps or tumors, the lesion is localized prior to docking the robot using a 5 mm laparoscope, which is always available. The table is then positioned in 10–20° of reverse Trendelenburg and 20–30° of right side up to allow the small intestine to fall away from the midline. The robot is docked from the patient's right side or over the right shoulder. The robotic camera is inserted through the 8.5 mm periumbilical port. The assistant surgeon uses a lateral 12 mm port to introduce laparoscopic instruments, energy devices, and endoscopic staplers and suction as needed. Using the bipolar fenestrated grasper (R2) and the hot shears (R1), a medial-to-lateral dissection is realized. First, the assistant surgeon grasps the ileocecal junction to place the ileocolic vascular pedicle on tension. It is critical to identify the cecum and ileocecal junction; this step cannot be overemphasized. A small window is created posteriorly near the origin of the ileocolic vessels. The dissection is continued for 2–3 cm to reveal the duodenum. Typically, the duodenum identifies the origin of the ileocolic artery. A second window is created to isolate the base of the vascular pedicle. It is divided at the level of the duodenum with a vascular stapler, clips, or energy device, which are brought in through the left lateral 12 mm assistant port.

The medial-to-lateral dissection is continued. The right mesocolon is mobilized off the retroperitoneum. This dissection is mostly blunt and accomplished by pushing the mesocolon anteriorly and the retroperitoneum posteriorly. This can be advanced to the lateral attachments, to the liver and hepatic attachments, and to the duodenal sweep as needed. The ileal mesentery is divided with an energy source or cautery to a point 8–10 cm from the ileocecal valve. Typically, two small vessels or branches will be encountered and can be divided with the energy device. The mesocolic mobilization is then carried up to the duodenum and the transverse mesocolon. The terminal ileum is transected with an endoscopic stapler. Next the right branch of the middle colic is identified and transected with the energy device or stapler. The ascending colon can be left attached to the right paracolic gutter to keep it from falling medially or completely detached and the specimen placed above the liver for later retrieval (if the resection is for cancer, the specimen is placed in a bag). Lateral mobilization begins at the ileocecal junction along the right paracolic gutter and advanced to the hepatic flexure and along the right transverse colon. Sometimes omentum is removed with the specimen. Usually, the omentum is partially detached from the colon by dividing the gastrocolic ligament. The transverse colon is isolated by creating a mesenteric window and then divided with the endoscopic stapler.

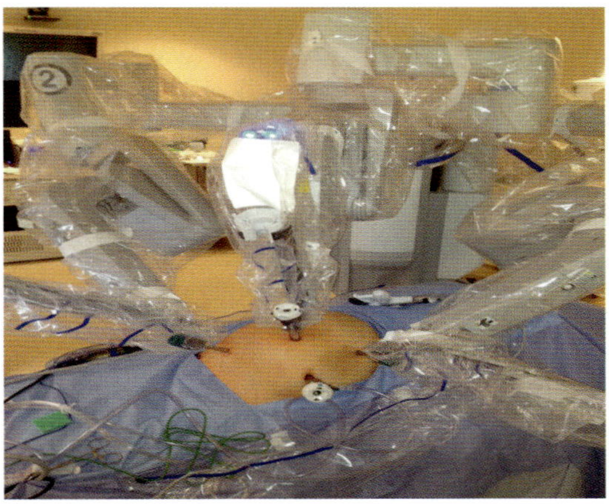

Fig. 17.1 Room setup

Next, attention is turned to construction of an isoperistaltic, side-to-side anastomosis. For this purpose, the terminal ileum and the transverse colon stump are brought together side by side as shown in Fig. 17.4a, b.

A 20 cm nonabsorbable suture on a Keith needle is used to put a stay suture approximating the transverse colon and terminal ileum up to the abdominal wall to provide tension and elevate the site of the anastomosis (Fig. 17.5).

Prior to creating the enterotomies, an endoscopic intestinal clamp (bulldog) can be placed on the terminal ileum to prevent spillage. Using an energy device or hot shears, a colotomy and ileotomy are created (Fig. 17.6) through which the jaws of the endoscopic linear stapler are introduced to construct the common channel (Fig. 17.7).

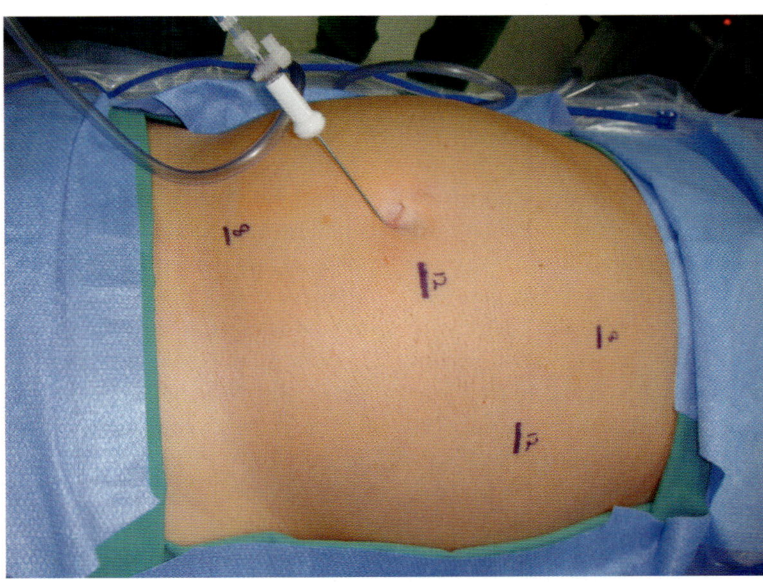

Fig. 17.2 Trocar placement for robotic right colectomy

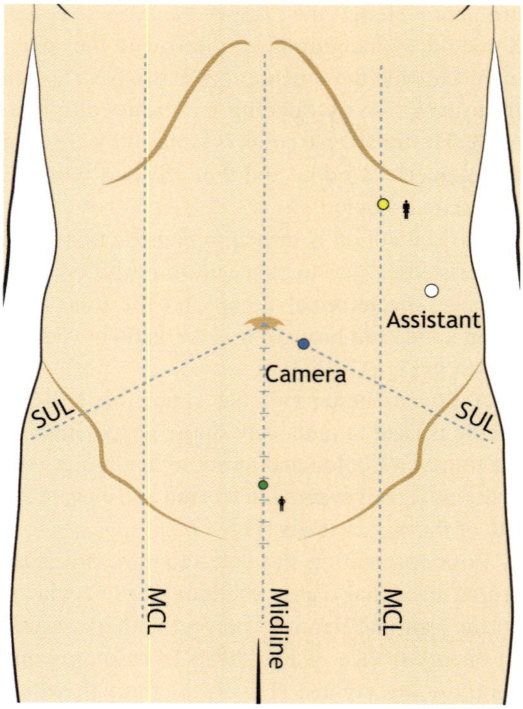

Fig. 17.3 Trocar placement for robotic right colectomy

The remaining common enterotomy is then closed with 2-0 Vicryl in two running layers using robotic suturing techniques (Fig. 17.8a, b).

Once complete, the stay suture is cut, and then attention is directed again to the specimen. As an alternative, a complete robotic-sewn anastomosis can be fashioned. If necessary, the remaining lateral and hepatic attachments are freed. A grasper with teeth or endoloop is introduced through the 12 mm left lateral port to hold the specimen (usually by the transected terminal ileum), and the robot is undocked. The 12 mm assistant port incision is then enlarged. Usually a 3–5 cm incision is necessary depending on the size of the pathology. A wound retractor is placed to protect the skin, and the specimen is extracted. The extraction incision site can be placed in the suprapubic region or at any site per surgeon's choice as shown in Fig. 17.9a, b.

Finally, laparoscopy can be performed to visualize the anastomosis and confirm hemostasis. It is not necessary to close the mesentery defect in most cases. The extraction site is closed in two layers. Any 12 mm port site incisions are closed. The skin is closed in subcuticular fashion (Fig. 17.10).

A summary of the critical steps is shown in Table 17.1.

(See Figs. 17.11, 17.12, 17.13a, b, 17.14, 17.15, and 17.16a, b.) The first robotic right colectomies described were hybrid, in other words, an extracorporeal anastomosis was utilized. When we perform a robotic-assisted right colectomy with an extracorporeal anastomosis, the mobilization, devascularization, and transection are performed under robotic guidance. The specimen is brought out through an extraction site, and the anastomosis is realized through this same wound. We found it useful to perform right colectomies in hybrid fashion early in our learning curve. Specifically, our first four right colectomy cases were performed in this fashion emulating our laparoscopic technique. However, inspired by the robotic platform, we have since performed 50 robotic colectomies with intracorporeal anastomosis. Table 17.2 summarizes our experience with robotic colectomy with intracorporeal anastomosis.

We would like to comment on patient positioning. The lithotomy position may be considered in particular circumstances. For example, if intraoperative colonoscopy is necessary in order to check the anastomosis or confirm adequate removal of the pathology, access to the perineum is necessary. Another example is when transrectal or transvaginal extraction of the specimen will be performed. Finally, when the possibility of avoiding a resection exists, as in colotomy and polypectomy, laparoscopic-guided polypectomy, or wedge resection of a benign lesion, the lithotomy position is used.

With robotic colectomy, specimen extraction is typically transabdominal. As mentioned, intracorporeal anastomosis allows the surgeon to choose the extraction site as shown in Fig. 17.9a, b.

Morcellation of specimen is a technique that has not been widely studied and may have a roll in specimen management in the future, the goal being (as with intracorporeal anastomosis, tran-a

b

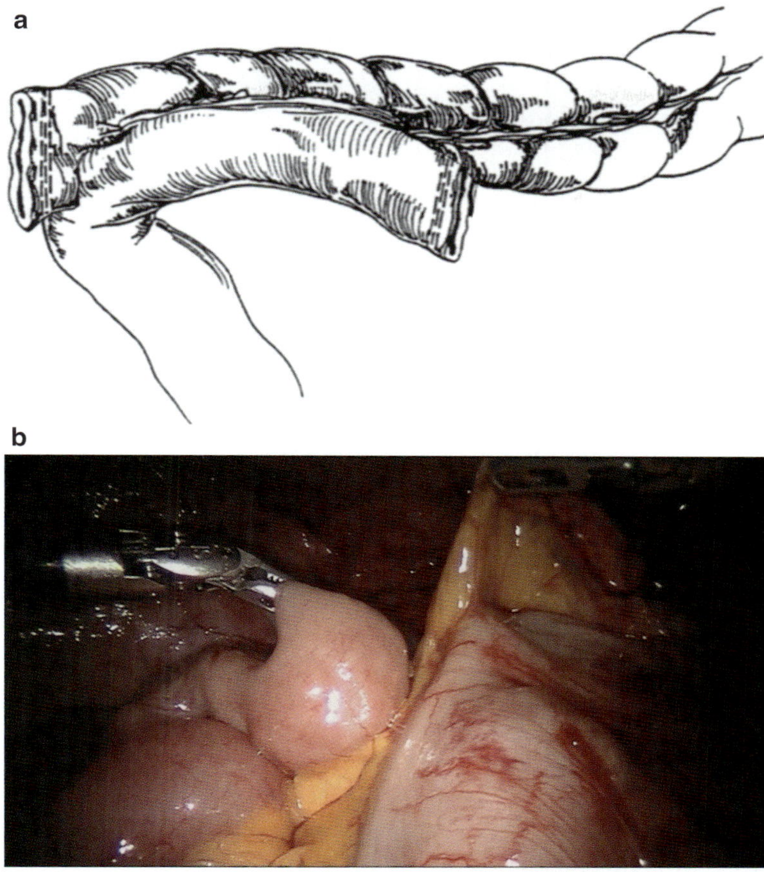

Fig. 17.4 (**a** and **b**) The terminal ileum and the transverse colon stump are brought together side by side

srectal, and transvaginal removal) smaller extraction site incisions.

One final note: although this chapter describes a three-arm technique, a fourth arm can be added intraoperatively if needed (Fig. 17.11). In select cases, particularly in the obese patient, it may be advantageous to start with a four-arm technique to facilitate the procedure.

Outcomes

In their systematic review of the literature, Antoniou et al. identified 39 series, which reported a total of 210 robotic right colectomies [6]. The mean operative time for these cases was 167 min (range, 152–228). These series included right colectomies with both extracorporeal and intracorporeal anastomotic techniques. Conversion rate was very low, 1.1 % to laparoscopic and 1.1 % to open. Intraoperative complications occurred in one patient (0.7 %). Overall postoperative morbidity was 12.7 %.

Table 17.3 summarizes the techniques, dissection, anastomosis, operative times, and conversion rate for the largest published series to date [17, 19, 22–24]. In 2011, we published our series comparing 25 laparoscopic to 22 robotic right colectomies [22]. Outcomes were similar and no conversions to open were necessary. Operative

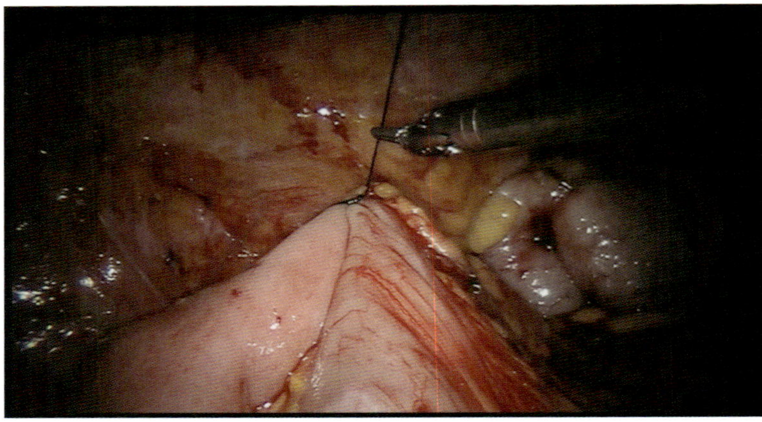

Fig. 17.5 A 20 cm nonabsorbable suture on a Keith needle is used to put a stay suture approximating the transverse colon and terminal ileum up to the abdominal wall to provide tension and elevate the site of the anastomosis

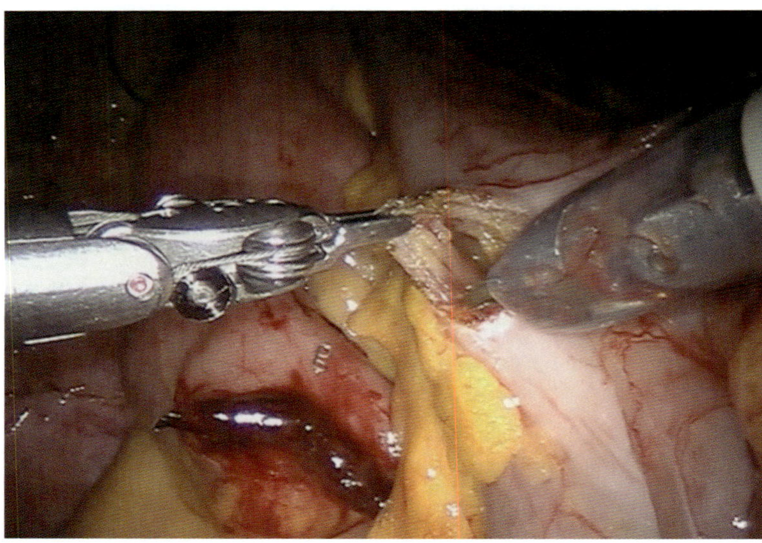

Fig. 17.6 Prior to creating the enterotomies, an endoscopic intestinal clamp (bulldog) can be placed on the terminal ileum to prevent spillage. Using an energy device or hot shears, a colotomy and ileotomy are created

times were longer in the robotic group; however, intracorporeal anastomosis was used in the robotic group, whereas an extracorporeal technique was used in the laparoscopic group. We used a three-arm robotic colectomy technique from the start of our learning curve initially to simplify the setup and decrease arm collisions (Fig. 17.17).

By only utilizing three robotic arms, port placement is easier because there is less concern with arm collisions. This is especially useful during the initial experience when the surgeon is challenged with multiple nuances of a new technique. As experience is gained, a fourth arm can be used selectively. We have found it advantageous to use the fourth robotic arm in right

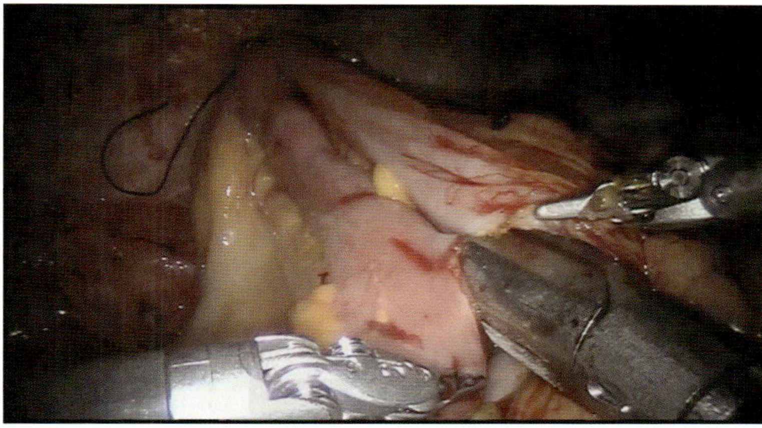

Fig. 17.7 The jaws of the endoscopic linear stapler are introduced to construct the common channel

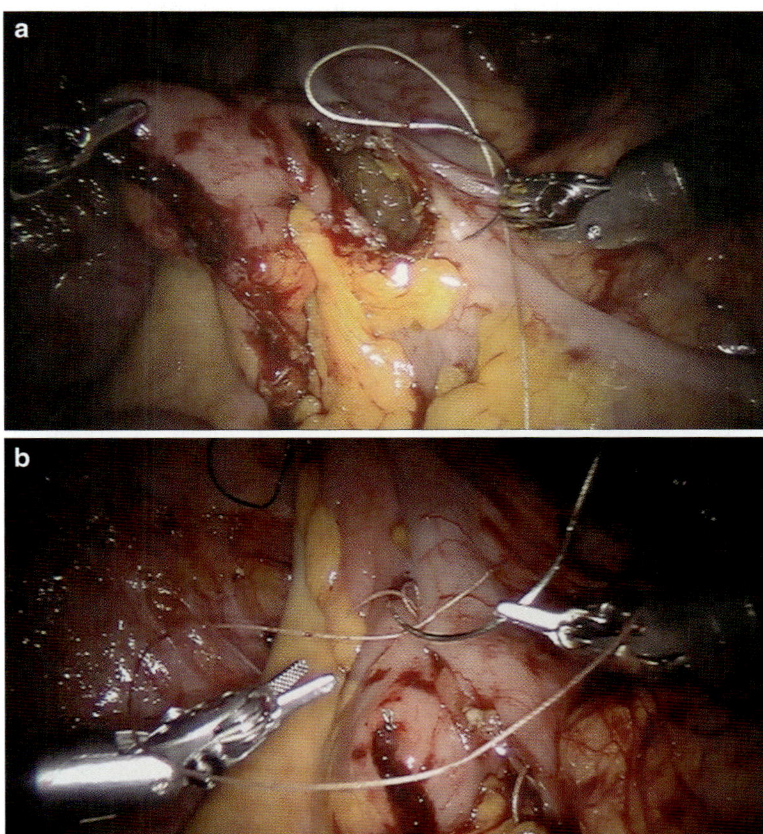

Fig. 17.8 (**a** and **b**) The remaining common enterotomy is then closed with 2-0 Vicryl in two running layers using robotic suturing techniques

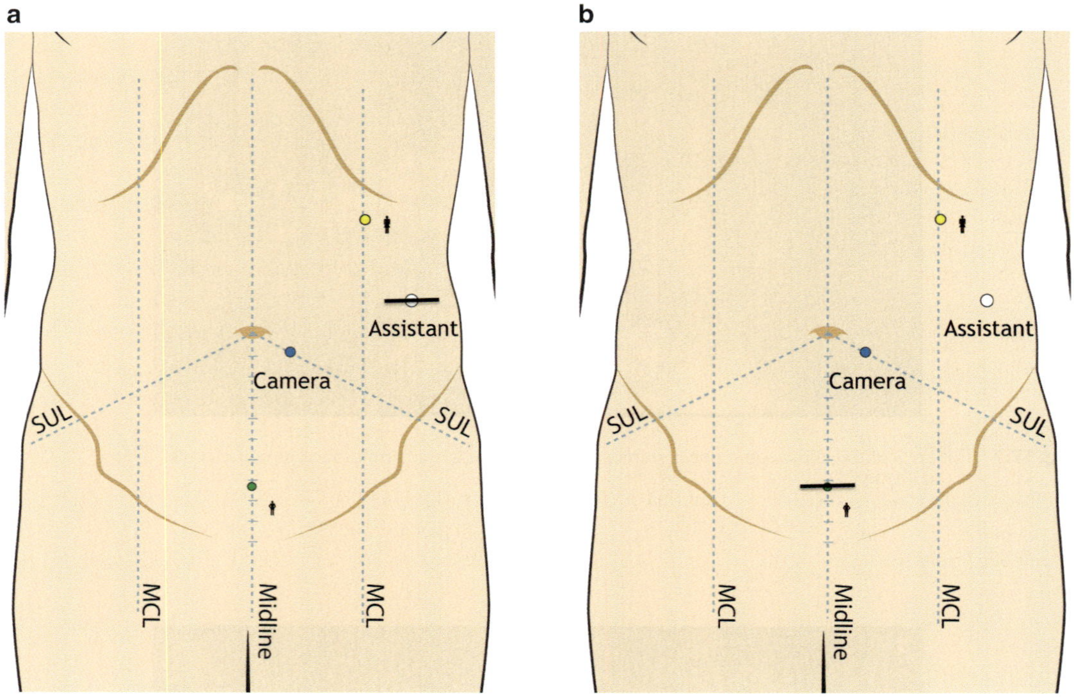

Fig. 17.9 (**a**) Extraction site placement for three-arm robotic right colectomy with intracorporeal anastomosis. The 12 mm assistant trocar site is extended as shown. (**b**) Alternative extraction site placement for three-arm robotic right colectomy with intracorporeal anastomosis. The 8 mm suprapubic R2 trocar site is extended as shown

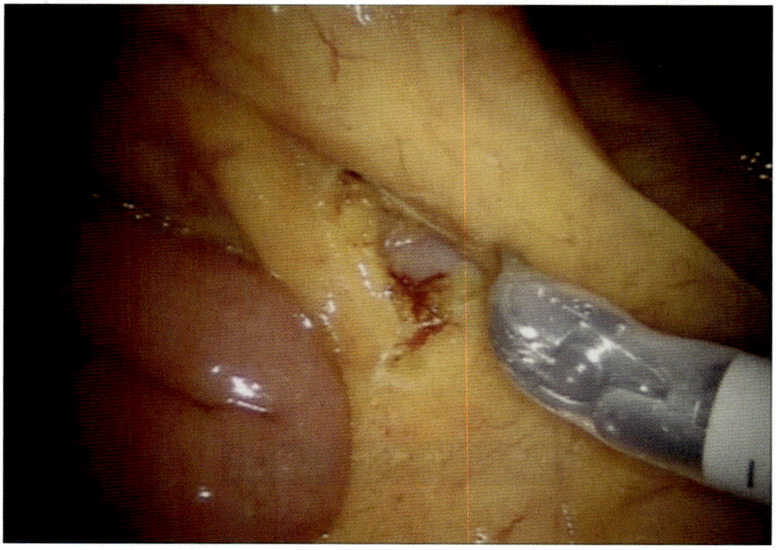

Fig. 17.10 The skin is closed in subcuticular fashion

Table 17.1 Critical steps of robotic right colectomy with intracorporeal anastomosis

	Figures
1. Identification of ileocecal junction (IJ)	17.10
2. Traction on IJ to expose the ileocolic vessels at their origin	17.10
3. Identify duodenum	17.10
4. Transect ileocolic vessels at their origin	17.11
5. Medial-to-lateral dissection	17.12
6. Transect terminal ileum	17.13a, b
7. Identify and divide right colic and right branch of middle colic	17.14
8. Transect transverse colon	17.15
9. Intracorporeal side-to-side isoperistaltic anastomosis	17.4a, b, 17.5, 17.6, 17.7, and 17.8a, b
10. Specimen extraction (wound protector)	17.16a, b

colectomies in the obese patient and when the dissection is challenging.

We believe the technique as we described above can be used in most cases and decreases time-consuming exchanges of instruments to the robotic arms. A 12 mm left lateral port allows the assistant to quickly do the necessary exchanges of graspers, suction, harmonic scalpel, suture transfer, and laparoscopic staplers. The assistant is kept actively involved in the procedure, and robotic arm exchanges are minimized. This is useful when the assistant is teaching the procedure to the console surgeon. It may also make the operation more efficient.

In general, a medial-to-lateral dissection technique is the preferred approach [25]. However, in some cases, because of anatomical variations, we start with a lateral-to-medial dissection. At this

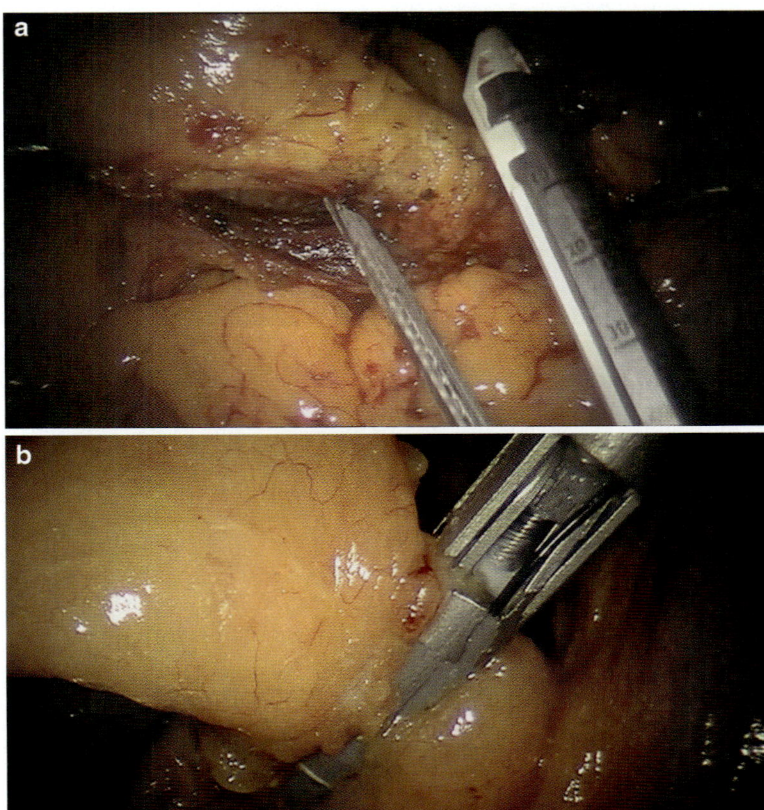

Fig. 17.11 If needed, an additional port (R3) can be added to the right lower quadrant

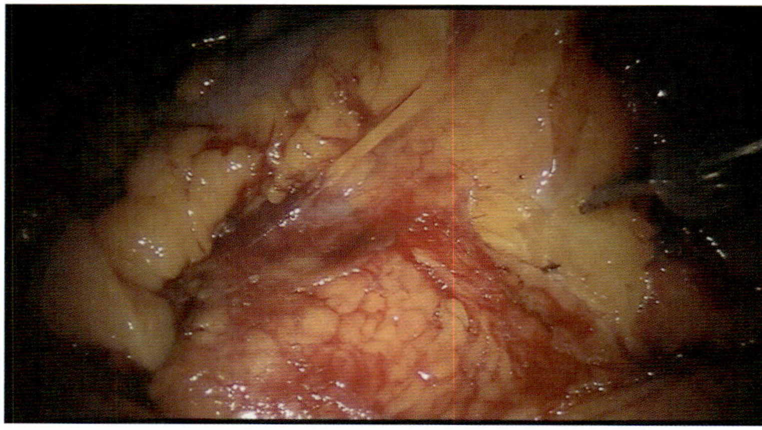

Fig. 17.12 Medial-to-lateral dissection

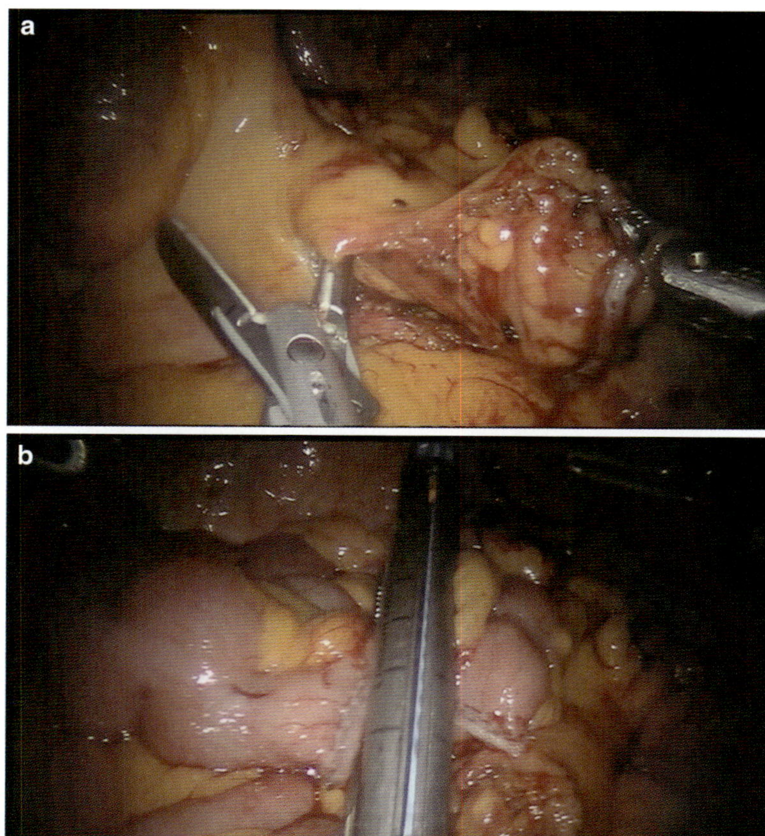

Fig. 17.13 (**a** and **b**) Transect terminal ileum

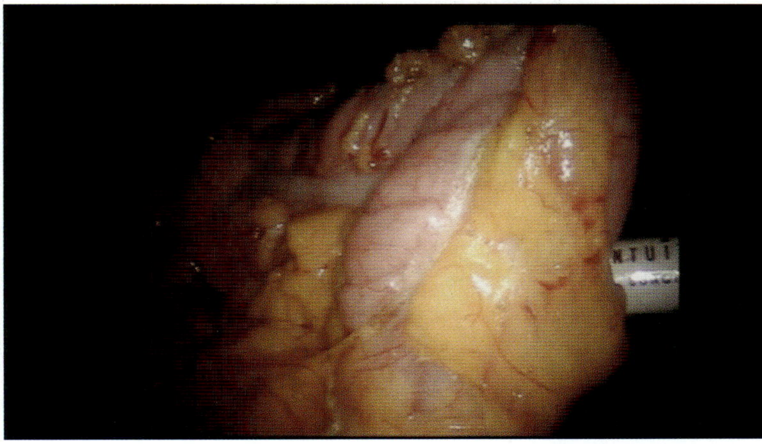

Fig. 17.14 Identify and divide right colic and right branch of middle colic

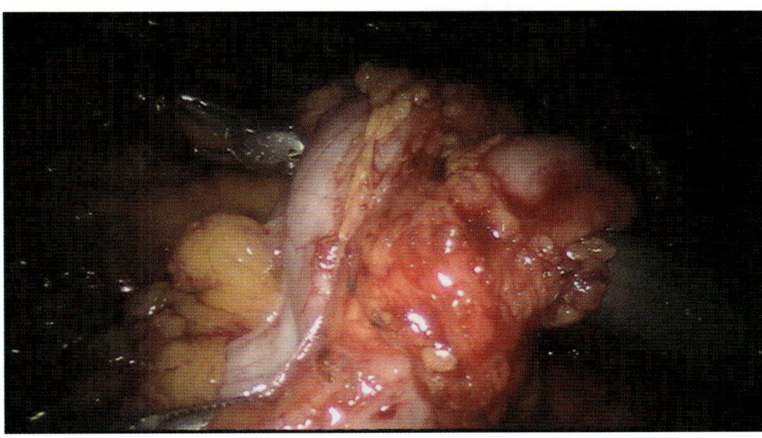

Fig. 17.15 Transect transverse colon

point, we recommend starting with a medial-to-lateral dissection; however, the surgeon's ability to apply either approach is useful and both seem to be effective. We found that lateral-to-medial dissection is often necessary, feasible, and does not require patient repositioning. For example, in the obese patient, it may first be necessary to get adequate length of mesentery, in order to identify, isolate, and transect the ileocolic vessels at their origin.

The mean operative time for a laparoscopic right colectomy as reported in the literature varies from 85 to 214 min [19]. In the systematic review mentioned above, the mean operative time for robotic right colectomy was 167 min ($N=210$) [6]. If we limit the data to laparoscopic right colectomy with intracorporeal anastomosis, the mean operative times as reported in the literature range from 136 to 190 min [26, 27, 28, 29]. Our operative times for a robotic right colectomy with intracorporeal anastomosis averaged 189 min ($N=50$) "skin-to-skin." Thus, our robotic operative times compare favorably with laparoscopic

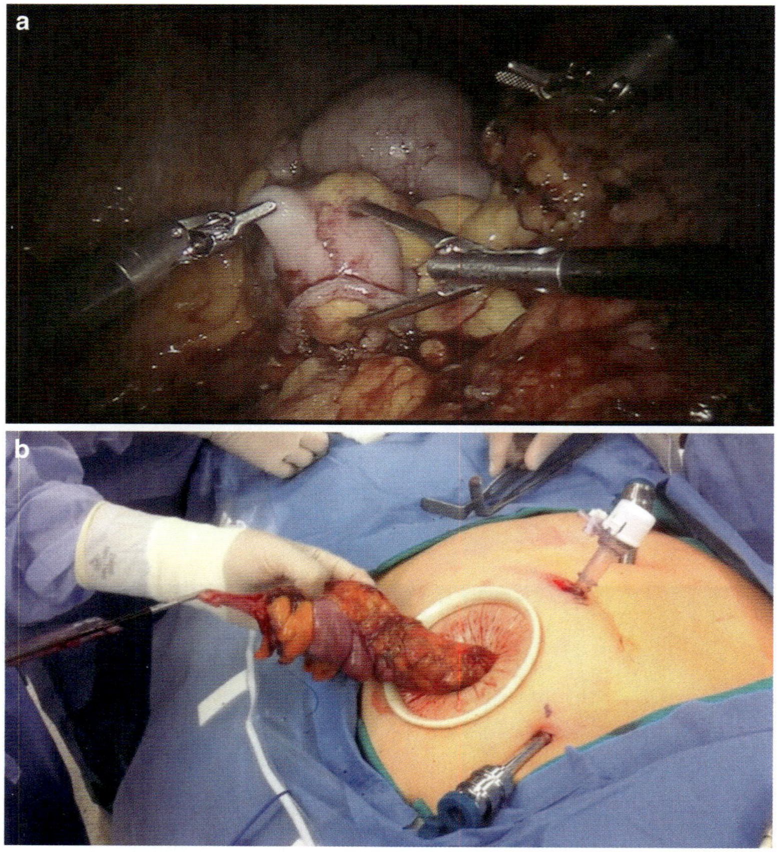

Fig. 17.16 (**a** and **b**) Specimen extraction (wound protector)

right colectomy times reported in the literature despite being early in our experience [22].

Additionally, we found that the transition from an extracorporeal to intracorporeal anastomosis was facilitated by the robotic platform. The improved surgical dexterity makes the switch to an intracorporeal anastomosis easier, and this may lead to a higher adoption rate for intracorporeal anastomosis, which is not very commonly used in laparoscopic right colectomy today. With an extracorporeal technique, the surgeon is often extracting, transecting, and creating an anastomosis through a small incision. Trying to accomplish this is sometimes difficult especially in the obese patient with a thick abdominal wall. There is probably less traction and tension applied to the colon and the mesentery during an intracorporeal anastomosis, as well as less trauma to the incision, which may translate into less postoperative ileus and fewer complications. Some studies have supported this potential benefit of the intracorporeal anastomosis [26, 27]. Grams et al. reported earlier return of bowel function, shorter length of hospital stay, and fewer complications [26]. Hellan et al. found similar outcomes with intracorporeal and extracorporeal anastomosis, but shorter incisions with intracorporeal anastomosis [27]. We found this to be true in our experience as well, with the mean extraction site excision measuring 4.6 cm

Table 17.2 Summary of our experience with robotic right colectomy with intracorporeal anastomosis

Demographic	Robotic right colectomy ($n=50$)
Mean age (range)	71.1 (52–89)
Mean BMI (range)	29.3 (19.4–68.8)
Gender	Female 23
	Male 27
Indication[a]	
Adenocarcinoma	28
Adenoma	20
Diverticulitis (right-sided)	1
Crohn's	1

Variable studied	Robotic right colectomy ($n=50$)
Mean operative time (range)	189.2 min (123–288)
Mean total operative time (range)	256.6 min (182–376)
Mean estimated blood loss (range)	48.6 ml (10–300)
Mean extraction site length (range)	4.3 cm (3–6.4)
Conversions to open surgery	0

Variable studied	Robotic right colectomy ($n=50$)
Intracorporeal anastomosis	50
Mean specimen length (range)	18.5 (10–37)
Mean lymph node harvest (range)	18.3 (0–40)
Length of stay (range)	Mean 3.7 days (1–21)
	Median 3 days

Complication	Robotic right colectomy ($n=50$)
Urinary retention	2
Wound infection	1
Nausea/vomiting	2
Ileus	4
Dehydration	1
Atelectasis	1
UTI	1
Pneumonia	1
Pleural effusion	1
Hypotension	1
Acute coronary syndrome	1
Postoperative rectal bleeding	1
Transfusion	2
Intra-abdominal abscess	2
Anastomotic leak[b]	1
30-Day mortality	0

Stage	$N=28$
0	4
I	5
II	10
III	8
IV	1

[a]Elective surgery
[b]Only reoperation requiring diverting loop ileostomy

versus 5.3 cm for the intracorporeal versus extracorporeal anastomosis [22]. Other practical advantages of the intracorporeal anastomosis include flexibility in choosing the extraction site since it is not determined by the anastomosis and the ability to prevent twisting of the mesentery by direct visualization prior to completion of the anastomosis.

Finally, there are very few studies to date addressing the oncologic outcomes with robotic techniques. It is likely that for robotic right colectomy and partial colectomy, results will be similar to laparoscopic colectomy. In their study of 50 consecutive right colectomies for cancer, D'Annibale et al. reported similar pathologic parameters and similar lymph node harvest in both groups [23]. They concluded robotic right colectomy was safe and provided adequate oncologic resection with acceptable short-term results. Because the da Vinci robot is a tool to perform laparoscopic surgery, studies will likely show no difference and no untoward effects as has been demonstrated with laparoscopic right colectomy for cancer. Future studies will reveal recurrence rates and long-term survival.

Conclusion

In conclusion, as several authors and we have demonstrated, robotic right colectomy is safe and feasible [2, 17, 19, 22–25]. Operative times actually seem to be comparable to laparoscopic col-

Table 17.3 Data of the largest published series of robotic right colectomy

Study (reference)	Year	*N*	Technique	# of ports (Robot arms)	Anastomosis	Operative time (min)
Rawlings et al. [17]	2007	17	MtL	5 (4)	IC	Mean 219
Spinoglio et al. [24]	2008	18	MtL	5 (4)	NR	267[a]
deSouza et al. [19]	2010	40	MtL > LtM	4 (3)	EC	Mean 159
D'Annibale et al. [23]	2010	50	MtL	5 (4)	IC	Median 224
Lujan et al. [22]	2011	22	MtL > LtM	4 (3)	IC	Mean 189

N = number of patients, # = number, MtL = medial-to-lateral, LtM = lateral-to-medial, IC = intracorporeal, EC = extracorporeal, NR = not reported
[a]Only last case reported

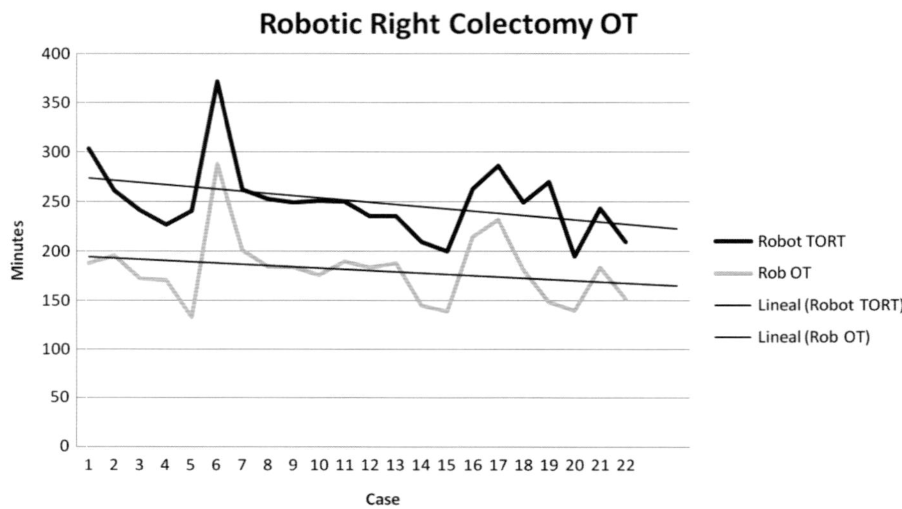

Fig. 17.17 Robotic right colectomy operative times and total operating room times: our published experience with the first 22 cases with intracorporeal anastomosis

ectomy. The true advantage of robotics may lie in its ability to simplify complex tasks, and robotics may facilitate the adoption of minimally invasive techniques, intracorporeal anastomosis, and promote associated advantages.

References

1. Maeso S, Reza M, Mayol JA, et al. Efficacy of the Da Vinci surgical system in abdominal surgery compared with that of laparoscopy: a systematic review and meta-analysis. Ann Surg. 2010;252:254–62.
2. Weber P, Merola S, Wasielewski A, Ballantyne GH. Telerobotic-assisted laparoscopic right and sigmoid colectomies for benign disease. Dis Colon Rectum. 2002;45(12):1689–96.
3. D'Annibale A, Morpurgo E, Fiscon V, et al. Robotic and laparoscopic surgery for colorectal diseases. Dis Colon Rectum. 2004;47:2162–8.
4. Mehran A, Daniel WB, Fahad B, Robert G, Trevor C. Robotic-assisted laparoscopic colorectal surgery. Surg Laparosc Endosc Percutan Tech. 2004;14(6):311–5.
5. Baik SH. Robotic colorectal surgery. Yonsei Med J. 2008;49(6):891.
6. Antoniou SA, Antoniou GA, Koch OO, Pointner R, Granderath FA. Robotic assisted laparoscopic surgery of the colon and rectum. Surg Endosc. 2012; 26:1–11.
7. Shabbir A, Rosiani A, Wong K-S, Tsang CB, Wong H-B, Cheong W-K. Is laparoscopic colectomy as cost beneficial as open colectomy? ANZ J Surg. 2009;79:265–70.

8. Fleshman J, Sargent DJ, Green E, et al. Laparoscopic colectomy for cancer is not inferior to open surgery based on 5-year data from the COST study group trial. Ann Surg. 2007;246(4):655–64.
9. Schwenk W, Haase O, Neudecker J, Muller JM. Short term benefits for laparoscopic colorectal resection. Cochrane Database Syst Rev. 2005;20(3):CD003145.
10. Romano G, Gagliardi G, Bianco F, Parker MC. Laparoscopic colorectal surgery: why it is still not the gold standard and why it should be. Tech Coloproctol. 2008;12:185–8.
11. Bordeianou L, Rattner D. Is laparoscopic sigmoid colectomy for diverticulitis the new gold standard? Gastroenterology. 2010;138:2213–6.
12. Lauter DM, Froines EJ. Initial experience with 150 cases of laparoscopic assisted colectomy. Am J Surg. 2001;181(5):398–403.
13. Jacobs M, Verdeja MC, Goldstein HS. Minimally invasive colon resection (laparoscopic colectomy). Surg Laparosc Endosc. 1991;1(3):144–50.
14. Carmichael JC, Masoomi H, Mills S, Stamos MJ, Nguyen NT. Utilization of laparocopy in colorectal surgery for cancer at academic medical centers: does site of surgery affect rate of laparoscopy? Am Surg. 2011;77(10):1300–4.
15. Kang CY, Halabi WJ, Luo R, Pigazzi A, Nguyen NT, Stamos MJ. Laparoscopic colorectal surgery: a better look into the latest trends arch surg. Surg. 2012; 147(8):724–31.
16. Pigazzi A, Garcia-Aguilar J. Robotic colorectal surgery: for whom and for what? Dis Colon Rectum. 2010;53:969–70.
17. Rawlings AL, Woodland JH, Vegunta RK, Crawford DL. Robotic versus laparoscopic colectomy. Surg Endosc. 2007;21(10):1701–8.
18. Zimmern A, Prasad L, deSouza A, Marecik S, Park J, Abcarian H. Robotic colon and rectal surgery: a series of 131 cases. World J Surg. 2010;34(8):1954–8.
19. DeSouza AL, Prasad LM, Park JJ, Marecik SJ, Blumetti J, Abcarian H. Robotic assistance in right hemicolectomy: is there a role? Dis Colon Rectum. 2010;53:1000–6.
20. Delaney CP, Lynch AC, Senagore AJ, Fazio VW. Comparison of robotically performed and traditional laparoscopic colorectal surgery. Dis Colon Rectum. 2003;46(12):1633–9.
21. Mutch M, Cellini C. Surgical management of colon cancer In: Beck DE, Roberts PL, Saclarides TJ, Senagore AJ, Stamos MJ, Wexner SD, eds. The ASCRS textbook of colon and rectal surgery. Second Edition, New York, NY: Springer Science + Business Media, LLC., 2011;711–20.
22. Lujan HJ, Maciel VH, Romero R, Plasencia G. Laparoscopic versus robotic right colectomy: a single surgeon's experience. J Robotic Surg. 2013;7:95.
23. D'Annibale A, Pernazza G, Morpurgo E, Monsellato I, Pende V, Lucandri G, et al. Robotic right colon resection: evaluation of first 50 consecutive cases for malignant disease. Ann Surg Oncol. 2010;17:2856–62.
24. Spinoglio G, Summa M, Priora F, Quarati R, Testa S. Robotic colorectal surgery: first 50 cases experience. Dis Colon Rectum. 2008;51:1627–32.
25. Ballantyne GH, Ewing D, Pigazzi A, Wasielewski A. Telerobotic-assisted laparoscopic right hemicolectomy: lateral to medial or medial to lateral dissection? Surg Laparosc Endosc Percutan Tech. 2006;16(6): 406–10.
26. Grams J, Tong W, Greenstein AJ, Salky B. Comparison of intracorporeal versus extracorporeal anastomosis for laparoscopic-assisted hemicolectomy. 2010;24: 1886–91.
27. Hellan M, Anderson C, Pigazzi A. Extracorporeal versus intracorporeal anastomosis for laparoscopic right hemicolectomy. JSLS. 2009;13:312–7.
28. Franklin ME, Gonzalez JJ, Miter DB, Mansur JH, Trevino JM, Glass JL, et al. Laparoscopic right hemicolectomy for cancer: 11-year experience. Rev Gastroenterol Mex. 2004;69 Suppl 1:65–72.
29. Scatizzi M, Kroning KC, Borrelli A, Andan G, Lenzi E, Feroci F. Extracorporeal versus intracorporeal anastomosis after laparoscopic right colectomy for cancer: a case–control study. World J Surg. 2010;34:2902–8.

Robotic Left Colectomy

18

Eduardo Parra-Davila and Carlos M. Ortiz-Ortiz

Introduction

Laparoscopic colorectal surgery has increased all over the world due to its known benefits such as less pain, shorter stay, reduced recovery time, early ambulation, and decreased associated comorbidities. However, laparoscopic colectomies have been a challenge due to steep learning curves, limited dexterity of laparoscopic instruments, and suboptimal visualization. With the use of a surgical robot, laparoscopic limitations can be overcome offering the patient a good alternative for a minimally invasive procedure.

The robotic platform has several advantages over conventional laparoscopy. It provides a magnified full high definition 3D camera that is always under the surgeon's control with instruments that have a free articulating endowrist and arms that facilitate the dissection and retraction of the specimen in complex surgeries. The movements of the robotic arms are precise with complete elimination of tremors produced by surgeon's hand. The ergonomic position of the surgeon while working on the console reduces the muscle strain on the surgeon in the difficult and long procedures [1].

The da Vinci system has been used for different types of general surgery procedures, and there has been increased interest in the last few years in colorectal surgery; however, there is still no standardized technique. For left colon resection several procedures have been described:

1. Hybrid technique: Mainly consists of laparoscopic mobilization of splenic flexure followed by docking for pelvic dissection and completion of procedure.
2. Single-docking technique [1]: Incorporates mobilizing the second and third robotic arm for different parts of the procedure.
3. Double-docking technique: Incorporates docking from left upper quadrant for dissection of the splenic flexure and then changing the docking to the left lower quadrant.

Recently the introduction of an articulating vessel sealer has allowed mobilization of the splenic flexure with minimal changes in the current port placement of a single-docking technique.

Patient Selection

Robotic-assisted left colectomy is recommended for small T0 (unable to be removed by colonoscopy), T1 tumors with invasion to submucosa,

E. Parra-Davila, M.D., F.A.C.S., F.A.S.C.R.S. (✉)
Director of Minimally Invasive and Colorectal Surgery, Director of Hernia and Abdominal Wall Reconstruction, Celebration Health-Florida Hospital, 410 Celebration Place, Suite 401, Celebration, FL 34747, USA
e-mail: eparradavila@gmail.com

C.M. Ortiz-Ortiz, M.D.
Department of General Surgery, Florida Hospital—Celebration, 410 Celebration Place, Suite 401, Celebration, FL 34747, USA
e-mail: zurdo_jc@hotmail.com

K.C. Kim (ed.), *Robotics in General Surgery*, DOI 10.1007/978-1-4614-8739-5_18,

and certain T2–T4 tumors that have an approach feasible for minimally invasive surgery.

Absolute and relative contraindications for robotic-assisted left colectomy include bulky disease with invasion to adjacent organs, colonic obstruction that needs emergent decompression, or patient with contraindications for pneumoperitoneum.

Ideal patients to start a robotic colorectal program include the following:

1. No previous medical conditions
2. BMI < 30
3. No previous intra-abdominal surgery
4. No previous radiotherapy
5. Low TNM status

Patient Preparation

Bowel preparation is based on surgeon preferences. In our patients we prepare the bowel with milk of magnesia unless the exact location of the lesion is unknown, in which case full bowel cleansing is ordered. We follow the guidelines for perioperative intravenous antibiotics [2].

Intraoperative preparation includes [2]:

1. Foley catheter
2. Orogastric tube for stomach decompression
3. DVT prophylaxis with bilateral sequential compression devices and subcutaneous low molecular weight heparin
4. Warmer to avoid hypothermia

OR Configuration

The operation room setup is shown in Fig. 18.1. The patient's left side of the table is kept clear to permit adequate docking of the robotic cart. During the procedure, the robotic cart is approached toward the left side of the table at the left upper or lower quadrant depending on whether splenic flexure mobilization is needed or not. The surgical assistant is located on the patient's right side, and the scrub nurse is at the lower right side.

Patient Positioning

The patient is positioned in modified lithotomy position with legs abducted and slightly flexed. The patient's arms are tucked along the side of the body, and pads are placed in possible pressure points. This position is fixed with a vacuum-assisted mattress device. Once the patient is secure, the patient is placed with a 15°–20° Trendelenburg position and with a tilt of 15° to the right side of the patient. After adequate patient positioning, we perform the robotic cart docking.

Port Placement and Robotic Position

Currently we are performing the robotic left colectomy with the following options depending on case selection and body habitus.

1. Trocar placement for single docking (Fig. 18.2a, b)

   This trocar placement configuration is best when using the da Vinci vessel sealer, which is wristed and provides the range of motion for the splenic flexure to be reached from the first and the third arms.
2. Trocar placement for hybrid technique (Fig. 18.3a, b)

   This trocar placement is used when anticipating pelvic adhesions and/or rectal surgery. The first portion of the procedure (splenic flexure takedown) is done laparoscopically, and then the second portion (pelvic dissection) is done with the robot docked from the left side.
3. Trocar placement for double docking totally robotic approach (Fig. 18.4a, b).

   With this trocar configuration the robot is docked at the left upper quadrant to start the mobilization of the splenic flexure. Once that is accomplished the robot is then docked at the left lower quadrant for the pelvic portion of the procedure.

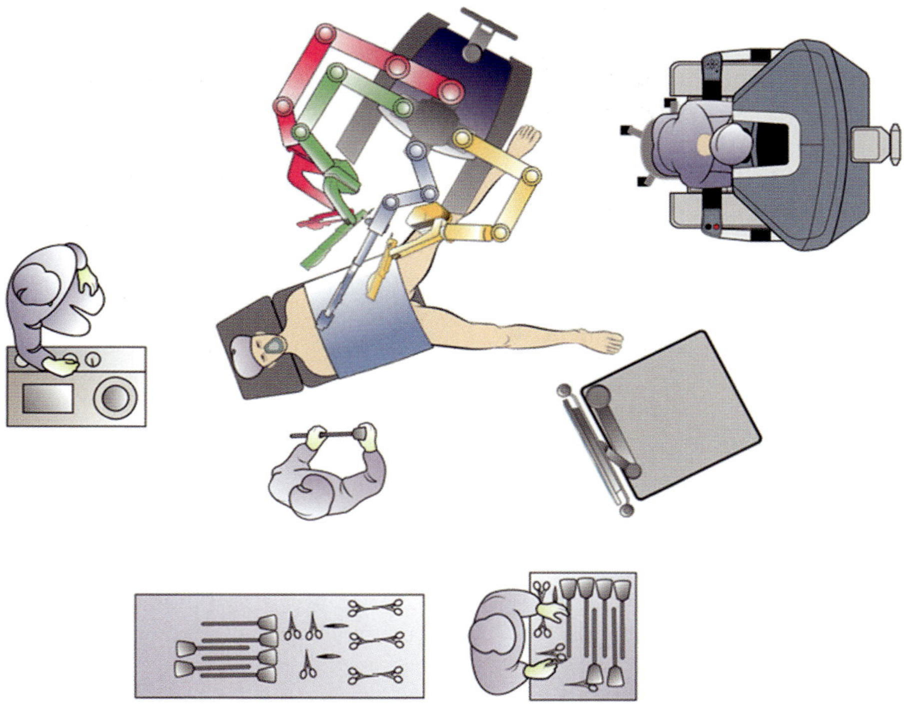

Fig. 18.1 Configuration of operating room for robot, console, and instrument table

Instrument Allocation to the Robotic Arms

- Instrument arm 1 with monopolar curved scissors or da Vinci vessel sealer: docked to the RLQ port as a surgeon's right hand
- Instrument arm 2 with Maryland bipolar forceps: docked to the LUQ port as a surgeon's left hand
- Instrument arm 3 with bowel grasper: docked to the RUQ port as a surgeon's second left hand

Initially, the surgeon makes an assessment of what seems easier either the medial or lateral approach. If the medial approach is chosen, the mesocolon over the inferior mesenteric artery (IMA) is retracted upwardly with the bowel grasper forceps. The peritoneum around the base of the IMA is incised and dissected with monopolar scissors. The periaortic hypogastric nerve plexus is carefully preserved. The left gonadal vessels and the ureter are identified and preserved. The IMA is divided near the root with Hem-o-lok® clips (Weck Closure System, Research Triangle Park, NC, USA) or with the da Vinci vessel sealer. The inferior mesenteric vein is identified by dissecting superiorly toward the ligament of Treitz and is divided near the inferior border of the pancreas.

The medial dissection continues laterally until the left colon is separated from the retroperitoneum and superiorly over the pancreas until the lesser sac is entered. Lateral detachment is initiated along the white line, while the sigmoid colon is retracted medially by the robotic arm 2 or the assistant. The lateral dissection continues cephalad to the mid portion of the descending colon. The splenic flexure is mobilized if necessary to achieve a tension-free anastomosis. The transverse mesocolon is opened just above the body of the pancreas to enter the lesser sac. Dissection of the transverse mesocolon continues toward the distal transverse colon and the

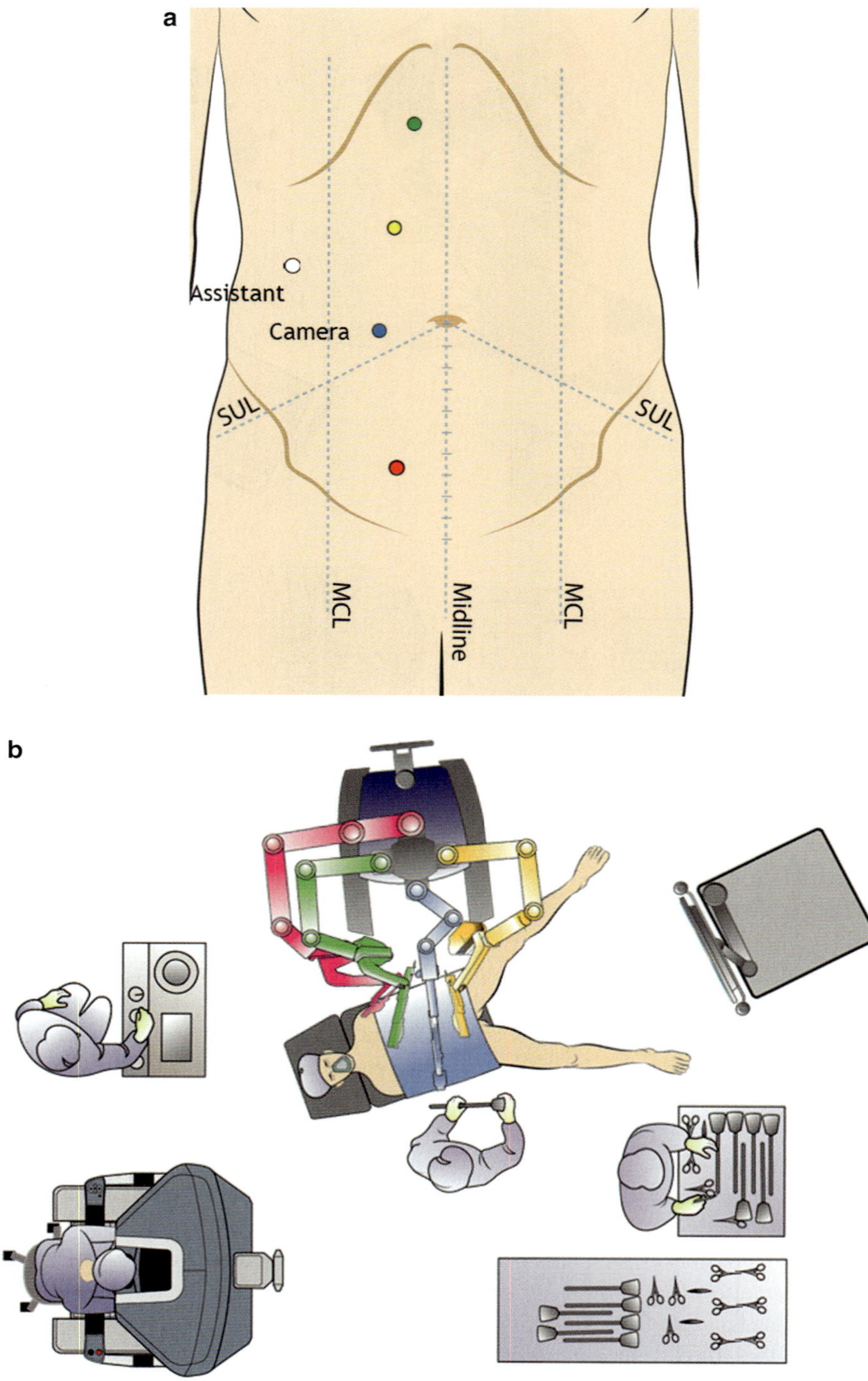

Fig. 18.2 (**a**) Trocar placement for single-docking technique. (**b**) Configuration of operating room for robot, console, and instrument table for single-docking technique

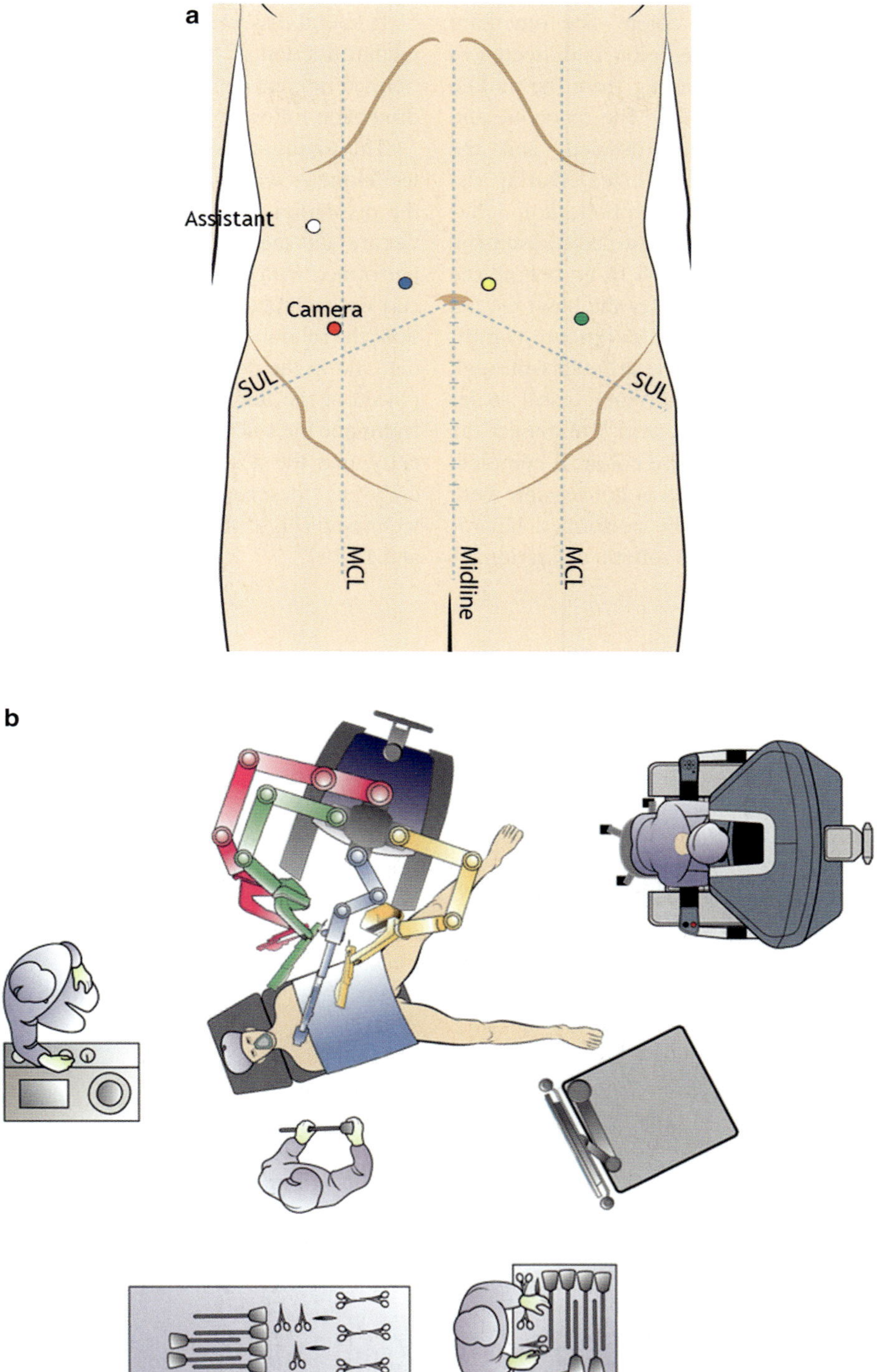

Fig. 18.3 (**a**) Trocar placement for hybrid technique. (**b**) Configuration of operating room for robot, console, and instrument table for hybrid technique

base of the descending colon. The omentum attached to the transverse colon is dissected in the avascular plane, beginning from the middle third of the transverse colon. The renocolic and splenocolic ligaments are divided, and the splenic flexure is fully mobilized. During the splenic flexure mobilization, robotic arm 1 has the da Vinci vessel sealer, and we take advantage of its wristed range of motion to go behind the lateral attachments and also for the blunt medial dissection. The assistant can contribute significantly by inserting his/her instruments through the remaining port. The da Vinci vessel sealer can also be used on robotic arm 3 to dissect the omentum from the transverse colon. If complete splenic flexure mobilization is not feasible with the robot docked, it can be performed laparoscopically at the end of the robotic dissection.

If lateral dissection is chosen, the first step is medial traction of the colon starting the dissection laterally as described above, and the medial dissection follows once the colon is up in the air.

This sequence works for the double-docking technique as well, and the only difference is that the dissection is done in two steps: the splenic flexure and the descending colon dissection are performed with a different location of the robotic cart for each phase. In the splenic flexure dissection, the robotic cart is placed over the left shoulder, and in the descending colon dissection, it is placed at the left lower quadrant. In the hybrid technique the splenic flexure is done laparoscopically, and the descending colon is done robotically as described for the double-docking technique (Figs. 18.5a, b, 18.6, 18.7, 18.8, 18.9, and 18.10).

a

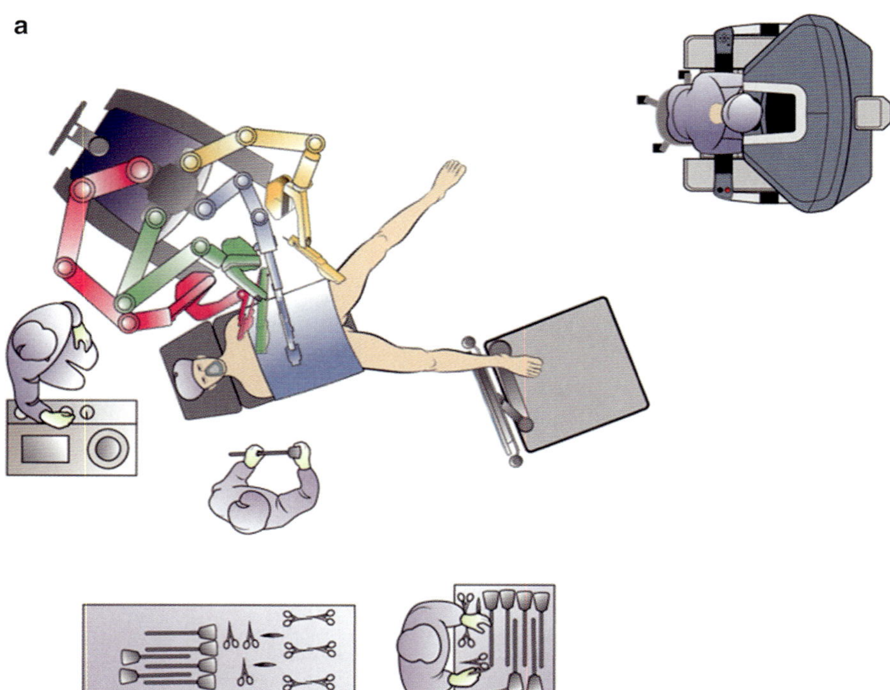

Fig. 18.4 (**a**) Trocar placement for double-docking technique. (**b**) Configuration of operating room for robot, console, and instrument table for double-docking technique

b

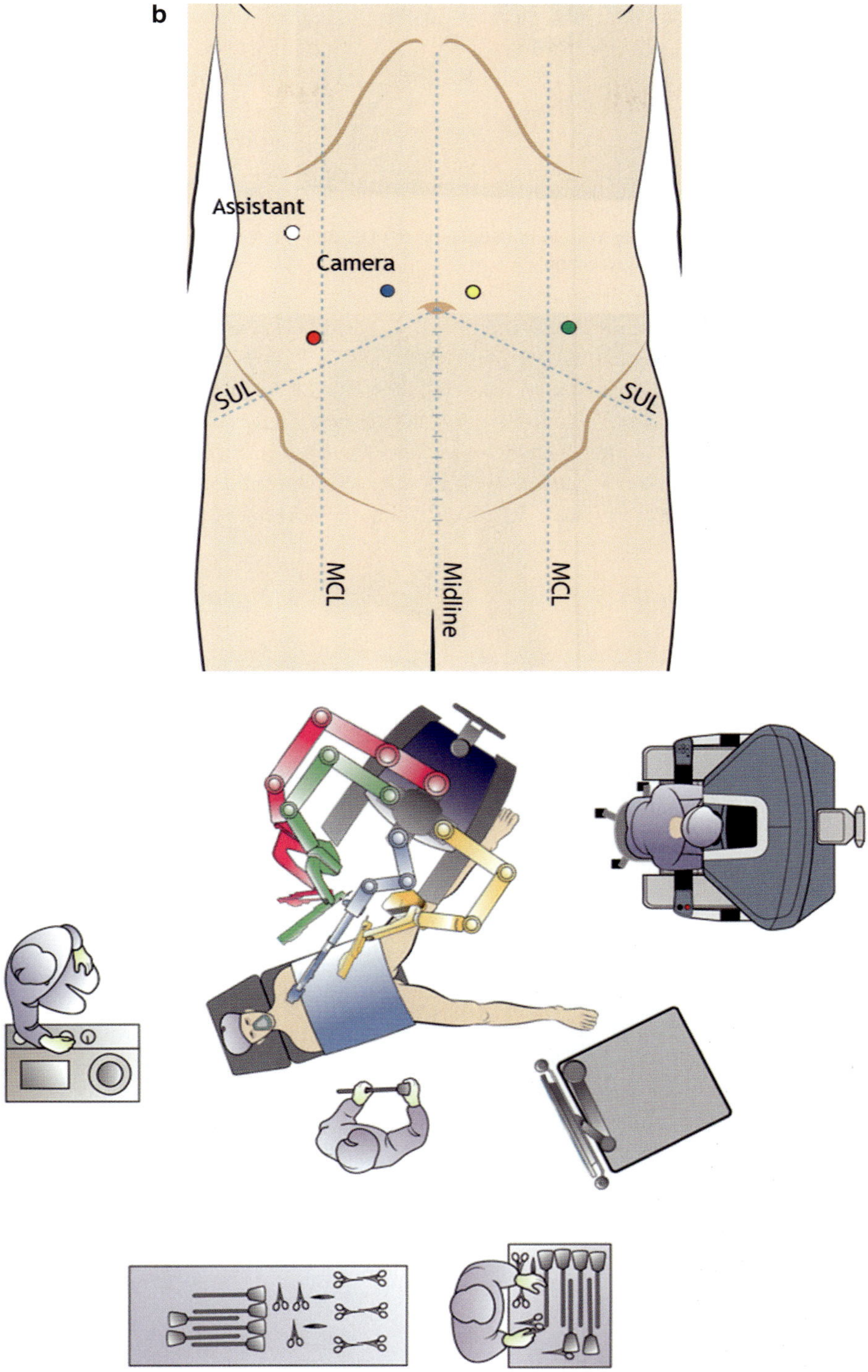

Fig. 18.4 (continued)

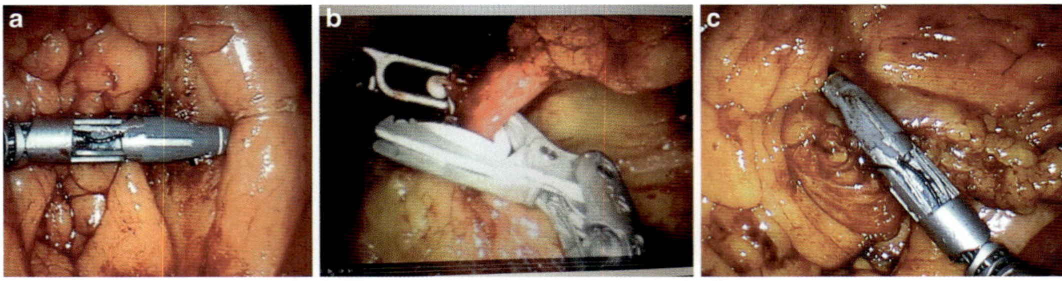

Fig. 18.5 (**a**) Vessel sealer-controlling vessels in mesentery. (**b**) Dividing IMA with robotic clip applier. (**c**) Vessel sealer cleaning mesentery at proximal resection

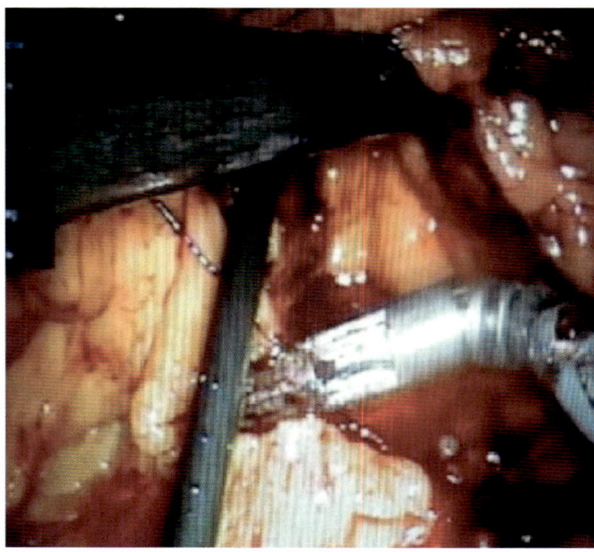

Fig. 18.6 Vessel sealer during medial dissection toward splenic flexure

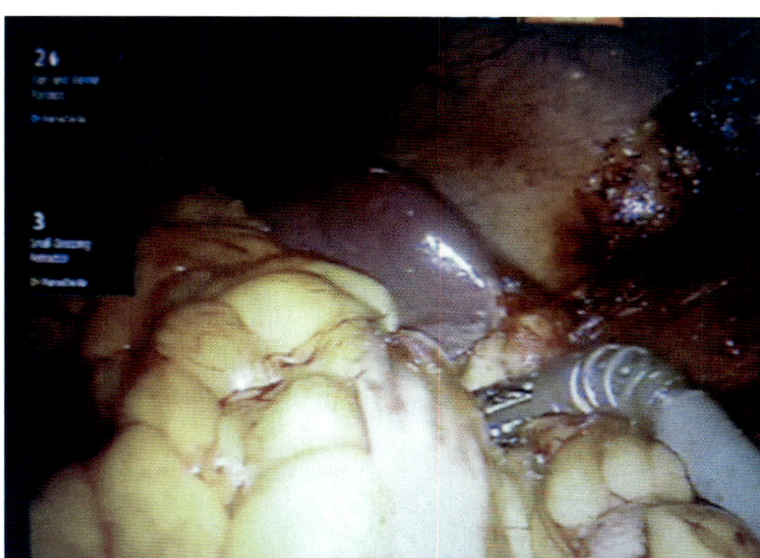

Fig. 18.7 Lateral mobilization of splenic flexure with vessel sealer

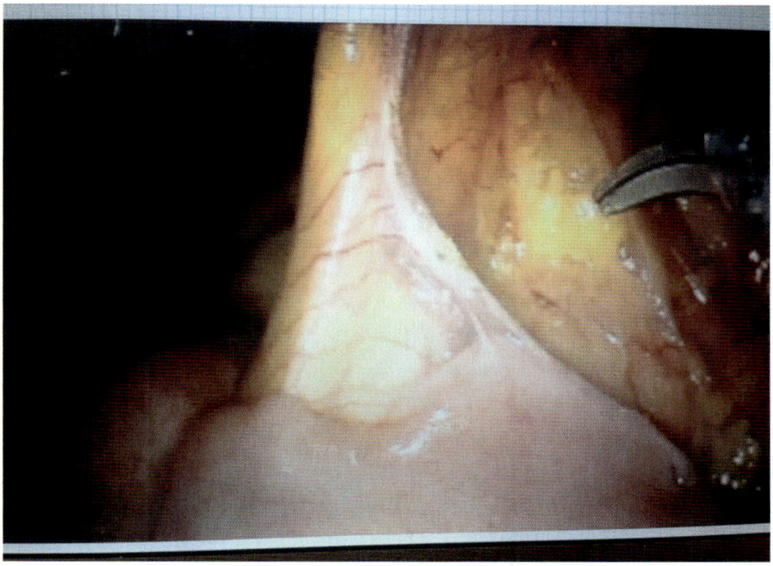

Fig. 18.8 Medial mobilization toward ligament of Treitz

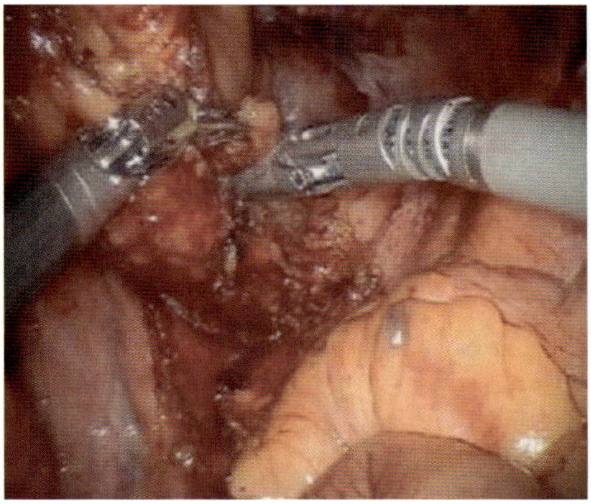

Fig. 18.9 Vessel sealer preparing rectum for stapler transaction

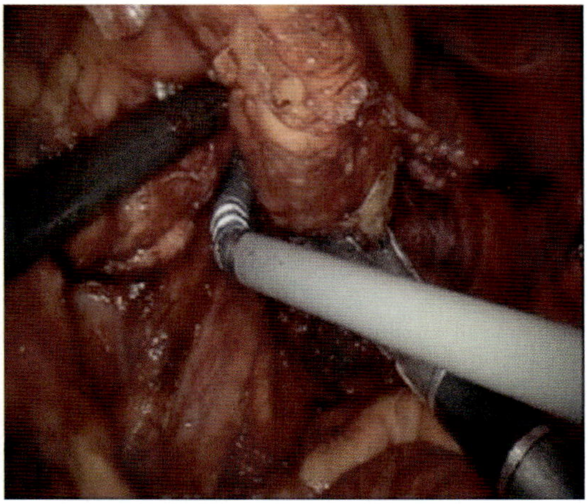

Fig. 18.10 Dissection of distal margin (rectum) with stapler

Limitations

Clinical outcomes of robotic left colectomies are quite comparable with those of the laparoscopic technique. The safety and feasibility of both hybrid and totally robotic colon surgery have already been established, and the only difference in approach appears to be longer operative times with the totally robotic approach [3–6].

Compared to laparoscopic surgery, the robotic system is not able to transmit tactile sensation to the surgeon in the console. Additionally, there are limitations in the instruments that are available, particularly the stapler (recently FDA approved), that require the assistant at the bedside to perform some components of the procedure. The nature of the instrument exchange required in robotic surgery can also add to the operative time and to potential injury to the patient. Lastly, accessing all the parts of the abdominal cavity necessary to perform a left colectomy can be a challenge requiring more than one docking, adding to the complexity of the procedure and the operative time.

Conclusions

Robotic left colectomy has been proven to be feasible and can be expected to have additional advantages from the enhanced visualization and maneuverability of instruments and precision in dissection over laparoscopic surgery especially in complicated procedures. Comparative studies are needed to determine whether these advantages will translate into improved clinical outcomes. This technology continues to evolve to add to the complement of tools that will increasingly make this platform a part of the armamentarium of the colorectal surgeon in order to provide better care for the patient.

References

1. Choi DJ, Kim SH, Lee PJ, et al. Single stage totally robotic dissection for rectal cancer surgery: technique and short term outcome in 50 consecutive patients. Dis Colon Rectum. 2009;52(11):1824–30.
2. Parra-Davila, Eduardo MD, Diaz-Hernandez, Juan MD. J Robot Surg 2011;5(1):57–64.
3. Weber PA, Merola S, Wasielewski A, Ballantyne GH. Telerobot-assisted laparoscopic right and sigmoid colectomies for benign disease. Dis Colon Rectum. 2002;45:1689–94.
4. D'Annibale A, Morpurgo E, Fiscon V, Trevisan P, Sovernigo G, Orsini C, Guidolin D. Robotic and laparoscopic surgery for treatment of colorectal diseases. Dis Colon Rectum. 2004;47:2162–8.
5. Anvari M, Birch DW, Bamehriz F, Gryfe R, Chapman T. Robotic-assisted laparoscopic colorectal surgery. Surg Laparosc Endosc Percutan Tech. 2004;14:311–5.
6. Rawlings AL, Woodland JH, Vegunta RK, Crawford DL. Robotic versus laparoscopic colectomy. Surg Endosc. 2007;21:1701–8.

Totally Robotic Low Anterior Resection

19

Jung Myun Kwak and Seon Hahn Kim

Introduction

Since the first robot-assisted colectomy was reported by Weber et al. [1] in 2002, robotic surgery has been performed in a variety of operations and embraced a wide range of diseases, including those benign and those malignant [2–4]. At present, given the particular advantage of utilizing robotics in pelvic procedure, there is a great interest in the application of a robotic surgical system for total mesorectal excision (TME). The majority of recent studies have been focusing on robotic TME for rectal cancer [5–12].

The surgical procedure for low anterior resection (LAR) involves more than one abdominal quadrant. Even when omitting the splenic flexure mobilization, the operator should mobilize a wide operative field from the left colon to the bottom of the pelvic floor. This limits the application of the current robotic system, which has a limited range of arm movement secondary to a fixed position of the patient cart. Due to this limitation, the complete robotic rectal resection initially required movement of the patient cart during the operation, which was troublesome and time consuming [2, 13]. A hybrid technique for rectal resections has therefore evolved and is currently being widely adopted [6–10].

Since we started using the da Vinci® robotic system to perform surgery for rectal cancers in July 2007, we have developed a single-stage totally robotic technique that does not require movement of the patient cart during the entire dissection of the LAR [5]. We have improved this technique during the course of more than 200 operations to further facilitate easy and safe operations. In this chapter, we describe the surgical technique of totally robotic LAR currently used at our institute and review short-term clinical, pathological, and oncological outcomes based on the literature.

J.M. Kwak, M.D., Ph.D. (✉) • S.H. Kim, M.D. Ph.D.
Department of Surgery, Korea University Anam Hospital, Anam-dong 5-Ga, Seongbuk-Gu, Seoul 136-705, Republic of Korea
e-mail: drkimsh@korea.ac.kr

Procedure Overview

Patient Positioning for Totally Robotic LAR

Proper positioning of the patient is an essential first step for total robotic LAR procedures. Without proper patient positioning and port placement, robotic-assisted procedures are tedious to perform and patient outcomes can be compromised. Attention should be placed not only on patient safety issues but also on safe docking of the robot and good exposure of the surgical field.

After the induction of general anesthesia, the patient is placed in a modified lithotomy position with a beanbag mattress to prevent sliding.

K.C. Kim (ed.), *Robotics in General Surgery*, DOI 10.1007/978-1-4614-8739-5_19,

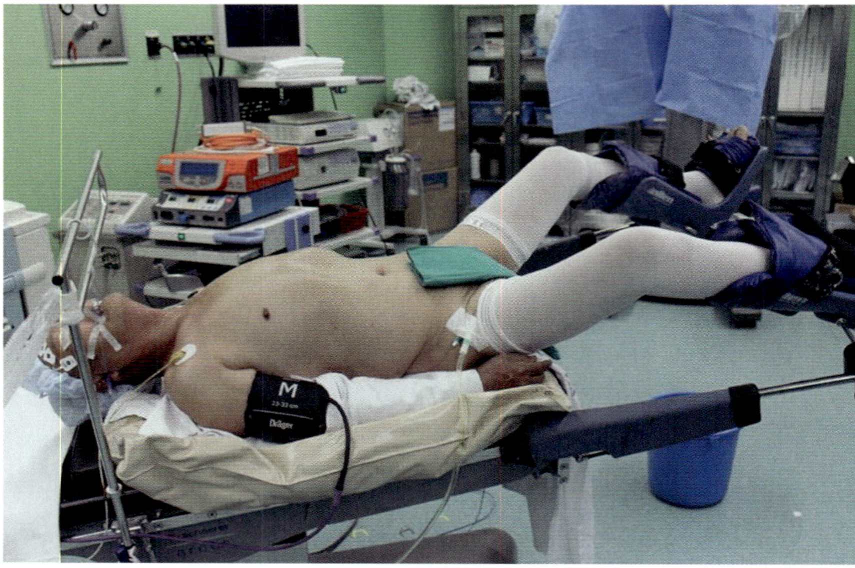

Fig. 19.1 Patient positioning for totally robot-assisted low anterior resection

A body warmer to prevent hypothermia and a sequential compression device to prevent deep vein thrombosis on the legs can be applied. Legs are placed in adjustable stirrups with the knees flexed. The left leg is less abducted as compared to the right one so as not to interfere with the approach of the robotic system. After positioning as seen in Fig. 19.1, the angle of Trendelenburg position and the angle of right side down tilting can be adjusted during the initial exposure step.

Trocar Placement

Proper port placement is crucial since the current da Vinci® system is rather bulky and requires sufficient room between arms, not only to avoid external collision but to also maximize internal movement.

Six ports are used, namely, one 12-mm camera port, four 8-mm robotic working ports, and one 5-mm port for the assistant. After pneumoperitoneum is achieved by either an open technique or a Veress needle, a 12-mm trocar is placed through an incision around the umbilicus for the robotic camera. Since there is an ideal distance (about 15 cm) between the scope and the target anatomy, the camera port should be shifted a few centimeters lateral to the umbilicus if the patient has a small body size. The intra-abdominal pressure is maintained at 8–12 mmHg. The first da Vinci® 8-mm port is placed on the right lower quadrant (RLQ), approximately at the McBurney point. The second 8-mm robotic port is inserted in the right upper quadrant (RUQ), mostly on the midclavicular line (MCL). The third 8-mm port is placed in the left upper quadrant (LUQ), approximately 1–2 cm above the camera port at the crossing of the MCL. The fourth port is inserted in the left lower quadrant (LLQ), approximately one to two centimeters lateral to the MCL. These four ports are used for the robotic instrument arms and are separated from each other by at least 8 cm. To allow the assistant access, a 5-mm trocar is placed in the right flank area, near the anterior axillary line at the umbilicus level. This is used for suction/irrigation, clipping of vessels, and retraction of tissues. The port placement is shown in Fig. 19.2. The port position can be altered according to the patient's physique. However, there are several principles when placing

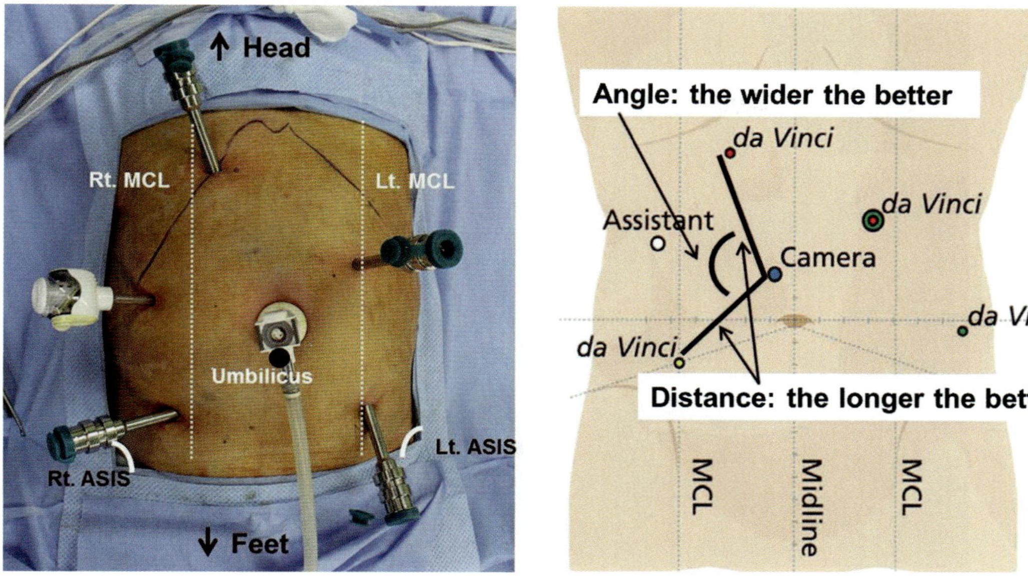

Fig. 19.2 (**a**) Trocar arrangement for totally robot-assisted low anterior resection. (**b**) Schematic figure showing desirable trocar placement which has a longer distance and a wider angle between the two right side trocars. *ASIS* anterior superior iliac spine; *MCL* midclavicular line

the trocars. Since the anterior iliac spine and the 12th rib are fixed in position, the RLQ port should always be placed first at McBurney point, and then the RUQ port is positioned close to the right costal margin. The camera port is placed around the umbilicus in order to be positioned at the same distance from the RLQ and RUQ ports. If possible, it is better to have a longer distance and a wider angle between the two right trocars, as shown in Fig. 19.2.

Initial Exposure

The first step of robotic LAR involves optimizing exposure and exploring the abdominal cavity laparoscopically. A zero-degree robotic camera or a conventional laparoscope is used. The whole abdominal cavity is inspected carefully for metastatic disease. The operating table is tilted to provide initial exposure of the operating field, by shifting the small bowel loops into the RUQ (Fig. 19.1). In general, inadequate exposure, which makes robotic surgery difficult, is mainly caused by distended small bowel with fatty mesentery. The right-sided omentum should be repositioned over the liver to create more space in the RUQ, then to maximally displace the small bowels to this space. This step is achieved with conventional laparoscopic instruments.

Robot Positioning and Docking

Once initial exposure has been achieved, the patient cart is brought in for docking. The patient cart is positioned obliquely at the LLQ of the abdomen along the imaginary line from the camera port to the left anterior superior iliac spine. The robotic arms are then docked to the trocars. When using all three da Vinci® instrument arms, setup joint of the camera arm should be positioned towards the patient's side to allow space for the instrument arms ② and ③. Before starting the console activity, the robotic arms should be adjusted to create maximal space in between, shown as a well-spread fan (Fig. 19.3).

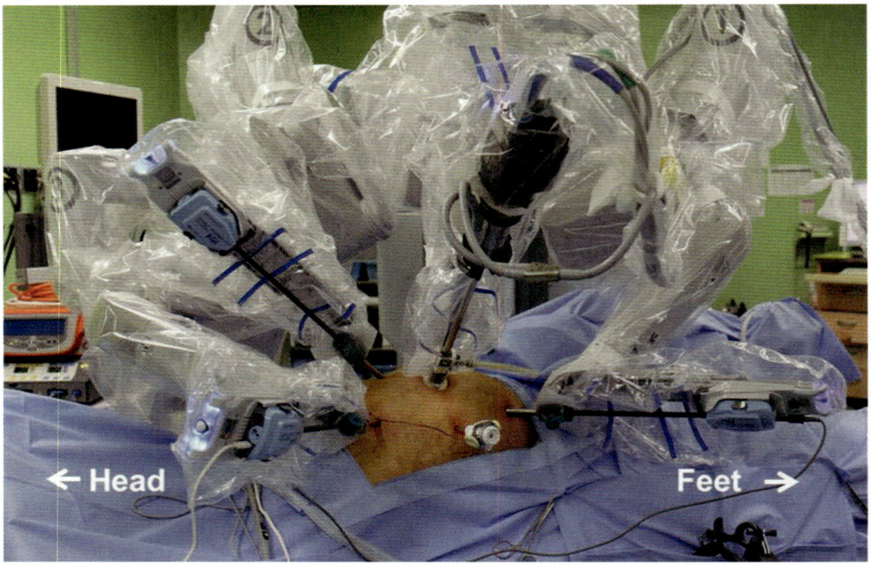

Fig. 19.3 The robot docked to the patient for totally robot-assisted low anterior resection. The patient cart is positioned obliquely at the LLQ of the patient

Vascular Ligation and Sigmoid Colon to Splenic Flexure Mobilization

- Instrument arm ① with monopolar curved scissors: Docked to the RLQ port as a surgeon's right hand
- Instrument arm ② with Cadiere forceps: Docked to the LUQ port as a surgeon's second left hand
- Instrument arm ③ with Maryland bipolar forceps: Docked to the RUQ port as a surgeon's left hand

Initially, the mesocolon over the IMA is retracted upwardly with the Cadiere forceps. The peritoneum around the base of the IMA is incised and dissected with monopolar scissors. The periaortic hypogastric nerve plexus is carefully preserved. The IMA is divided near the root with Hem-o-lok® clips (Weck Closure System, Research Triangle Park, NC, USA) (Fig. 19.4). The inferior mesenteric vein is identified by dissecting superiorly toward the ligament of Treitz and is divided near the inferior border of the pancreas.

The medial dissection continues laterally until the left colon is separated from the retroperitoneum and superiorly over the pancreas until the lesser sac is entered. The left gonadal vessels and the ureter are identified and preserved. Lateral detachment is initiated along the white line while the sigmoid colon is retracted medially by the assistant. Lateral countertraction by the instrument arm ② facilitates safe dissection. The lateral dissection continues cephalad to the middle portion of the descending colon. Splenic flexure is mobilized if necessary to achieve a tension-free anastomosis. The transverse mesocolon is opened just above the body of the pancreas to enter the lesser sac. Dissection of the transverse mesocolon continues towards the distal transverse colon and the base of the descending colon. Then omentum attached to the transverse colon is then dissected in the avascular plane, beginning from the middle third of the transverse colon. The renocolic and splenocolic ligaments are divided and the splenic flexure is fully mobilized. During splenic flexure mobilization, only robotic arms 1 and 3 are aligned to minimize external collision; however, the assistant can contribute significantly by inserting his/her instruments through the remaining ports. If complete splenic flexure mobilization is not feasible with whatever rea-

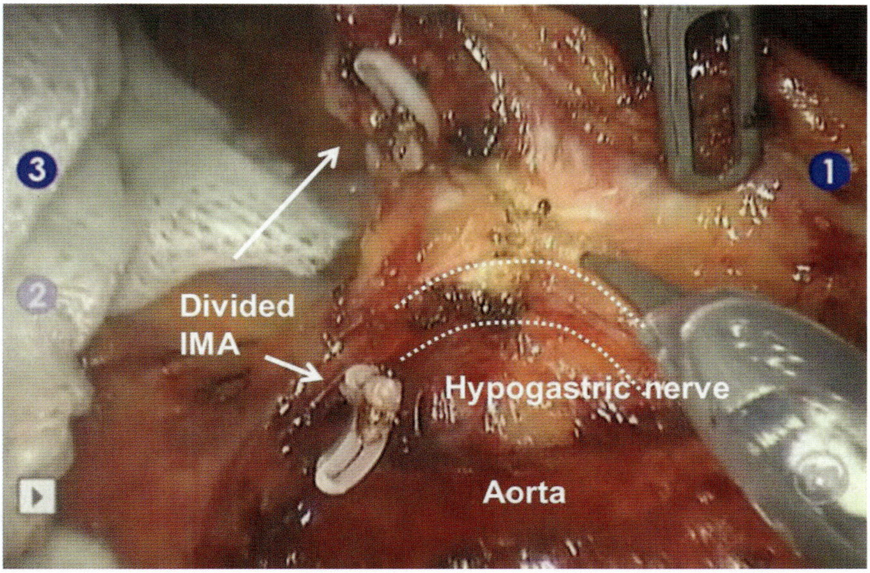

Fig. 19.4 IMA is clipped and divided at its origin. The periaortic hypogastric nerve is identified and swept down

sons, it can be performed lastly, after completion of robotic pelvic dissection.

Pelvic TME

- Instrument arm ① with monopolar curved scissors: Docked to the RLQ port as a surgeon's right hand
- Instrument arm ② with Cadiere forceps: Docked to the LLQ port as a surgeon's second left hand
- Instrument arm ③ with Maryland bipolar forceps: Docked to the LUQ port as a surgeon's left hand

The robotic instruments of the RUQ and LUQ ports are dedocked and redocked to the LUQ and LLQ ports, respectively. Before beginning the console activity, the robotic arms should again be adjusted to create maximal space in between, shown as a well-spread fan. The assistant then uses the RUQ port to retract the rectosigmoid cephalad and the 5-mm assistant port for suction and/or retraction (Fig. 19.5). Therefore, five instruments are used in the operative field (three robotic and two handheld), maximizing assistance by using both hands for TME. The assistant applies cephalic traction using a cotton tie around the sigmoid colon. The robotic Cadiere grasper retracts the rectum anteriorly, thus exposing the plane between the mesorectal fascia and the inferior hypogastric nerves. The avascular space between the mesorectal fascia and the presacral fascia is sharply dissected with monopolar scissors. The inferior hypogastric nerves and, distally, the pelvic nerve plexus are identified and preserved. Further posterior dissection down to the levator ani muscle is approached from the left lateral plane, while the rectum is lifted up using the Cadiere forceps. The left lateral dissection is performed while the rectum is drawn to the right side by the assistant. Then, the right lateral dissection is completed in the reverse order used for rectal retraction. Finally, anterior dissection is performed by incising the peritoneal reflection. Sharp dissection is continued until the correct plane between the rectum and vagina/seminal vesicles/prostate is achieved. The rectum is retracted downward with the instrument attached to robotic arm 3 (Maryland grasper), and the vagina/prostate is counter-retracted upward with the instrument

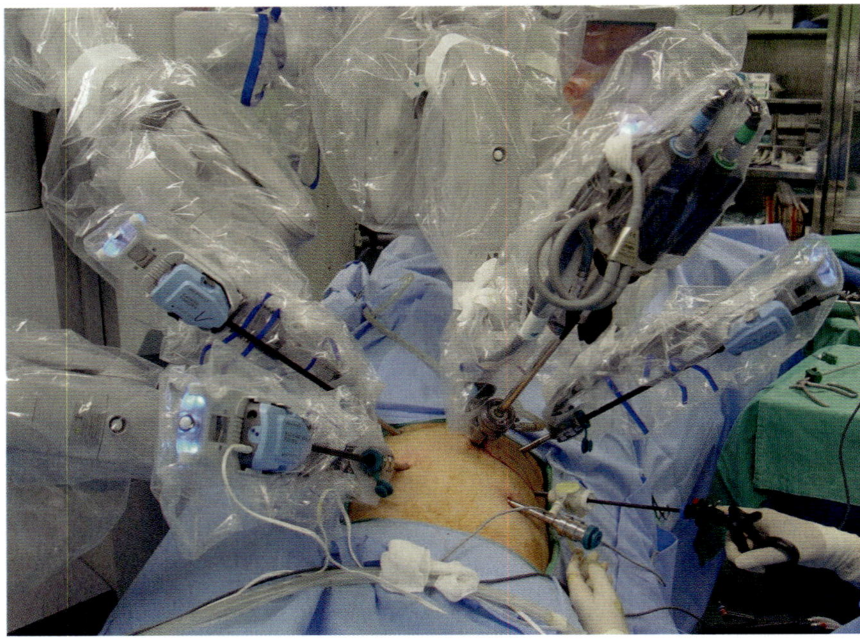

Fig. 19.5 The assistant is using both his hands through the RUQ port and the assistant port in the pelvic phase

attached to robotic arm 2 (Cadiere forceps). During the pelvic dissection stage, the assistant uses the RUQ port as well, therefore maximizing assistance by use of both hands.

An effective method to enhance the exposure of the pelvic cavity in postmenopausal women is suspension of the uterus from the abdominal wall using a suture (Fig. 19.6). A similar suspension can be made with a suture around the thick, fatty peritoneum to retract the bladder in obese patients.

Rectal Division and Anastomosis

Robotic stapling devices are currently unavailable. Therefore, after adequate TME down to the pelvic floor, undocking of the robotic arms, movement of the patient cart away from the operating table, and a switch to a laparoscopic setting are necessary for rectal transection using an endostapler. The remaining steps are performed using conventional laparoscopic methods. After extending the robotic 8-mm port on RLQ to a 12-mm port, an articulating linear endostapler loaded with a gold cartridge (4.2 mm) is used via the RLQ port. A distal rectal washout is then performed, and the rectum is divided using an endostapler to achieve at least a 2-cm distal margin. The specimen is delivered through a small incision at the LLQ port, and the wound is covered with an impermeable protector. Transection of the proximal bowel is performed extracorporeally. The anastomosis is performed intracorporeally using a standard double stapling technique. A diverting ileostomy is selectively constructed in cases with air leaks, incomplete doughnuts, preoperative radiation, extreme difficulty in pelvic dissection, or coloanal anastomosis.

Recently, we modified our technique to maximize the advantages that we could gain from using a robotic system. After TME, the instrument

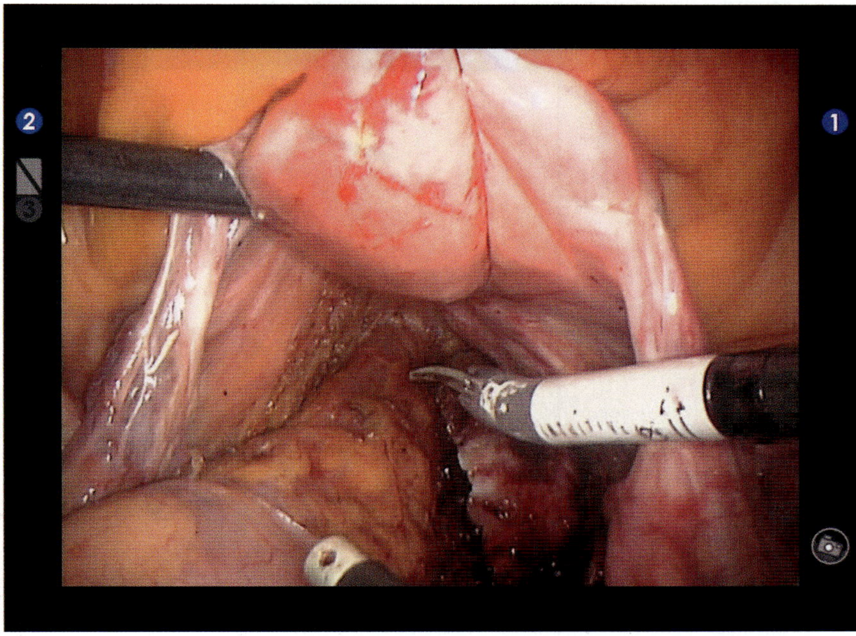

Fig. 19.6 The uterus is lifted up to the anterior abdominal wall using a suture to enhance the exposure of the pelvic cavity in postmenopausal woman

arms ① and ③ are dedocked; however, the robotic camera and the instrument arm ② are left in place to provide stable and constant upward traction with Cadiere forceps and a stable camera view (Fig. 19.7), both of which make it easier to apply and fire the endostapler.

Potential Advantages of Totally Robotic LAR

Once a surgeon's preference is established, it is hard to adapt a new surgical approach to his/her practice. Because most experienced laparoscopic colorectal surgeons feel quite comfortable when they perform laparoscopic mobilization of the left and sigmoid colon, they don't contemplate the introduction of a totally robotic procedure into their practice.

However, a hybrid technique may have some limitations. First, it has no advantage from robotic technology, neither at the phase of IMA dissection nor at the phase of splenic flexure mobilization. Robotic third arm controlled by the surgeon can provide effective lifting up of IMA. Because not only the pelvic nerves but also the periaortic nerves are important for voiding/sexual functions [14, 15], we believe that robotic dissection around the IMA pedicle is a critical step. The three-dimensional magnified view and EndoWrist function could be helpful in identifying and preserving the periaortic hypogastric nerve plexus. Also, these technical advantages could enable easier mobilization of a difficult splenic flexure than conventional laparoscopic approach.

Second, it may be inconvenient to perform an intraoperative colonoscopic examination because the bulky patient cart is located between the patient's legs. Under the hybrid setting, it is impossible to apply our modified stapling technique.

Unfortunately, it may be very difficult to demonstrate the clinical benefits of these potential advantages of totally robotic LAR. In the present

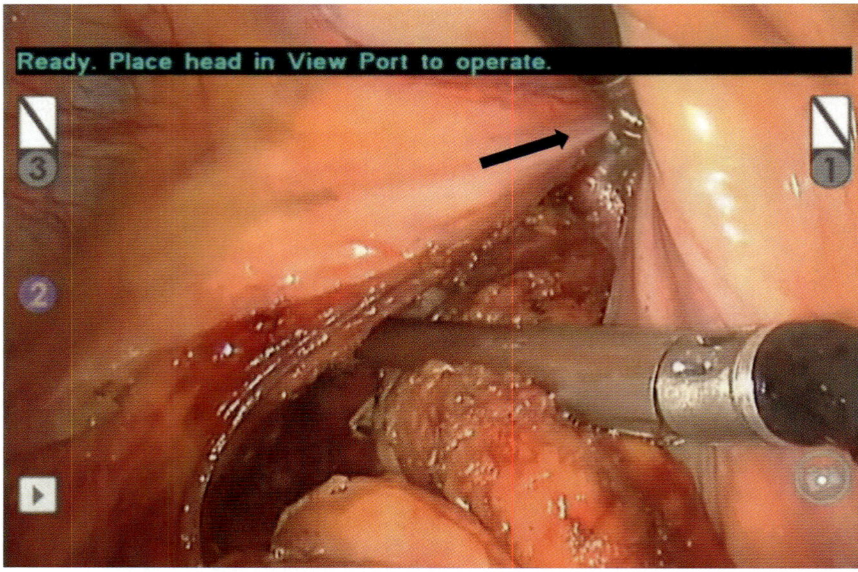

Fig. 19.7 During rectal transection with an endostapler, the undocked robotic camera and robotic arm ② (Cadiere forceps, *arrow*) provide more stable vision and better exposure

situation in which more stringent scientific evaluations in the setting of multicentre, randomized clinical trials are required to verify the benefits of the robot-assisted rectal cancer surgery, it is far too early to talk about the superiority between the totally robotic and hybrid approach. Nonetheless, we should be concerned how we can maximize this advanced technology in every step of the procedure.

Limitations

Very few limitations specific to fully robotic LAR exist. As shown in Table 19.1, the clinical outcomes of our fully robotic LAR technique are quite comparable with those of our laparoscopic counterpart or other series performed using hybrid technique. No intraoperative complication related to robotic vascular ligation and sigmoid colon mobilization was recorded. As the safety and feasibility of the various types of robotic colon surgery are already proven in previous studies, there is no issue arguing about fully robotic approach except longer operating time [1–4].

If the patient has had previous abdominal surgery, the initial creation of the pneumoperitoneum should be carefully planned and executed. Once the peritoneal cavity is entered, it is more convenient to resolve any adhesions laparoscopically that can interrupt dissection or bowel repositioning prior to docking of the robotic arms. If the adhesions are too extensive or dense to perform adhesiolysis using laparoscopic instruments, a longer incision is made to lyse the adhesions under direct visualization. Air leaks do not matter once the fascia is closed properly.

The current robotic surgical system has limited instruments and bulky arms and lacks tactile feedback. However, improvements in robotic engineering will undoubtedly contribute to the evolution of instruments, which will translate into expansion of the applications of surgical robotic systems. Recently developed new technologies such as a fluorescent image or robotic stapler seem promising. We hope that incorporation of sensors into the tips of instruments, which can provide a degree of "tactile" sensation, would be developed in the near future. These technological advancements are expected to overcome the current pitfalls of the robotic system.

Table 19.1 Comparison of clinical outcomes between the robotic and the laparoscopic surgery for rectal cancer

Study	Country (year)	Study design	Surgery	Number	Operation time (min)	Conversion (%)	Hospital stay (days)	Total complication (%)
Kwak et al. [11][a]	Korea (2011)	Case matched	Robot, total	59	270 (241–325)*	0.0	NA	32.2
			Lap	59	228 (177–254)	3.4	NA	27.1
Park et al. [10]	Korea (2011)	Case matched	Robot, hybrid	41	231.9 ± 61.4 *	0.0	9.9 ± 4.2	29.3
			Lap	82	168.6 ± 49.3	0.0	9.4 ± 2.9	23.2
Baek et al. [9]	USA (2011)	Case matched	Robot, hybrid	41	296 (150–520)	7.3	6.5 (2–33)	22.0
			Lap	41	315 (174–584)	22.0	6.6 (3–20)	26.8
Bianchi et al. [8]	Italy (2010)	Comparative	Robot, mixed	25	240 (170–420)	0.0	6.5 (4–15)	16.0
			Lap	25	237 (170–545)	4.0	6.0 (4–20)	24.0
Patriti et al. [7]	Italy (2010)	Comparative	Robot, hybrid	29	202 ± 12	0.0*	11.9 ± 7.5	30.6
			Lap	37	208 ± 7	29.2	9.6 ± 6.9	18.9
Baik et al. [6]	Korea (2009)	Comparative	Robot, hybrid	56	190.1 ± 45.0	0.0*	5.7 ± 1.1*	5.4*
			Lap	57	191.1 ± 65.3	10.5	7.6 ± 3.0	19.3

NA not available
**P* value <0.05
[a]Values in parentheses are interquartile range

Preferable Indications and Relative Contraindications

Our indications for robotic rectal cancer resection are identical to those for laparoscopic surgery. There are no contraindications applied solely to robotic rectal cancer surgery. Proper training, whether in vivo or in vitro, or even virtual reality, is required prior to attempting robotic surgery to ensure that this novel technology is applied correctly. A well-trained team approach is also an important factor to reduce the operating time and ensure that the surgery goes smoothly. There is a steep learning curve before operating time, lower morbidity, and the surgeon's comfort comparative to those obtained by conventional laparoscopic surgery can be achieved.

Some cases may prove to be more difficult to operate on using robot-assisted surgery before the surgeon has gained experience with this technology. These include morbidly obese patients, male patients, and low-lying rectal cancer cases. Surgeons should be selective about which cases they perform robotically at the beginning of their learning curves. However, as experience is gained, the factors listed above could change preferable indications for using robot-assisted surgery.

Contraindications are largely contingent on the experience of the surgeon. Intestinal obstruction, severe adhesion with/without previous surgery, and marked obesity are relative contraindications. Absolute contraindications include carcinoma with direct invasion into adjacent structures, perforation, and mid- or lower rectal carcinoma greater than 5 cm in diameter. Systemic factors that contraindicate a laparoscopic approach, such as severely impaired cardiovascular or respiratory functions and uncorrectable coagulopathy, apply equally to conventional and robot-assisted laparoscopy.

Outcomes

Short-Term Outcomes of Safety and Feasibility

Short-term clinical outcomes for robot-assisted rectal surgery for rectal cancer have been reviewed and compared with laparoscopic surgery in Table 19.1.

In general, longer operating time is widely considered to be one of the downsides of robotic surgery, along with higher cost and lack of tactile sense, as compared with conventional laparoscopic procedure. Notably, although it is just a numerical difference, some authors have reported even shorter operating time for robotic rectal cancer resections using a hybrid technique [6, 7, 9]. From these results, it can be inferred that the technical advantages of the robot can make difficult pelvic dissection easier and shorten the operating time. As we overcome the learning curve and standardize every step of the procedure, the operating time can be expected to decrease further.

The excellent conversion rate has been reported consistently in several series of robot-assisted rectal cancer surgery, and this is promising and encouraging when considering reported conversion rates in laparoscopic rectal cancer surgery ranged from 12 to 20 % [16, 17]. Since converted patients may have higher complication rates and worse oncological outcomes, this result can lead to better postoperative course, as well as improved oncological and functional outcomes [18, 19].

In terms of postoperative recovery, similar outcomes were reported in most series. Postoperative complications after robot-assisted rectal cancer resection seem to be equivalent to laparoscopic surgery. When comparing our data with other series performed by hybrid technique, no significant differences are observed in operating time, conversion rate, and morbidity. To the best of our knowledge, there was no report of patient injury or mortality from device malfunction.

As most studies are based on data from highly experienced laparoscopic colorectal surgeons, there is a definitive difference in the surgeon's expertise between the two operative techniques. This difference may attenuate the benefits of robotic surgery, resulting in similar clinical outcomes rather than superior results due to its technological advantages. In view of the results achieved so far, skillful laparoscopic surgeons can perform robot-assisted rectal cancer surgery safely and feasibly.

Table 19.2 Pathologic outcomes between the two groups

Study	Country (year)	Study design	Surgery	Number	LN harvested (number)	DRM (cm)	CRM (% involved)
Kwak et al. [11][a]	Korea (2011)	Case matched	Robot, total	59	20 (12–27)	2.2 (1.5–3.0)	1.7
			Lap	59	21 (14–28)	2.0 (1.2–3.5)	0.0
Park et al. [10]	Korea (2011)	Case matched	Robot, hybrid	41	17.3±7.7	2.1±1.4	4.9
			Lap	82	14.2±8.9	2.3±1.5	3.7
Baek et al. [9]	USA (2011)	Case matched	Robot, hybrid	41	13.1 (3–33)	3.6 (0.4–10)	2.4
			Lap	41	16.2 (5–39)	3.8 (0.4–11)	4.9
Bianchi et al. [8]	Italy (2010)	Comparative	Robot, mixed	25	18 (7–34)	2 (1.5–4.5)	0.0
			Lap	25	17 (8–37)	2 (1.8–3.5)	4.0
Patriti et al. [7]	Italy (2010)	Comparative	Robot, hybrid	29	10.3±4	2.1±0.9	0.0
			Lap	37	11.2±5	4.5±7.2	0.0
Baik et al. [6]	Korea (2009)	Comparative	Robot, hybrid	56	18.4±9.2	4.0±1.6	7.1
			Lap	57	18.7±12	3.6±1.7	8.8

LN lymph node, *DRM* distal resection margin, *CRM* circumferential resection margin
**P* value <0.05
[a]Values in parentheses are interquartile range

Oncological Outcomes

There is increasing evidence that the number of harvested lymph nodes has an important impact on survival [20]. Table 19.2 showed no significant differences regarding this issue, and the reported mean/median numbers are acceptable considering a recommendation from the College of American Pathologist for a 12-node minimum [21]. Also, other parameters such as distal resection margin length or circumferential resection margin involvement rate, which can be an index of surgical quality, were not different between the two groups in rectal cancer surgery.

Evidence of the oncological outcomes of robot-assisted rectal cancer surgery is very limited, as shown in Table 19.3. In a multicenter study for robotic TME by Pigazzi et al., the 3-year overall survival rate was 97 % in 143 consecutive patients with rectal cancer undergoing robotic surgery, and isolated local recurrences were not found during the mean follow-up period of 17.4 months [12]. In that study, the absence of a control group, relatively short follow-up period, and extensive use of neoadjuvant chemoradiation could have been barriers to reaching definitive conclusions. Nevertheless, their excellent results suggest that a robotic surgical system is likely to improve local disease control.

In our study, we compared the short-term surgical and oncological outcomes of robot-assisted rectal cancer surgery with those of laparoscopic surgery [11]. Both the short-term surgical and oncological outcomes were comparable between the groups. Although the mean follow-up period (17 months in robotic group versus 13 months in laparoscopic group) was not long enough to allow a definitive assessment, the pattern of cancer recurrence was not different between the two groups. Expectation of improvement in local disease control by robotic dissection will be evaluated with follow-up research.

Only prospective clinical trials with long-term follow-up can clearly answer whether the technological advantages of robotic surgical system can translate into favorable surgical or oncological outcomes. Currently, several multicenter, randomized controlled trials of robot-assisted versus conventional laparoscopic resection for rectal cancer have been undertaken. Attention is now focused on how these trials will develop and their overall results.

Functional Outcomes

A current issue of great interest in robot-assisted TME for rectal cancer is whether it can preserve

Table 19.3 Short- and midterm oncological outcomes of robot-assisted proctectomy for rectal cancer

Study	Patient	Surgery	Number	Mean F/up (month)	Oncological outcome
Kwak et al. [11][a]	Korea (2011)	Robot, total	55	17 (11–25)	1 locoregional recurrence/ 2 distant metastasis
		Lap	54	13 (9–22)	1 locoregional recurrence/ 2 distant metastasis
Pigazzi et al. [12]	USA (2010)	Robot, hybrid	143	17.4	3-year DFS 77.6 %/3-year OS 97 %/no isolated local recurrence
Patriti et al. [7]	Italy (2010)	Robot, hybrid	29	29.2 ± 14.0	0 % of local recurrence/no difference in OS and DFS
		Lap	37	18.7 ± 13.8	5.4 % of local recurrence

DFS disease-free survival, *OS* overall survival

[a]Values in parentheses are interquartile range

voiding and sexual function by avoiding injury to autonomic nerves following rectal resection. Because the incidence of postoperative voiding and sexual dysfunction is high even with incorporation of autonomic nerve-preserving techniques in TME and always results in poor quality of life, better functional outcomes with robotic approach can offset an indictment of its high cost.

In terms of laparoscopic TME with pelvic autonomic nerve preservation, there are two contrary hypotheses about the impact of laparoscopic approach on postoperative voiding and sexual function; one is that the magnified view of the pelvis afforded by the laparoscope may facilitate identification of the autonomic nerves and thus prevent inadvertent injury, while the other is that several technical pitfalls of laparoscopic surgery may predispose to nerve injury. However, Jayne et al. [14]. showed that laparoscopic rectal resection did not adversely affect voiding function, but there was a trend towards worse male sexual function from the MRC CLASICC trial's patients. They also found that TME and conversion to open surgery were independent predictors of postoperative male sexual dysfunction [14].

Several studies have reported low conversion rates of robotic resection for rectal cancer [6–11], and we can expect this to result in better preservation of voiding and sexual function. Recently, Kim et al. [22]. reported a comparative study of functional outcomes after TME for rectal cancer in laparoscopic and robotic surgery. They assessed functional outcomes using standardized, internationally approved multiple questionnaires and invasive urodynamic tests to provide the most objective results. Although the number of patients enrolled was relatively small, they demonstrated that robot-assisted TME was associated with early recovery of voiding and sexual function compared to laparoscopic TME. Well-designed studies should be followed to verify the benefit of robotic approach to preserve postoperative voiding and sexual function.

Conclusions

Single-stage totally robotic LAR is feasible and expected to have additional advantages from maximal use of advanced robotic technology. Our data shows equivalent clinical and pathological outcomes when compared to its laparoscopic counterpart and other studies performed by hybrid technique. Longer operating time is a shortcoming of totally robotic procedure, but partially caused by initial unfamiliarity.

A great deal of progress has occurred in the field of colorectal surgery over the last few years, and this has generated a great deal of interest in using robotic systems to perform rectal cancer surgery. Although the initial reports are promising, more stringent scientific evaluations in the setting of multicenter, randomized clinical trials are essential to verify the safety, efficacy, and long-term functional and oncological benefits of this new technology. Developing of adequate training program and high cost are real issues that must be solved. The future, however, looks very promising because of the great potential of robotic surgical systems to extend the capabilities of surgical performance beyond human limitations, and it will greatly improve the quality of surgical care.

References

1. Weber PA, Merola S, Wasielewski A, Ballantyne GH. Telerobot-assisted laparoscopic right and sigmoid colectomies for benign disease. Dis Colon Rectum. 2002;45:1689–94.
2. D'Annibale A, Morpurgo E, Fiscon V, Trevisan P, Sovernigo G, Orsini C, Guidolin D. Robotic and laparoscopic surgery for treatment of colorectal diseases. Dis Colon Rectum. 2004;47:2162–8.
3. Anvari M, Birch DW, Bamehriz F, Gryfe R, Chapman T. Robotic-assisted laparoscopic colorectal surgery. Surg Laparosc Endosc Percutan Tech. 2004;14:311–5.
4. Rawlings AL, Woodland JH, Vegunta RK, Crawford DL. Robotic versus laparoscopic colectomy. Surg Endosc. 2007;21:1701–8.
5. Choi DJ, Kim SH, Lee PJ, Kim J, Woo SU. Single-stage totally robotic dissection for rectal cancer surgery: technique and short-term outcome in 50 consecutive patients. Dis Colon Rectum. 2009;52:1824–30.
6. Baik SH, Kwon HY, Kim JS, Hur H, Sohn SK, Cho CH, Kim H. Robotic versus laparoscopic low anterior resection of rectal cancer: short-term outcome of a prospective comparative study. Ann Surg Oncol. 2009;16:1480–7.
7. Patriti A, Ceccarelli G, Bartoli A, Spaziani A, Biancafarina A, Casciola L. Short- and medium-term outcome of robot-assisted and traditional laparoscopic rectal resection. JSLS. 2009;13:176–83.
8. Bianchi PP, Ceriani C, Locatelli A, Spinoglio G, Zampino MG, Sonzogni A, Crosta C, Andreoni B. Robotic versus laparoscopic total mesorectal excision for rectal cancer: a comparative analysis of oncological safety and short-term outcomes. Surg Endosc. 2010;24:2888–94.
9. Baek JH, McKenzie S, Garcia-Aguilar J, Pigazzi A. Oncologic outcomes of robotic-assisted total mesorectal excision for the treatment of rectal cancer. Ann Surg. 2010;251:882–6.
10. Park JS, Choi GS, Lim KH, Jang YS, Jun SH. Robot-assisted versus laparoscopic surgery for Low rectal cancer: case-matched analysis of short-term outcomes. Ann Surg Oncol. 2010;17:3195–202.
11. Kwak JM, Kim SH, Kim J, Son DN, Baek SJ, Cho JS. Robotic vs. laparoscopic resection of rectal cancer: short-term outcomes of a case control study. Dis Colon Rectum. 2011;54:151–6.
12. Pigazzi A, Luca F, Patriti A, Valvo M, Ceccarelli G, Casciola L, Biffi R, Garcia-Aguilar J, Baek JH. Multicentric study on robotic tumor-specific mesorectal excision for the treatment of rectal cancer. Ann Surg Oncol. 2010;17:1614–20.
13. Spinoglio G, Summa M, Priora F, Quarati R, Testa S. Robotic colorectal surgery: first 50 cases experience. Dis Colon Rectum. 2008;51:1627–32.
14. Jayne DG, Brown JM, Thorpe H, Walker J, Quirke P, Guillou PJ. Bladder and sexual function following resection for rectal cancer in a randomized clinical trial of laparoscopic versus open technique. Br J Surg. 2005;92:1124–32.
15. Quah HM, Jayne DG, Eu KW, Seow-Choen F. Bladder and sexual dysfunction following laparoscopically assisted and conventional open mesorectal resection for cancer. Br J Surg. 2002;89:1551–6.
16. Delgado S, Momblán D, Salvador L, Bravo R, Castells A, Ibarzabal A, Piqué JM, Lacy AM. Laparoscopic-assisted approach in rectal cancer patients: lessons learned from >200 patients. Surg Endosc. 2004;18:1457–62.
17. Dulucq JL, Wintringer P, Stabilini C, Mahajna A. Laparoscopic rectal resection with anal sphincter preservation for rectal cancer: long-term outcome. Surg Endosc. 2005;19:1468–74.
18. Delgado S, Momblán D, Salvador L, Bravo R, Castells A, Ibarzabal A, Piqué JM, Lacy AM. Short-term endpoints of conventional versus laparoscopic-assisted surgery in patients with colorectal cancer (MRC CLASICC trial): multicentre, randomised controlled trial. Lancet. 2005;365:1718–26.
19. Rottoli M, Bona S, Rosati R, Elmore U, Bianchi PP, Spinelli A, Bartolucci C, Montorsi M. Laparoscopic rectal resection for cancer: effects of conversion on short-term outcome and survival. Ann Surg Oncol. 2009;16:1279–86.
20. Sigurdson ER. Lymph node dissection: is it diagnostic or therapeutic? J Clin Oncol. 2003;21:965–7.
21. Compton CC, Fielding LP, Burgart LJ, Conley B, Cooper HS, Hamilton SR, Hammond ME, Henson DE, Hutter RV, Nagle RB, Nielsen ML, Sargent DJ, Taylor CR, Welton M, Willett C. Prognostic factors in colorectal cancer. College of American Pathologists Consensus Statement 1999. Arch Pathol Lab Med. 2009;124:979–94.
22. Kim JY, Kim NK, Lee KY, Hur H, Min BS, Kim JH. A comparative study of voiding and sexual function after total mesorectal excision with autonomic nerve preservation for rectal cancer: laparoscopic versus robotic surgery. Ann Surg Oncol. 2012;19(8):2485–93.

20 Robotic Hybrid Low Anterior Resection

Eric M. Haas and Rodrigo Pedraza

Background

Laparoscopic surgery is considered by many to be the surgical approach of choice for disease processes requiring colon resection. Laparoscopic colectomy has been widely recognized as a safe alternative for curative resection for colon cancer [1] and has steadily gained adoption. Currently it is estimated that in high-volume institutions, 50 % of all colectomies for cancer are performed with the laparoscopic approach [2]. This enthusiasm, however, has not been reflected when approaching patients requiring rectal resection with curative intent for rectal cancer. As such, it is currently estimated that approximately only 10 % of rectal resections for rectal cancer are performed with the utilization of a minimally invasive surgical approach.

Early experience of laparoscopic surgery for the treatment of rectal cancer resulted in a prolonged procedure with high conversion rate, high morbidity rate, and jeopardized oncological outcomes [3]. Therefore, the routine utilization of the laparoscopic approach for the management of rectal cancer is cautioned. Accordingly, the rationale for robotic-assisted laparoscopic surgery for the treatment of rectal cancer is based on achieving the advantages of a minimally invasive platform without high conversion rates and without compromising oncological and pathological outcomes.

The concept of a robotic hybrid procedure was first popularized by Pigazzi et al. [4]. The hybrid approach utilizes conventional laparoscopy to achieve parts of the procedure and the robotic platform to achieve the portions related to pelvic dissection. In this approach, the abdominal portion of the procedure is performed laparoscopically, whereas the pelvic portion is accomplished robotically. The rationale for the utilization of this approach is based on the premise that this hybridization enhances the surgeon ability to complete the procedure with the various minimally invasive approaches to maximize the benefits while minimizing the intrinsic limitations of both techniques.

During the non-pelvic portions of the procedures, the intrinsic advantages of the robotic platform such as enhanced optics and dexterity are not as much as a beneficial factor as it when operating in the confined anatomy of the rectum. Furthermore, colon dissection and mobilization usually requires multiple quadrant

E.M. Haas, M.D. (✉) • R. Pedraza, M.D.
Division of Minimally Invasive Colon and Rectal Surgery, Department of Surgery, The University of Texas Medical School at Houston, Houston, TX 77030, USA

Colorectal Surgical Associates, Ltd, LLP, 7900 Fannin, Suite 2700, Houston, TX 77054, USA
e-mail: ehaasmd@houstoncolon.com; rpedraza@houstoncolon.com

K.C. Kim (ed.), *Robotics in General Surgery*, DOI 10.1007/978-1-4614-8739-5_20,

maneuvers thus resulting in potential re-docking of the robot leading to procedure interruption and longer operative times. In addition, the utilization of advanced platforms such as the robotic technique may be precluded, as the limitations of conventional laparoscopic surgery are not exposed during abdominal procedures. As such, we perform the abdominal portion of the procedure with conventional laparoscopic technique and the pelvic portion with the robotic assistance. This hybridization avoids the robotic cart re-docking and optimizes the attributes of each minimally invasive surgical approach. While conventional laparoscopic technique serves ideally for multi-quadrant procedures and for variable anatomy, the robotic approach performs optimally for a fixed segment and confined spaces such as the pelvic cavity.

Surgical Technique

Patient Positioning

The patient is placed on modified lithotomy position with moderate Trendelenburg and both arms tucked. It is imperative to ensure correct patient positioning and proper techniques to secure the patient to the operating table, as portions of the procedure will require extreme tilt and angulation. There are several appropriate techniques to secure the patient depending on the size of the patient, available equipment, and surgeon preference. We prefer to use a wrapped technique, in which a 3 in. tape is utilized to secure the patient at the level of the chest, in such a fashion to prevent movement, yet avoiding excessive tension as to restrict airway flow (Fig. 20.1).

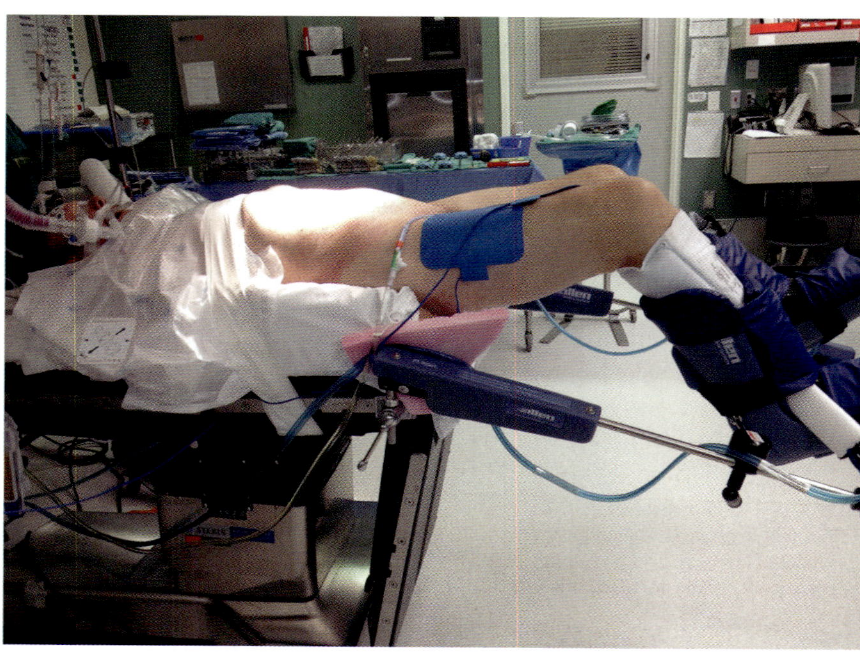

Fig. 20.1 Patient positioning. The patient is placed on modified lithotomy position with moderate Trendelenburg and both arms tucked. The patient is secured to the operating table using a wrapped technique

Port Placement

It is best to choose port placement based on ideal location for the utilization for the robotic platform. Although such placement may result in suboptimal location during the laparoscopic portions, it is most important to ensure proper placement for the robotic arms to optimize the range of motion of the robotic instruments and to avoid collision during the pelvic portions of the procedure. The exact port placement varies based on patient body habitus; thus, the following should be use as a general reference. The frame of reference in the vertical plane is adjusted based on the distance between the umbilicus and the pubic symphysis, whereas the frame reference in the horizontal plane is based on the distance between the midline and the anterior superior iliac spines. The port placement consists of a 12-mm camera port, which is located 2 cm above and 2 cm lateral to the umbilicus. We prefer direct abdominal entry utilizing the OptiView® (Ethicon Endo-Surgery, Cincinnati, OH) bladeless trocar; however, the use of the Veress needle or other entry techniques is appropriate based on surgeon experience and preference. The additional ports are not placed until pneumoperitoneum is established and laparoscopic exploration is performed. This is important for three reasons: first, unexpected findings such as metastatic disease can be evaluated; second, adhesions at proposed port sites can be taken down before port placement; third, by establishing the pneumoperitoneum and enlarging the surface area of the abdominal wall, the port placement will be optimized. A total of three 8-mm ports for the robotic arms are then placed and the assistant 12-mm port as shown in Fig. 20.2. Port 1 is placed along in the right lower quadrant along a line between the anterior superior iliac spine and the camera port, at distance of 8 cm of separation from the midline in the horizontal plane (Fig. 20.2). Port 2 is placed at a variable height above the level of the camera port 1–2 cm above the camera port at the level of 8 cm in the horizontal plane. Port 3 is ideally placed 2 cm above the anterior superior iliac spine and 8 cm from port 2 in the horizontal plane (Fig. 20.2). However, the latter is the most

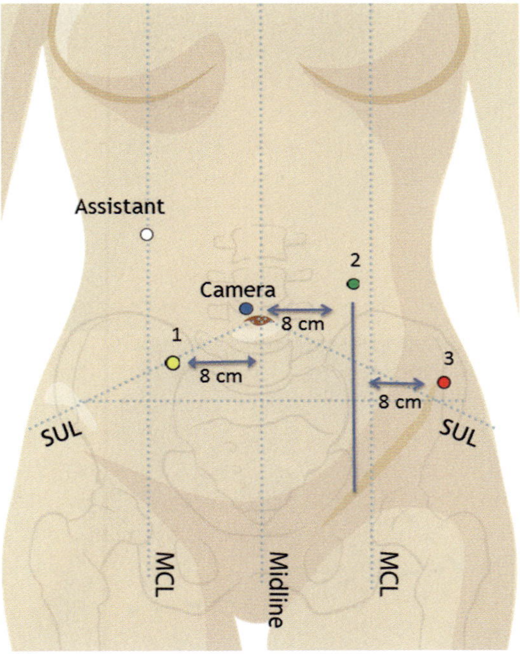

Fig. 20.2 Layout of port placement for robotic hybrid rectal resection. One umbilical 12-mm camera port, one 12-mm assistant port in the right hypochondrium, and three (1, 2, and 3) 5-mm ports for the robotic arms are placed as depicted

difficult port placement to master and the one with highest variability: on one hand it has to be placed laterally in order to provide 8 cm of horizontal clearance with respect to port 2; on the other hand if placed far laterally, the iliac bone will impede instrument reach into the pelvis.

Laparoscopic-Assisted Abdominal Dissection

In our institution, we perform the left colon mobilization utilizing a medial-to-lateral approach. The lateral attachments of the colon help with retraction and dissection in the retroperitoneal plane, which allows early identification of the ureter and vascular structures. The procedure commences with laparoscopic exploration and, if needed, lysis of adhesions. The small bowel is retracted to the right of the midline and ligament of Treitz is identified. This is the

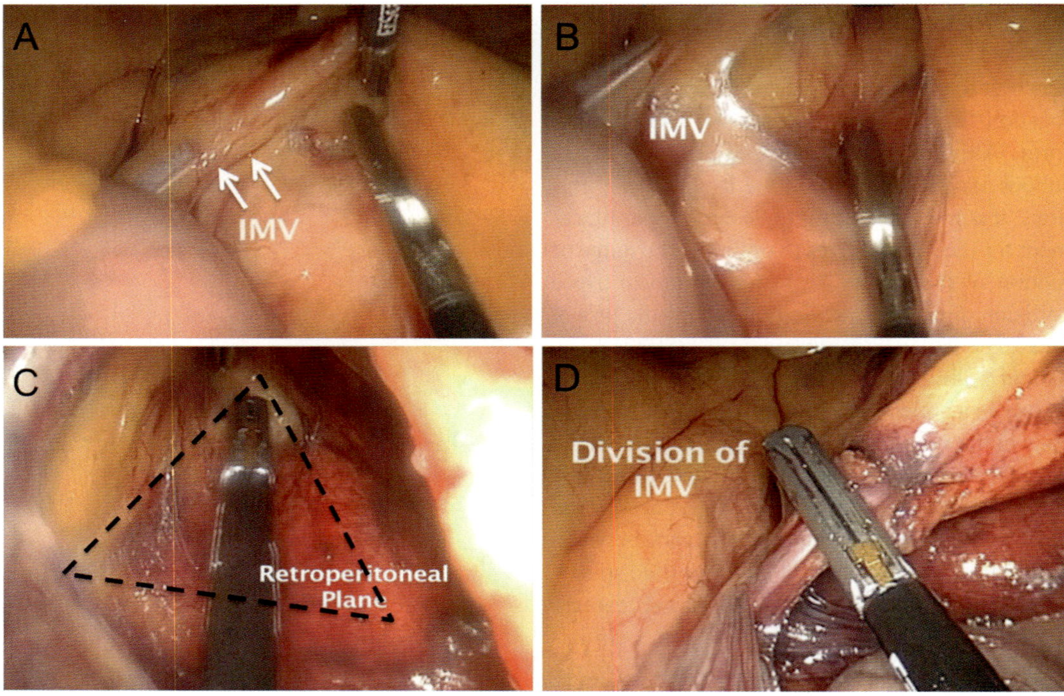

Fig. 20.3 Once the small bowel is retracted to right and superior, the inferior mesenteric vein (IMV) is readily identified (**a**). The medial peritoneum is incised inferior to the vein, and the retroperitoneal plane is established using a triangulation lift technique (**a**, **b**, and **c**). The inferior mesenteric vein is divided (**d**)

initial stem and can be cumbersome, especially in the obese; however, this exposure is essential and must be performed to successfully initiate the procedure. Exposure is facilitated with right tilt (left side elevation) and slight Trendelenburg with traction of the small bowel superiorly out of the pelvis as well. With this exposure, the inferior mesenteric vein is readily identified running parallel to the ligament of Treitz before it enters deep to the pancreatic body (Fig. 20.3a). At this level, the medial peritoneum is incised just inferior to the vein, and the retroperitoneal plane is established using a triangulation lift technique (Fig. 20.3a, b, c). The inferior mesenteric vein is divided (Fig. 20.3d) and the retroperitoneal plane fully developed (Fig. 20.4a). Proper dissection in the retroperitoneal plane of dissection is carried superiorly along the inferior border of the pancreas, laterally to the white line of Toldt, and inferiorly to the level of the takeoff of the left colic artery from the inferior mesenteric artery. One will often be able to identify the ureter in this plane as well.

Once the retroperitoneal plane is fully developed (Fig. 20.4a), attention is then drawn to the gastrocolic ligament, which is detached from the colon at the level of the distal transverse colon (Fig. 20.4b). The lesser sac is entered and the splenic flexure takedown is performed (Fig. 20.4b, c, d). When maximum exposure and reach have been achieved, attention is drawn to the descending colon (Fig. 20.5a, b), which is released from the peritoneal attachments (white line of Toldt) in a caudal to cranial direction and the splenic flexure mobilization is then completed in this direction.

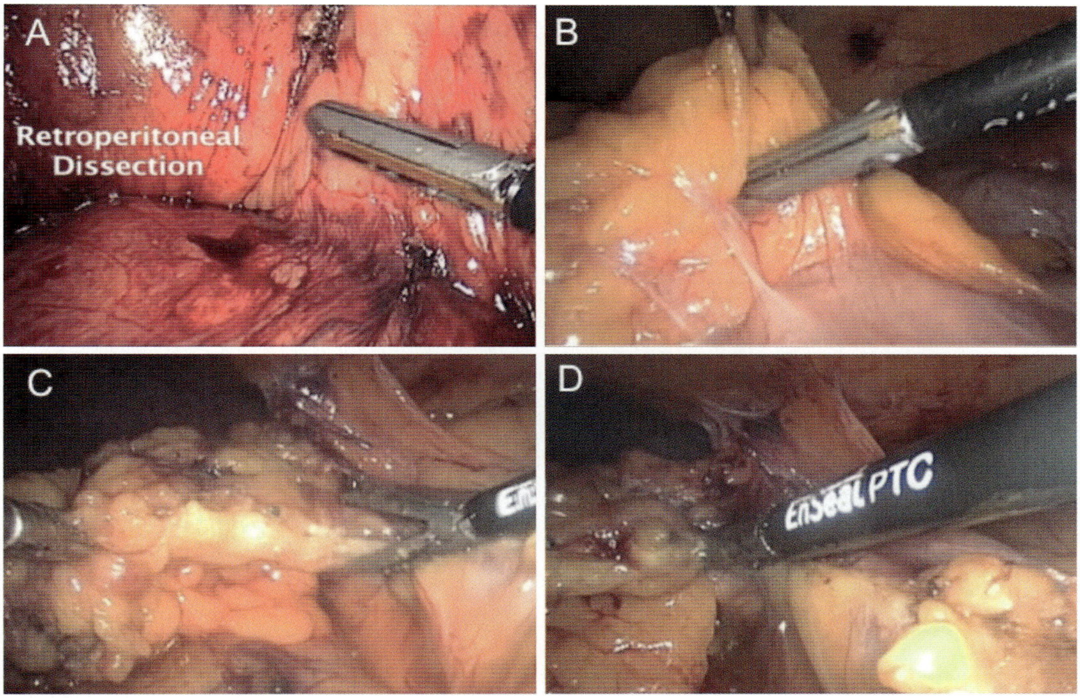

Fig. 20.4 With the retroperitoneal plane is fully developed (**a**), attention is then drawn to the gastrocolic ligament, which is detached from the colon at the level of the distal transverse colon (**b**). The lesser sac is entered and the splenic flexure takedown is performed (**b**, **c**, and **d**)

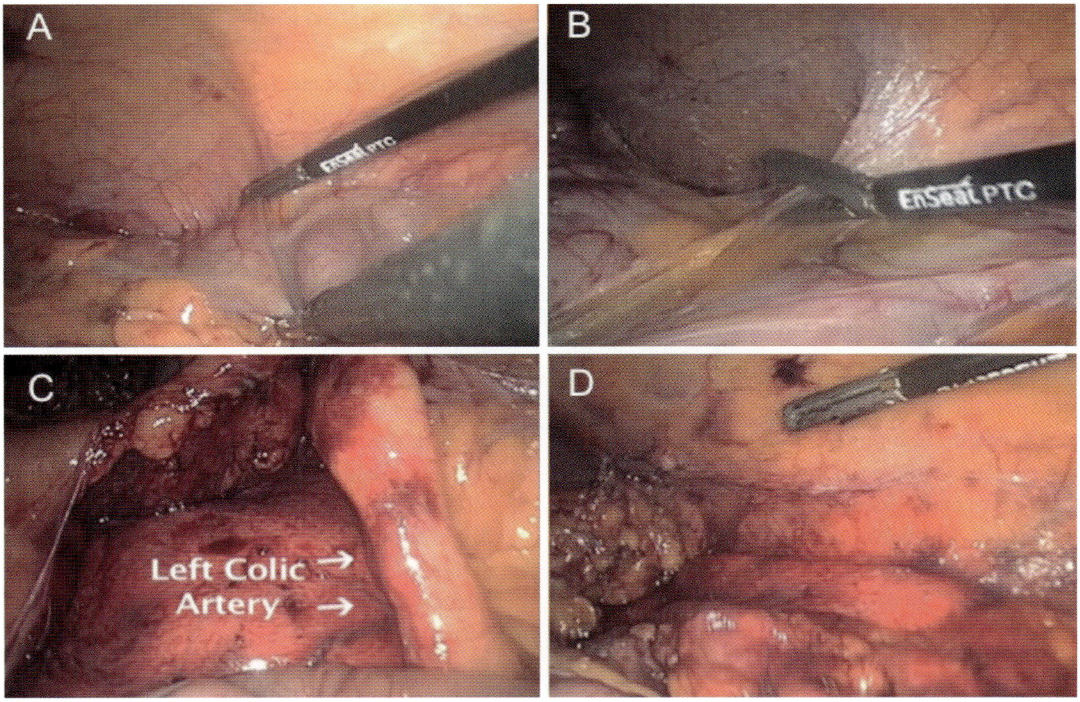

Fig. 20.5 Takedown of lateral attachments of the descending colon in a caudal to cranial fashion with the splenic flexure mobilization in this direction (**a** and **b**). Retroperitoneal plane is fully developed and the left colon fully mobilized (**c** and **d**)

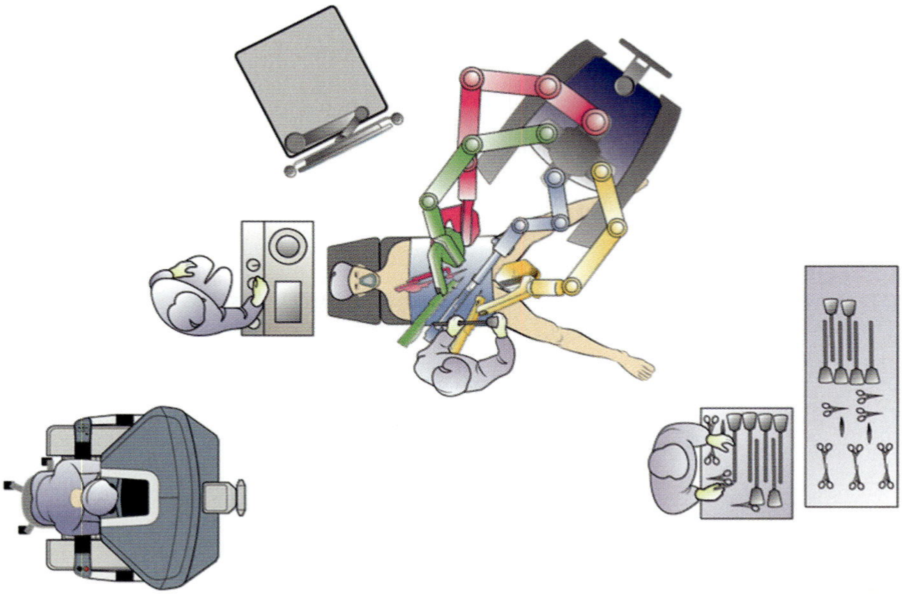

Fig. 20.6 Operative room configuration. The robotic cart is ideally docked in left side of the patient, in an acute angle. Robotic docking between the patient's legs hinders access to the perineum, which is required for a transanal approach or specimen extraction

Robotic Docking

Once the left colon is mobilized, the patient is placed in steep Trendelenburg position with the left side elevated, the laparoscopic instruments are removed and the robotic instruments are placed and the robotic cart is then docked. It is important to recognize that once the robotic cart is docked, further patient position modifications are precluded.

The robotic cart is ideally docked in left side of the patient, in an acute angle (Fig. 20.6). Alternatively, some prefer robotic docking between the patient's legs; however, this patient-cart configuration hinders access to the perineum, which is needed for a transanal approach or transanal specimen extraction, unless the robot is undocked. Furthermore, we do not recommend complete robotic undocking as we favor to perform the anastomosis under direct robotic visualization, since the dexterity and maneuverability provided by the robotic instrumentation would afford a more reliable suture repair in cases in which an anastomotic defect is encountered.

Robotic-Assisted Pelvic Dissection

The robotic pelvic segment of the procedure is commenced with retraction of the small bowel superiorly out of the pelvic cavity. The rectosigmoid is retracted anteriorly with the utilization of the third robotic instrumentation arm, and the peritoneum is incised medially at the level of the sacral promontory, and the retroperitoneal plane is identified (Fig. 20.7). Careful and meticulous dissection in this plane is paramount to remain in the proper plain and avoid injury to the hypogastric nerves and iliac vessels. Once the plane is developed, the left ureter is identified and the tissue planes are further developed. The superior rectal artery is readily visualized and is lifted to facilitate ongoing dissection in the retroperitoneal plane (Fig. 20.7d). The extent of the plane is carried out laterally to the peritoneal reflection, inferiorly to the presacral plane, and superiorly to the confluence of the superior rectal and inferior mesenteric artery (Fig. 20.8). At this level, continuity is established with previously exposed

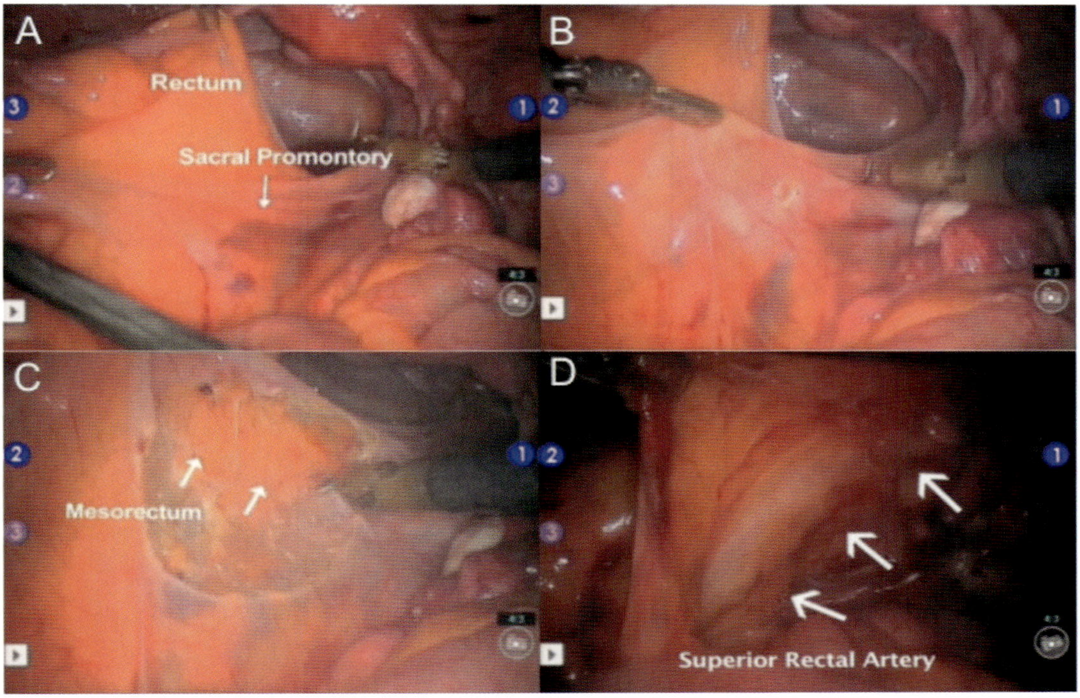

Fig. 20.7 The rectosigmoid is retracted anteriorly with the utilization of the third robotic instrumentation arm, and the peritoneum is incised medially at the level of the sacral promontory, and the retroperitoneal plane is identified (**a**, **b**, and **c**). The superior rectal artery is readily visualized and is lifted to facilitate ongoing dissection in the retroperitoneal plane (**d**)

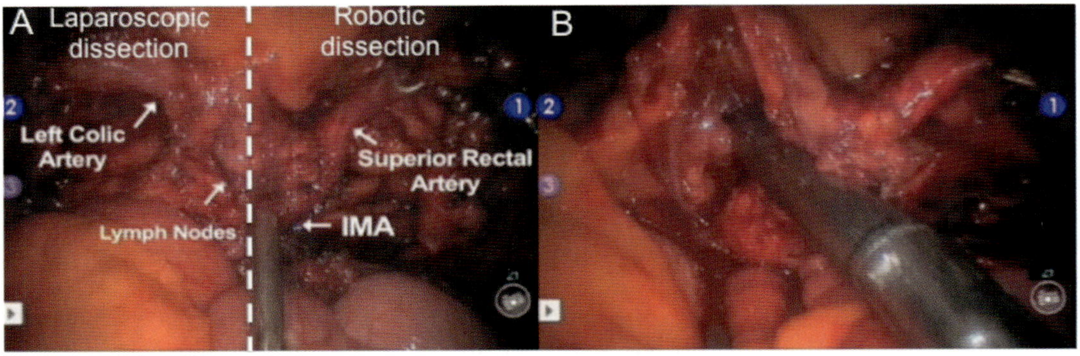

Fig. 20.8 *The eagle sign*. Continuity is established with previously exposed retroperitoneal plane during the laparoscopic portion of the procedure, exposing the anatomy of the vascular pedicle (**a**). The "eagle sign" is exposed: the left colic artery represents the superior "wing," the superior rectal artery represents the inferior "wing," and the inferior mesenteric artery represents the "body" of the "eagle" (**a**). The division of the inferior mesenteric artery is then carried out with an endoscopic stapling or energy device placed via the assistant port or with robotic application of clips (**b**)

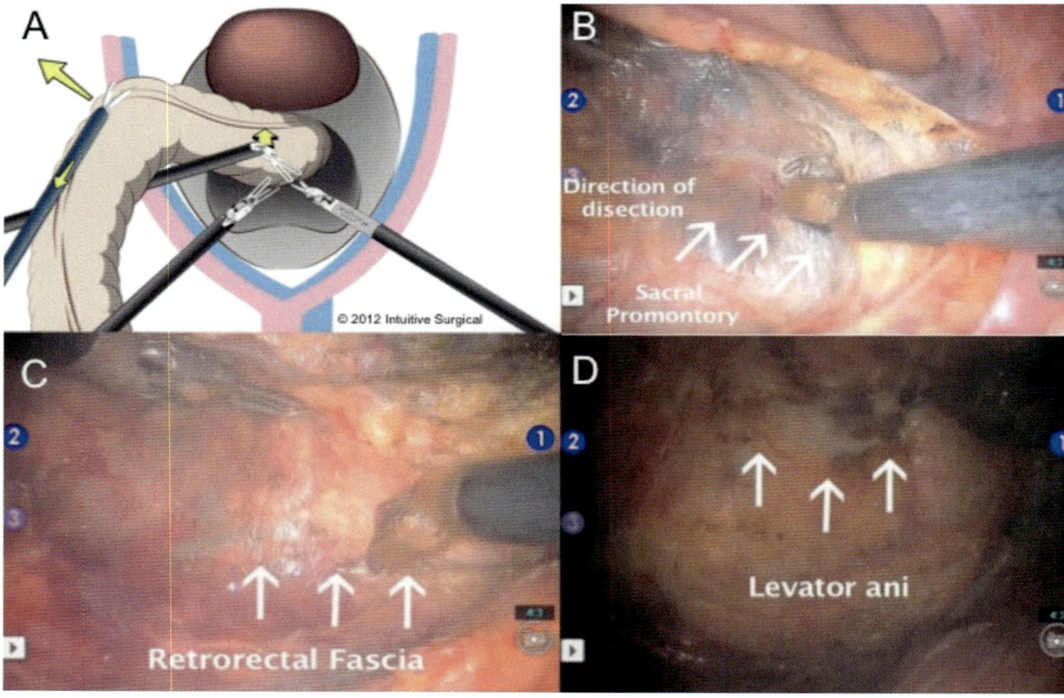

Fig. 20.9 Presacral plane dissection. The second robotic instrument arm serves to gently retract the mesorectum without grasping (**a**), while the first arm dissects to the alveolar plane (**b** and **c**). Dissection in the presacral plane continues through the retrorectal fascia and to the level of the levator ani muscles (**c** and **d**)

retroperitoneal plane during the laparoscopic portion of the procedure, thus fully exposing the anatomy of the pedicle. This exposure results in the "eagle sign" with the superior "wing" representing the left colic artery, the inferior "wing" representing the superior rectal artery, and the "body" representing the inferior mesenteric artery (Fig. 20.8a). The inferior mesenteric artery is then divided with the use of an endoscopic stapler or energy device placed through the assist port or with robotic application of clips (Fig. 20.8b). The third arm now elevates the divided portion of the pedicle to expose any remaining retroperitoneal attachments, which are then readily divided. Attention is then drawn to the lateral attachment, which is then divided from the level of the laparoscopic dissection to the upper portion of the rectum.

During the pelvic portion of the procedure, the avascular presacral plane is entered, and the dissection is continued in this plane carefully preserving the fascia propria of the rectum in an effort to accomplish a proper mesorectal excision. The second robotic instrument arm (typically the bipolar cautery) serves to gently elevate the mesorectum without grasping, while the first arm (typically the scissors with electrocautery) readily dissects to the alveolar plane (Fig. 20.9a). This serves to avoid traumatic tearing of the fascia propria and maintains an intact mesorectal envelop. The third arm facilitates this dissection by initially retracting on the rectosigmoid in a cephalad fashion. Once the upper and middle portions of the presacral plane are developed using cautery and sharp dissection typically with the robotic shears, the third arm is repositioned deep to the upper third of the mesorectum and then elevates this portion to further assist in exposure (Fig. 20.9b, c). Dissection in the presacral plane then continues through the retrorectal fascia and to the level of the levator ani muscles (Fig. 20.9c, d).

Once the full extent of the posterior dissection has been achieved to the level of the levator

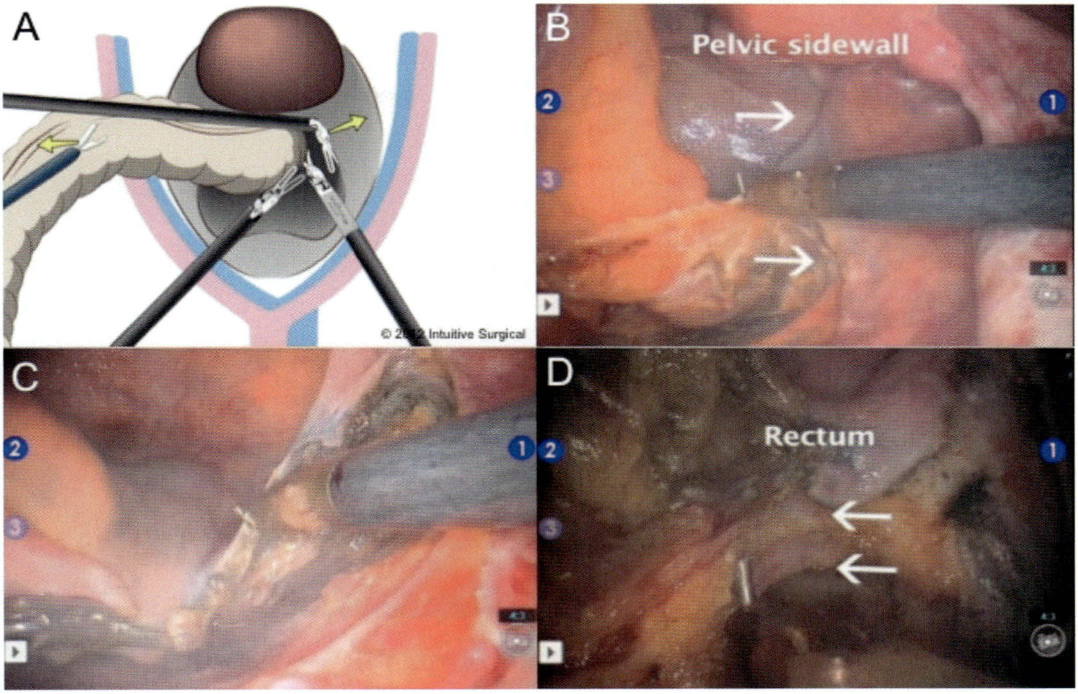

Fig. 20.10 The right lateral rectal dissection, which is carried down through the lateral stalks (**a**, **b**, **c**, and **d**)

ani, attention is then drawn to lateral and anterior dissection (Figs. 20.10, 20.11, and 20.12). The lateral dissection is carried down through the lateral stalks, which contain the middle rectal vessels (Figs. 20.10 and 20.11). It is important to maintain the dissection close to the rectum so as to avoid inadvertent injury to the nerve plexus. The final portion of the rectal dissection involves entrance to the anterior cul-de-sac with the establishment of the rectovaginal plane in women and Denonvilliers' fascia in men (Fig. 20.12).

For the purposes of an oncological procedure, the rectum has to be dissected, mobilized, and resected with the entirety of the mesorectal envelope (Fig. 20.13a, b). For low anterior resections we perform the rectal division with surgical stapler (Fig. 20.13c, d) and then extracorporealize the bowel via a small Pfannenstiel incision (Fig. 20.14a, d). Bowel continuity is established via an end-to-end anastomosis using a circular stapling device under robotic visualization (Fig. 20.14b, c). In this fashion, any small leaks noted during the air insufflation test can be oversewn using the aid of the robotic platform.

In cases in which the rectal pathology is located in close proximity to the anal verge, an "ultralow" anterior resection may be warranted. In such cases, we favor a combined approach with distal transection performed through a perineal approach with the aid of a Lone Star retractor (CooperSurgical, Inc., Trumbull, CT) (Fig. 20.15). Through the perineal approach, the distal margin is achieved, the rectum is divided, and the planes are met with the ones established during the robotic dissection. The rectum is extracted transanally and the anastomosis is performed with hand-sewn technique from the perineum (Fig. 20.15).

Outcomes

Robotic hybrid rectal resection is a safe and feasible surgical technique for the management of benign and malignant rectal diseases. Current literature

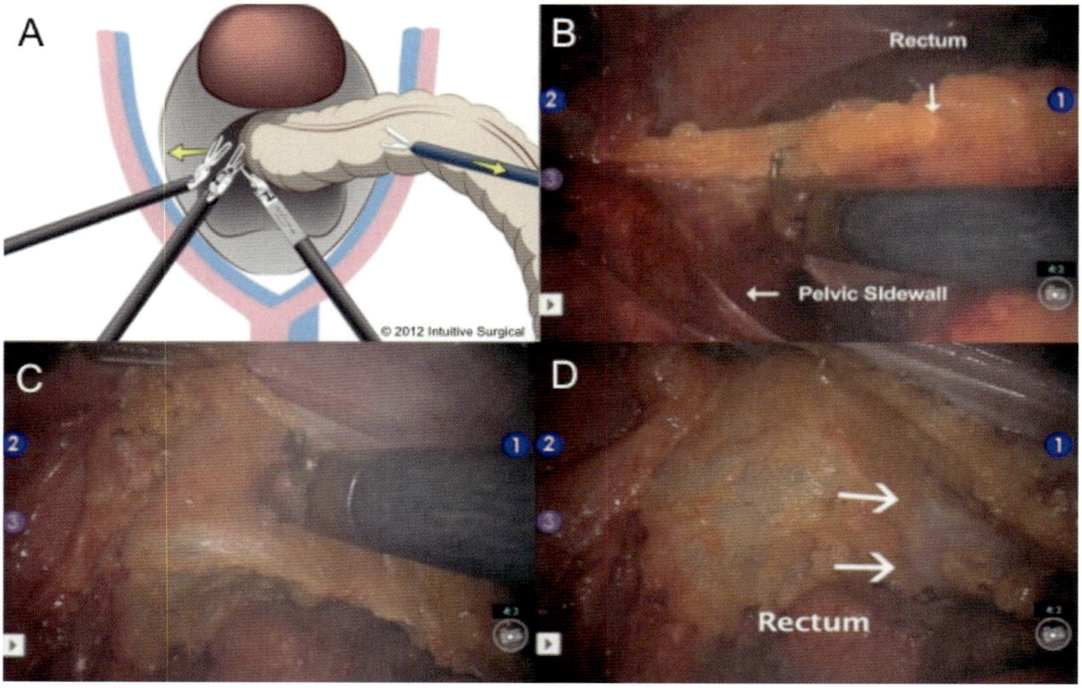

Fig. 20.11 The left lateral rectal dissection. Carried down through the lateral stalks (**a**, **b**, **c**, and **d**)

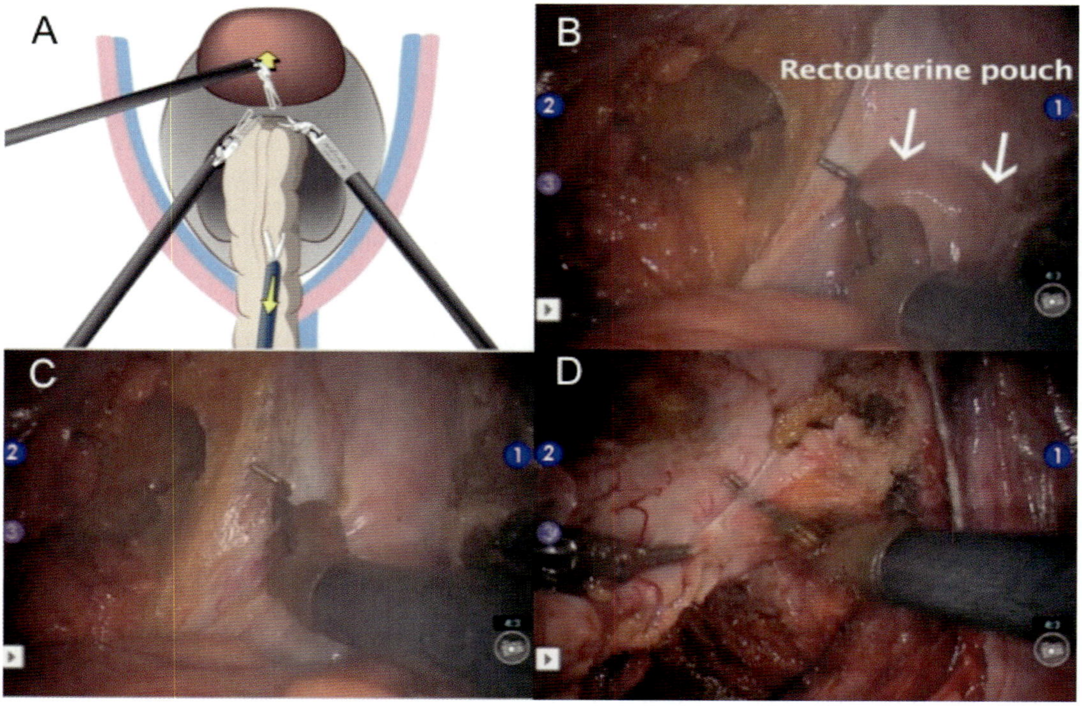

Fig. 20.12 Anterior rectal dissection. The entrance to the cul-de-sac is accomplished and the rectovaginal plane in women or Denonvilliers' fascia planes in men are established

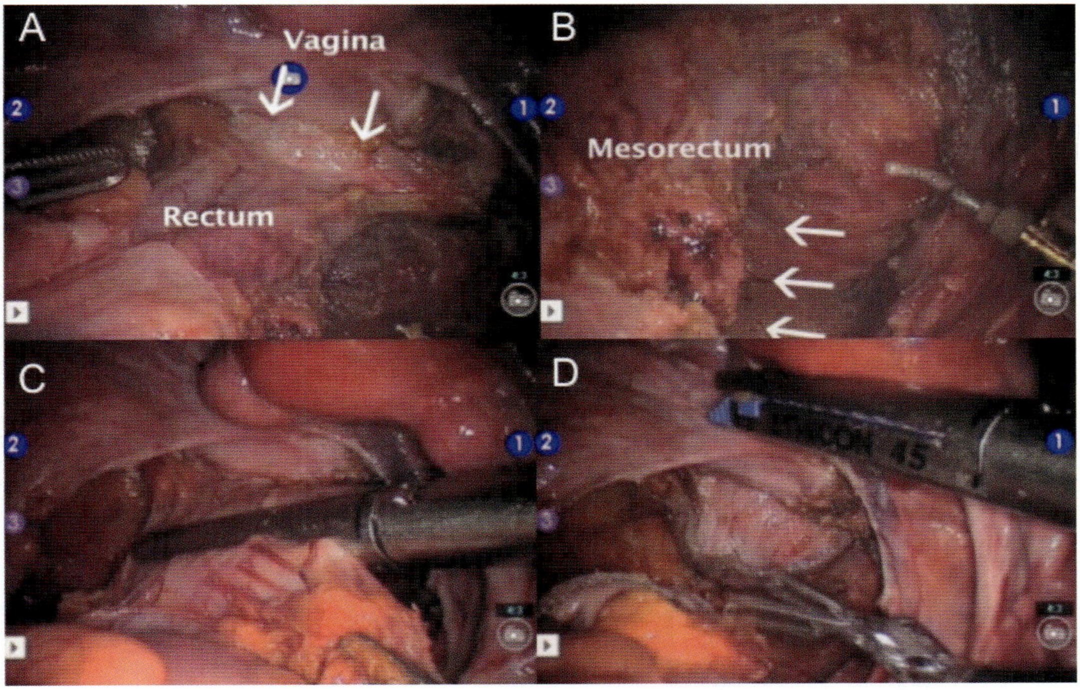

Fig. 20.13 Completion of robotic rectal dissection. For the purposes of an oncological procedure, the rectum has to be dissected, mobilized, and resected with the entirety of the mesorectal envelope (**a** and **b**). The rectal division is carried out with a surgical stapler (**c** and **d**)

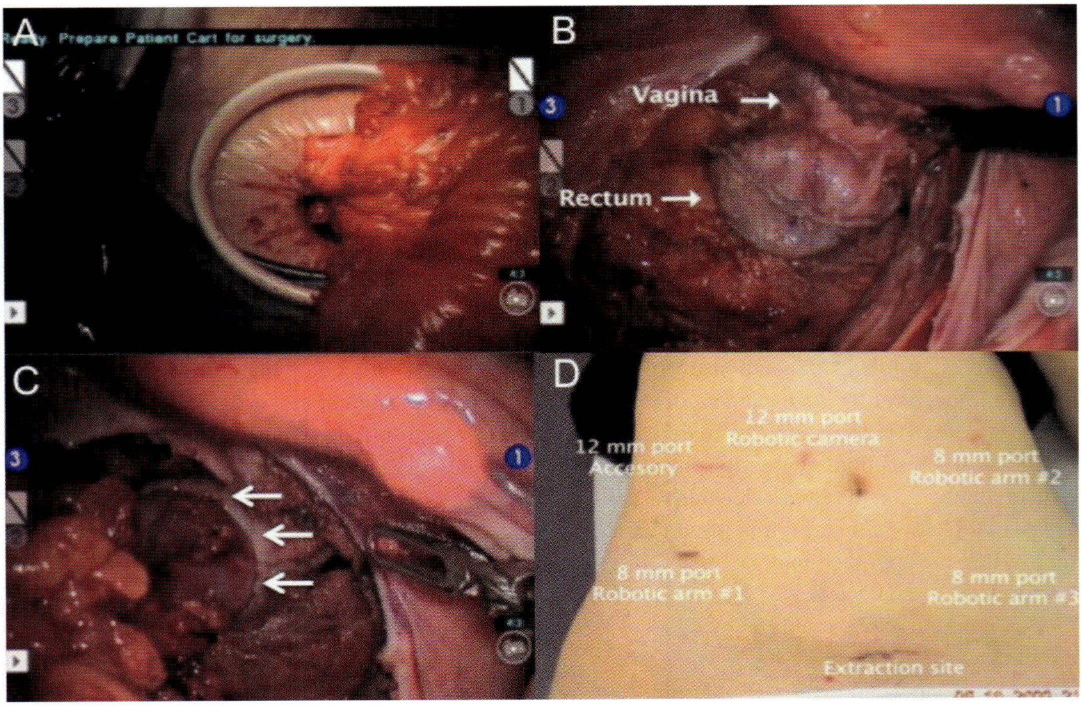

Fig. 20.14 Specimen extracorporealization via a small Pfannenstiel incision (**a** and **d**). The bowel continuity is established via an end-to-end anastomosis using a circular stapler, under robotic visualization (**b** and **c**)

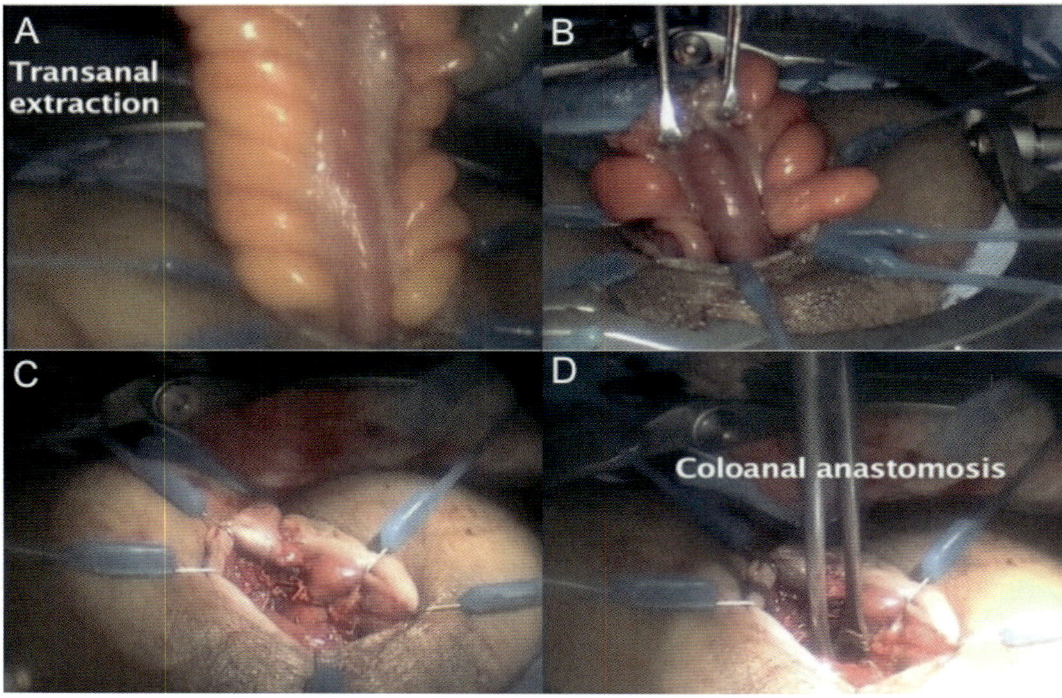

Fig. 20.15 Perineal approach with transanal extraction for "ultralow" robotic rectal resection. A hand-sewn anastomosis is performed in such cases

evaluates outcomes following the hybrid technique in comparison to those following conventional laparoscopic rectal resection. In general, these available data demonstrate that the robotic hybrid approach results in similar clinical and pathological outcomes as compared to conventional laparoscopy (Table 20.1) [5–9]. While totally robotic rectal surgery, also referred to as single-stage robotic rectal surgery, has demonstrated to be a viable approach for the management of rectal diseases, we tend to approach the majority of the robotic rectal resections with a hybrid technique. Our preference for the hybrid technique is based on several factors; however, it is important to recognize that the approach may be altered based on individual case characteristics.

Learning curve represents a key concept when adopting and implementing a new surgical modality. It has been estimated that the learning curve in robotic colorectal surgery is achieved after two phases comprising 25 surgical cases [10]. For laparoscopic surgeons attempting to adopt robotic surgery as part of their minimally invasive surgical armamentarium, we believe that the hybrid approach may be the most practical way to obtain exposure during the learning curve phases of one's experience. This hybrid technique affords the completion of a significant portion of the procedure laparoscopically and the remaining segment performed robotically. Thus, the transition from conventional laparoscopy to robotic surgery is facilitated and accomplished more readily.

The hybrid approach affords a safe abdominal cavity entry, but most importantly the entry is performed through an approach that all laparoscopic surgeons are accustomed to. The initial laparoscopic exploration allows a thorough four-quadrant abdominal exploration, which is imperative in oncological cases. Furthermore, it

Table 20.1 Studies comparing outcomes following robotic hybrid and pure laparoscopic rectal resection for rectal cancer

Author	Technique	*N*	Operative time (min)	Conversion rate	Postoperative complication rate	Hospital stay (days)	CRM involvement	Lymph node extraction
Baik et al. [6]	Lap	57	191.1 ± 65.3	10.5 %	19.3 %	7.6 ± 3.0[a]	8.8 %	18.7 ± 12
	Hybrid RALS	56	190.1 ± 45.0	0	10.7 %	5.7 ± 1.1[a]	7.1 %	18.4 ± 9.2
Bianchi et al. [7]	Lap	25	237 (170–545)[b]	4 %	24 %	6 (4–20)[b]	4 %	17 (8–37)[b]
	Hybrid RALS	25	240 (170–420)[b]	0	16 %	6.5 (4.15)[b]	0	18 (7–34)[b]
Park et al. [8]	Lap	82	168.6 ± 49.3[a]	0	23.2 %	9.4 ± 2.9	3.7 %	14.2 ± 8.9
	Hybrid RALS	41	231.9 ± 61.4[a]	0	29.3 %	9.9 ± 4.4	4.9 %	17.3 ± 7.7

Data are reported as mean ± standard deviation
CRM circumferential resection margin, *Hybrid RALS* hybrid robotic-assisted laparoscopic surgery, *Lap* laparoscopic technique, *N* number of cases
[a]Statistically significant difference
[b]Data are reported as median (range)

additionally facilitates takedown of intra-abdominal adhesions in an expeditious fashion. Moreover, the hybrid technique allows expeditious laparoscopic splenic flexure takedown and left colon mobilization. In the hybrid approach, the robotic cart docking typically represents a onetime event during the procedure, whereas re-docking may be required while performing a totally robotic approach [11]. Ultimately, the overriding benefit of the hybrid technique is found in the ability to utilize both the laparoscopic and robotic platform at particular portions of the procedure such that the merits of each approach are optimized.

References

1. Clinical Outcomes of Surgical Therapy Study G. A comparison of laparoscopically assisted and open colectomy for colon cancer. N Engl J Med. 2004;350:2050–9.
2. Fox J, Gross CP, Longo W, Reddy V. Laparoscopic colectomy for the treatment of cancer has been widely adopted in the United States. Dis Colon Rectum. 2012;55:501–8.
3. Guillou PJ, Quirke P, Thorpe H, et al. Short-term endpoints of conventional versus laparoscopic-assisted surgery in patients with colorectal cancer (MRC CLASICC trial): multicentre, randomised controlled trial. Lancet. 2005;365:1718–26.
4. Pigazzi A, Ellenhorn JD, Ballantyne GH, Paz IB. Robotic-assisted laparoscopic low anterior resection with total mesorectal excision for rectal cancer. Surg Endosc. 2006;20:1521–5.
5. Baik SH, Ko YT, Kang CM, et al. Robotic tumor-specific mesorectal excision of rectal cancer: short-term outcome of a pilot randomized trial. Surg Endosc. 2008;22:1601–8.
6. Baik SH, Kwon HY, Kim JS, et al. Robotic versus laparoscopic low anterior resection of rectal cancer: short-term outcome of a prospective comparative study. Ann Surg Oncol. 2009;16:1480–7.
7. Bianchi PP, Ceriani C, Locatelli A, et al. Robotic versus laparoscopic total mesorectal excision for rectal cancer: a comparative analysis of oncological safety and short-term outcomes. Surg Endosc. 2010;24:2888–94.
8. Park JS, Choi GS, Lim KH, Jang YS, Jun SH. Robotic-assisted versus laparoscopic surgery for low rectal cancer: case-matched analysis of short-term outcomes. Ann Surg Oncol. 2010;17:3195–202.
9. Patriti A, Ceccarelli G, Bartoli A, Spaziani A, Biancafarina A, Casciola L. Short- and medium-term outcome of robot-assisted and traditional laparoscopic rectal resection. JSLS. 2009;13:176–83.
10. Bokhari MB, Patel CB, Ramos-Valadez DI, Ragupathi M, Haas EM. Learning curve for robotic-assisted laparoscopic colorectal surgery. Surg Endosc. 2011;25:855–60.

Robotic-Assisted Extralevator Abdominoperineal Resection

21

Kang Hong Lee, Mehraneh D. Jafari, and Alessio Pigazzi

Current Applications of Robotic Abdominoperineal Resection

The evolution of surgical technique, instrumentation, and superior outcomes of minimally invasive surgery has made laparoscopy the standard of care for colon cancer treatment. The feasibility and the advantages of laparoscopic colectomy in terms of faster recovery, lower postoperative pain, and shorter hospital stay have been demonstrated by large prospective studies [1–5].

Laparoscopic abdominoperineal resection (APR) with total mesorectal excision (TME) for low rectal cancer has been shown to be safe and effective. It is associated with several advantages including lower morbidity, shorter duration of hospital stay, reduced cost, and reduced intensive care unit admissions [6]. However, laparoscopy has some limitations secondary to the anatomical structure of pelvis, rigid visualization system, instrument length, and articulation. The da Vinci robot has the potential to overcome some of the limitations of laparoscopy by providing improved three-dimensional vision, enhanced ergonomics, articulated instruments, and tremor elimination [7–9]. Early experiences with robotic rectal resection highlight the potential for decreased conversion rates, lower blood loss, and superior mesorectal grade compared to conventional laparoscopy [8–11].

Robotic APR can be performed utilizing a fully robotic technique or a hybrid laparoscopic–robotic technique whereby the robot is docked after mobilizing the sigmoid colon and dividing the vessels with conventional laparoscopic techniques.

Indications

Currently the most common indications for APR in the era of minimally invasive surgery are:

- Rectal cancer invading the sphincter complex
- Rectal cancer in patients who are not candidate for sphincter preservation because of poor functional status or comorbidities
- Recurrent rectal cancer
- Anal cancer, which recurs after or does not respond to chemoradiotherapy

K.H. Lee, M.D., Ph.D.
Department of Surgery, Hanyang University College of Medicine, 17 Haengdang-dong, Seongdong-gu, Seoul 133-792, South Korea
e-mail: leekh@hanyang.ac.kr

M.D. Jafari, M.D.
Department of Surgery, University of California, Irvine School of Medicine, 333 City Blvd., West Suite 850, Orange, CA 92868, USA
e-mail: jafarim@uci.edu

A. Pigazzi, M.D., Ph.D. (✉)
Division of Colorectal Surgery, Department of Surgery, University of California, Irvine Medical Center, 333 City Blvd., West Suite 850, Orange, CA 92868, USA
e-mail: apigazzi@uci.edu

K.C. Kim (ed.), *Robotics in General Surgery*, DOI 10.1007/978-1-4614-8739-5_21,

Robotic Positioning and Docking

Room setup is standard as for any robotic colorectal procedure keeping in mind the necessary space requirements for the surgeon, the assistant, and the operating room personnel. The patient is positioned in modified lithotomy in Trendelenburg position with a degree of right-sided table tilt enough to keep the small intestine out of the pelvic cavity. The robot cart is docked utilizing a left hip approach, more or less aligning the main post of the cart with the left anterior iliac spine and the camera port (Fig. 21.1).

Trocar Placement

A total of six ports are inserted under direct visualization. The camera port (C) is placed halfway between the xiphoid process and symphysis pubis. A 12 mm trocar (R1) is inserted in the midclavicular line (MCL) halfway in between C and the right anterior superior iliac spine (ASIS). This port can be used for ileostomy placement and will be used for the insertion of the stapler, if necessary. A second 8 mm trocar (R2) is inserted as a mirror image of R1. The third 8 mm robotic trocar (R3) is inserted 10–12 cm lateral to R2, usually directly above the left ASIS. The first 5 mm laparoscopic port (L1) is inserted in the MCL about 12 cm superior to R1. The second 5 mm laparoscopic trocar (L2) is inserted halfway between MCL and midline a handbreadth superior to L1 (Fig. 21.2).

Operative and Technical Steps (Hybrid Technique)

Laparoscopic Mobilization of Sigmoid Colon and Ligation of Vessels

Both surgeon and assistant stand on the patient's right side. Medial to lateral dissection of the sigmoid colon is begun at the inferior mesenteric artery (IMA). The sigmoid mesocolon is retracted anteriorly and dissection is begun at the sacral promontory. The parietal peritoneum medial to

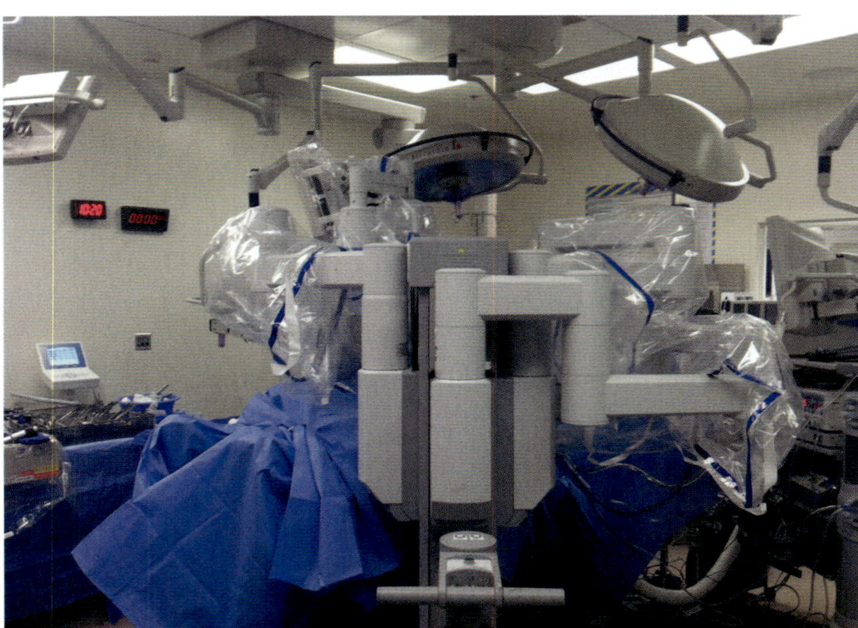

Fig. 21.1 The robot is docked from the left hip and the surgeon assistant stands on the right of the patient

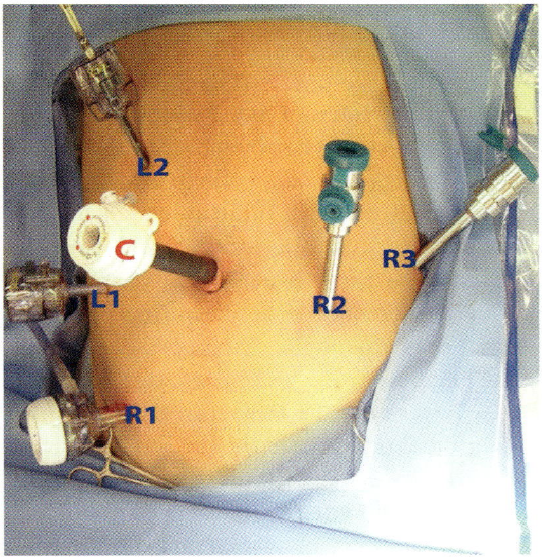

Fig. 21.2 Robotic laparoscopic port placement

the right common iliac artery at the sacral promontory is incised. A combination of sharp and blunt dissection is used to isolate the IMA avoiding injury to the hypogastric nerve plexus. The retroperitoneal structures including the left ureter are identified and swept posteriorly. The IMA (either at the origin or distal to the takeoff of the left colic artery) is skeletonized and divided via vessel sealer device and/or vascular stapler (Fig. 21.3). Atraumatic graspers are fundamental as with any laparoscopic bowel resection case to minimize injury.

In contrast with robotic low anterior resection, splenic flexure mobilization is not necessary in abdominoperineal resection. A shorter length of the colon is needed for creation of a colostomy in APR compared to the colorectal anastomosis in LAR. In general, the colon is able to reach the abdominal wall without the need of further mobilization. However, in certain patients, including patients with high BMI, further mobilization may be necessary. The lateral reflections of the left colon are taken down with a combination of blunt dissection and electrocautery. The colon is then divided above the IMA stump via an Endo GIA stapler.

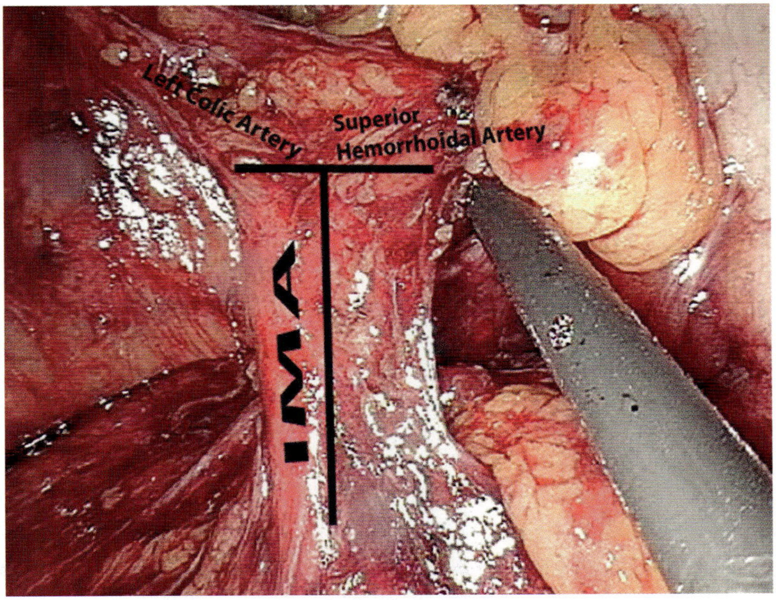

Fig. 21.3 The "T" configuration is visualized at the junction of the left colic artery and the superior hemorrhoidal artery

Robotic Setup and Instrument Selection

The four-arm da Vinci robot is docked using the left hip approach once the mobilization of the sigmoid colon is completed (Fig. 21.1). A 0° robotic camera is inserted in port C. Robotic arm 1 is docked to the R1 port; robotic arms 2 and 3 are docked to R2 and R3 trocar, respectively, in sequence. A monopolar scissors is inserted in R1. Alternatively a hook with monopolar energy source can be useful for dissection. A fenestrated bipolar forceps with bipolar energy source is inserted in R2 for holding, traction, and coagulation of vessels. A fenestrated forceps or a robotic suction irrigator devices inserted in R3 for traction. Grasping of the mesorectum should be avoided with the robotic graspers. The assistant uses the two laparoscopic ports. A laparoscopic grasper is used via the L2 port for retraction and manipulation of the sigmoid colon and rectum, and an irrigation and suction system is used via the L1 port for countertraction.

Total Mesorectal Excision

A total mesorectal excision is begun at the sacral promontory using only monopolar and bipolar cautery. The dissection begins posteriorly while the assistant surgeon retracts the rectum cephalad and anteriorly (Fig. 21.4). The avascular plane is between the presacral fascia and the mesorectum. The dissection is continued laterally around the rectum preserving both hypogastric nerves, which are located anterolaterally. Anteriorly, the rectovesical/rectovaginal fold of the peritoneum is incised to expose Denonvilliers' fascia or the rectovaginal septum. Maintaining a plane posterior to Denonvilliers' fascia prevents bleeding from the pampiniform plexus surrounding the seminal vesicles in men. The third arm allows for the retraction of the rectum during posterior dissection, the lateral sidewalls during lateral dissection, and the bladder/vagina during anterior dissection.

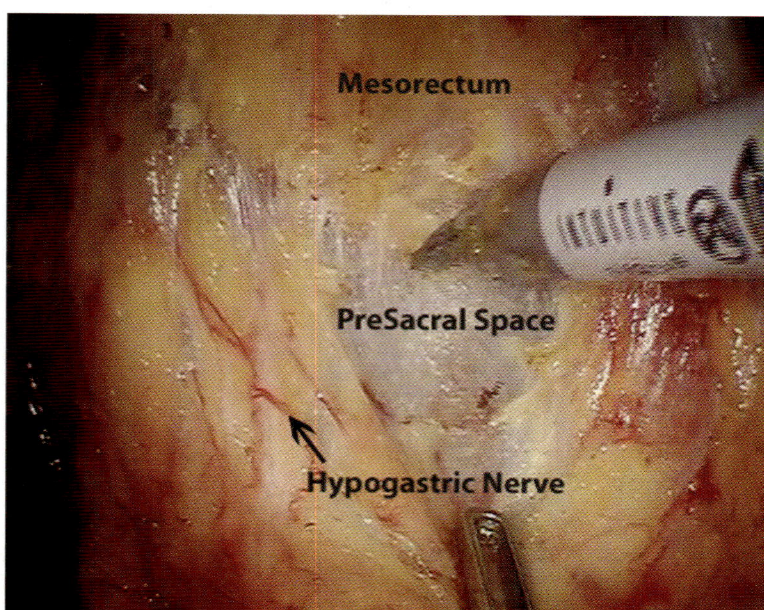

Fig. 21.4 Posterior dissection

Extralevator Abdominoperineal Resection

The dissection is continued distally, and a wide resection of the levators near their origin is carried out using robotic scissors in order to minimize the possibility of a positive circumferential margin (Fig. 21.5a). Care is taken not to lift the rectum off the levator muscle as in a conventional low anterior resection. Instead, the muscle will be taken widely at its origin along the bony structures of the deep pelvis, and the ischiorectal fat will be dissected en bloc using robotic instruments (Fig. 21.5b). The posterior limit of the rectal dissection can be decided by palpating the position of the coccyx tip via digital rectal examination from below while manipulating a robotic instrument on the coccyx from above.

The levator transection is continued posteriorly toward the midline and the anococcygeal ligament is transected (Fig. 21.6). The lateral limit of transection of the levator muscle is the medial edge of the obturator fascia, where autonomic nerve and vessels originating from the internal iliac artery and vein are found. Anteriorly, the levator transection is continued along the plane posterior to Denonvilliers' fascia/posterior wall of the vagina toward the perineum. Extreme care must be taken to avoid urethral injury in male patients. The dissection is continued distally into the ischiorectal fat as far as feasible just before encountering the perineal skin.

Robotic-assisted transabdominal resection of the levator muscles allows for a controlled transection of the pelvic floor and minimizes the risk of accidental injury to vascular structures under direct vision. This approach also renders the perineal resection very quick and simple, without the need to turn the patient prone and thus potentially improving the perineal wound healing rate [12]. In addition, this technique may offer the flexibility of varying the extent of levator muscle excision depending on the location of the tumor [12].

Perineal Procedure and Stoma Creation

Once the rectum is freed and hemostasis is achieved, the robot is undocked. The patient is placed in steep Trendelenburg, and a member of the surgical team via a perineal approach creates a circumferential incision around the anus from the perineal body to the coccyx. Because the levator muscles have been divided, the prior dissection plane is quickly encountered

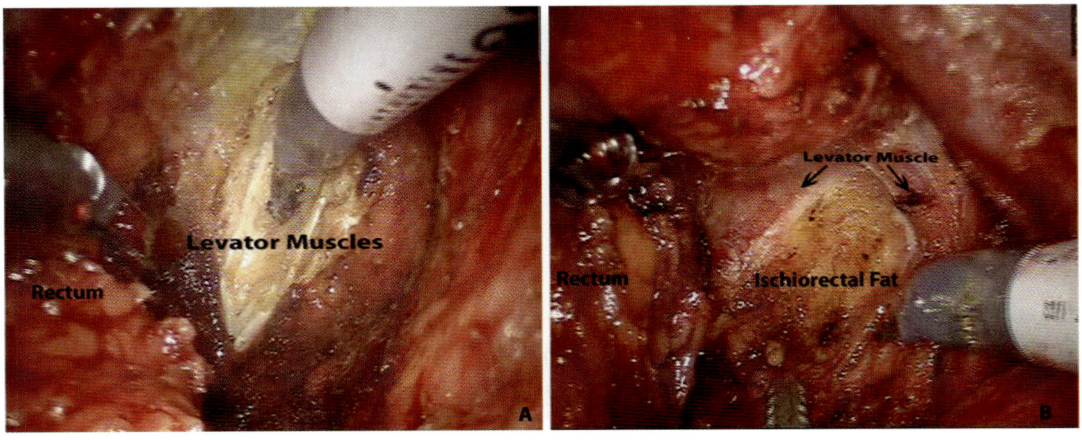

Fig. 21.5 (**a**) The division of the right levator muscles; (**b**) complete division of the levator muscles

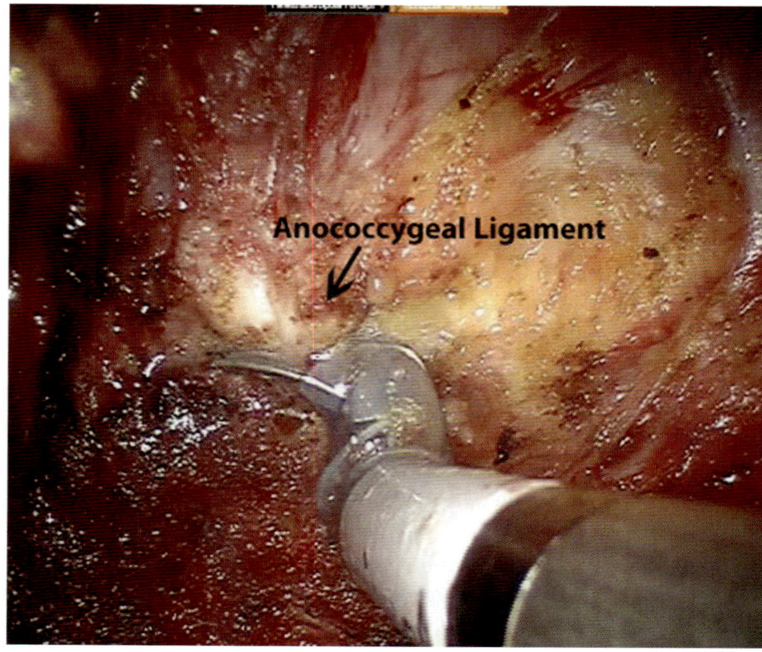

Fig. 21.6 Division of the anococcygeal ligament

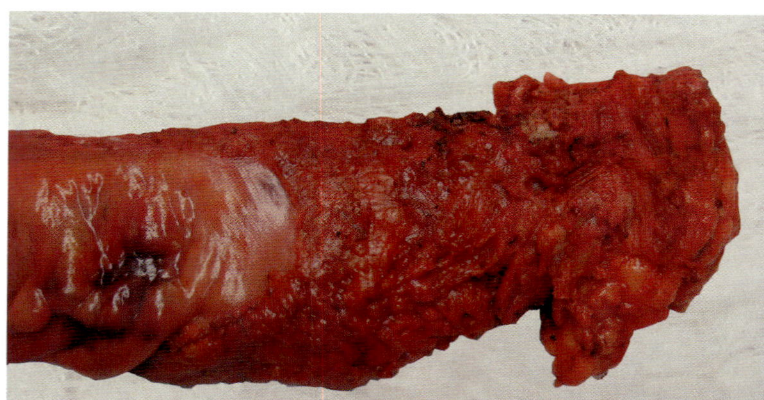

Fig. 21.7 Cylindrical APR specimen

and the "cylindrical"-shaped specimen is easily delivered through the perineum (Fig. 21.7). The perineal incision is closed in three layers. A transabdominopelvic drain is placed. The abdomen is re-insufflated and inspected; an end colostomy is brought out at an appropriate location.

Outcomes

Total mesorectal excision has been shown to dramatically reduce rates of local recurrence and is the accepted standard of care for rectal cancer [13–15]. However, the benefits of TME in LAR have not been reproduced in abdominoperineal resection. This has been thought to reflect, in part, a higher rate of circumferential resection margin (CRM) involvement leading to a higher rate of local recurrence, and lower survival rates after APR compared with LAR [13, 14, 16, 17]. A higher rate of positive CRMs can be attributed, in part, to the hourglass-shaped resection of the rectum seen with traditional APR techniques that exposes the tumor-bearing area around the anorectal ring. Extralevator abdominoperineal resection (EAPR) has been proposed in an effort to decrease the rate of CRM positivity, lower rectal perforation incidence, and lower local recurrence rates [18–22]. These beneficial results are achieved by wide resection of the levator muscles surrounding the tumor in the deep pelvis producing a cylindrical surgical specimen rather than an hourglass-shaped specimen and decreasing the chance of a close, or involved, surgical margin [22]. EAPR allows for en bloc resection of tissue and is associated with lower CRM positivity and lower chances of rectal perforation, resulting in lower rates of local recurrences. We believe this technique is especially suited for a robotic approach given the versatility of robotic surgical instruments in rectal cancer surgery [18–23].

References

1. Anderson C, Uman G, Pigazzi A. Oncologic outcomes of laparoscopic surgery for rectal cancer: a systematic review and meta-analysis of the literature. Eur J Surg Oncol. 2008;34(10):1135–42.
2. Aziz O, et al. Laparoscopic versus open surgery for rectal cancer: a meta-analysis. Ann Surg Oncol. 2006;13(3):413–24.
3. Liang Y, et al. Laparoscopic versus open colorectal resection for cancer: a meta-analysis of results of randomized controlled trials on recurrence. Eur J Surg Oncol. 2008;34(11):1217–24.
4. Pugliese R, et al. Laparoscopic resection for rectal adenocarcinoma. Eur J Surg Oncol. 2009;35(5): 497–503.
5. Kang CY, et al. Laparoscopic colorectal surgery: a better look into the latest trends. Arch Surg. 2012; 147(8):724–31.
6. Simorov A, et al. Comparison of perioperative outcomes in patients undergoing laparoscopic versus open abdominoperineal resection. Am J Surg. 2011;202(6):666–70. discussion 670-2.
7. Ballantyne GH. Robotic surgery, telerobotic surgery, telepresence, and telementoring. Review of early clinical results. Surg Endosc. 2002;16(10):1389–402.
8. deSouza AL, et al. A comparison of open and robotic total mesorectal excision for rectal adenocarcinoma. Dis Colon Rectum. 2011;54(3):275–82.
9. Pigazzi A, et al. Robotic-assisted laparoscopic low anterior resection with total mesorectal excision for rectal cancer. Surg Endosc. 2006;20(10):1521–5.
10. Baik SH, et al. Robotic versus laparoscopic low anterior resection of rectal cancer: short-term outcome of a prospective comparative study. Ann Surg Oncol. 2009;16(6):1480–7.
11. deSouza AL, et al. Total mesorectal excision for rectal cancer: the potential advantage of robotic assistance. Dis Colon Rectum. 2010;53(12):1611–7.
12. Marecik SJ, et al. Robotic cylindrical abdominoperineal resection with transabdominal levator transection. Dis Colon Rectum. 2011;54(10):1320–5.
13. Eriksen MT, et al. Inadvertent perforation during rectal cancer resection in Norway. Br J Surg. 2004; 91(2):210–6.
14. Heald RJ, et al. Abdominoperineal excision of the rectum–an endangered operation. Norman Nigro Lectureship. Dis Colon Rectum. 1997;40(7):747–51.
15. Kapiteijn E, et al. Preoperative radiotherapy combined with total mesorectal excision for resectable rectal cancer. N Engl J Med. 2001;345(9):638–46.
16. Nagtegaal ID, et al. Low rectal cancer: a call for a change of approach in abdominoperineal resection. J Clin Oncol. 2005;23(36):9257–64.
17. Wibe A, et al. Oncological outcomes after total mesorectal excision for cure for cancer of the lower rectum: anterior vs. abdominoperineal resection. Dis Colon Rectum. 2004;47(1):48–58.
18. Bebenek M. Abdominosacral amputation of the rectum for low rectal cancers: ten years of experience. Ann Surg Oncol. 2009;16(8):2211–7.
19. Bebenek M, et al. Therapeutic results in low-rectal cancer patients treated with abdominosacral resection are similar to those obtained by means of anterior resection in mid- and upper-rectal cancer cases. Eur J Surg Oncol. 2007;33(3):320–3.
20. Holm T, et al. Extended abdominoperineal resection with gluteus maximus flap reconstruction of the pelvic floor for rectal cancer. Br J Surg. 2007;94(2): 232–8.
21. West NP, et al. Multicentre experience with extralevator abdominoperineal excision for low rectal cancer. Br J Surg. 2010;97(4):588–99.
22. Kang CY, et al. Robotic-assisted extralevator abdominoperineal resection in the lithotomy position: technique and early outcomes. Am Surg. 2012;78(10): 1033–7.
23. West NP, et al. Evidence of the oncologic superiority of cylindrical abdominoperineal excision for low rectal cancer. J Clin Oncol. 2008;26(21):3517–22.

Robotic Single-Port Colorectal Surgery

22

Byung Soh Min, Sami Alasari, and Avanish Saklani

Introduction and History

Single-port surgery is an emerging technique in minimal access surgery, and its real benefit in its current form is debatable. This is because, while single-port surgery is not ergonomically efficient and requires high level of technical proficiency, its benefits seem limited to cosmesis and subjective patient satisfaction. This dilemma becomes more acute when it comes to oncologic surgery: can surgeons maintain the same quality of surgery with this new technique or is there trade-off/compromise between access ports and quality of surgery? In this chapter we will seek answers for these questions. We believe that the robotic surgical system for single-port colon surgery will enable more surgeons to perform single-port surgery without compromising oncologic integrity.

The first published report of single-port surgery, although it may be different from modern technique, came in 1971 [1]. The authors reported a successful series of tubal sterilizations using a special instrument specifically made for a single-port procedure. Then, in 1992 the laparoscopic single port emerged by Pelosi and Pelosi again in the field of gynecology. They reported a successful single-port subtotal hysterectomy [2]. With the increasing popularity of laparoscopic techniques, more and more surgeons have become interested in minimally invasive surgery (MIS). The increase in uptake of MIS led to an explosive increase in novel MIS techniques. Natural orifice transluminal endoscopic surgery (NOTES) was a revolutionary concept and succeeded in getting a lot of hype: however, its clinical application as an alternative to laparoscopic approach, at this moment, seems remote. One of the major obstacles in NOTES is technology, i.e., lack of instruments or system to enable surgeons to overcome technical and ergonomic challenges [3]. In contrast, laparoscopic single-port approach seems to have some benefits over NOTES in the sense that surgeons are able to perform this with available technology and conventional (multiport) laparoscopic instruments. A stepwise approach (i.e., from conventional multiport to reduced port and then to single port) seems to be rational and may help overcome the learning curve with reduced efforts. Moreover, some laparoscopic experts consider single-port surgery as a bridge between conventional (multiport) laparoscopic surgery and NOTES [4]. Starting from relatively simple procedures such as appendectomy and cholecystectomy, the application of single-port technique has been expanding to include procedures like hysterectomy, nephrectomy, and more complex general surgical procedures [5, 6]. In late 2008, Bucher et al.

B.S. Min, M.D., Ph.D. (✉) • S. Alasari, M.D.
Department of Surgery, Yonsei University College of Medicine, 50 Yonsei-ro Seodaemun gu, 120-752 Seoul, South Korea
e-mail: bsmin@yuhs.ac; SSS_ALLAH@hotmail.com

A. Saklani, M.S., F.R.C.S.
Colorectal Division, Tata Memorial Centre, Surgical Oncology, 402 Valencia B, Hiranandani Gardens, Powai, Mumbai 400076, Maharashtra, India
e-mail: asaklani@hotmail.com

K.C. Kim (ed.), *Robotics in General Surgery*, DOI 10.1007/978-1-4614-8739-5_22,

were the first to publish about the laparoscopic single port surgery right hemicolectomy [7]. Since then the number of articles published about laparoscopic singel-port colorectal surgery has increased exponentially, and each report describes different techniques and tips, which may raise an issue of standardization of the technique.

With the robotic era, the first robotic single-port surgery was reported in 2008 by Kaouk et al. [8]. He succeeded in performing a radical prostatectomy, pyeloplasty, and radical nephrectomy using the current da Vinci S(tm) surgical robotic system with conventional arms. Ostrowitz et al. published the first case report of robotic single-port right hemicolectomy at the end of 2009. They also used da Vinci S system with conventional two robotic arms and scope [9]. Since then, multiple robotic single-port surgeries have been published for cholecystectomy and hernia repair as well as colorectal surgery [10–13] using the da Vinci S or Si system either with conventional arms or the single-site platform.

Definitions and Terminologies

Several terminologies have been used in literature to describe single-port surgery. We reviewed the literature and summarize abbreviations that are currently used (see Table 22.1).

Table 22.1 Summary of the terminology definitions

Terminology	Abbreviation
Single-incision surgery	SIS
Single-port surgery	SPS
Single-access surgery	SAS
Laparoscopic Single-port surgery	SPLS
Robotic single-port surgery	SPRS
Single-incision laparoscopic surgery	SILS[a]
Single-incision robotic surgery	SIRS
Single access port	SPA
One-port umbilical surgery	OPUS
Laparoendoscopic single-site surgery	LESS
Single-site laparoscopy	SSL
Robotic single-site surgery	RSS
Natural orifice trans-umbilical surgery	NOTUS

[a]SILS is trademark of Covidien

Although the terminologies may be different, they all indicate a type of MIS that primarily introduces multiple (more than two) laparoendoscopic (or robotic) instruments through a single access port (usually through trans-umbilical incision) or skin incision. To avoid possible confusion, in this chapter we will use the terms "single-port surgery," "laparoscopic single-port surgery," and "robotic single-port surgery," unless otherwise defined by cited studies.

Access Ports for Single-Port Surgery

Different kinds of access ports are commercially available and include SILS port (Covidien; Mansfield, MA), R-Port (ASC, Wicklow, Ireland), homemade port using a surgical glove and Alexis wound retractor (Applied Medical, Santa Margarita, CA, USA), GelPort or GelPOINT (Applied Medical, Santa Margarita, CA, USA), OCTO Port (Dalim, Korea), TriPort and QuadPort (Olympus, Japan), and da Vinci SS platform (Intuitive, USA). Apart from da Vinci single-site platform, which is exclusively for robotic single-port surgery and is attached to da Vinci Si system, almost all of the access ports were originally for laparoscopic single-port surgery. A few of these access ports have been evaluated in literature. Thus far, among commercially available access ports, only SILS port [9] and GelPort [14] have been used in published literature on robotic single-incision surgery. Based on these reports, the SILS port seems to have limitations in the size of the whole access port. It tends to be too small for robotic instruments, which are bulkier than laparoscopic instruments, and spaces between the instruments are inadequate, which results in frequent arm collision and limitation of range of motion. Another limiting factor is that there is limited room for a third robotic arm or for an assistant. GelPort may be a better alternative because it allows the surgeon to design individual port configurations within the access port and may help overcome the limitations in space, crowding of robotic arms and external clashing.

Our preference is a homemade port using a surgical glove and Alexis wound retractor. The glove port offers multiple advantages over commercially available products. Its construction is simple and additional cost is negligible since the Alexis wound retractor would have been used in standard laparoscopic or multiport robotic colorectal surgery for specimen extraction. Other major benefits of this port include accommodation of variable abdominal wall thickness and the virtual absence of air leaks, which frequently hinder procedures involving standard MIS ports [12].

Laparoscopic Single-Port Colorectal Surgery Overview

Laparoscopic single-port surgery has been widely described for appendectomy and cholecystectomy. Although most reports have small numbers related to a single surgeon's experiences, information pooled from these series regarding access port evaluation and technical tips make a firm base for performing more complex and multiquadrant procedures like colorectal surgery.

Another factor that has facilitated single-port surgery has been the evolution in surgical tools such as advanced articulating or flexible instruments including even energy devices, staplers, and endoscopes.

In a large systematic review, Makino et al. in 2012 examined the safety and feasibility of laparoscopic Single-port colorectal surgery for both benign and malignant conditions [15]. He reviewed 23 studies including 378 patients. The conversion rate was 1.6 % (6 cases) to open, 1.6 % (6 cases) to hand-assisted laparoscopy colectomy (HALC), and 4 % (14 cases) to conventional multiport laparoscopy. Additional laparoscopic ports were required in 12 patients out of 247 (4.9 %). The overall mortality and morbidity rates were 0.5 % (2 cases) and 12.9 % (45 cases), respectively. The causes of death were pulmonary embolism and metastasis for a palliative case. Of the four case-matched studies two studies showed shorter hospital stay for the single-incision laparoscopy than HALC and multiport laparoscopy. One study reported lower postoperative pain in SPLS over multiport and HALC. The readmission rate reported in two studies were 6.3 and 13.8 %, and when compared to multiport surgery found not to be significantly different. The reported complications from laparoscopic single-port surgery in literature were ileus, wound infection/hematoma, and anastomotic bleeding/leakage, which also were observed in multiport surgery as well as conventional open. Makino in his review concluded that despite the technical difficulty, in early series of highly selected patients laparoscopic single-port colorectal surgery was found to be safe and feasible in the hands of highly skilled surgeons. However standardization of the technique, learning curve and long-term evaluation are still in its infancy and need to be evaluated in large randomized controlled trails.

Why Robotic Single-Port Surgery?

Robotic colorectal surgery was reported in 2002 by Weber et al. [16]. Since then this has been adopted by colorectal surgeons in high-volume specialized centers. Recently meta-analysis and several large systematic reviews have confirmed the safety and feasibility of robotic colorectal surgery without inferiority in oncological outcome. Furthermore, randomized controlled trials are ongoing to provide a better level of evidence for this procedure. The advantages of the robotic approach articulated in published robotic papers largely focus on better high-definition three-dimensional vision, filtration of physiologic tremor, human wrist-like motion of robotic instruments, stable camera control, better ergonomics, and reduction of the fatigue associated with conventional laparoscopy.

These advantages of the robotic interface help overcome many of the limitations of single-port surgery such as internal and external collisions, difficulty in achieving traction for triangulation, loss of ergonomics, body fatigue, instability of the camera, poor positioning with the assistant, and lack of stereotactic sense due to a two-dimensional view. Although efforts have been made to minimize the above limitations with use of articulated instruments and special cameras, the results have been less than perfect with limited adoption by laparoscopic surgeons. This is more so in colorectal surgery where multiquadrant access is required. By adopting the robotic system to single-port approach, theoretically surgeons can have stable and three-dimensional operative view and human wrist-like functioning robotic instruments that allow adequate traction and countertraction. Additionally, the surgeon can restore intuitive control of the instruments in the operative field despite the instruments being crossed by reassigning the hands at the console so that the instrument in the operative field corresponds to the appropriate hand on the console.

There are, however, some potential drawbacks of using the robotic system to perform single-port surgery. Because the robotic arms are bigger than laparoscopic instruments, a larger size skin incision may be necessary. Additionally, this may also limit the ability to introduce additional laparoscopic instruments through the access port, as is commonly done in laparoscopic single-port surgery.

Robotic Single-Port Colorectal Surgery Overview

The first robotic single-port surgery for radical prostatectomy was published by Kaouk et al. This was followed by pyeloplasty and nephrectomy; since then, several animal as well as human trials have been published for numerous benign and malignant procedures. In the colorectal field, robotic single-port surgery is still a novel technique and only a few surgeons have reported their results in literature (Tables 22.2 and 22.3).

Ostrowitz et al. was the first to publish about robotic single-port colectomy in 2009 [9]. He reported a three robotic single-port right hemicolectomy using da Vinci S system and 3 ports including a camera inserted through one incision. The incision was through or around the umbilicus with a 4-cm length incision. There were no reported complications. The average operative time was 152 min. The first case was converted to non-robotic single-incision right hemicolectomy during mobilization of the ascending colon, due to uncontrollable air leakage around the ports. The second and third cases were successfully completed without air loss by purse-stringing sutures around each individual port and the use of the SILS port, respectively.

Singh et al. in 2010 reported the first case of robotic single-port right hemicolectomy [14]. He performed the procedure using a GelPort as an access port through a 4-cm abdominal incision. Their operative time was 179 min and estimated blood loss was minimal. There were no reported intra-/postoperative complications. In 2012 Lim et al. published a multimedia article about robotic single-port anterior resection for sigmoid colon cancer [12]. They reported short-term results of 20 patients who underwent this procedure. The mean estimated blood loss was 24.5 ml (range 5–230). The mean operative time was 167.5 min (range 112–251), and there were no conversions. The median skin incision length was 4.7 cm (range 4.2–8). The mean proximal and distal resection margins were 12.9 (range 7.5–25.1) and 12.3 cm (range 4.5–19.2), respectively. The mean harvested lymph node was 16.8 (range 0–42). The immediate postoperative pain score was 2.8 (range 1–5) and 1.4 [1–3] on the first postoperative day. The mean length of hospital stay was 6 days (range 5–9). Obias et al. reported their comparative study

Table 22.2 Single-port colorectal operative outcome

Author	Study type	Patient no./procedure	Port type	Incision length[a] (cm)	OR time[a] (min)	EBL[a] (ml)	Con.
Ostrowitz	Case report	3 RHC	3 ports + SILS	4	152	75	1 to lap due to air leak
Singh	Case report	1 RHC	GelPort	4	179	Minimal	0
Lim	Retrospective	20 AR	Glove + Alexis	4.7	167.5	24.5	0

OR operative time, *EBL* estimated blood loss, *Con* conversion, *Lap* laparoscopic
[a]All results in mean

Table 22.3 Short-term outcome

Author	LOS (days)[a]	COMP	LN[a]	Margins	Mortality
Ostrowitz	3.6	0	22	Negative	0
Singh	4	0	14	Negative	0
Lim	6	0	16.8	Negative	0

LOS length of stay, *COMP* complication, *LN* lymph node
[a]All results in mean

between robotic and laparoscopic single-port colectomy [17]. They compared 11 patients having robotic single-port colectomy to 10 patients receiving laparoscopic single-port colectomy. In the robotic group all of the patients had single-port right hemicolectomy with three conversions to conventional laparoscopy. There were three cases of postoperative complications (ileus, anastomotic bleeding, and wound infection). The laparoscopic group consisted of hemicolectomies and ileocecectomies. One case was converted to open due to adhesions, and one case had postoperative bleeding requiring drainage. There was no statistically significant difference in measured clinical parameters between the two groups.

Technical Consideration

Laparoscopic single-port surgery is reported to be limited by the coaxial arrangement of the instruments. Although it may not be as frequent as in laparoscopy, arm collision is still a significant problem in robotic single-port surgery. Joseph et al. in 2010 reported a chopstick surgery technique to use the robotic arms through a single incision without collision [18]. He conducted an experimental study using the da Vinci S robot in a porcine model to perform cholecystectomy and nephrectomy with three laparoscopic ports introduced through a single incision. The chopstick arrangement crosses the instruments at the abdominal wall so that the right instrument is on the left side of the target and the left instrument on the right. This arrangement prevents collision of the external part of robotic arms. To correct for the change in handedness, the robotic console is instructed to drive the left instrument with the right hand effector and the right instrument with the left. Both procedures were satisfactorily completed with no external collision of the robotic arms in acceptable times and with no technical complications. He concluded that the chopstick surgery significantly enhances the functionality of the surgical robot when working through a small single incision.

In our experience, arm collision seems to be more complex than that can be resolved with a single solution. Theoretically to make an optimal chopstick arrangement, the crossing point should be the remote center of robotic arms and should be located at the level of skin incision. However, in procedures that deal with a wide range of motion in the peritoneal cavity, it is often difficult to keep the crossing point fixed at the ideal location. Inadequate location of the crossing point, subsequently, may result in arm collision. Choosing an adequate access port seems to be another key to success. Ostrowitz et al. reported that the very first case of robotic single-port surgery had to be converted due to air leak. He associated this with dilatation of the port site caused by external clashing of the large robotic arms when he was trying to use them parallel to each other without crossing [9]. According to the authors, they succeeded in subsequent cases using SILS port (Covidien) without an air leak. Singh et al. reported a successful case of robotic single-port right colectomy using GelPort as an access port [14]. They made a 4-cm-sized skin incision and put a GelPort into it. Because they didn't need to puncture abdominal fascia to insert individual ports, they could avoid excessive stretch of the wound and therefore could prevent air leak during the surgery and could reduce postoperative wound pain. Lim et al. demonstrated a glove-port technique and suggested similar advantages as GelPort [12]. An additional advantage of their technique is the availability of a third robotic arm and an assistant port through the five fingers of a glove port. The very low comparative cost of a glove is also an obvious advantage of this technique.

Robotic Single-Site Platform

The robotic single-port platform developed by Intuitive Surgical incorporates the principle of crossing the instrument arms internally with the ability of reassigning hands at the console (Fig. 22.1).

The set includes a multichannel access port with four cannulas and an insufflation valve. Two curved cannulas are for robotically controlled instruments, and the other two cannulas are straight; one cannula is 8.5 mm and accommodates the robotic endoscope, and the other cannula is a 5-mm bedside-assistant port. The curved cannulas are integral to the system, since their configuration allows the instruments to be positioned to achieve triangulation of the target anatomy. This triangulation is achieved by crossing the curved cannulas through the access port. Same-sided hand–eye control of the instruments is maintained through assignment of software of the Si system that enables the surgeon's right hand to control the screen right instrument even though the instrument is in the left robotic arm and, reciprocally, the left hand to control the screen left instrument even though the instrument is in the right robotic arm. The second part of the platform is a set of semirigid, nonwristed instruments with standard da Vinci instrument tips. The potential disadvantages of this set may be that it is limited to two arms while we need three arms in colorectal surgery. They do not have a wrist at the distal end of the instrument and that the traction and grasping power of the instruments are weaker than conventional ones. This platform reported to be helpful in relatively simple procedures like cholecystectomy and some minor urological procedures.

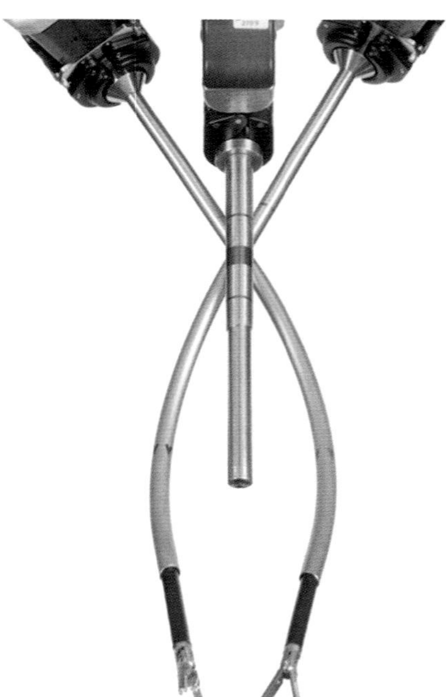

Fig. 22.1 Robotic single-port platform by intuitive

Surgical Technique

Patient Selection

Benign diseases including diverticular disease and inflammatory bowel disease-related conditions might be good indications for this technique. At this point, the efficacy of single-port surgery for malignant disease is controversial, and surgeons should consider its limitations and potential benefits that have been shown by current evidences seriously before they apply this technique to the patients. Early stages of colon cancer that confined to colon wall (T1–3) without lymph node metastasis (N0) may be candidates of this technique when the patients fully understand and when the informed consents are properly signed.

Technical limitation of the technique should be taken into consideration at the time of patient selection. Sigmoid colon diseases seem to be the best fit for the resection. Proximal descending colon may not be adequate because splenic flexure mobilization is sometimes limited especially when the patient is obese or/and tall. Rectum distal to peritoneal reflection may also be inadequate because of the limited reach of the instruments. Especially currently available laparoscopic staplers have limited angulation that proper resection of distal rectum can seldom be made. Robotic stapler, which is currently not available, may make difference in near future.

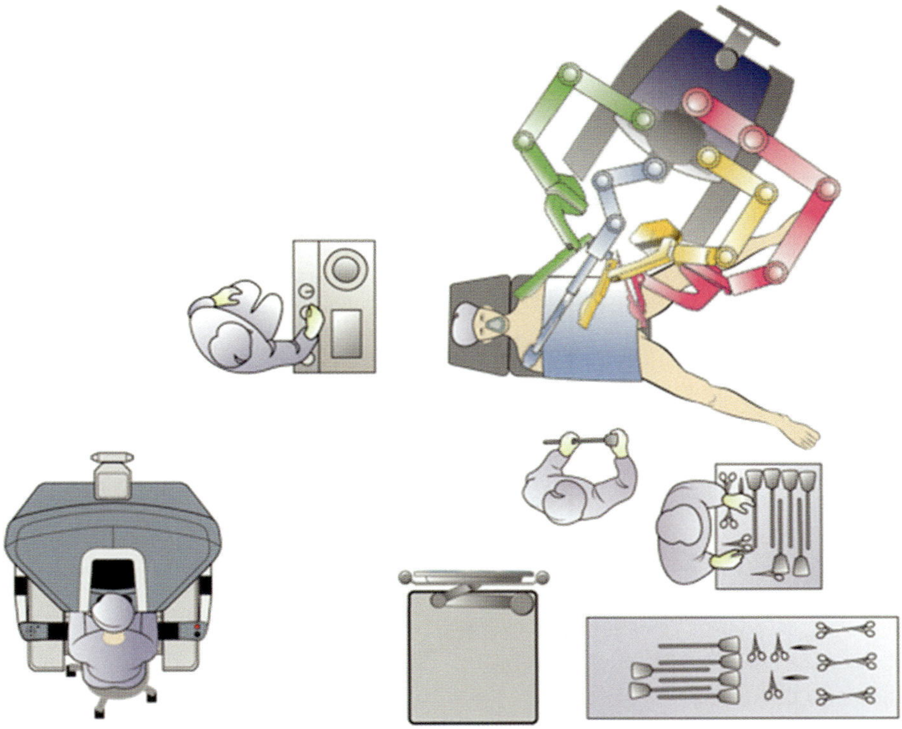

Fig. 22.2 Operating room setup

Patient Position and Operating Theater Setting

The patient is adequately padded and safely secured to the operating table in the Lloyd-Davis position with 15° Trendelenburg and 30° right side tilt. The patient-side robotic cart is positioned and locked in a 70° angle with the foot of the bed on the patient's left side at the level of the umbilicus and a 15° tilt toward the patient's head (Fig. 22.2).

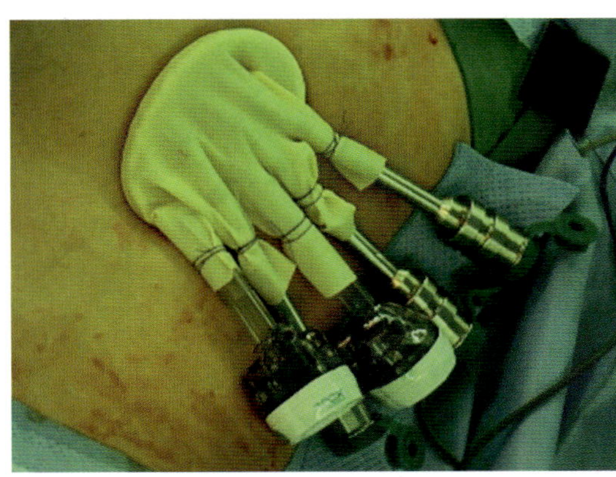

Fig. 22.3 Homemade glove port

Surgical Technique

The access device is a port constructed from a small size Alexis wound retractor manufactured by Applied Medical and a size 7 right-handed surgical glove. Initially, a 3.5-cm vertical transumbilical incision is made. Once the Alexis wound retractor is placed into the peritoneal cavity in the standard manner, the surgical glove is affixed to the outer ring and folded onto it to take up the slack of the plastic sleeve of the Alexis wound retractor. This ensures that the inner and outer rings fit snuggly against the abdominal wall preventing an air leak (Fig. 22.3).

Two 12-mm trocars are then inserted into the third and the fifth finger of the glove. Three 8-mm

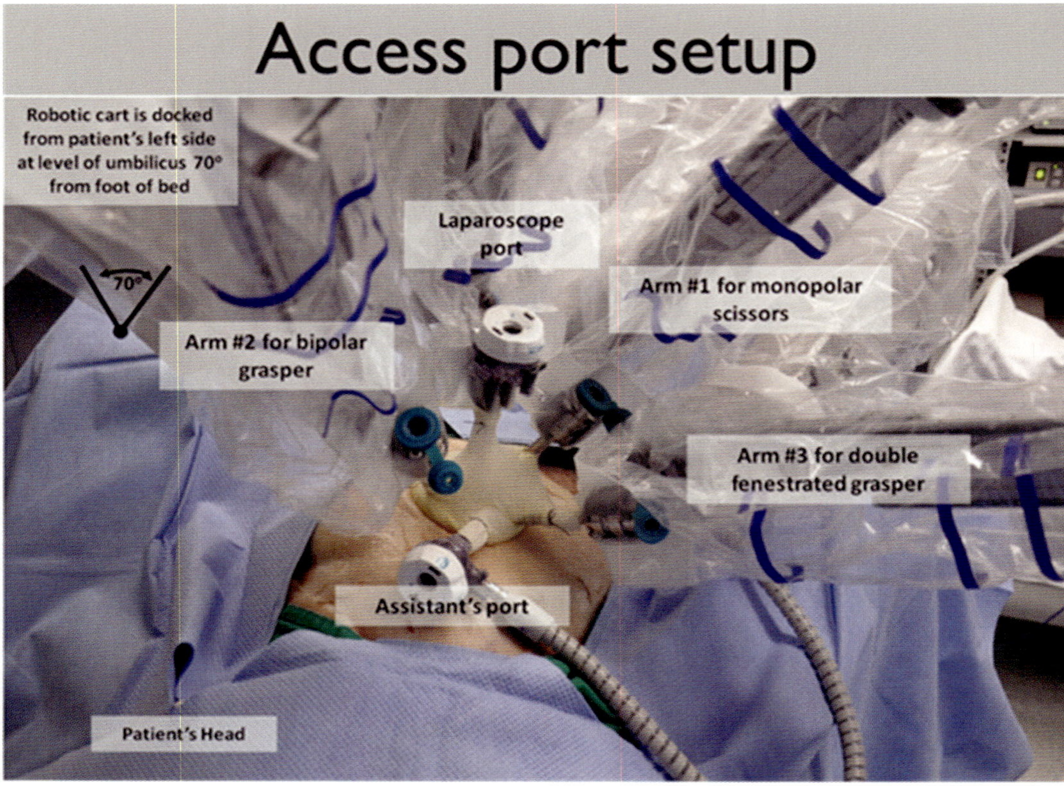

Fig. 22.4 Port setup after all robotic arms docked

robotic metal trocars are inserted into the remaining three fingers in the configuration depicted in Fig. 22.1. The trocars are secured to the glove with silk ties. The 30° up laparoscope is docked via the third finger 12-mm trocar. The other 12-mm trocar is for the assistant's use. The assistant stays directly at the patient's right side. The robotic arms are numbered 1–3 and are coupled with the three 8-mm robotic trocars. Arms #1–3 handle the monopolar scissors, the bipolar grasper, and the double fenestrated grasper, respectively. The da Vinci console-operating surgeon, using the right and left hands, respectively, controls instruments on arm #1 and arm #2. The double fenestrated grasper will be anchored to the robotic arm #3, which will be mainly used for static retraction and will be operated by surgeon's right hand when necessary (Fig. 22.4).

After pneumoperitoneum is established through the assistant's 12-mm port, the sigmoid colon mesentery is retracted supero-anteriorly using the double fenestrated grasper on arm #3. Peritoneum of the left mesocolon is incised superiorly from the sacral promontory, identifying the inferior mesenteric artery (IMA) along the way. After skeletonization, the IMA is ligated and divided at the root level with robotic Hem-o-lock clips, preserving the hypogastric nerve plexus. The peritoneal incision is then extended up to the duodenojejunal junction, exposing the inferior mesenteric vein (IMV). The IMV is temporarily spared, so as to utilize its "tenting effect," which is caused by the traction of the small bowel during the medial-to-lateral mobilization of colonic mesentery. Medial-to-lateral dissection is then performed until the lower border of pancreas superiorly and Toldt's line laterally, identifying and protecting vital structures such as the left ureter and gonadal vessels. The left colon is then freed laterally up to the splenic flexure.

The posterior side of upper rectum is mobilized to facilitate later application of circular stapler for anastomosis.

Following complete mobilization of the left colon, the mesentery and mesorectum are then divided using an energy-based device robotically or if preferred, by the patient-side assistant. The assistant then divides the distal resection margin using an articulating endo-stapler. One of the robotic instruments is usually disengaged, and the robotic arm uncoupled to make space for comfortable movement by the assistant. The robot is then undocked and the colon is exteriorized through the Alexis wound retractor. The IMV is ligated and the proximal margin is transected between a purse-string clamp and a bowel clamp. The anvil of the circular stapler is inserted into the proximal colonic segment and secured with a purse string. Finally, the port is reconstructed and the anastomosis is completed laparoscopically using a circular stapler.

Outcomes

Since single port is still in its early stages, there are no long-term results for this procedure published so far. We have been performing robotic single-port colectomies since 2009 and have thus far completed 73 cases. These have included the following procedures: right hemicolectomy (33 cases), anterior resection for sigmoid colon cancer (37 cases), and low anterior resection (2 cases). In our experience, we have been able to complete 96 % of the cases using the single-port technique. Conversions included one right hemicolectomy, one anterior resection, and one low anterior resection, and all these were conversions to multiport robotic colectomies. Two of the conversions, a right hemicolectomy and an anterior resection, occurred during our initial experience and were due to external arm collision and reach limitation. A recent conversion of a single-port low anterior resection was due to not being able to apply the endo-stapler properly from the umbilical port. The entire dissection except the distal rectal division had been completed using the single-port technique. Because currently available endo-staplers have limited flexion angles, we could not divide the distal rectum properly from the umbilical port and had to make an additional port in the suprapubic area from which we were able to apply the endo-stapler.

We have found that splenic flexure mobilization in tall obese patients and the pelvic dissection (total mesorectal excision) were the most challenging parts of our technique, and our patient selection is based on these technical limitations. However we look forward to technological advance in the near future including new staplers that will allow greater articulation, which will enable us to overcome current limitations (Table 22.4).

Table 22.4 Summary of our experience of robotic single-port colectomy

Parameter	Value
Gender	
Male	36
Female	37
Types of surgery	
Right hemicolectomy	33
Anterior resection	37
Low anterior resection	2
Age (mean, years)	54.3
Body mass index (mean, kg/m^2)	23.2
AJCC stage	
I	34
II	21
III	17
Lymph node harvest (mean)	19.8
Resection margin involvement	0
Conversion (to multiport)	3 (4.1 %)
Operation time (mean, min)	167.2
Estimated blood loss (mean, ml)	40.2
Mortality (within postoperative 30 days)	0
Overall morbidity (within postoperative 30 days)	13 (17.8 %)
Length of stay (mean, days)	6.2

Learning Curve

Because the procedure is not well standardized and is relatively new, no single study has been published about the learning curve. Currently available reports are all from robotic/laparoscopic experts who already have passed their learning curves in either robotic or laparoscopic multiport surgery. Possible issues regarding the learning curve of robotic single-port surgery are as follows: whether training in multiport robotic surgery is mandatory, whether training in single- or multiport laparoscopic surgery is mandatory, and how do we shorten the learning curve.

Future Innovation for Robotic Single-Port Surgery

The ideal robotic platform for single-port surgery should have a low external profile, the possibility of being deployed through a single access site, and the possibility of restoring intra-abdominal triangulation while maintaining the maximum degree of freedom for precise maneuvers and strength for reliable traction.

Several robotic prototypes for single-port surgery are being tested.

The Single-Port lapaRoscopy bImaNual roboT (SPRINT) is part of a major Array of Robots Augmenting the KiNematics of Endoluminal Surgery (ARAKNES) program coordinated by Dario and Cuschieri and funded by the EU Framework 7 program [19]. This robot has a three-dimensional high-definition television imaging system and is operated through a console in the sterile field so that the surgeon is not remote from the patient. This robot comprises of two arms with 6 degrees of freedom that can be individually inserted and removed in a 30–35-mm diameter umbilical access port. The system is designed to leave a central lumen free during operations, thus allowing the insertion of other laparoscopic tools [20]. Preliminary in vitro testing by Sanchez et al. [21] from Italy suggested that in the near future, the robot could become a reliable system in the field of robotic single-port surgery.

The group of Oleynikov from the USA is also developing a multi-dexterous miniature in vivo robotic platform that is completely inserted into the peritoneal cavity through a single incision [22]. The platform consists of a multifunctional robot and a remote surgeon interface. The robot has two arms and specialized end effectors that can be interchanged to provide monopolar cautery, tissue manipulation, and intracorporeal suturing capabilities. Its use has been demonstrated in multiple non-survival porcine studies.

Moreover, another new surgical robot is being developed and tested by investigators from Japan [23]. The robot consists of a manipulator for vision control, and dual tool tissue manipulators can be attached at the tip of a sheath manipulator. The group of Simaan described a novel insertable robotic effectors platform with integrated stereovision and surgical intervention tools for SPRS. This design provides can be inserted through a single 15-mm access port. Dexterous surgical intervention and stereovision are achieved by the use of two snakelike continuum robots and two controllable charge-coupled device cameras [24].

Conclusion

Rrobotic single-port colorectal surgery is still in its infancy. While robotic single-port colorectal surgery is feasible in selected cases, further evolution of technique and technology will be required for complex procedures (rectal cancer) for universal adoption. Research and development is ongoing to develop appropriate platforms for robotic single-port surgery. It is possible that the platforms for robotic single-port surgery may evolve to be organ specific, i.e., the robotic platform for gall bladder may be different from the one for colorectal surgery.

References

1. Thompson B, Wheeless RC. Outpatient sterilization by laparoscopy. A report of 666 patients. Obstet Gynecol. 1971;38(6):912–5.

2. Pelosi MA, Pelosi III MA. Laparoscopic supracervical hysterectomy using a single-umbilical puncture (mini-laparoscopy). J Reprod Med. 1992;37(9):777–84. PubMed PMID: 1453397.
3. Rattner D, Kalloo A, Group ASW. ASGE/SAGES Working Group on Natural Orifice Translumenal Endoscopic Surgery. October 2005. Surg Endosc. 2006;20(2):329–33.
4. Abe N, Takeuchi H, Ueki H, Yanagida O, Masaki T, Mori T, et al. Single-port endoscopic cholecystectomy: a bridge between laparoscopic and translumenal endoscopic surgery. J Hepatobiliary Pancreat Surg. 2009;16(5):633–8. PubMed PMID: 19373428.
5. Jung YW, Kim YT, Lee DW, Hwang YI, Nam EJ, Kim JH, et al. The feasibility of scarless single-port transumbilical total laparoscopic hysterectomy: initial clinical experience. Surg Endosc. 2010;24(7):1686–92. PubMed PMID: 20035346.
6. Ponsky LE, Cherullo EE, Sawyer M, Hartke D. Single access site laparoscopic radical nephrectomy: initial clinical experience. J Endourol. 2008;22(4):663–6. PubMed PMID: 18324901.
7. Bucher P, Pugin F, Morel P. Single port access laparoscopic right hemicolectomy. Int J Colorectal Dis. 2008;23(10):1013–6. PubMed PMID: 18607608.
8. Kaouk JH, Goel RK, Haber GP, Crouzet S, Desai MM, Gill IS. Single-port laparoscopic radical prostatectomy. Urology. 2008;72(6):1190–3. PubMed PMID: 19041022.
9. Ostrowitz MB, Eschete D, Zemon H, DeNoto G. Robotic-assisted single-incision right colectomy: early experience. Int J Med Robot. 2009;5(4):465–70. PubMed PMID: 19806602.
10. Kroh M, El-Hayek K, Rosenblatt S, Chand B, Escobar P, Kaouk J, et al. First human surgery with a novel single-port robotic system: cholecystectomy using the da Vinci single-site platform. Surg Endosc. 2011;25(11):3566–73. PubMed PMID: 21638179.
11. Tran H. Robotic single-port hernia surgery. JSLS. 2011;15(3):309–14. PubMed PMID: 21985715. Pubmed Central PMCID: 3183567.
12. Lim MS, Melich G, Min BS. Robotic single-incision anterior resection for sigmoid colon cancer: access port creation and operative technique. Surg Endosc. 2013;27:1021. PubMed PMID: 23052525.
13. Trastulli S, Cirocchi R, Desiderio J, Guarino S, Santoro A, Parisi A, et al. Systematic review and meta-analysis of randomized clinical trials comparing single-incision versus conventional laparoscopic cholecystectomy. Br J Surg. 2013;100(2):191–208. PubMed PMID: 23161281.
14. Singh J, Podolsky ER, Castellanos AE, Stein DE. Optimizing single port surgery: a case report and review of technique in colon resection. Int J Med Robot. 2011;7(2):127–30. PubMed PMID: 21394870.
15. Makino T, Milsom JW, Lee SW. Feasibility and safety of single-incision laparoscopic colectomy: a systematic review. Ann Surg. 2012;255(4):667–76. PubMed PMID: 22258065.
16. Weber PA, Merola S, Wasielewski A, Ballantyne GH. Telerobotic-assisted laparoscopic right and sigmoid colectomies for benign disease. Dis Colon Rectum. 2002;45(12):1689–94. PubMed PMID: 12473897; discussion 95–6.
17. Obias V, editor. Robotic versus laparoscopic single port right hemicolectomy. Chesapeake Colorectal Society meeting. Apr 2011.
18. Joseph RA, Salas NA, Johnson C, Goh A, Cuevas SP, Donovan MA, et al. Video. Chopstick surgery: a novel technique enables use of the Da Vinci Robot to perform single-incision laparoscopic surgery. Surg Endosc. 2010;24(12):3224.
19. Tang B, Hou S, Cuschieri SA. Ergonomics of and technologies for single-port laparoscopic surgery. Minim Invasive Ther Allied Technol. 2012;21(1):46–54. PubMed PMID: 22066862.
20. Piccigallo M, Scarfogliero U, Quaglia C, Petroni G, Valdastri P, Menciassi A, et al. Design of a novel bimanual robotic system for single-port laparoscopy. IEEE-ASME Trans Mechatron. 2010;15(6):871–8. PubMed PMID: WOS:000285361700006. English.
21. Sanchez LA, Petroni G, Piccigallo M, Scarfogliero U, Niccolini M, Liu C, et al. Real-time control and evaluation of a teleoperated miniature arm for single port laparoscopy. Conf Proc IEEE Eng Med Biol Soc. 2011;2011:7049–53. PubMed PMID: 22255962.
22. Dolghi O, Strabala KW, Wortman TD, Goede MR, Farritor SM, Oleynikov D. Miniature in vivo robot for laparoendoscopic single-site surgery. Surg Endosc. 2011;25(10):3453–8. PubMed PMID: 21487861.
23. Kobayashi Y, Tomono Y, Sekiguchi Y, Watanabe H, Toyoda K, Konishi K, et al. A surgical robot with vision field control for single port endoscopic surgery. Int J Med Robot. 2010;6(4):454–64. PubMed PMID: 20949430.
24. Ding JXK, Goldman R, et al. Design, simulation and evaluation of kinematic alternatives for insertable robotic effectors platforms in single port access surgery. In: EEE International Conference on Robotics and Automation; Anchorage, AK, USA, May 3–8, 2010.

Robotic Transanal Surgery

23

Sam Atallah and Matthew Albert

Introduction

Over recent years, new techniques for local excision of benign- and early-stage, well-selected neoplasms of the rectum have been developed. Transanal minimally invasive surgery (TAMIS) was pioneered in 2009 as a method for local excision of rectal neoplasia, and preliminary experience shows that TAMIS provides high-quality local excision, comparable to transanal endoscopic microsurgery (TEM) [1–4].

TAMIS uses ordinary laparoscopic instruments to perform intraluminal full-thickness local excision in combination with FDA-approved single ports, such as the SILS Port (Covidien, Mansfield, MA) or the GelPOINT path transanal access platform (Applied Medical, Inc.). The success with this approach was met with such enthusiasm that soon after its development, investigation began into the use of robotics with the TAMIS platform.

In 2010, it was learned that the da Vinci Robotic Surgical System (Intuitive Surgical, Inc., Synnyvale, CA) could be used to perform transanal surgery. Initial experiments were conducted in a dry lab and using a cadaveric model [5]. This approach was also shown to be feasible using a specialized glove port [6]. Subsequent to this, robotic transanal surgery (RTS) was successfully performed for local excision of a rectal neoplasm in a live patient [7].

S. Atallah, M.D., F.A.C.S., F.A.S.C.R.S. (✉)
Center for Colon and Rectal Surgery, Florida Hospital, 242 Loch Lomond Drive, Winter Park, FL 32792, USA
e-mail: atallah@post.harvard.edu

M. Albert, M.D., F.A.C.S., F.A.S.C.R.S.
Center for Colon and Rectal Surgery, Florida Hospital, 661 E. Altamonte Drive, Suite 309, Altamonte, FL 32701, USA
e-mail: matthew.albert.md@flhosp.org

Patient Selection

The indications for RTS are the same as for TAMIS and TEM. They include resection of benign rectal neoplasms and, for curative-intent surgery, well-selected T1 carcinomas, with histologically favorable features, where the risk of nodal metastasis is low [8]. The indication for RTS may also be broadened to include local excision of cT0 lesions in patients with locally advanced rectal cancer after neoadjuvant therapy for the purpose of confirming mural cPR (ypT0). This can be considered a valid option since the risk of occult node positivity for ypT0 lesions is low, at 3–6 % [9–14]. While most segments of the rectum can be reached with RTS, this approach is most suited for mid-rectal lesions (5–10 cm from the anal verge).

RTS should not be considered as an alternative to standard oncologic resection for locally advanced tumors. The lesion should not occupy more than 40 % of the luminal diameter. RTS may have special applications beyond local excision, such as for transanal repair of complex fistulae, such as for

K.C. Kim (ed.), *Robotics in General Surgery*, DOI 10.1007/978-1-4614-8739-5_23,

repair of a rectourethral fistula. This, in fact, has been attempted with limited success.

Preoperative Workup

All patients who have been selected to undergo RTS resection must have also undergone colonoscopy to assess for synchronous lesions and to obtain a biopsy of the rectal lesion. For malignant, early-stage tumors of the rectum, endorectal ultrasound is performed to determine preoperative T and N stage. Pelvic 3-Tesla (3 T) MRI is a valid alternative. Currently, only patients with histologically favorable, early-stage malignancy (uTis or uT1uN0M0 cancer) are considered candidates for TAMIS. More advanced lesions require standard resection (APR vs. LAR) except in patients who are not medically fit to undergo major surgery. CEA level and CT body imaging is also performed to assess for tumor metastasis. Patients with stage IV disease or locally advanced lesions are not candidates for RTS unless the objective is palliation.

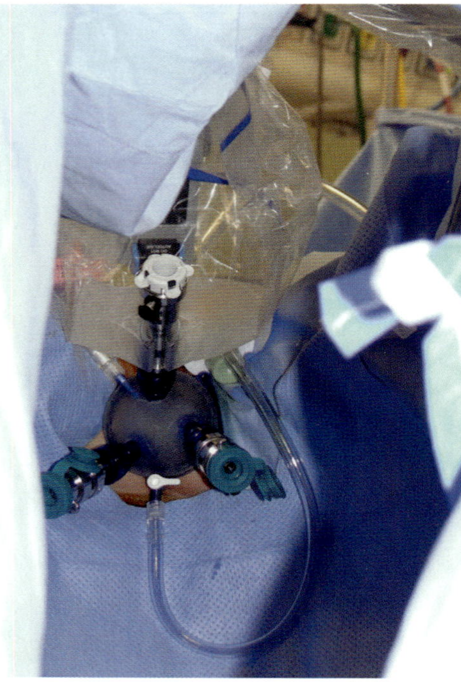

Fig. 23.1 The robotic trocar is introduced into the GelPOINT Path TAMIS port via three cannulas. The cannulas are placed into the TAMIS port gelatinous lid which is then placed and secured onto its sheath (not shown)

Operating Room

The patient is brought into the operating theater and positioned modified lithotomy in Allen stirrups. This position is recommended based on initial, cadaveric studies, which have demonstrated this position to be optimal for robotic access [5]. This is preferred, regardless of the position of the lesion in the rectal wall. A downward-angled lens is preferred for posterior lesions, and an upward-angled lens is preferred for anterior lesions.

The operating room should be fitted with standard laparoscopic equipment, including light source, video monitor, and CO_2 insufflator, as well as the da Vinci Robotic System. We strongly recommend general anesthesia with muscle paralysis to avoid collapse of the rectal wall, which often occurs with diaphragmatic excursion.

Parenteral antibiotics are administered 30 min prior to incision (our preference is single-dose ertapenem 1 g intravenously). The patient must undergo mechanical bowel prep preoperatively as well. The patient is then prepped and draped in the usual fashion. The abdomen should also be prepped, in the event that the lesion cannot be excised locally, or should abdominal access become necessary.

For RTS, the GelPOINT path transanal access platform is used (Applied Medical, Rancho Santa Margarita, CA). The device consists of a rigid cylindrical sleeve, which helps protect against injury to the sphincter mechanism. The sleeve is lubricated with petroleum jelly and introduced into the anal canal using an obturator provided by the manufacturer. Once seated above the anorectal ring, the sleeve is sutured to the skin with 2-0 silk stay sutures.

For both TAMIS and RTS, patients are pharmacologically paralyzed to prevent rectal lumen collapse, and humidified CO_2 is used with the pressure set to 15 mmHg. With the GelPOINT path port seated in place and pneumorectum established, a laparoscope is introduced to perform cursory visualization of the target lesion and to assess the rectum for luminal expansion.

Next, three GelPOINT path cannulas are introduced at an equilateral distance (Fig. 23.1). The

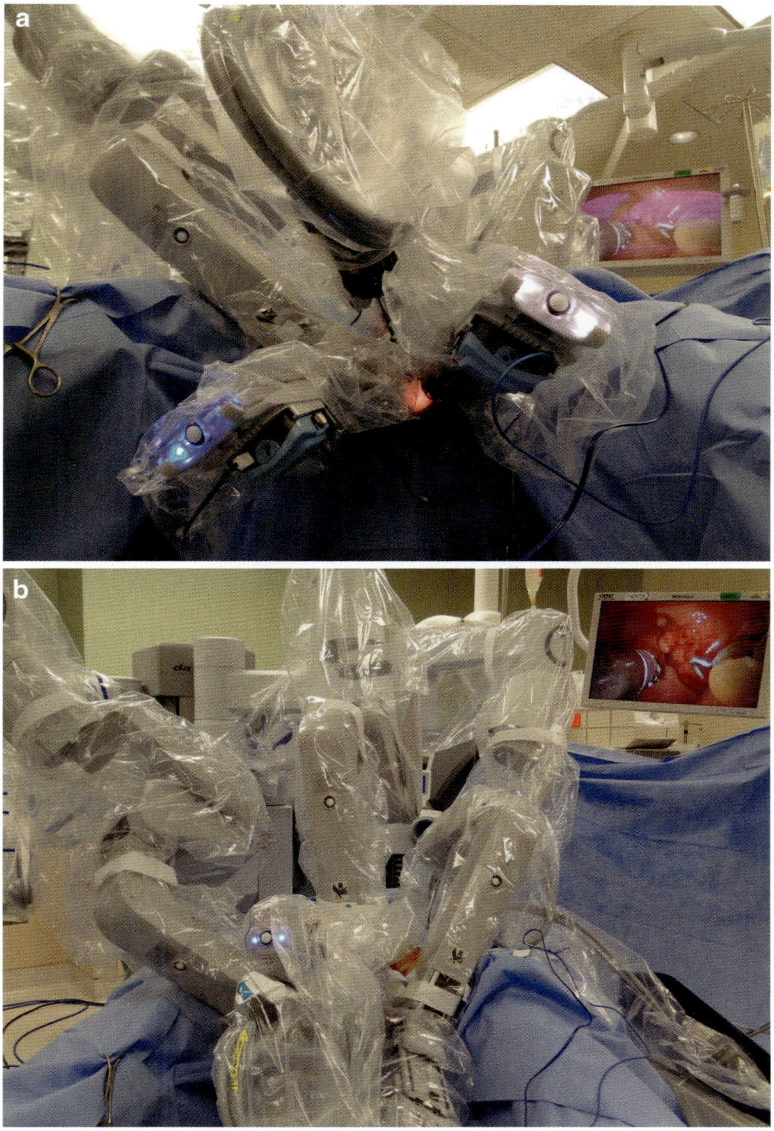

Fig. 23.2 The setup for RTS. The robotic cart is docked over the left (or right) shoulder with the patient positioned modified lithotomy in Allen stirrups. A bedside assistant operates a suction irrigator device to assist with smoke evacuation. The robotic arms are configured using either an 8-mm or 15-mm lens with 8-mm working arms

da Vinci robotic 8-mm trocars are then placed into these cannulas. The GelPOINT path lid is next placed onto the sleeve, which had already been seated in position, and the robotic cart is then docked over the patient's right shoulder (Fig. 23.2a, b). Next, a robotic hook cautery and Maryland grasper are secured (Fig. 23.3). The console surgeon then performs a full-thickness local excision. Resection using RTS is typically performed by demarcating the perimeter of the lesion, providing an appropriate margin. This is done using thermal energy. For evacuation of smoke, a bedside assistant uses a 5-mm laparoscopic suction-irregator device; this is passed directly into the GelPOINT path lid, without the need for a trocar (Fig. 23.4). We find that a simple

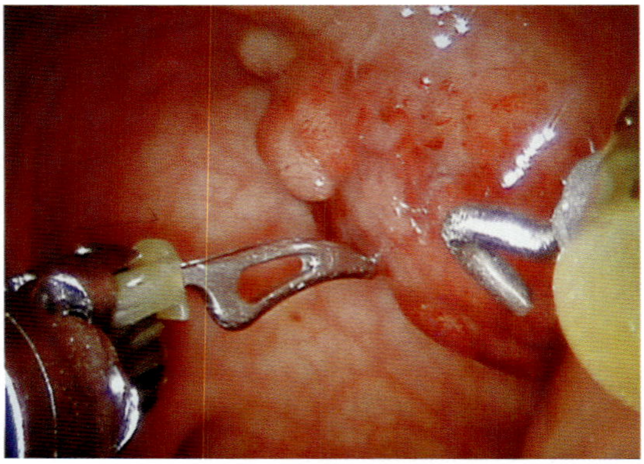

Fig. 23.3 A T1 well-differentiated adenocarcinoma arising from a tubulovillous adenoma measure 3 cm is shown being removed during RTS for local excision

short burst of suction maintains image clarity without collapsing the rectal lumen. The specimen may be tented gently using a robotic Maryland grasper while hook cautery allows for full-thickness excision (Fig. 23.5). Importantly, the CO_2 insufflation provides a natural "pneumodissection" thereby augmenting the ease and clarity of local excision using RTS.

To retrieve the resected specimen, the robot must be dismounted from the GelPOINT path interface. The lesion can be retrieved with a 5-mm grasper, the lid to the port simply removed allowing for specimen extraction.

The next step is closure of the full-thickness rectal wall defect, which is always recommended.

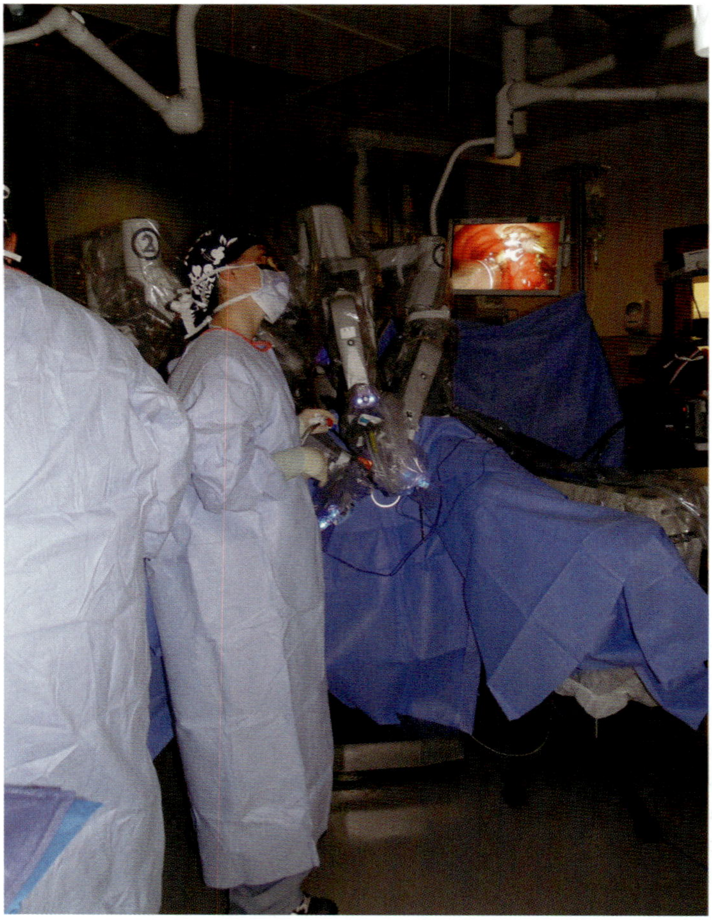

Fig. 23.4 The robot is now docked transanally. The console surgeon performs the excision, assisted only by the need for periodic smoke evacuation. A 5-mm laparoscopic smoke evacuator can be operated by a bedside assistant

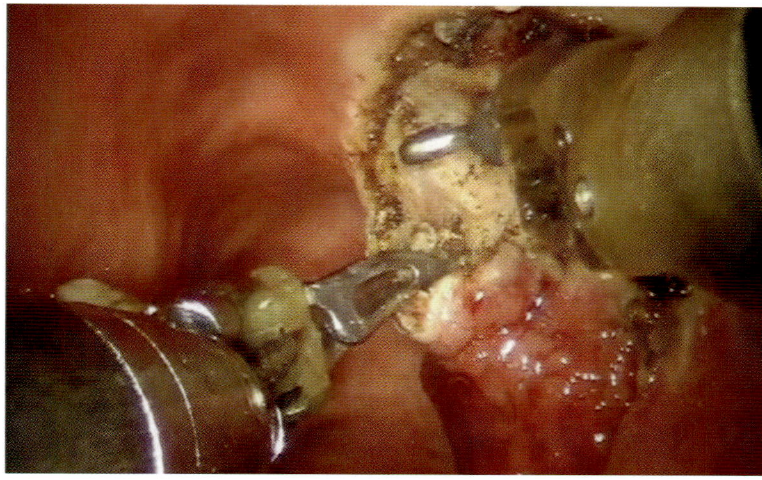

Fig. 23.5 The tumor is now visible and a hook cautery and Maryland grasper are all that are needed to complete the RTS local excision of rectal neoplasm

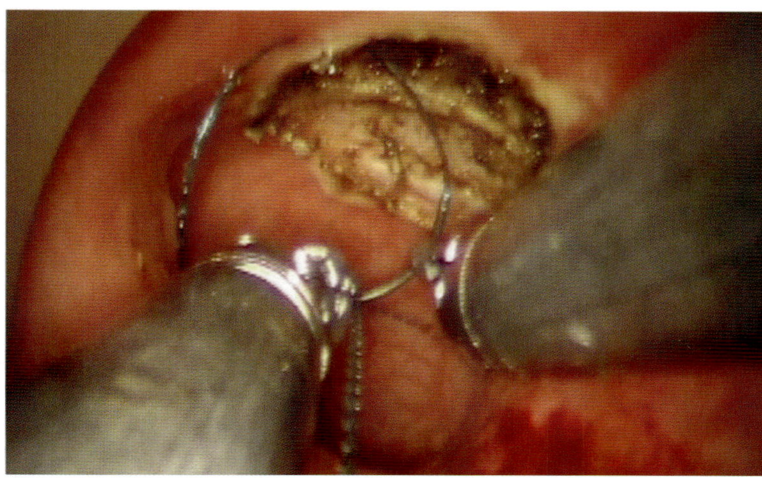

Fig. 23.6 Once local excision has been completed, the full-thickness defect is closed using needle drivers and a V-Loc suture, obviating the need for knot tying

To do this, the hook cautery and Maryland grasper are exchanged with two robotic needle drivers. Robotic intraluminal suturing is then carried out using a V-Loc 180 Absorbable Wound Closure Device (Covidien, Mansfield, MA). This allowed for suturing without the need for intraluminal knot tying, since the unidirectional barbs on the suture self-lock as they pass through the rectal wall. The defect can be closed with a single running V-Loc stitch, thereby completing the operation (Fig. 23.6).

Discussion

RTS illustrates a novel approach to the resection of well-selected and appropriately staged rectal neoplasia. A key advantage of RTS over TAMIS or TEM is that the console surgeon is able to perform intricate surgery more easily within the narrow, cylindrical lumen. The EndoWrist movement allows for greater intraluminal dexterity. This, together with magnified 3D optics, enhances the surgeon's ability to perform transanal local excision with improved precision. This also improves the ability to successfully complete complex tasks, such as intraluminal suturing. RTS is a new approach to transanal access, and its ability to accomplish intricate tasks with ease makes this method suitable for complex cases, where local excision or other advanced transanal procedures (such as transanal repair of rectourethral fistulae) may prove difficult with TAMIS or TEM.

Although greatly advantageous, RTS increases operative cost substantially, and therefore this approach should be reserved for more complex cases, where standard TAMIS and TEM are not possible. RTS is a technique still in its infancy, and its application for rectal surgery has not yet been fully defined. RTS is currently undergoing further investigation, and more data are necessary to establish its efficacy and practicality. A comparative analysis of the available platforms for advanced transanal surgery would be useful.

References

1. Atallah S, Larach S, Albert M. Transanal minimally invasive surgery: a giant leap forward. Surg Endosc. 2010;24(9):2200–5.
2. Lim SB, Seo SI, Lee JL, Kwak JY, Jang TY. Feasibility of transanal minimally invasive surgery for mid-rectal lesions. Surg Endosc. 2012;26(11):3127–32.
3. Barendse RM, Doornebosch PG, Bemelman WA, Fockens P, Dekker E, de Graaf EJ. Transanal employment of single access ports is feasible for rectal surgery. Ann Surg. 2012;256(6):1030–3.
4. Lorenz C, Nimmesgern T, Back M, Langwieler TE. Transanal single port microsurgery (TSPM) as a modified technique of transanal microsurgery (TEM). Surg Innov. 2010;17:160–3.
5. Atallah SB, Albert MR, deBeche-Adams TH, Larach SW. Robotic transanal minimally invasive surgery in a cadaveric model. Tech Coloproctol. 2011;15(4):461–4.
6. Hompes R, Rauh SM, Hagen ME, Mortensen NJ. Preclinical cadaveric study of transanal endoscopic da Vinci® surgery. Br J Surg. 2012;99(8):1144–8. doi:10.1002/bjs.8794.
7. Atallah S, Parra-Davilla E, deBeche-Adams T, Albert M, Larach S. Excision of a rectal neoplasm using robotic transanal surgery (RTS): a description of the technique. Tech Coloproctol. 2012;16(5):389–92.
8. Nascimbeni R, Burgart LJ, Nivatvongs S, Larson DR. Risk of lymph node metastasis in T1 carcinoma of the colon and rectum. Dis Colon Rectum. 2002;45(2):200–6.
9. Garcia-Aguilar J, Shi Q, Thomas Jr CR, Chan E, Cataldo P, Marcet J, Medich D, Pigazzi A, Oommen S, Posner MC. A phase II trial of neoadjuvant chemoradiation and local excision for T2N0 rectal cancer: preliminary results of the ACOSOG Z6041 trial. Ann Surg Oncol. 2012;19(2):384–91.
10. Kundel Y, Brenner R, Purim O, Peled N, Idelevich E, Fenig E, et al. Is local excision after complete pathological response to neoadjuvant chemoradiation for rectal cancer an acceptable treatment option? Dis Colon Rectum. 2010;53(12):1624–31.
11. Kim CJ, Yeatman TJ, Coppola D, Trotti A, Williams B, Barthel JS, Dinwoodie W, et al. Local excision of T2 and T3 rectal cancers after downstaging chemoradiation. Ann Surg. 2001;234(3):352–8. discussion 358–9.
12. Bedrosian I, Rodriguez-Bigas MA, Feig B, Hunt KK, Ellis L, Curley SA, et al. Predicting the node-negative mesorectum after preoperative chemoradiation for locally advanced rectal carcinoma. J Gastrointest Surg. 2004;8(1):56–62.
13. Bujko K, Nowacki MP, Nasierowska-Guttmejer A, Kepka L, Winkler-Spytkowska B, Suwaski R, et al. Prediction of mesorectal nodal metastases after chemoradiation for rectal cancer: results of a randomised trial: implication for subsequent local excision. Radiother Oncol. 2005;76(3):234–40.
14. Yeo SG, Kim DY, Kim TH, Chang HJ, Oh JH, Park W, Choi DH, Nam H, et al. Pathologic complete response of primary tumor following preoperative chemoradiotherapy for locally advanced rectal cancer: long-term outcomes and prognostic significance of pathologic nodal status (KROG 09–01). Ann Surg. 2010;252(6):998–1004.

Part VIII

Surgical Techniques: *Endocrine*

Robotic Thyroidectomy and Radical Neck Dissection Using a Gasless Transaxillary Approach

24

Jandee Lee and WoongYoun Chung

General Overview of Robotic Thyroidectomy

History and Development of Robotic Thyroidectomy

The open method of thyroid surgery, first described in the nineteenth century, originally required an 8–10 cm transverse skin incision. Since then, the length of the incision has been greatly reduced, and an incision between 4 and 6 cm in length has become standard [1]. Although the open method is quick, provides adequate access, and leaves a scar that is often well hidden in the skin crease, the possibilities of scar hypertrophy and neck discomfort due to sensory changes after surgery have resulted in the development of minimally invasive techniques as well as endoscopic methods.

The potential benefits of minimally invasive surgery include reduced trauma to adjacent tissues, decreased postoperative discomfort, and better cosmetic outcomes. Various types of minimally invasive operative techniques have been introduced, including mini-incision, video-assisted, endoscopic, and laparoendoscopic single-site surgery (LESS). Endoscopic thyroid surgery was first described in 1997 [2]; this was a totally endoscopic approach requiring carbon dioxide insufflation of the neck. Since then, complete endoscopic approaches to the thyroid have been further divided into cervical approaches, with port placements in the neck and extra cervical approaches, with the latter introduced to hide neck scars. These include port placements in the axilla and incisions through the breast, chest wall, and even the postauricular region [3–5]. The results of recent cadaveric experiments have suggested a completely scarless technique, known as natural orifice transluminal endoscopic surgery (NOTES™), in which the thyroid is approached from the oral cavity [5].

With recent advances, cancer surgery is moving toward the goals of adequate resection with minimum collateral damage. In neck surgery, however, where vital structures are in close proximity to each other and the operative field is a deep and narrow space, these minimally invasive approaches can be especially challenging [5, 6]. The advent of the da Vinci robot system (Intuitive Inc., Sunnyvale, California, USA) has further revolutionized the surgical management of thyroid disease within the endoscopic environment. These technical advances have increased understanding of the essential neck anatomy and have improved surgical techniques. Robotic surgery addresses some of these issues,

J. Lee, M.D., Ph.D.
Department of Surgery, Eulji University College of Medicine, Hagye 1-dong, Nowon-gu, Seoul, South Korea
e-mail: ljd0906@hanmail.net

W. Chung, M.D., Ph.D. (✉)
Department of Surgery, Yonsei University College of Medicine, 134 Shinchon-dong, Seodaemun-ku, Seoul, South Korea
e-mail: woungyounc@yuhs.ac

K.C. Kim (ed.), *Robotics in General Surgery*, DOI 10.1007/978-1-4614-8739-5_24,

with better visualization and a range of manipulators that can fit within deep and narrow spaces during neck operations. The optical channels of the robotic system can replace two-dimensional with three-dimensional imaging, thus enhancing the precision of anatomic dissection. Furthermore, the computer provides motion scaling and tremor elimination, facilitating more difficult surgical procedures. One of the most significant advantages of this robotic system is its three-dimensional view, which improves visualization of the surgical field and allows greater precision and accuracy. Another advantage is the wrist-like motion of the robotic arm, which provides finer and more dexterous movements, enabling surgical procedures that were impossible by conventional endoscopic methods. Robotic surgery has been found to eliminate many problems encountered with conventional endoscopic techniques [6–8].

The history of robotic thyroidectomy is short and the technique is still developing. The first series, published in 2009, included 100 patients [9]. The shift toward robotic thyroidectomy has reshaped the surgical approach to thyroid disease in South Korea and some parts of Asia. Its impact in the USA and Europe, however, has been somewhat delayed and less widespread than in Asian countries [4, 10–17]. In thyroid surgery, the da Vinci robotic system is being used in a wide range of specialties, including surgery for thyroid cancer and benign thyroid disease. Its aims are identical to those of conventional surgery, although its postoperative outcomes are better and cosmetic satisfaction is improved. Therefore, for patients, the potential advantages of robotic surgery compared with conventional endoscopic procedures include greater precision, lower error and bleeding rates, shorter hospital stay, more rapid recovery, and less pain. For surgeons, the use of a robot, controlled via a master–slave interface, may improve visualization and surgical ergonomics. For example, a surgeon may remain seated during the operation [4, 6–8].

Complete oncologic resection of a tumor with minimal disruption of the surrounding healthy tissue is the overall aim of cancer surgery. The development of new technologies has brought this goal closer. Robotic methods can aid surgery in traditionally hard-to-reach places in the neck area via an axillary approach. Several studies comparing the efficacy of complete thyroid resection and the extent of cervical lymph node (LN) dissection by robotic and conventional open techniques found that short-term oncologic effectiveness, as determined by postoperative [^{131}I] iodine (^{131}RI) scanning, serum thyroglobulin (Tg) concentration, and the number of harvested cervical LNs, was similar. By comparison, robotic thyroidectomy has shown excellent oncologic results and low complication rates when performed by experienced surgeons [4, 17–22]. Moreover, functional outcomes increasingly emphasize high scores on validated quality-of-life (QOL) instruments. Several large-volume centers have reported that the "functional and QOL" benefits of robotic thyroidectomy include excellent cosmetic outcomes, and reduced pain and voice and swallowing discomfort, when compared with conventional open surgery [23–26].

Robotic thyroidectomy, at present, compares favorably with open thyroidectomy in surgical completeness, safety, and QOL outcomes, including cosmetic results. Further analyses of surgeons' experience with long-term follow-up, as well as randomized controlled trials, remain important. In this chapter, we review the recent surgery literature, with a focus on how the refinement of surgical techniques in robotic thyroidectomy and the development of robotic surgical training will alter the future direction of these procedures. We also discuss the impact of these developments on thyroid cancer management, including oncologic, safety, and QOL outcomes.

Indications and Contraindications for Robotic Thyroidectomy

Patient selection is of the utmost importance when considering the use of newly developed techniques. Although there are no established guidelines on the limitations of robotic thyroidectomy, most experienced specialized surgeons would consider a robotic approach for the removal of a thyroid benign nodule <5 cm in size and for resecting a differentiated thyroid cancer without locally advanced features.

We have found that preoperative patient evaluation, including accurate tumor staging, was the most important factor in choosing a surgical method. Thyroid nodules were diagnosed preoperatively based on the results of ultrasonography (US)-guided fine needle aspiration biopsy. Patient workup consisted of a physical examination and imaging analyses, including high-resolution US and neck-computed tomography (CT). Staging US was also utilized for preoperative clinical staging, influencing patient selection and surgical extent. Tumor characteristics assessed included diameter, site, presence of extrathyroidal invasion, multiplicity, bilaterality, and presence of cervical LN metastasis.

Patients were considered eligible for robotic surgery if they had (a) follicular proliferation with a tumor size ≤5 cm and (b) differentiated thyroid cancer without the following contraindications. Patients were excluded if they had (a) a history of previous head-and-neck surgery, (b) severe thyrotoxicosis, (c) locally advanced thyroid cancers featuring definite invasion to adjacent structures, (d) distant metastasis, or (e) lesions located in the dorsal thyroid area, especially in the region adjacent to the tracheoesophageal groove, because of possible injury during surgery to the trachea, esophagus, or recurrent laryngeal nerve (RLN).

The extent of thyroidectomy was determined based on American Thyroid Association Guidelines [27]. All patients with thyroid cancers also underwent prophylactic central compartment node dissection (CCND).

Overview of the Procedure

Robotic Thyroidectomy Procedure

Refinements in the surgical technique during the established steps of thyroid surgery have led to improved operative outcomes following robotic thyroidectomy. We use three robotic arms and a single camera and recently formulated a standard template for robotic thyroidectomy (two-incision technique and single-incision technique) [4, 5, 9, 28–30]. Since it is important to avoid collisions among robot instruments but also to provide free access to the thyroid bed, robot docking and port (cannula) placement is of major concern for robot thyroidectomy. We briefly describe the main features of the technique (Fig. 24.1).

Patient Positioning

Patient Preparation. The patient under general anesthesia is placed in a supine position on a small shoulder roll with the neck slightly extended. The arm is extended and a 5- and 6-cm vertical incision is marked in the anterior aspect of the ipsilateral axilla (Fig. 24.2a).

The arm is then replaced into its natural position to ensure that the incision will be hidden after the procedure is completed. The arm of the lesion side is raised straight superiorly but naturally within the range of shoulder motion to avoid brachial plexus paralysis. The arm is fixed to afford the shortest distance between the axilla and the anterior neck. This setup rotates the clavicle, lowering its medial aspect and providing excellent access to the thyroid. The alternative patient positing has been developed in the USA especially for the patients with some obstacles originated by a large body habitus [10–15]. The lesion-side arm was extended to expose his/her axillary area at the shoulder and then flexed at the elbow an approximately 90° angle such that the wrist is over the patient's forehead with the palm facing the ceiling. The arm is then padded and fixed to an arm board overlying the forehead (Fig. 24.2b).

Creation of Working Space. After the patient is prepped and draped, a 5- to 6-cm vertical skin incision along the lateral border of the pectoralis major muscle is made in the axilla, and a working space is then created in the plane between the subcutaneous tissue and the pectoralis major muscle by electrical cautery under direct vision. After exposure of the medial border of the sternocleidomastoid (SCM) muscle, the dissection is approached through the avascular space of the SCM branches (between the sternal head and the

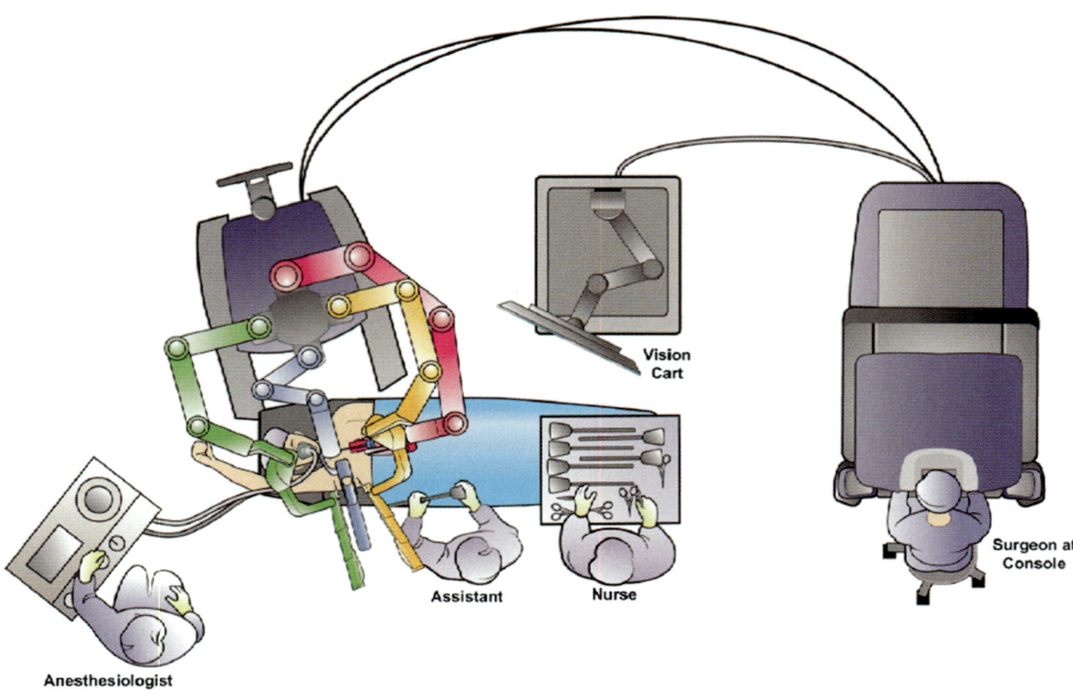

Fig. 24.1 Operating room set up (for a *right-sided lesion*): An overhead view of the recommended operating room configuration for a da Vinci thyroidectomy. The patient cart should always be placed contralateral to the location of the thyroid lesion. For a *left-sided lesion*, the patient and anesthesiologist should be rotated 180° and the scrub nurse should be on the left side of the assistant

clavicular head). The carotid sheath is separated down from the strap muscle, taking care not to injure the internal jugular vein (IJV) and the common carotid artery (CCA), and the omohyoid muscle is retracted superficially and posterolateral. Then, the strap muscles are elevated muscle until the medial one-third portion of the contralateral lobe of the thyroid is exposed. To maintain a working space, a spatula-shaped external retractor (Chung's thyroid retractor) with a table mount lift is placed under the strap muscles and secured to the lift. To achieve an adequate working space, the incision entrance should be maintained to provide a height of >4 cm and the retractor blade should be >1 cm from the anterior surface of the thyroid gland (Fig. 24.3a, b).

Robot Positioning and Docking

Robot Positioning and Cannula Placement. The camera arm is positioned set-up joint toward the patient's head to insure maximum clearance for instrument arm. For the camera arm should be positioned in the middle of the incision of the patient's axilla, the camera arm is in line with the camera cannula and center column of the patient cart. The "sweet spot" should be confirmed to maximize the range of motion for the instrument arms prior to docking. We have to align the blue arrow within the blue marker on the second joint or assure a ~90° angle between the first and third joints on the camera arm. We also achieve a straight line by aligning the clutch button, the third joint of the camera arm, and the gray dot in "da Vinci" on the center column. After then, the patient cartwheel is locked once the correct location of the camera arm within its "sweet spot" is reached. The cart's arms are extended over the patient, and the cannulas are placed in the incision site with the remote centers located just inside the skin edge.

Docking Stage (Two-Incision Technique). The novel method of robotic thyroidectomy using a gasless transaxillary approach requires

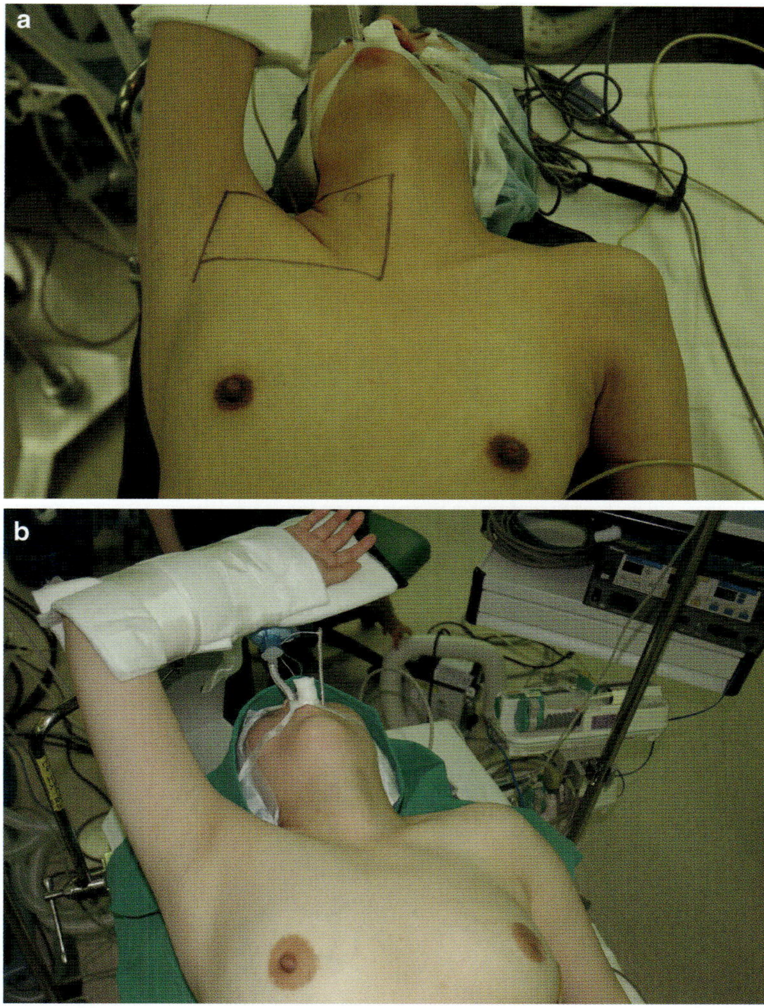

Fig. 24.2 (**a**) Patient position and skin incision line. The incision was made along the axillary skin crease on the lateral border of the pectoralis major muscle (**b**) Modified arm position. The lesion-side arm was extended to expose the axillary area at the shoulder and flexed at the elbow at an approximately 90° angle to avoid brachial plexus neuropraxia

two skin incisions, axillary incision for camera, first and second robot arm access, and an anterior chest incision for the third robotic arm [4, 5, 28, 29]. In two-incision robotic thyroidectomy, a second skin incision (0.6–0.8 cm long) is made on the medial side of the anterior chest wall to insert the third robot arm, 2 cm superiorly and 6–8 cm medially from the nipple. A dual-channel telescope is placed on the central arm, and harmonic curved shears, together with a Maryland dissector, are placed on both lateral sides of the scope. A ProGrasp forceps is inserted through the anterior chest wall incision (Fig. 24.4a, b) [4, 30]. It is important that the angle and position of the da Vinci arm joints are optimized during this setup. The camera arm starts parallel with the retractor and centered above the thyroid. The instrument arms should come in at the edges of the incision and angle out away from the camera. Once the thyroid is visualized with the endoscope, the back end of the camera arm will form an inverted triangle with the instrument arms, while the instrument tips and endoscope tips will form a normal triangle at the surgical site. During the procedure, the robot arms and camera may need slight adjustments during the most extreme

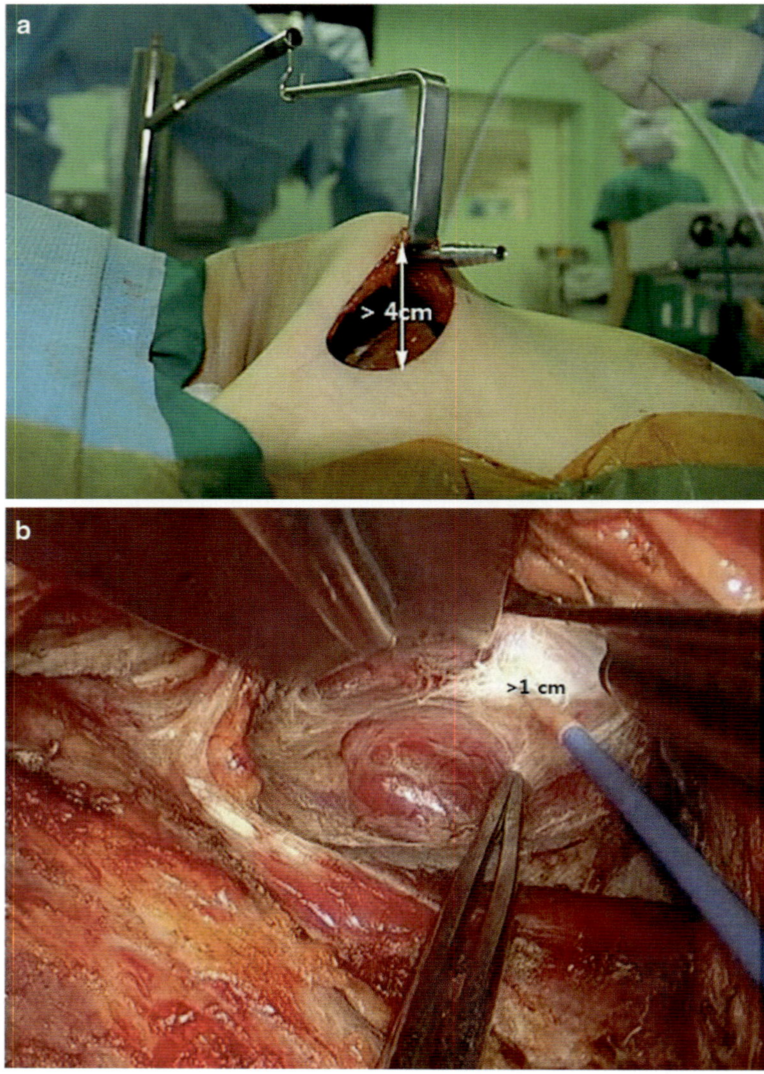

Fig. 24.3 To achieve an adequate working space after retractor blade positioning, (**a**) the axillary incision entrance should be maintained to provide a height of at least 4 cm and (**b**) the retractor blade should be >1 cm from the anterior surface of the thyroid gland to provide enough space for movement of the robotic instrument

upper and lower pole dissections. After docking procedure, we should check for any external collisions and tweak arm position as necessary to ensure that there is full access to the target anatomy. Our initial robotic thyroidectomy procedures (about 700 cases) were performed using this novel method using two-incision approach.

Docking Stage (Single-Incision Technique). After performing more than 700 robotic thyroidectomies via a two-incision technique, we found that we were able to perform robotic thyroidectomy without the second incision. According to single-incision technique, all robotic arms with camera are inserted through an axillary single incision. To prevent collision between robotic arms, we realize several tips and rules about there to place the ProGrasp forceps and how to introduce the robotic arms at appropriate angles and inter arm distances. For the conduit of the right-side robotic thyroidec-

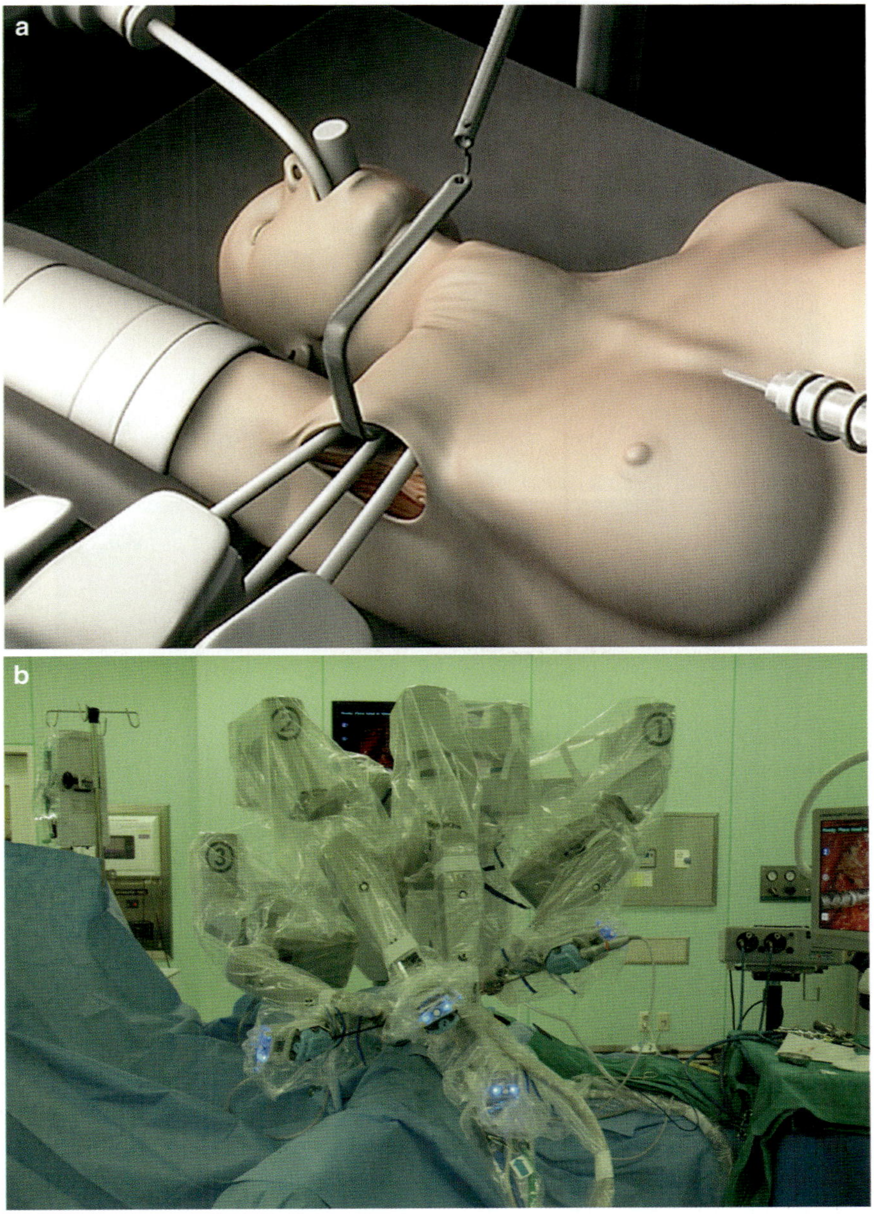

Fig. 24.4 Two-incision robotic thyroidectomy. (**a**) Schematic of a two-incision thyroidectomy docking. A second 0.6–0.8 cm skin incision was created on the tumor side of the anterior chest wall to allow insertion of the fourth robotic arm (with ProGrasp forceps). (**b**) External view after port placement and instrument insertion

tomy via a single axillary incision, a 12-mm cannula for the 30° dual-channel endoscopic camera is placed in the center of the axillary incision. The edge of camera cannula is inserted in an upward direction and centered at the bottom of the incision. The tip of the camera is positioned to view the target anatomy by clutching the camera and extending tilting the back of the arm toward the floor. With the 30° down scope, this provides a good view of the thyroid. Before the 8-mm cannula is positioned in the incision, attach the ProGrasp to the robot arm and insert the

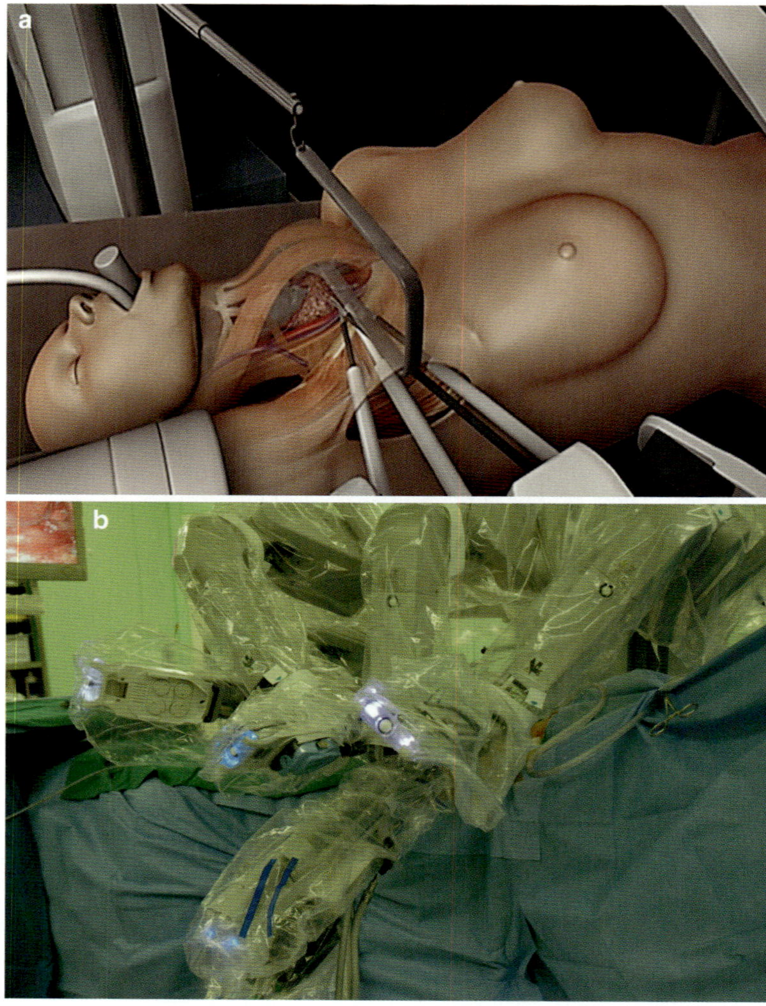

Fig. 24.5 Single-incision robotic thyroidectomy. (**a**) Schematic of a single-incision thyroidectomy docking. All four robotic instruments and the camera were inserted through the axillary incision. (**b**) External view after port placement and instrument insertion. All instruments should be as far from each other as possible

instrument through the cannula until it is at full insertion. The tip of ProGrasp forceps is then positioned as parallel and just to the right side of the retractor blade at the top of the incision just above the thyroid. The 5-mm cannula of a Maryland dissector is then positioned on the left edge of the incision and the 5-mm cannula for the Harmonic curved shears at the right side of the camera. Therefore, all three instruments and the camera are inserted through the axillary incision (Fig. 24.5a, b) [4, 30].

If the setup has been performed correctly, the Maryland dissector arm, the Camera arm, and the ProGrasp forceps arm will form an inverted triangle externally with the insertion axis and make a triangle internally with the instrument tips. At this point, the ProGrasp forceps must be located as close as possible to the ceiling of the working space (the retractor blade). Instruments should be as far apart as possible. The arms must be spaced and positioned in a manner minimizing collisions between the instruments and the camera. If most movements could not be at the wrists during single-incision technique, large internal movements may cause external collisions.

Step-by-Step Review of Critical Elements of the Robotic Thyroidectomy

Console Stage. The general principle of operation proceeding for robotic thyroidectomy was the same manner as a conventional open thyroidectomy. The thyroid gland is retracted using a ProGrasp forceps on the fourth robotic arm, and dissection is performed employing a Harmonic curved shears and a Maryland dissector. This procedure allows the surgeon to use three robotic arms during thyroidectomy. We initiate the dissection of superior pole of the thyroid gland using the ProGrasp forceps to retract the thyroid downward and Maryland dissector to create traction on the thyroid tissue. The superior thyroid gland vessels are identified and individually ligated close to the thyroid gland to avoid injury of the external branch of superior laryngeal nerve using Harmonic curved shears. The upper pole of thyroid gland is separated from the cricopharyngeal and cricothyroid muscles until the superior parathyroid gland is exposed and preserved (Fig. 24.6a).

The thyroid gland is then pulled in a superior and medial direction using the ProGrasp forceps, and the lateral side of the CCND is performed from the CCA artery to the inferior thyroid artery superiorly and to the substernal notch inferiorly. All dissections and ligations of vessels are performed using the Harmonic curved shears. After exposing the CCA to the inferior thyroid artery, soft tissue and central compartment nodes are detached to the substernal notch until the anterior surface of trachea is exposed (Fig. 24.6b). The inferior thyroid artery is divided close to the thyroid gland using the Harmonic curved shears, and the whole cervical course of the RLN is traced. In the Berry ligament area, the thyroid gland is meticulously detached from the trachea to avoid direct or indirect thermal injury of the RLN. In cases of bilateral total thyroidectomy, contralateral lobectomy was usually performed after completing ipsilateral lobectomy. The removal of the contralateral lobe was done by capsular dissection through the thyroid capsule with adequate retraction of the thyroid lobe and trachea. The blood vessels were divided close to the thyroid capsule. The contralateral Berry's ligament was divided by Harmonic curved shear close to the thyroid capsule while retracting the contralateral lobe laterally and taking care to preserve the contralateral RLN. In patients with a prominent trachea and a deeply located contralateral thyroid, the surgical table can be tilted by 10–15°, which provides optimal exposure of the contralateral trachea-esophageal groove. The resected specimen is removed through an axillary skin incision. A 3-mm closed suction drain is inserted through a separate skin incision under the axillary skin incision. Wounds are closed cosmetically. The axillary incision scar is completely covered when the arm is in its natural position (Fig. 24.7a, b). Apart from docking of the robotic arms, during console stage, the two-incision and single-incision robotic thyroidectomy procedures are the same.

Robotic Radical Neck Dissection Procedure

Although the papillary thyroid cancer (PTC) usually has shown a favorable prognosis and relatively mild biological behavior, but frequently, more than 30 %, metastasizes to regional LNs [31–33]. In PTC patients with lateral neck node metastases (N1b) should undergo total thyroidectomy with modified radical neck dissection (MRND). Standard guidelines for thyroid cancer treatment recommend that comprehensive neck dissection for DTC patients with lateral cervical LN metastasis is essential to address all levels (levels II–V) due to the possibility of skip metastasis. Recently, we described in detail robotic MRND using a gasless transaxillary approach for PTC and demonstrated its feasibility and provided details of operative techniques and short-term operative outcomes [4, 5, 34, 35]. In robotic MRND technique, the complete anatomical neck LN dissection, matching that of the open method, was found to be possible using excellent robotic instruments, such as magnified and three-dimensional operative field, a stable camera platform, multi-articulated and tremor filtering system, and three accessible robotic arms.

a

b

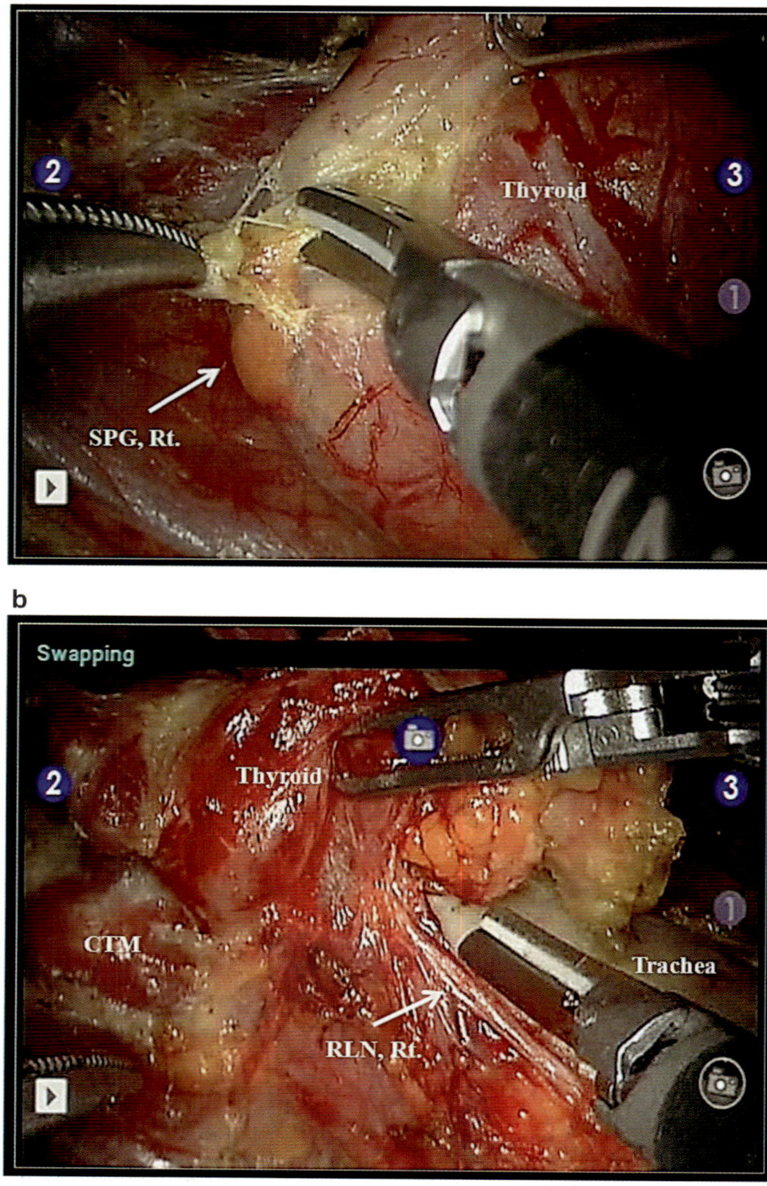

Fig. 24.6 Operative findings for robotic thyroidectomy. (**a**) Dissection around the superior parathyroid gland (SPG) and its vessels using a Maryland dissector and dissection with Harmonic curved shears. (**b**) Division of Berry's ligament to free the recurrent laryngeal nerve (RLN) from the trachea and CTM (cricothyroid muscle)

Patient Positioning

Patient Preparation. With the patient in the supine positions and under general anesthesia, the neck is extended slightly by inserting a soft pillow under the shoulder and the face is turned away from the lesion. The lesion-side arm is abducted by 80° from body to expose axilla and lateral neck, and the head is tilted and rotated to face the non-lesion side (Fig. 24.8) [4, 5, 34]. The landmarks for flap dissection are bounded by the

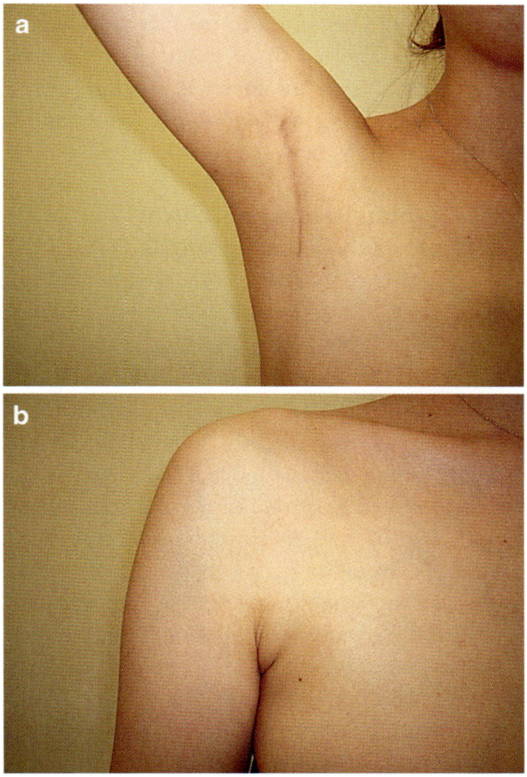

Fig. 24.7 Postoperative outcomes. (**a**) Operative scar 3 months after robotic thyroidectomy. (**b**) Concealment of an axillary scar by a patient arm by her side in the normal position

sternal notch and the midline of the anterior neck medially, the anterior border of the trapezius muscle laterally, and the submandibular gland superiorly.

Creation of Working Space. A 7–8 cm vertical skin incision is made in the axilla along the anterior axillary fold and the lateral border of the pectoralis major muscle. The subcutaneous flap from the axilla to the midline of the anterior neck is dissected over the anterior surface of the pectoralis major muscle and clavicle by electrical cautery under direct vision. After exposing the clavicle, subplatysmal flap dissection proceeds to the midline of the anterior neck medially, to the upper point where the external jugular vein and greater auricular nerve cross the lateral border of the SCM muscle superiorly. The external jugular vein is ligated at the crossing point of the SCM muscle. Laterally the trapezius muscle is identified and dissected upward along its anterior border. During the flap dissection in the posterior neck area, the spinal accessory nerve is identified and exposed along its course. After subplatysmal flap dissection, the clavicular head of the SCM is divided at the level of its attachment to the clavicle to expose the junction area between the IJV and the subclavian vein, and the dissection proceeds upward

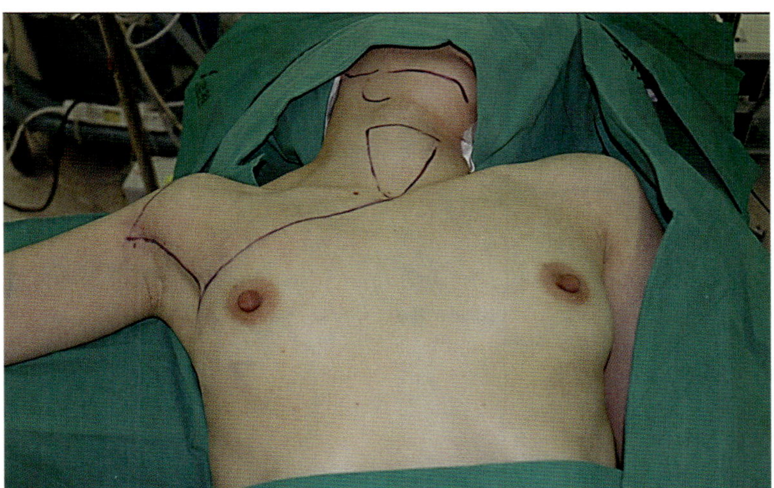

Fig. 24.8 Patient position for robotic MRND. The neck was extended slightly and the face was turned away from the lesion. The lesion-side arm was abducted 80° from the body to expose the axilla and lateral neck, and the head was tilted and rotated to face the non-lesion side

along with the posterior surface of the SCM to expose the submandibular gland and the posterior belly of the digastric muscle. The proximal external jugular vein is then clipped and divided at the crossing point of the SCM lateral border, and soft tissue detachment from the posterior surface of the SCM is continued lateral to medial until the IJV and CCA are exposed. After flap dissection, the patient's head is returned to the neutral position. A spatula-shaped wide external retractor (Chung's retractor) is then used to raise and tent the skin flap at the anterior chest wall, the SCM, and the strap muscles to create a working space. The entire neck levels (level IIa, III, IV, Vb, and VI areas) are fully exposed by elevating the SCM muscle and the strap muscles. A second skin incision (0.6–0.8 cm long) is then made on the medial side of the anterior chest wall to allow the fourth robotic arm to be inserted (2 cm superiorly and 6–8 cm medially from the nipple).

Robot Positioning and Docking

Robot Positioning and Docking Stage. The robotic column is placed on the lateral side of the patient contralateral to the main lesion, and the operative table is positioned slightly obliquely with respect to the direction of the robotic column to allow direct alignment between the axis of the robotic camera arm and the operative approach. Proper introduction angles are important to prevent collisions between robotic arms. Four robotic arms are used during the operation. Three arms are inserted through the axillary incision. A 30° dual-channel camera is placed on the camera arm through a 12-mm cannula which should be placed in the center of the axillary skin incision. In particular, the camera arm has to be inserted to face upward which means the external third joint should be placed in the lower portion (floor) of the incision entrance, and the camera tip should be directed upward. The 5-mm Maryland dissector is installed on the left side of the camera and the Harmonic curved shears on the right side through 8-mm cannula. A ProGrasp forceps is placed on the fourth arm and inserted through the 8-mm anterior chest cannula. The Harmonic curved shear and the Maryland dissector arms should be inserted in the opposite manner to the camera arm (to face downward). Finally, the external three joints of the robotic arms should form an inverted triangle. These proper positioning of angles are important to prevent collisions between robotic arms.

Step-by-Step Review of Critical Elements of the Robotic MRND

Console Stage. Actually, the robotic modified radical neck dissection procedure is similar to conventional open technique. Lateral neck dissection is initiated from the level III and IV area around the IJV. The IJV is handled medially using the ProGrasp forceps, and soft tissues and LNs are pulled laterally using a Maryland dissector. Careful dissection is needed during the detachment of the LNs from the posterior aspect of the IJV to avoid injury to the CCA and the vagus nerve. Smooth, sweeping, lateral movements of a Harmonic curved shears can establish a proper plane and allow vascular structures to be differentiated from specimen tissues. The dissection of the IJV is progressed upward from level IV to the upper level III area. During this procedure, the superior belly of the omohyoid muscle is cut at the thyroid cartilage level. Bundle of LNs are then drawn superiorly using the ProGrasp forceps, and the LNs are meticulously detached from the junction of the IJV and subclavian vein. In general, the transverse cervical artery as a branch of the thyrocervical trunk courses laterally across the anterior scalene muscle, anterior to the phrenic nerve. Using this anatomic landmark, the phrenic nerve and transverse cervical artery can be preserved without injury or ligation. Further dissection is followed along the subclavian vein laterally. The inferior belly of omohyoid muscle is cut where it meets the trapezius muscle. The distal external jugular vein is then clipped and divided at its connection with the subclavian vein. Level VB dissection in the posterior neck area proceeds along the spinal accessory nerve in the superomedial direction, and is followed by level IV dissection, while preserving the brachial nerve plexus, the phrenic nerve, and the thoracic duct. The dissection proceeds by making turns at levels VB, IV, and III and then by proceeding upward to the level IIA area. The individual nerves of the cervical plexus are sensory nerves, and when encountered during dissection, some of them might be sacrificed to ensure complete node dissection, while preserving the phrenic nerve and ansa cervicalis.

After performing the level III, IV, and VB node dissection, re-docking is needed for a better operating view to dissect the level II LN. The external retractor is then reinserted through the axillary incision and directed toward the submandibular gland. The operating table should also be repositioned more obliquely with respect to the direction of the robotic column to allow the same alignment between the axis of the robotic camera arm and the direction of retractor blade insertion. Drawing the specimen tissue inferolaterally, soft tissues and LNs are detached from the lateral border of the sternohyoid muscle, the submandibular gland, and the anterior surfaces of the carotid artery and the IJV. Level IIA dissection is advanced until the posterior belly of the digastric muscle is exposed superiorly. After removing the specimen, fibrin glue is sprayed around the area of the thoracic duct and minor lymphatics, and a 3-mm closed suction drain is inserted just under the axillary skin incision. Wounds are closed cosmetically. The incision scar in the axilla is completely covered when the arm is in its neutral position (Fig. 24.9a, b) [5, 35].

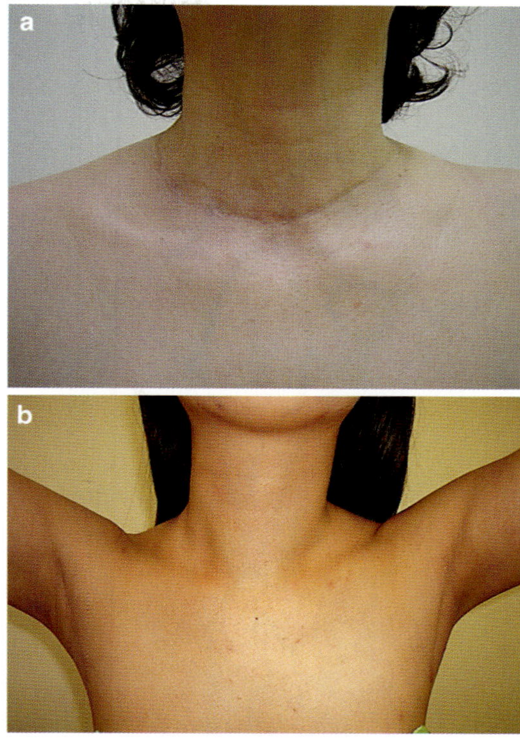

Fig. 24.9 Comparison of postoperative scars 6 months after (**a**) conventional unilateral (*right*) open MRND and (**b**) bilateral robotic MRND

Review of Perioperative Outcomes

Perioperative Outcome

Over the past decade, robotic thyroidectomy has gained considerable traction in thyroid surgery, both locally in South Korea and abroad. Perioperative results, including operation time, volume of blood loss, length of hospital stay, occurrence of perioperative complications, and recurrence rates following robotic thyroidectomy, are summarized in Table 24.1 [9, 11–14, 16, 17, 21, 28–30, 34–45]. The operative safety and feasibility of robotic thyroidectomy were demonstrated in studies of 100, 200, 338, and 1,000 procedures performed by a single surgeon [9, 28, 29, 38] and of 1,043 procedures performed at several centers [40]. The major complication rate following 1,000 consecutive robotic thyroidectomies performed by a single surgeon was 0.8 %, whereas the rate following robotic thyroidectomy in 1,043 consecutive patients in several centers was 1.0 % [38, 40]. These complication rates are comparable to those following open thyroidectomy performed in experienced centers of excellence. However, these results come from centers with the largest worldwide experience with robotic thyroidectomy and may not be generalizable to less experienced centers, especially during their early adoption of this technique.

A recent multicenter trial of 2,014 patients with thyroid cancers showed that robotic thyroidectomy yielded excellent postoperative outcomes, including minimal complication rates, a high degree of oncological safety, and superior ergonomic benefits for surgeons [40]. In this study, surgeons completed a survey about neck, shoulder, and back muscle discomfort after open, endoscopic, and robotic thyroidectomies. These

Table 24.1 Clinical outcomes after robotic thyroidectomy (or robotic modified radical neck dissection) using a gasless transaxillary approach

Author (year)	Cases	Pathology (patients)	Operation type	Operative time (Mean[±SD], min)	Major complications[a] (Conversion to open)	Hospital stay (Mean[±SD], days)	Recurrence	Character
Robotic thyroidectomy with/without central compartment node dissection								
Kang et al. [9]	100	PTMC (100)	TT and CCND (16) LTT and CCND (84)	Total:136.5 ± 36.6	0/80(0 %)	3.0 ± 0.45 Console:59.9 ± 25.9	None (None)	Single surgeon experience (Chung's data)
Kang et al. [28]	200	PTC (200)	TT and CCND (45) LTT and CCND (155)	Total:141.1 ± 38.8	1/200(0.5 %)	3.2 ± 0.6 Console:57.6 ± 23.8	None (None)	Single surgeon experience (Chung's data)
Kang et al. [29]	338	PTC (332) Benign (6)	TT and CCND (104) TT and CCND (234)	Total:144.0 ± 43.5	5/338 (1.5 %)	3.3 ± 0.8 Console:59.1 ± 25.7	None (None)	Single surgeon experience (Chung's data)
Ryu et al. [30]	1,047	PTC (1042) FTC (2) MTC (3)	TT and CCND (371) LTT and CCND (676)	Total:114.94 ± 27	5/1047 (0.5 %)	3.13 ± 0.58 Console:48.26 ± 11.88	None (None)	Single surgeon experience; single-incision technique (Chung's data)
Landry et al. [11]	12	PTC (1) FTC (1) Benign (9)	LTT (12) Completion TT (1)	Total:142	0/12 (0 %)	1	None (None)	M.D. Anderson surgery group; initial experience
Lewis et al. [12]	5		LTT (5)	Total: 30–90				M.D. Anderson ENT group; cadaver dissection
Berber et al. [13]	2		TT (1) LTT (1)		0/2 (0 %)	1	(None)	Cleveland surgery group; initial experience
Berber et al. [36]	1	PTC (1)	TT and CCND (1)		0/1 (0 %)	1	(None)	Cleveland surgery group; Surgical completeness
Brunaud et al. [37]	1	Benign (1)	TT (1)		0/1 (0 %)	1	(None)	France; initial experience

Kang et al. [38]	1,000	PTC (996) FTC (1) HCC (1) MTC (2)	TT and CCND (337) TT and MRND (36) LT and CCND (627)	Total: 136.7 ± 44.4	8/1000 (0.8 %)	3.0 ± 0.45	None (None)	Single center in Korea
Lee et al. [39]	1,043	PTC (1041) FTC (2)	TT (366) LTT (677) CCND (940) MRND (35)	Total: 132.4 ± 48.5	10/1043 (1.0 %)	2.9 ± 0.8 Console:63.9 ± 39.5	None (None)	Multicenter study in Korea
Lee et al. [40]	2,014	PTC (1947) FTC (6) HTC (1) MTC (5) Benign (55)	TT (740) LTT (1274) CCND (1865) MRND (61)	Total:119.7 ± 61.8	21/2014 (1.0 %)	3.4 ± 2.3 Console:65.8 ± 29.2 (Conversion: one case)	None [(1/2014) (0.05 %)]	Multicenter study in Korea; surgeon's ergonomic consideration
Kuppersmith et al. [14]	31	PTC (3) Benign (28)	TT (11), LTT(20)	Total:196 → 109	0/31 (0 %)	1 Console:131 → 51	None (None)	M.D. Anderson ENT group
Ishikawa et al. [16]	1	PTC (1)	LT and CCND (1)	Total:228	0/1 (0 %)	2	(None)	Japan; initial experience
Lang et al. [17]	7	DTC (1) Benign (6)	TT (4), LTT(3)	Total:149	1/7 (14.3 %)	2 Console:80	None (None)	Hong Kong; initial experience
Kandil et al. [41]	5	Graves' disease (5)	TT (5)	Total:159 ± 17.82	0/5 (0 %)	1	(None)	New Orleans: Graves disease
Kandil et al. [42]	50	TT (13), LTT(37)	Total: 122.5	0/50 (0 %)	1	Console: 55.5	None (None)	New Orleans
Massasati et al. [43]	1	Benign	LTT (1)	Total: 69	0/1 (0 %)	1 Console: 21	(None)	New Orleans; video clip-neuromonitoring
Kandil et al. [44]	100	TT (22), LTT (69)	Total: 108.1 ± 60.5	1/100 (1 %)	1 Completion TT (9)	(Conversion: two cases)	None	New Orleans; BMI, learning curve
Tae et al. [21]	113	Benign (21) DTC (92)	TT (44), LTT (69) CCND (72)	TT (total): 184.5 ± 42.3 LTT (total): 147.9 ± 33.1	0/100 (0 %)	5.9	None (None)	Single Surgeon in Korea

(continued)

Table 24.1 (continued)

Author (year)	Cases	Pathology (patients)	Operation type	Operative time (Mean[±SD], min)	Major complications[a] (Conversion to open)	Hospital stay (Mean[±SD], days)	Recurrence	Character
Kiriakopoulos et al. [45]	8	Toxic adenoma (3) Multinodular goiter (2) PTC (3)	TT (42), LTT (3) TT and CCND (1)	Total: 211	0/8 (0 %)	1.5 Console: 166	None	Greece; initial experience, postoperative visual analogue score, cost
Robotic modified radical neck dissection								
Kang et al. [34]	33	PTC (33)	TT and MRND (33)	Total:280.8 ± 40.6	0/33(0 %)	5.4 ± 1.6	None (None)	Single surgeon (Chung's data); initial experience of robotic MRND
Kang et al. [35]	56	PTC (56)	TT and MRND (56)	Total:277.4 ± 43.2	0/56(0 %)	6.0 ± 2.5	None (None)	Single center experience (Chung's data) Robotic MRND

PTMC papillary thyroid microcarcinoma, *TT* total or near-total thyroidectomy, *CCND* central compartment node dissection, *LTT* less than total thyroidectomy, *PTC* papillary thyroid carcinoma, *FTC* follicular thyroid carcinoma, *MTC* medullary thyroid carcinoma, *MRND* modified radical neck dissection, *HTC* hurthle cell carcinoma, *DTC* differentiated thyroid carcinoma

[a]Major complications were defined as those causing permanent damage, such as recurrent laryngeal nerve injury, permanent hypocalcemia, hematoma of the muscle flap requiring reoperation, hemorrhage of a major vessel requiring reoperation, tracheal injury, Honor's syndrome, major chyle leakage, and brachial plexus neuropraxia, but did not include minor complications such as transient hypocalcemia, transient hoarseness, wound seroma, wound infection, and hematoma of the muscle flap requiring conservative management

three approaches involve different physical tasks, and the type and magnitude of musculoskeletal stress vary. The results of the survey showed that use of the robotic technique reduced musculoskeletal discomfort, compared with that experienced during open or endoscopic thyroidectomy.

Operation Time and Surgical Learning Curve

Any new technology requires a learning curve and a period of adaptation. Moreover, the rising cost of health care requires a determination of whether the advantages of a new technique merit any increases in cost and time. Assessment of the learning curve for robotic thyroidectomy by a single pioneering surgeon showed that the actual operation (console) time for robotic thyroidectomy reached a standard of around 60 min after approximately 40–45 operations [29]. A comparison of perioperative outcomes and surgical learning curves for robotic and endoscopic thyroidectomy by a single surgeon showed that robotic thyroidectomy resulted in a shorter operation time and a more rapid learning curve (35–40 operations) than conventional endoscopic thyroidectomy (55–60 operations) [22].

The learning curves for robotic thyroidectomy were evaluated in a multicenter trial by analyzing a range of perioperative parameters, including operation time, complication rate, intraoperative blood loss, length of hospital stay, number of dissected LNs, and extent of complete resection [46, 47]. The study results indicated that to become proficient in robotic total thyroidectomy with CCND and subtotal thyroidectomy with CCND, a surgeon must perform 50 and 40 operations, respectively. Moreover, beginning surgeons had acquired the necessary technical skills, similar to those of experienced surgeons, once the learning curve was overcome.

Oncologic Efficacy and Outcome

Short-term oncologic data from large numbers of patients have established the oncologic efficacy of robotic surgery. Table 24.2 summarizes the results of studies comparing robotic and open (or endoscopic) thyroidectomy, as well as any notable outcomes of these studies [17–26, 35, 45, 48, 49]. Early measures of oncologic success, including postoperative 131RI scan and Tg concentrations, as well as the number of harvested cervical LNs, were similar in large groups of patients who underwent robotic versus conventional thyroidectomy. Several recent reports showed that robotic thyroidectomy with or without radical neck dissection, when performed by experienced surgeons, yielded excellent postoperative oncologic outcomes compared with conventional techniques.

A retrospective comparison of 192 patients who underwent robotic total thyroidectomy with 266 who underwent open thyroidectomy [20] showed no differences in oncologic outcomes, including postoperative 131RI scan and Tg concentrations, and number of harvested cervical LNs. Moreover, a comparison of 580 consecutive patients who underwent robotic thyroidectomy with 570 who underwent conventional endoscopic thyroidectomy found that the real operation time tended to be shorter and the mean number of retrieved central LNs greater in the robotic than in the endoscopic group [18]. Another retrospective comparison of 96 thyroid cancer patients who underwent conventional endoscopic and 163 who underwent robotic thyroidectomy, all performed by a single surgeon, showed the number of retrieved cervical LNs was greater, the operation time was shorter, and the surgical learning curve was shorter, for robotic than for conventional endoscopic thyroidectomy [22]. Together, these findings indicate that the robotic technique was superior to conventional endoscopy in thyroid cancer patients. Another retrospective comparison of robotic and endoscopic thyroidectomies by a single surgeon in South Korea found that the oncologic outcomes were better after robotic than after conventional endoscopic thyroidectomy in patients with thyroid cancer [21].

Patient Perception and Satisfaction After Robotic Thyroidectomy

Several recent studies have evaluated patient perception of and satisfaction with robotic thyroidectomy (Table 24.2). Questionnaires evaluating

Table 24.2 Postoperative outcomes in patients undergoing robotic and endoscopic (or open) thyroidectomy

Author (year)	Cases	Operation time	Complication rate	Oncologic safety[a]	Functional outcomes	Comments
Open thyroidectomy (OT) vs. robotic thyroidectomy (RT)						
Lee et al. [23]	OT (43) vs. RT (41)	Operation time (RT>OT)	No difference	No difference	Cosmetic satisfaction (RT>OT), hyper or paresthesia on neck (OT>RT) Voice handicap index (OT=RT) Swallowing impairment score (OT>RT)	First comparative study of functional outcomes Cosmetic outcomes, sensory change Swallowing discomfort: RT>OT
Tae et al. [25]	RT (41) vs. OT (163)	Operation time (RT>OT)	No difference	No difference	Cosmetic satisfaction (RT>OT), Pain (OT=PT)	Cosmetic outcomes RT>OT
Tae et al. [19]	RT (75) vs. OT (226)	Operation time (RT>OT)	Transient - hypoparathyroidism (OT>RT)	No difference	Cosmetic satisfaction (RT>OT), hyper or paresthesia on neck (OT>RT), hyper or paresthesia on chest (RT>OT)	Cosmetic outcomes, sensory change RT>OT
Lee et al. [20]	RT (192) vs. OT (266)	Operation time (OT>RT)	No difference	No difference	No data	Oncologic safety, complication rates: RT=OT
Landary et al. [48]	RT (25) vs. OT (25)	Operation time (RT>OT)	Brachial plexus injury (RT>OT)	No difference	No data	Oncologic safety: RT=OT
Foley et al. [49]	RT (11) vs. OT (16)	Operation time (RT>OT)	No difference	No difference	No data	Safety: RT=OT
Tae et al. [26]	RT (50) vs. OT (61)	Operation time (RT>OT)	No difference	No difference	Voice function (RT>OT) Swallowing function (RT=OT)	Voice function: RT>OT
Lee et al. [24]	RT (42) vs. OT (46)	No data	No difference	No difference	Objective voice function (RT=OT)	Voice function recovery: RT=OT
Endoscopic thyroidectomy (ET) vs. robotic thyroidectomy(RT)						
Lee et al. [22]	RT (163) vs. ET (96)	Operation time (ET>RT) Learning curve (ET>RT) Advanced cancer (RT>ET)	No difference	Retrieved LN (RT>ET)	No data	First comparative study of RT and ET, showing that RT was superior in operation time, LN retrieval, and learning curve
Lang et al. [17]	RT (7) vs. ET (39)	Operation time (RT>ET)	No difference	No data	No data	Reported initial experience of RT in Hong Kong

Lee et al. [18]	RT (580) ET (570)	Operation time (ET > RT) Advanced cancer (RT > ET)	Transient - hypoparathyroidism	Retrieved LN (RT > ET) (RT > ET)	No data	RT was superior to ET in operation time, and number of LNs retrieved
Kiriakopoulos et al. [45]	RT (8) ET (4)	Operation (ET > RT)	No difference	No data	Visual analogue scale (RT = ET) Cost (RT > ET)	Comparative study of visual analogue scale and cost between RT vs. ET
Tae et al. [21]	RT (113) ET (105)	Operation time (RT > ET)	No difference	Retrieved LN (RT = ET)	Neck and anterior chest pain (RT = ET) Cosmesis (RT = ET)	RT was superior to ET for performing TT, bilateral CCND. In terms of cost effectiveness, ET was comparable to RT in performing LTT
Open MRND vs. *robotic MRND*						
Kang et al. [35]	Robot (56) vs. operation time (RT > OT) Open (109)	No difference Advanced stage (OT > RT)	No difference	No data		First comparative study of robotic MRND and open MRND, showing that robotic MRND was superior in cosmetic outcome, and no difference in complication rate and oncologic safety between two groups

LN lymph node

[a]Oncologic safety: Surgical completeness and radicality, representing the results of ^{131}RI scans, serum thyroglobulin level, postoperative neck ultrasound, and number of retrieved lymph nodes

Table 24.3 Advantages and disadvantages of robotic compared with open (or endoscopic) thyroidectomy

	Robotic thyroidectomy	vs.	Open thyroidectomy	Robotic thyroidectomy	vs.	Endoscopic thyroidectomy
Operation time		Worse than			Better than or similar to	
Cost		Worse than			Worse than	
Morbidity		Similar to			Better than or similar to	
Cosmetic satisfaction		Much better than			NA*	
Pain		Better than or similar to			NA	
Neck discomfort		Better than			NA	
Swallowing discomfort		Better than or similar to			NA	
Voice change		Better than or similar to			NA	
Learning curve		NA			Better than	
Surgeon's ergonomic consideration		Better than			Much better than	

**NA* no available data

patient satisfaction and regret found that robotic thyroidectomy yielded better patient outcomes, including reduced pain, increased cosmetic satisfaction, and improved QOL [21–26]. Moreover, robotic thyroidectomy resulted in better postoperative functional outcomes, as shown by lower rates of hyperesthesia, paresthesia, and swallowing discomfort. Robotic thyroidectomy does not involve midline dissection of the strap muscle and is associated with a reduction in traction over the paraesophageal area; this may prevent the development of postoperative swallowing problems and voice impairment [4, 23].

Patients undergoing open surgery experienced higher levels of dissatisfaction and regret than those undergoing robotic surgery, as shown by the analysis of multiple QOL measurements [23]. Moreover, studies of early postoperative voice changes showed that patients undergoing robotic thyroidectomy had improved short-term voice and swallowing outcomes than those undergoing conventional open thyroidectomy [21–26], with the most obvious difference being satisfaction with the postoperative scar. A systemic review of prospective trials comparing robotic thyroidectomy and open (or endoscopic) surgery found that QOL measurements, including pain, neck discomfort, voice changes, swallowing changes, and cosmetic measurements, favored robotic thyroidectomy [4].

The relative advantages and disadvantages of robotic and open thyroidectomy on patient QOL remain unclear. Moreover, because the robotic technique was first introduced in late 2007, long-term surgical outcomes are yet undetermined. Efforts continue to be made to modify the technique to further improve patient satisfaction and QOL. Additional scientific studies are needed to critically compare the effectiveness of robotic, open, and endoscopic thyroidectomy, with results of these studies helping to define the role of robotic thyroidectomy in patients with thyroid disease. Endocrine surgeons are central to this process and should honestly counsel patients, providing a realistic forecast of outcomes, based on our experience and specific to each patient's unique situation.

Due to the current refinements of the conventional method, not all physicians will find robotic techniques worthwhile to pursue. Although the literature addressing the merits and demerits of robotic thyroidectomy is extensive, diversity of opinion predominates over consensus. Table 24.3

summarizes the published results comparing the advantages and disadvantages of robotic thyroidectomy with conventional open and endoscopic thyroidectomy.

Robotic Modified Radical Neck Dissection Procedure

Our initial evaluation of outcomes after robotic modified radical neck dissection (MRND) in 33 patients with papillary thyroid carcinoma (PTC) and lateral neck node metastasis (N1b) showed that robotic MRND was satisfactory, with no serious postoperative complications observed and that use of axillary incisions yielded maximal cosmetic effects [34]. This technique allowed the precise manipulation of robotic instruments and complete compartment-oriented dissection without injuring major vessels or nerves or compromising surgical oncologic principles. Recently, early postoperative outcomes were compared in 56 patients who underwent robotic MRND and 165 who underwent open MRND [35]. In that study, the mean tumor size was smaller, the mean age was lower, and the disease stage was earlier in the robotic MRND group. Although the mean operation time was significantly longer in robotic than in open MRND, the complication rates were similar. Taken together, the short-term oncologic effectiveness of thyroid surgery, as assessed by serum Tg concentration, 131RI scan, and cervical LNs retrieved, appears to show that robotic and open thyroidectomy are equivalent, whereas mean hospital stay after robotic MRND was shorter. In contrast, long-term effectiveness, evaluated as lack of tumor recurrence, cannot yet be determined due to the relatively short time the robotic technique has been in use. Together, these findings indicate that the oncologic outcomes and safety of robotic and conventional open MRND were similar, whereas robotic MRND provides more satisfactory cosmetic outcomes compared with the long neck scar resulting from open MRND. However, robotic MRND remains at an early stage, and the advantages and disadvantages of this new technique require further evaluation.

Limitations and Future Directions in Robotic Thyroidectomy

Endoscopic thyroid surgery, although becoming more popular in parts of Asia, has not been widely used because of limited technical feasibility. The limitations of conventional endoscopic thyroidectomy led to the development of robotic surgical systems, and future telerobotic surgery is not far away, enabling a surgeon to operate at a distance from the operating table. Although experience with robotics is very recent, it has great potential in many areas of medicine. Moreover, due to increased awareness of these techniques by clinicians and patients, the popularity of robotics may become patient driven. As robotic approaches to other types of general and urologic surgery become more feasible, robotic thyroidectomy and neck dissection will be more widely used and become accepted as an alternative to traditional open surgery.

Before the widespread acceptance of this technology in thyroid surgery, however, its benefits to patients must be carefully evaluated and proven. In the absence of clear guidelines and without proper training of operators, the applications of robotic surgery will be limited. A steep learning curve, the relatively high costs of equipment and consumables, and the absence of a clear cost-benefit analysis hamper the widespread use of robotic surgery. The loss of tactile sensation is often cited as a disadvantage of working with robotic systems. Although most surgeons are able to compensate using the improved visual feedback afforded by the 3-D display, the absence of tactile feedback and the high cost of the technology remain limitations to its adoption. New generations of robotic surgical systems should address these defects.

Nations differ widely in financial models of health care. South Korea has a combined model, involving both national and private insurance. Recognition of the worth of robotic systems, and agreement by insurance companies to reimburse charges associated with its use, will significantly affect its utilization, as reflected by the expansion of its use in South Korea. Regardless of financial model, however, only centers with substantial patient volumes can reduce the average cost of robotic surgery procedures to more affordable levels. The sustainability of robotic systems in some publicly funded systems and in many private care systems remains very challenging.

It is unrealistic to expect that patients will have a complete understanding of the literature and the results of QOL outcome analysis and reporting. It remains the responsibility of clinicians to help patients gain a deeper appreciation of outcomes specific to their age, body habitus, disease grade and stage, relevant comorbidities, and safety. This may be accomplished by more thoughtful discussions with patients, especially of quantitative and qualitative postoperative results, based on patient-specific parameters and intraoperative challenges. Furthermore, these discussions should be conducted in the context of outcomes specific to the counseling surgeon and his or her own experience and not based solely on published data from more experienced centers.

Conclusion

Robotic thyroidectomy is becoming more widespread in endocrine surgery, but its ultimate impact remains uncertain. We found that robotic thyroidectomy and MRND using a gasless transaxillary approach were both safe and feasible in thyroid cancer patients, yielding excellent cosmetic effects, a reduction in pain, improvements in sensory changes, and decreased postoperative voice changes and swallowing discomfort. Moreover, this technique shows the same oncologic outcomes as conventional open surgery, as determined by postoperative 131RI scans, Tg concentrations, and number of retrieved cervical LNs. For surgeons, the use of robotic thyroidectomy offers a shorter operation time and the need for a shorter learning curve than conventional endoscopic thyroidectomy. Robotic thyroidectomy also causes less musculoskeletal discomfort to surgeons than open or endoscopic thyroidectomy. However, the clear guidelines of this procedure and the proper training curriculum of operators are limited. Therefore, large-volume studies with long-term follow-up periods are needed to determine whether the robotic procedure is superior to endoscopic or open thyroidectomy in terms of patient satisfaction and QOL outcomes.

Author Disclosures All authors including Drs. Lee and Chung have no conflicts of interest or financial ties to disclose.

References

1. Goh HK, Ng YH, Teo DT. Minimally invasive surgery for head and neck cancer. Lancet Oncol. 2010; 11:281–6.
2. Hüscher CS, Chiodini S, Napolitano C, Recher A. Endoscopic right thyroid lobectomy. Surg Endosc. 1997;11:877.
3. Ikeda Y, Takami H, Sasaki Y, Kan S, Niimi M. Endoscopic neck surgery by the axillary approach. J Am Coll Surg. 2000;191:336–40.
4. Lee J, Chung WY. Current status of robotic thyroidectomy and neck dissection using a gasless transaxillary approach. Curr Opin Oncol. 2012;24:7–15.
5. Lee J, Chung WY. Advanced developments in neck dissection technique: perspectives in minimally invasive surgery. In: Kummoona R, editor. Neck dissection – clinical application and recent advances. InTech; 2012. ISBN: 978-953-51-0104-8. Available from http://www.intechopen.com/books/neck-dissection-clinical-application-and-recent-advances/advanced-developments-in-neck-dissection-technique-perspectives-in-minimally-invasive-surgery
6. Maan ZN, Gibbins N, Al-Jabri T, D'Souza AR. The use of robotics in otolaryngology-head and neck surgery: a systemic review. Am J Otolaryngol. 2012; 33:137–46.
7. Maeso S, Reza M, Mayol JA, Blasco JA, Guerra M, Andradas E, et al. Efficacy of the Da Vinci surgical system in abdominal surgery compared with that of laparoscopy: a systematic review and meta-analysis. Ann Surg. 2010;252:254–62.
8. Chen CC, Falcone T. Robotic gynecologic surgery: past, present, and future. Clin Obstet Gynecol. 2009; 52:335–43.
9. Kang SW, Jeong JJ, Yun JS, Sung TY, Lee SC, Lee YS, et al. Robot-assisted endoscopic surgery for thyroid cancer: experience with the first 100 patients. Surg Endosc. 2009;23:2399–406.
10. Holsinger FC, Terris DJ, Kuppersmith RB. Robotic thyroidectomy: operative technique using a transaxillary endoscopic approach without CO_2 insufflation. Otolaryngol Clin North Am. 2010;43:381–8.
11. Landry CS, Grubbs EG, Perrier ND. Bilateral robotic-assisted transaxillary surgery. Arch Surg. 2010;145:717–20.

12. Lewis CM, Chung WY, Hosinger FC. Feasibility and surgical approach of transaxillary robotic thyroidectomy without CO_2 insufflation. Head Neck. 2010; 32:121–6.
13. Berber E, Heiden K, Akyildiz H, Milas M, Mitchell J, Siperstein A. Robotic transaxillary thyroidectomy: report of 2 cases and description of the technique. Surg Laparosc Endosc Percutan Tech. 2010; 20:e60–3.
14. Kuppersmith RB, Holsinger FC. Robotic thyroid surgery: an initial experience with North American patients. Laryngoscope. 2011;121:521–6.
15. Perrier ND, Randolph GW, Inabnet WB, Marple BF, VanHeerden J, Kuppersmith RB. Robotic thyroidectomy: a framework for new technology assessment and safe implementation. Thyroid. 2010;20: 1327–13326.
16. Ishikawa N, Kawaguchi M, Moriyama H, Tanaka N, Watanabe G. First robot-assisted thyroidectomy in Japan performed using a standard da Vinci surgical system. Artif Organs. 2012;36:496–8.
17. Lang BH, Chow MP. A comparison of surgical outcomes between endoscopic and robotically assisted thyroidectomy: the authors' initial experience. Surg Endosc. 2011;25:1617–23.
18. Lee S, Ryu HR, Park JH, Kim KH, Kang SW, Jeong JJ, et al. Excellence in robotic thyroid surgery; a comparative study of robot-assisted versus conventional endoscopic thyroidectomy in papillary thyroid microcarcinoma patients. Ann Surg. 2011;253:1060–6.
19. Tae K, Ji YB, Cho SH, Lee SH, Kim DS, Kim TW. Early surgical outcomes of robotic thyroidectomy by a gasless unilateral axillo-breast or axillary approach for papillary thyroid carcinoma: 2 years' experience. Head Neck. 2012;34:617–25.
20. Lee S, Ryu HR, Park JH, Kim KH, Kang SW, Jeong JJ, et al. Early surgical outcomes comparison between robotic and conventional open thyroid surgery for papillary thyroid microcarcinoma. Surgery. 2012; 151:724–30.
21. Tae K, BaeJi Y, HyeokJeong J, Rae Kim K, Hwan Choi W, HernAhn Y. Comparative study of robotic versus endoscopic thyroidectomy by a gasless unilateral axillo-breast or axillary approach. Head Neck. 2013;35(4):477–84.
22. Lee J, Lee JH, Nah KY, Soh EY, Chung WY. Comparison of endoscopic and robotic thyroidectomy. Ann Surg Oncol. 2011;18:1439–46.
23. Lee J, Nah KY, Kim RM, Ahn YH, Soh EY, Chung WY. Differences in postoperative outcomes, function, and cosmesis: open versus robotic thyroidectomy. Surg Endosc. 2010;24:186–94.
24. Lee J, Na KY, Kim RM, Oh Y, Lee JH, Lee J, et al. Postoperative functional voice changes after conventional open or robotic thyroidectomy: a prospective trial. Ann Surg Oncol. 2012;19(9):2963–70.
25. Tae K, Ji YB, Jeong JH, Lee SH, Jeong MA, Park CW. Robotic thyroidectomy by a gasless unilateral axillo-breast or axillary approach: our early experiences. Surg Endosc. 2011;25:221–8.
26. Tae K, Kim KY, Yun BR, Ji YB, Park CW, Kim DS, et al. Functional voice and swallowing outcomes after robotic thyroidectomy by a gasless unilateral axillo-breast approach: comparison with open thyroidectomy. Surg Endosc. 2012;26:1871–7.
27. Cooper DS, Doherty GM, Haugen BR, Kloos RT, Lee SL, Mandel SJ, et al. Management guidelines for patients with thyroid nodules and differentiated thyroid cancer. Thyroid. 2006;16:109–42.
28. Kang SW, Jeong JJ, Nam KH, Chang HS, Chung WY, Park CS. Robot-assisted endoscopic thyroidectomy for thyroid malignancies using a gasless transaxillary approach. J Am Coll Surg. 2009;209:e1–7.
29. Kang SW, Lee SC, Lee SH, Lee KY, Jeong JJ, Lee YS, et al. Robotic thyroid surgery using a gasless, transaxillary approach and the da Vinci S system: the operative outcomes of 338 consecutive patients. Surgery. 2009;146:1048–55.
30. Ryu HR, Kang SW, Lee SH, Rhee KY, Jeong JJ, Nam KH, et al. Feasibility and safety of a new robotic thyroidectomy through a gasless, transaxillary single-incision approach. J Am Coll Surg. 2010;211:e13–9.
31. Hay ID, Bergstralh EJ, Goellner JR, Ebersold JR, Grant CS. Predicting outcome in papillary thyroid carcinoma: development of a reliable prognostic scoring system in a cohort of 1779 patients surgically treated at one institution during 1940 through 1989. Surgery. 1993;114:1050–7.
32. Lin JD, Huang MJ, Juang JH, Chao TC, Huang BY, Chen KW, et al. Factors related to the survival of papillary and follicular thyroid carcinoma patients with distant metastases. Thyroid. 1999;9:1227–35.
33. Schlumberger MJ. Diagnostic follow-up of well-differentiated thyroid carcinoma: historical perspective and current status. J Endocrinol Invest. 1999; 22:3–7.
34. Kang SW, Lee SH, Ryu HR, Lee KY, Jeong JJ, Nam KH, et al. Initial experience with robot-assisted modified radical neck dissection for the management of thyroid carcinoma with lateral neck node metastasis. Surgery. 2010;148:1214–21.
35. Kang SW, Lee SH, Park JH, Jeong JS, Park S, Lee CR, et al. A comparative study of the surgical outcomes of robotic and conventional open modified radical neck dissection for papillary thyroid carcinoma with lateral neck node metastasis. Surg Endosc. 2012;26(11):3251–7.
36. Berber E, Siperstein A. Robotic transaxillary total thyroidectomy using a unilateral approach. Surg Laparosc Endosc Percutan Tech. 2011;21:207–10.
37. Brunaud L, Germain A, Zarnegar R, Klein M, Ayav A, Bresler L. Robotic thyroid surgery using a gasless transaxillary approach: cosmetic improvement or improved quality of surgical dissection? J Visc Surg. 2010;147:e399–402.
38. Kang SW, Park JH, Jeong JS, Lee CR, Park S, Lee SH, et al. Prospects of robotic thyroidectomy using a gasless, transaxillary approach for the management of thyroid carcinoma. Surg Laparosc Endosc Percutan Tech. 2011;21:223–9.

39. Lee J, Yun JH, Nam KH, Choi UJ, Chung WY, Soh EY. Perioperative clinical outcomes after robotic thyroidectomy for thyroid carcinoma: a multicenter study. Surg Endosc. 2011;25:906–12.
40. Lee J, Kang SW, Jung JJ, Choi UJ, Yun JH, Nam KH, et al. Multicenter study of robotic thyroidectomy: short-term postoperative outcomes and surgeon ergonomic considerations. Ann Surg Oncol. 2011;18: 2538–47.
41. Kandil E, Noureldine S, Abdel Khalek M, Alrasheedi S, Aslam R, Friedlander P, et al. Initial experience using robot-assisted transaxillary thyroidectomy for Graves' disease. J Visc Surg. 2011;148:e447–51.
42. Kandil E, Abdelghani S, Noureldine SI, Friedlander P, Abdel Khalek M, Bellows CF, et al. Transaxillary gasless robotic thyroidectomy: a single surgeon's experience in North America. Arch Otolaryngol Head Neck Surg. 2012;138:113–7.
43. Massasati S, Noureldine S, Aslam R, Kandil E. Robotic transaxillary thyroid lobectomy of a follicular neoplasm. Ann Surg Oncol. 2012;19:2310.
44. Kandil EH, Noureldine SI, Yao L, Slakey DP. Robotic transaxillary thyroidectomy: an examination of the first one hundred cases. J Am Coll Surg. 2012; 214:558–64.
45. Kiriakopoulos A, Linos D. Gasless transaxillary robotic versus endoscopic thyroidectomy: exploring the frontiers of scarless thyroidectomy through a preliminary comparison study. Surg Endosc. 2012; 26(10):2797–801.
46. Lee J, Yun JH, Nam KH, Soh EY, Chung WY. The learning curve for robotic thyroidectomy: a multicenter study. Ann Surg Oncol. 2011;18:226–32.
47. Chung WY, Lee JA. Defining the learning curve for a new surgical technique: considering recent advances in robotic surgery. In: Berjardt LV, editor. Advances in medicine and biology, vol. 31. Nova Science Publisher Inc.; 2012. ISBN: 978-7-61324-714-3. Available from https://www.novapublishers.com/catalog/productinfo.php?products_id=33131&osCsid=be410bfe49edb2ea0ea3239891d33244
48. Landry CS, Grubbs EG, Morris GS, Turner NS, Holsinger FC, Lee JE, et al. Robot assisted transaxillary surgery (RATS) for the removal of thyroid and parathyroid glands. Surgery. 2011;149: 549–55.
49. Foley CS, Agcaoglu O, Siperstein AE, Berber E. Robotic transaxillary endocrine surgery: a comparison with conventional open technique. Surg Endosc. 2012;26(8):2259–66.

25 Robotic Adrenalectomy

Halit Eren Taskin and Eren Berber

General Overview

After the initial reports by Gagner et al. [1] and Mercan et al. [2], the laparoscopic techniques have been standard in the removal of adrenal tumors. Although accepted as a safe and effective procedure, laparoscopic approach has certain disadvantages including the two-dimensional view, unstable camera platform, and rigid instrumentation. Robotic technology can potentially provide a solution to these drawbacks of minimally invasive surgery, owing to the three-dimensional view, wristed instrument, and stable camera platform [3].

The first published robotic adrenalectomy (RA) was by Piazza et al. [4], as a right adrenalectomy in a patient with Conn's syndrome using the ZEUS AESOP system. In the same year, Hubens et al. also reported a case that was performed as a left adrenalectomy using AESOP [5]. While these studies were reported from Europe, the first application of robotic system for adrenalectomy was reported in pigs at the Cleveland Clinic in the USA [6]. After the FDA approval of da Vinci system for use in general surgical procedures in July 2000, Horgan et al. reported 34 advanced general surgical cases (including single bilateral adrenalectomy) that were performed with using this system [3]. Since then, numerous studies and case reports describing RA have been published in the literature (Table 25.1) [7–25].

Both posterior retroperitoneal (PR) and lateral transabdominal (LT) adrenalectomies have been described robotically and demonstrated to be feasible and safe [4, 7]. The indications for robotic adrenalectomy are the same as the laparoscopic procedure and comprise hormonally active adrenal tumors, including pheochromocytoma, aldosteronoma, and Cushing's, as well large (>4–6 cm) or enlarging tumors suspicious for malignancy [4, 8].

Robotic Lateral Transabdominal Adrenalectomy

Positioning

After intubation and administration of general anesthesia the patient is placed in a lateral right or left decubitus position according to the side of the mass (Fig. 25.1).

H.E. Taskin, M.D.
Research Fellow at Endocrine Surgery Division, Cleveland Clinic, 9500 Euclid Avenue/F20, Cleveland, OH 44195, USA

Department of General Surgery, Cleveland Clinic, 9500 Euclid Avenue/F20, Cleveland, OH, USA
e-mail: taskinh@ccf.org

E. Berber, M.D., F.A.C.S. (✉)
Department of General Surgery, Cleveland Clinic, 9500 Euclid Avenue/F20, Cleveland, OH, USA
e-mail: berbere@ccf.org

K.C. Kim (ed.), *Robotics in General Surgery*, DOI 10.1007/978-1-4614-8739-5_25,

Table 25.1 Robotic adrenalectomy cases involving >30 patients reported in the literature

Author	Year published	Approach	*n*	Mean OR time (min)	Conversions (%)	Average tm size (cm)	Complications (%)	Hospital stay (days)
Winter et al. [14]	2006	LT	30	185	0	2.4	7	2 (median)
Brunaud et al. [11]	2008	LT	100	99	5	2.9 ± 1.9	10	6.4 ± 3 (mean)
Giulianotti et al. [8]	2010	AT	42	118 ± 46	0	5.5	4.8	4 (median)
Raman et al. [23]	2011	LT–AT	40	117 ± 50	4	6.97	10	3.2 ± 1.2 (mean)
Nordenstrom et al. [22]	2011	LT	100	113	7	5.3	13	–
Agcaoglu et al. [24]	2012	PR	31	163.2	0	3.1	0	1 (median)
Karabulut et al. [25]	2012	LT–PR	50	166 ± 7	1	3.9 ± 0.3	1	1.1 ± 0.3 (mean)

LT lateral transperitoneal, *PR* posterior retroperitoneal, *AT* anterior transperitoneal, *VHL* von hippel lindau, *IVC* inferior vena cava

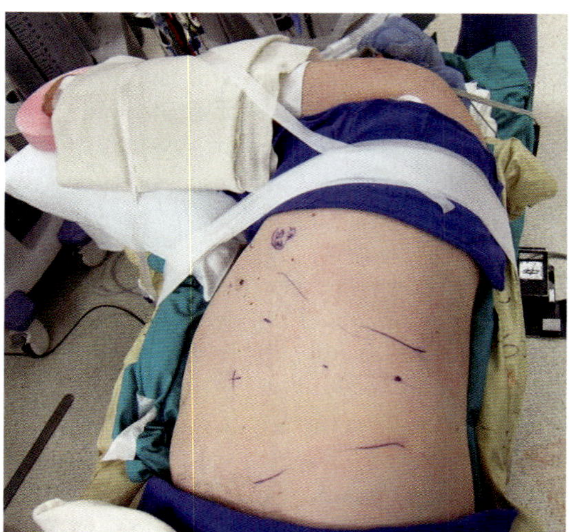

Fig. 25.1 Intraoperative photo showing the position of the patient in robotic left LT adrenalectomy

Trocar Placement

The first optical 12 mm trocar is introduced midway between the umbilicus and the costal margin. After CO_2 insufflation, two 8 mm and one 15 mm robotic trocars are placed beneath the costal margin. The trocar placement should be configured to give enough space for the first assistant to use the suction-irrigator and the clip applier when necessary (Fig. 25.2). This is usually the most medial port for right-sided and the most lateral port for left-sided masses. In special circumstances such as obese individuals, or patients with short stature, the position of the first assistant port might need to be changed depending on the anatomy.

Robot Positioning and Docking

The robot is docked coming to position from the ipsilateral shoulder of the patient and robotic trocars are connected (Fig. 25.3). The table might need to be rotated clockwise according to the patient's anatomy. Close cooperation with an experienced anesthesia team is very important for a fast docking.

Steps of the Operation

For right adrenal tumors, first, the liver is mobilized by dividing the right triangular ligament. For left-sided tumors, the splenocolic and splenorenal ligaments are divided using electrocautery (Fig. 25.4a, b). Then, laparoscopic ultrasound is performed to identify the lesion

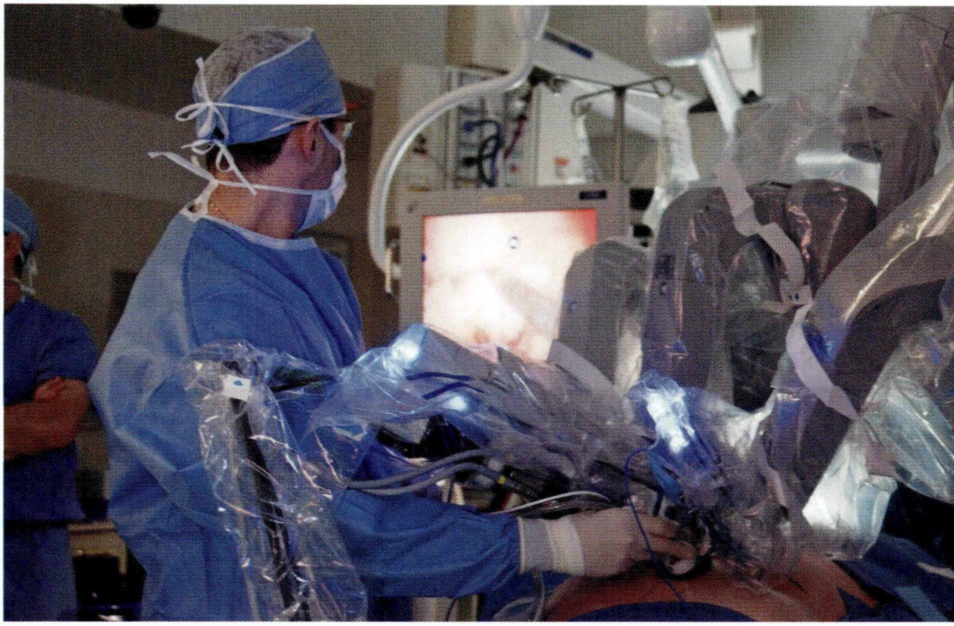

Fig. 25.2 Intraoperative photo showing the position of the robotic trocars and first assistant port for a left LT adrenalectomy

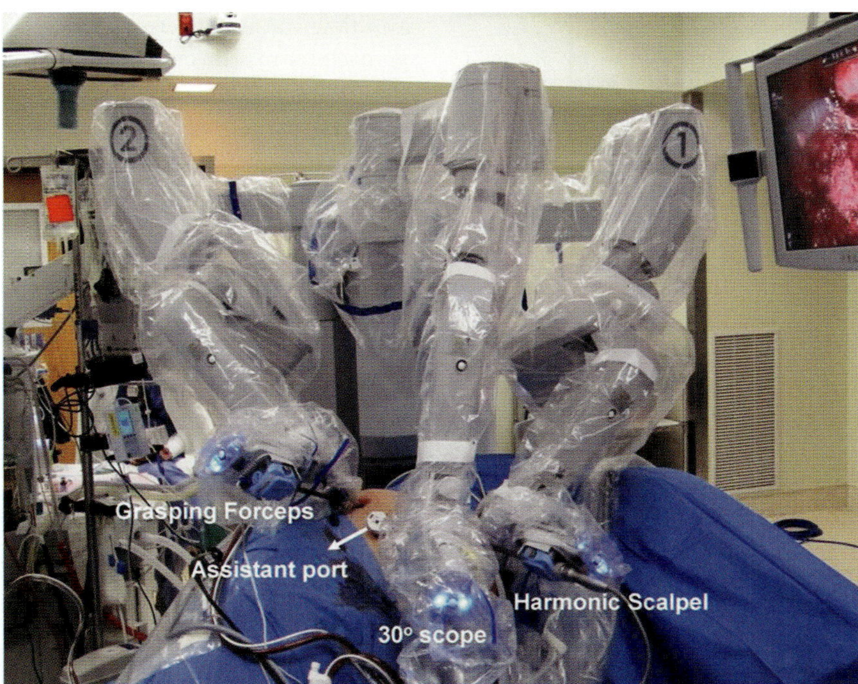

Fig. 25.3 Intraoperative image depicting the position of the robotic system in a robotic right LT adrenalectomy

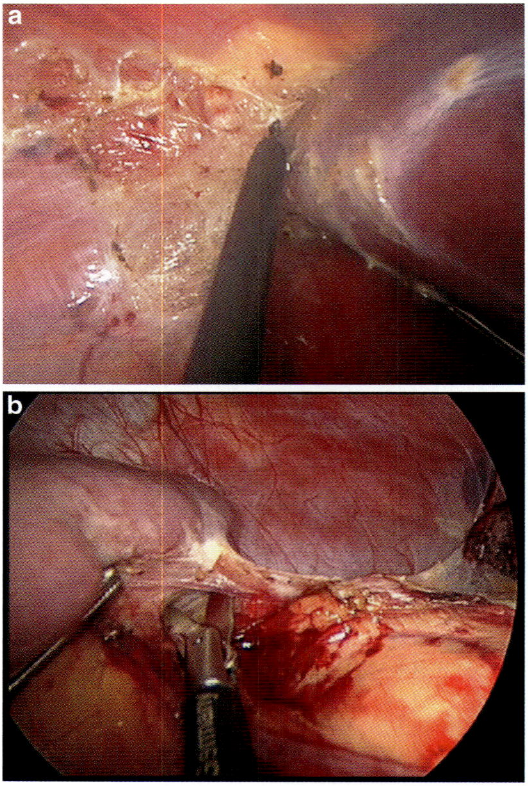

Fig. 25.4 Intraoperative figure showing the division of the right triangular ligament on the right (**a**) and splenocolic ligament on the left (**b**) for robotic LT adrenalectomy

and establish its relationship with adjacent organs. These steps are done laparoscopically. Then the robot is docked. The dissection is performed along the lateral and superior borders of the mass initially, followed the inferior and medial dissection (Fig. 25.5). The adrenal vein is divided either using the harmonic scalpel or between clips based on its size (Fig. 25.6). After the dissection is completed, the robot is undocked. The tumor is removed using a specimen retrieval bag and morcellated if >3 cm (Fig. 25.7). The operative site is irrigated and suctioned laparoscopically. Then, the trocars are removed. Fascial holes for the 12 mm trocar sites are closed, followed by skin closure.

Hybrid Versus Totally Robotic Approach

The laparoscopic portion of the case includes the hepatic/splenic mobilization and extraction of the specimen steps. The robot is used for the dissection of the mass. We believe that this approach saves time and also determines the exact angle of approach for robotic docking.

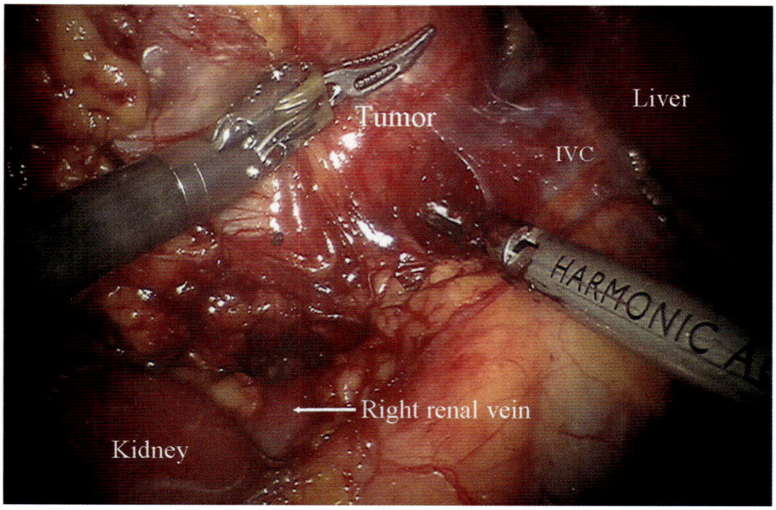

Fig. 25.5 Intraoperative picture showing the robotic dissection of a right-sided pheochromocytoma via LT approach

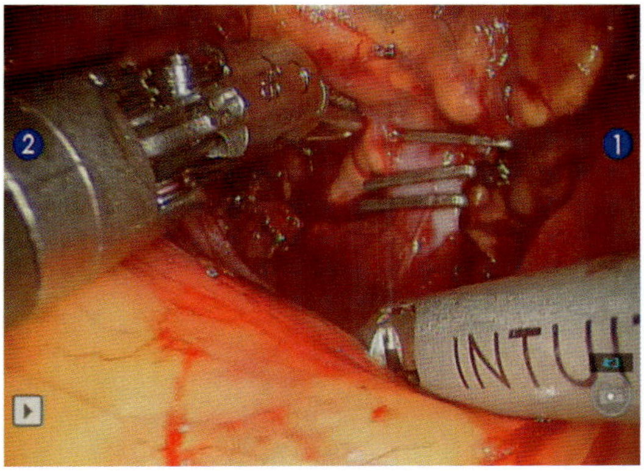

Fig. 25.6 Intraoperative photo showing the division of the adrenal vein in a robotic left LT adrenalectomy

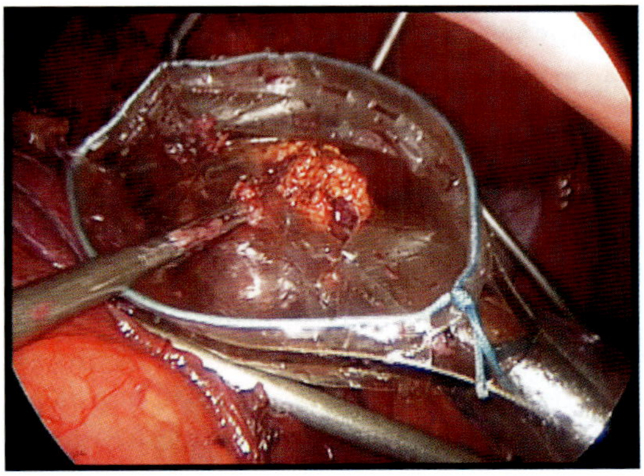

Fig. 25.7 Intraoperative figure showing extraction of the specimen in a robotic right LT adrenalectomy

Robotic Posterior Retroperitoneal Adrenalectomy

Positioning

After the intubation and administration of anesthesia on a gurney, the patient is placed in prone jackknife position on a Wilson frame (Fig. 25.8).

Trocar Placement

First, an optical trocar is inserted inferior to the 12th rib through a cm incision. Once in the Gerota's space, this optical trocar is replaced by a balloon trocar and a potential space is created by inflating this trocar under direct vision (Fig. 25.9). The balloon dissector is then removed and this space is insufflated with CO_2. Two 5 mm trocars are inserted medial and lateral to the initial trocar.

Robot Positioning and Docking

The robot is brought in from the head of the table, between the shoulders, with the final alignment depending on the location of the adrenal gland (Fig. 25.10). The operating table might need to be rotated, depending on the patient's anatomy.

Steps of the Operation

We use a robotic grasper from the lateral port and the robotic Harmonic scalpel from the medial port. Depending on the progress of the case, these instruments may need to be swapped. The dissection is started superiorly and laterally first. The inferior border is dissected next and the medial border last (Fig. 25.11). The adrenal vein is identified and divided either using the Harmonic scalpel or between 5-mm clips placed by the first assistant through the medial port (Fig. 25.12). This requires removal of the Harmonic scalpel temporarily. Suctioning is also performed by the first assistant through the same port when necessary. The robot is undocked after the completion of adrenalectomy. The specimen is extracted using a specimen retrieval bag (Fig. 25.13). The fascial incision for the 12-mm port and the skin incisions are closed.

Hybrid Versus Totally Robotic Approach

In this approach, after the trocars are placed and the retroperitoneal space is exposed, the procedure is finished robotically.

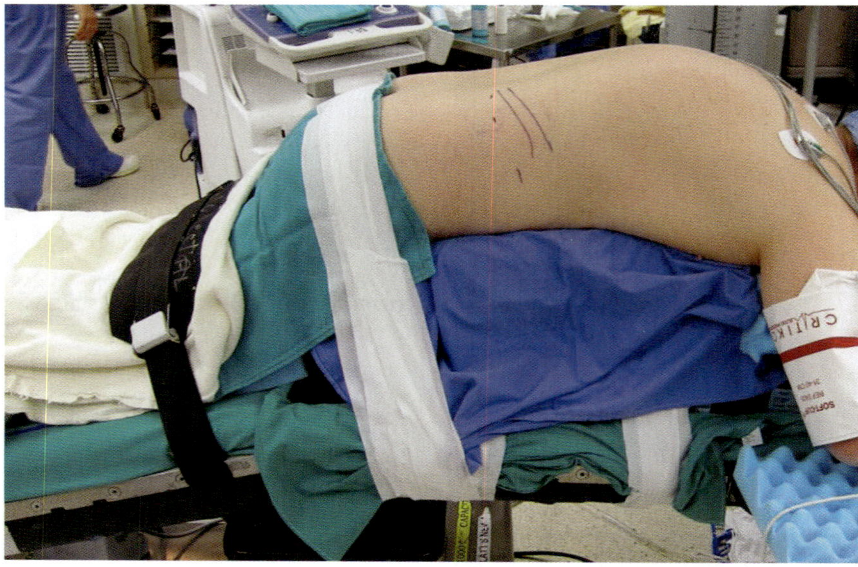

Fig. 25.8 Intraoperative photo showing the patient position in a robotic right PR adrenalectomy

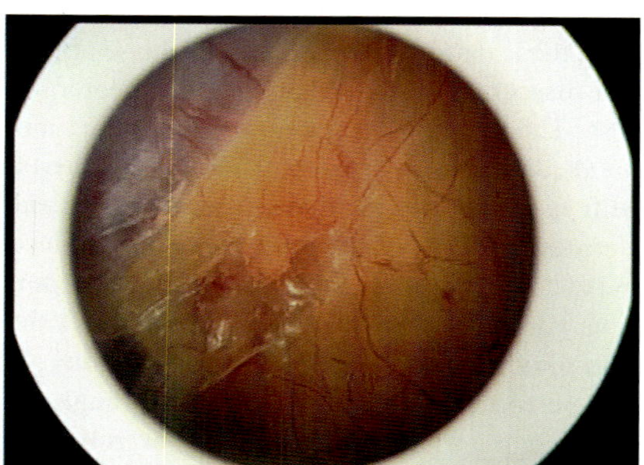

Fig. 25.9 Intraoperative image showing the retroperitoneal space dissected using a balloon trocar

Discussion

Although both the LT and PR techniques are viable options for removing adrenal glands, there is still controversy and bias among surgeons about the procedure of choice in a given patient. In our practice we utilize the LT technique in patients presenting with tumors >6 cm. In those patients with tumors <6 cm, we prefer the PR approach if the distance between the skin and the Gerota's space is 7 cm and the 12th rib is rostral to the renal hilum [26]. In these patients, there would be ergonomic manipulation of the trocars to perform the adrenalectomy. Also, in patients with bilateral tumors and extensive upper abdominal scarring from previous operations, we prefer the PR approach. If these principles are adhered to, the outcomes of PR and LT adrenalectomy will be similar, as shown by us as well as other groups [25, 27].

Review of the Literature

The first randomized prospective trial comparing laparoscopic approach to robotic counterpart was reported by Morino et al. in 2004. There were 40 patients randomized to laparoscopic versus robotic surgery groups. Operative time was longer in the robotic group (169 vs. 115 min). There were no conversions to open; however, conversion to laparoscopy was necessary in 4 of 10 robotic patients. Perioperative morbidity was also higher in the robotic group (20 % vs. 0 %), but hospital stay was similar. The cost of the

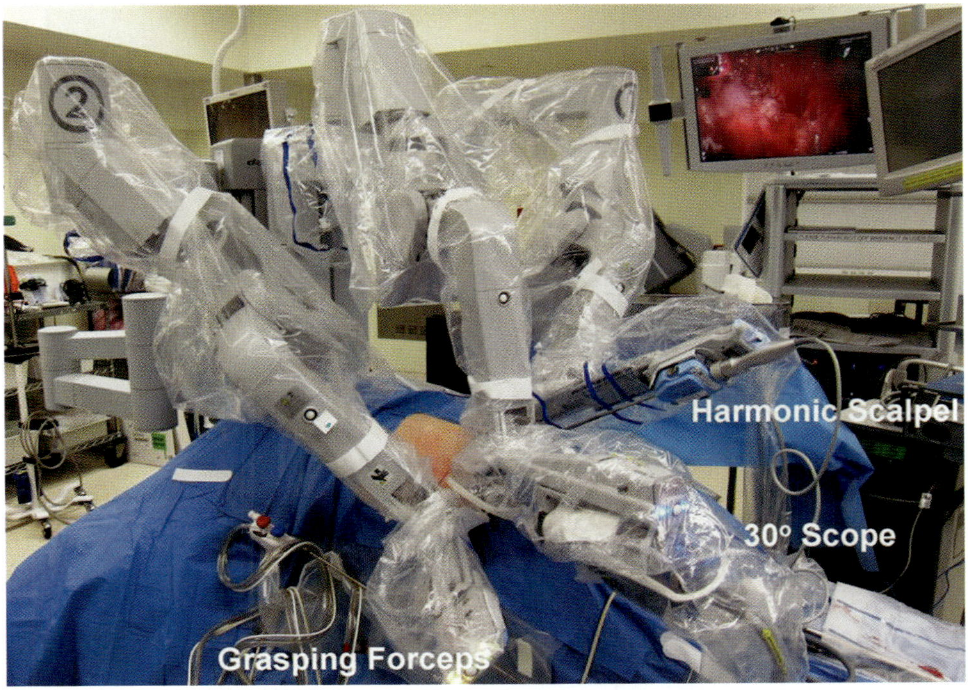

Fig. 25.10 Intraoperative photo depicting the position of the robot in a left robotic PR procedure

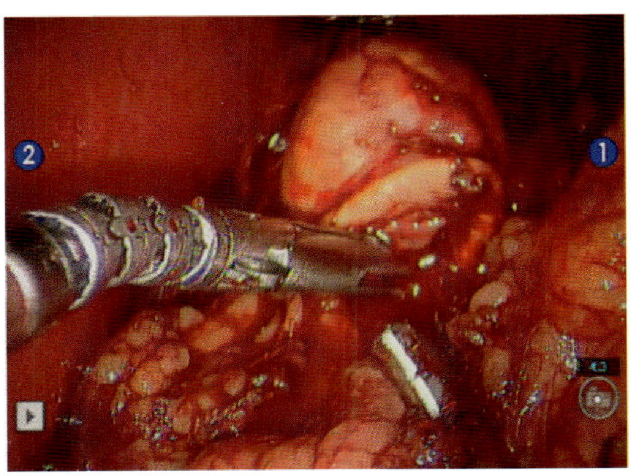

Fig. 25.11 Intraoperative photo showing dissection of an adrenal mass in a right robotic PR adrenalectomy

robotic procedure was significantly higher than the laparoscopic counterpart ($3,467 vs. $2,737). The authors concluded that laparoscopic adrenalectomy was superior to robot-assisted in terms of feasibility, morbidity, and cost [17].

On the other hand, Branaud et al. evaluated 100 patients who underwent robotic LT adrenalectomy. The mean operative time for robotic-assisted adrenalectomy was 95 min and conversion rate was 5 %. Pathology was aldosteronoma ($n=39$), pheochromocytoma ($n=24$), nonfunctional adenoma ($n=19$), Cushing adenoma or hyperplasia ($n=16$), and cyst ($n=2$). Morbidity and mortality rates were 10 % and 0 %, respectively. The mean operative time decreased by 1 min every 10 cases. Operative time improved more for junior surgeons than for senior surgeons ($P=0.006$) after the first 50 cases. By multiple regression analysis, surgeon's experience (-18.9 ± 5.5), first assistant level (-7.8 ± 3.2), and tumor size (3 ± 1.4) were independent predictors of operative time ($P<0.001$ each). The robotic procedure was 2.3 times more costly than lateral transperitoneal laparoscopic adrenalectomy (4,102 vs. 1,799€). In conclusion, they commented that robotic

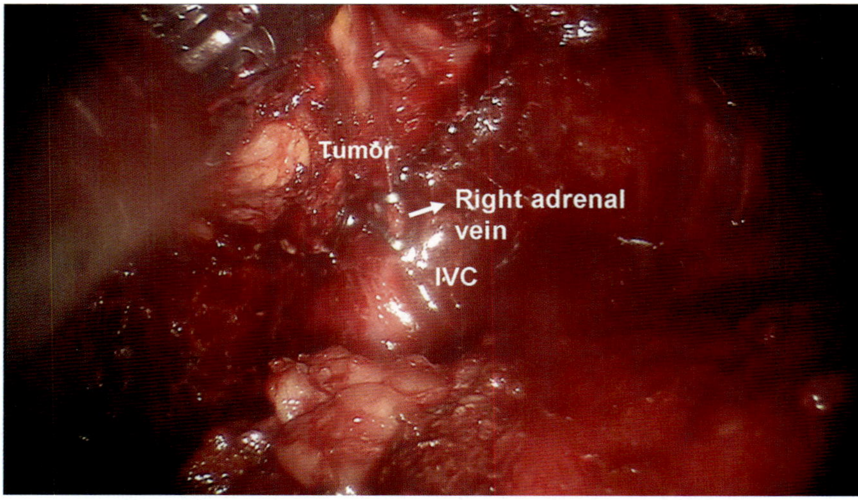

Fig. 25.12 Intraoperative image depicting the division of adrenal vein in a left robotic PR adrenalectomy. *IVC* inferior vena cava

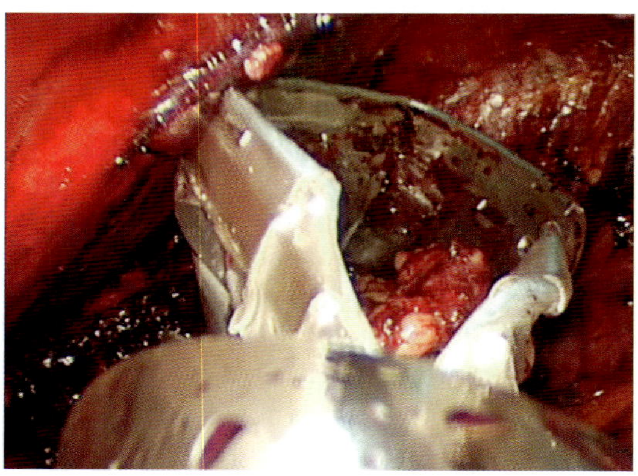

Fig. 25.13 Intraoperative image showing extraction of the specimen in a robotic right PR adrenalectomy

approach provided significant advantages to the surgeon, such as more ergonomics and better image quality, although it was not cheaper or safer than the laparoscopic counterpart [11]. The same group also evaluated the perioperative quality of life in patients after laparoscopic versus RA, and reported similar results between two groups [28].

Our group reported the first case series of robotic posterior adrenalectomy in 2010. In this study, 23 patients underwent robotic adrenalectomy and in eight of these patients PR approach was preferred. There were no conversions to either laparoscopy or open surgery. The mean operative time was 214.8 min. There were no complications and patients are discharged on first 24 h. In this study, we believed that the robot overcame the limitations of laparoscopic surgery and was a refinement of the technique [9].

Giulianotti et al. also later reported that robotic adrenalectomy could be a safe and feasible option in high volume centers. In their series of 42 patients who underwent robotic LT adrenalectomy, the mean lesion size was 5.5 cm, with a median blood loss of 27 mL. The postoperative morbidity was 2.4 % and mortality 2.4 %. Median hospital stay was 4 days. They had no conversions but one intraoperative complication due to capsular tear in a case of 6 cm pheochromocytoma. They also underscored that robotic adrenalectomy can be good option for patients with higher BMI. They did not have any technical challenges in their series where the patients had a mean BMI of 30 kg/m^2 [8].

We have recently published our perioperative outcomes of robotic adrenalectomy compared to the laparoscopic approach. Fifty patients who underwent robotic adrenalectomy (both LT=32 and PR=18 approaches) were compared with 50 (LT=32, PR=18) consecutive patients who underwent laparoscopic adrenalectomy. For the LT approach, despite larger tumor size in the robotic versus the laparoscopic group (4.7±0.4 vs. 3.8±0.4 cm, P=0.05), the operative times were similar (168 min vs. 159 min, P=0.5). Regarding the time spent for the individual steps of the operation, the results were similar between both approaches. In the PR approach, with similar tumor sizes (2.7 cm vs. 2.3 cm, P=0.4), operative time was equivalent (166 min vs. 170±15 min; P=0.8). Also, time spent intraoperatively for each step was similar, except for shorter hemostasis time in the robotic group (23 min vs. 42 min, P=0.03). Interestingly, the presence of two staff surgeons versus a staff and a fellow decreased operative time for the robotic LT (P<0.02), but not the robotic PR approach. The morbidity was 10 % and 2 %, respectively, for laparoscopic and robotic procedures. We concluded that the intra-operative time use was similar between two groups for both LT and PR approaches; however, the robotic procedures were more favorable because of lesser morbidity and shorter hospital stay over the laparoscopic counterpart [25].

Another study from our group compared the use of robot versus standard laparoscopy in the resection of adrenal tumors >5 cm. Perioperative outcomes of 24 patients with 25 tumors who underwent robotic adrenalectomy were compared with those of 38 patients with 38 tumors who had laparoscopic adrenalectomy. Tumor size was similar in both groups [6.5 (robotic) vs. 6.2 (laparoscopic), P=0.661]. Operative time was shorter for the robotic versus laparoscopic group (159.4 vs. 187.2 min, respectively, P=0.043), while estimated blood loss was similar (P=0.147). The conversion rate to open was less in the robotic (4 %) versus the laparoscopic (11 %) group; P=0.043. Hospital stay was shorter for the robotic group (1.4 vs. 1.9 days, respectively, P=0.009). The 30-day morbidity was 0 in robotic and 2.7 % in laparoscopic group. As a result we concluded that the robot facilitated the resection of large adrenal tumors >5 cm and that it could shorten operative time and decrease the rate of conversion to open surgery [29].

In another study, we compared the perioperative outcomes of robotic PR adrenalectomy versus laparoscopic PR adrenalectomy. Thirty-one patients who underwent robotic PR adrenalectomy were compared with 32 consecutive laparoscopic patients. The mean tumor sizes for the robotic and laparoscopic groups were similar (3.1 vs. 3.0 cm, respectively; P=0.48). For all patients, the mean skin-to-skin operative times were similar in both groups (163.2 vs. 165.7 min, respectively; P=0.43). When the last 21 patients who underwent robotic PR adrenalectomy were compared with the 31 patients from the laparoscopic series, it was seen that the mean operative time was shorter for the robotic group than for the laparoscopic group (139.1 vs. 166.9 min; P=0.046). The mean estimated blood losses and hospital stays were similar between the groups. The mean pain score on postoperative day 1 was lower in the robotic group than in the laparoscopic group (2.5 vs. 4.2; P=0.008); however, the mean pain scores for the groups were similar on postoperative day 14 (P=0.53). There were no deaths or cases of morbidity in either group. In conclusion, we commented that once beyond the learning curve, robotic posterior retroperitoneal adrenalectomy could shorten the operative time compared to the laparoscopic approach [24].

Robotic cortical-sparing partial adrenalectomy can be used in bilateral adrenalectomy cases where patients would require lifelong steroid supplementation. Julien et al. reported a case of robotic cortical-sparing adrenalectomy in a patient with VHL disease who developed a right-sided pheochromocytoma at age 18, 9 years after his initial open adrenalectomy for left-sided pheochromocytoma. This tumor was managed by robot-assisted cortical-sparing adrenalectomy, and the patient was gradually weaned off the steroid replacement following 1 year after the operation [30]. Asher et al. also reported on 12 patients undergoing 15 robotic partial adrenalectomy procedures for pheochromocytoma. They had one conversion to open where an inferior venacaval injury ocured due to severe adhesions to the liver. During their follow-up of 17.5 months, there were no recurrences and only one patient has required steroid supplementation [31].

Robotic adrenalectomy can also be feasible in the setting of pregnancy. Podolsyky et al. reported a case of robotic LT adrenalectomy for a right-sided pheochromocytoma in a patient during second trimester of her pregnancy. The reported operative time was 270 min and the estimated blood loss was 350 mL. The hemodynamic parameters of the patient were stable during the operation. They reported an uneventful postoperative course, and the patient had a successful cesarean delivery at 39 weeks of gestation [32].

Conclusion

Over the last decade feasibility and safety of robotic adrenalectomy both through lateral transabdominal and posterior retroperitoneal approaches has been reported. Although these studies were unable to demonstrate a benefit of using robot in terms of patient outcomes, more recent studies have documented advantages over the laparoscopic technique for the PR approach and also for removing large adrenal tumors. In our opinion, the robotic approach is safe and feasible in centers experienced both in laparoscopic adrenalectomy and robotic surgery. Currently, training and cost are two major drawbacks for robotic adrenalectomy. Future studies involving larger case series and randomized trials will determine the exact benefit and role of robotics in adrenal surgery. Further innovations in robotic technology will also provide more advanced robotic systems that can render this approach preferable over conventional laparoscopy.

References

1. Gagner M, Lacroix A, Bolte E. Laparoscopic adrenalectomy in Cushing's syndrome and pheochromocytoma. N Engl J Med. 1992;327:1033.
2. Mercan S, Seven R, Ozarmagan S, Tezelman S. Endoscopic retroperitoneal adrenalectomy. Surgery. 1995;118:1071–5.
3. Horgan S, Vanuno D. Robots in laparoscopic surgery. J Laparoendosc Adv Surg Tech A. 2001;11:415–9.
4. Piazza L, Caragliano P, Scardilli M, Sgroi AV, Marino G, et al. Laparoscopic robot-assisted right adrenalectomy and left ovariectomy (case reports). Chir Ital. 1999;51:465–6.
5. Hubens G, Ysebaert D, Vaneerdeweg W, Chapelle T, Eyskens E. Laparoscopic adrenalectomy with the aid of the AESOP 2000 robot. Acta Chir Belg. 1999;99:125–7.
6. Gill IS, Sung GT, Hsu TH, Meraney AM. Robotic remote laparoscopic nephrectomy and adrenalectomy: the initial experience. J Urol. 2000; 164:2082–5.
7. Choi KH, Ham WS, Rha KH, Lee JW, Jeon HG. Laparoendoscopic single-site surgeries: a single-center experience of 171 consecutive cases. Korean J Urol. 2011;52:31–8.
8. Giulianotti PC, Buchs NC, Addeo P, Bianco FM, Ayloo SM, et al. Robot-assisted adrenalectomy: a technical option for the surgeon? Int J Med Robot. 2011;7:27–32.
9. Berber E, Mitchell J, Milas M, Siperstein A. Robotic posterior retroperitoneal adrenalectomy: operative technique. Arch Surg. 2010;145:781–4.
10. Boris RS, Gupta G, Linehan WM, Pinto PA, Bratslavsky G. Robot-assisted laparoscopic partial adrenalectomy: initial experience. Urology. 2010;77(4):775–80. doi:10.1016/j.urology.2010.07.501.
11. Brunaud L, Ayav A, Zarnegar R, Rouers A, Klein M, et al. Prospective evaluation of 100 robotic-assisted unilateral adrenalectomies. Surgery. 2008;144: 995–1001.
12. Wu JC, Wu HS, Lin MS, Chou DA, Huang MH. Comparison of robot-assisted laparoscopic adrenalectomy with traditional laparoscopic adrenalectomy – 1 year follow-up. Surg Endosc. 2008;22:463–6.
13. Krane LS, Shrivastava A, Eun D, Narra V, Bhandari M, et al. A four-step technique of robotic right adrenalectomy: initial experience. BJU Int. 2008; 101:1289–92.
14. Winter JM, Talamini MA, Stanfield CL, Chang DC, Hundt JD, et al. Thirty robotic adrenalectomies: a single institution's experience. Surg Endosc. 2006; 20:119–24.
15. Miyake O, Kiuchi H, Yoshimura K, Okuyama A. Urological robotic surgery: preliminary experience with the Zeus system. Int J Urol. 2005;12:928–32.
16. Corcione F, Esposito C, Cuccurullo D, Settembre A, Miranda N, et al. Advantages and limits of robot-assisted laparoscopic surgery: preliminary experience. Surg Endosc. 2005;19:117–9.
17. Morino M, Benincà G, Giraudo G, Del Genio GM, Rebecchi F, et al. Robot-assisted vs laparoscopic adrenalectomy: a prospective randomized controlled trial. Surg Endosc. 2004;18:1742–6.
18. Hanly EJ, Talamini MA. Robotic abdominal surgery. Am J Surg. 2004;188(4A Suppl):19S–26.
19. Talamini MA, Chapman S, Horgan S, Melvin WS. Academic robotics group. A prospective analysis of 211 robotic-assisted surgical procedures. Surg Endosc. 2003;17:1521–4.

20. Desai MM, Gill IS, Kaouk JH, Matin SF, Sung GT, et al. Robotic-assisted laparoscopic adrenalectomy. Urology. 2002;60:1104–7.
21. Bentas W, Wolfram M, Bräutigam R, Binder J. Laparoscopic transperitoneal adrenalectomy using a remote-controlled robotic surgical system. J Endourol. 2002;16:373–6.
22. Nordenstrom E, Westerdahl J, Hallgrimsson P, Bergenfelz A. A prospective study of 100 robotically assisted laparoscopic adrenalectomies. J Robot Surg. 2011;5:127–31.
23. Raman SR, Shakov E, Carnevale N, Yiengpruksawan A. Robotic adrenalectomy by an open surgeon: are outcomes different? J Robot Surg. 2011;5:1–6.
24. Agcaoglu O, Aliyev S, Karabulut K, Siperstein A, Berber E. Robotic vs laparoscopic posterior retroperitoneal adrenalectomy. Arch Surg. 2012;147:272–5.
25. Karabulut K, Agcaoglu O, Aliyev S, Siperstein A, Berber E. Comparison of intraoperative time use and perioperative outcomes for robotic versus laparoscopic adrenalectomy. Surgery. 2012;151:537–42.
26. Agcaoglu O, Sahin DA, Siperstein A, Berber E. Selection algorithm for posterior versus lateral approach in laparoscopic adrenalectomy. Surgery. 2012;151:731–5.
27. Lee CR, Walz MK, Park S, Park JH, Jeong JS, et al. A comparative study of the transperitoneal and posterior retroperitoneal approaches for laparoscopic adrenalectomy for adrenal tumors. Ann Surg Oncol. 2012; 19:2629–34.
28. Brunaud L, Bresler L, Zarnegar R, Ayav A, Cormier L, et al. Does robotic adrenalectomy improve patient quality of life when compared to laparoscopic adrenalectomy? World J Surg. 2004;28:1180–5.
29. Agcaoglu O, Aliyev S, Karabulut K, Mitchell J, Siperstein A, Berber E. Robotic versus laparoscopic resection of large adrenal tumors. Ann Surg Oncol. 2012;19:2288–94.
30. St Julien J, Ball D, Schulick R. Robot-assisted cortical-sparing adrenalectomy in a patient with Von Hippel-Lindau disease and bilateral pheochromocytomas separated by 9 years. J Laparoendosc Adv Surg Tech A. 2006;16:473–7.
31. Asher KP, Gupta GN, Boris RS, et al. Robot-assisted laparoscopic partial adrenalectomy for pheochromocytoma: The National Cancer InstituteTechnique. Eur Urol. 2011;60:118–24.
32. Podolsky ER, Feo L, Brooks AD, Castellanos A. Robotic resection of pheochromocytoma in the second trimester of pregnancy. JSLS. 2010;14:303–8.

Part IX

Surgical Techniques: *Solid Organ*

Robot-Assisted Splenectomy

26

Luciano Casciola, Alberto Patriti, and Graziano Ceccarelli

Introduction

Laparoscopic splenectomy (LS) was first described in 1991 by Delaitre, and in the last two decades, it has progressively become the procedure of choice for nontraumatic splenic lesions [1, 2].

LS can be performed with times comparable to those required for open splenectomy, as well as minimal morbidity and less postoperative pain. The postoperative length of stay is also significantly reduced following LS, which in turn can lead to decreased hospital costs [3].

Laparoscopy does, however, have some disadvantages, including two-dimensional vision and rigid instrumentation, which can make splenectomy for splenomegaly challenging. Robotic surgery (da Vinci®; Intuitive Surgical, Sunnyvale, CA) can overcome these limitations providing "wrist-like" action of the instruments and three-dimensional visualization, resulting in high-resolution binocular view of the surgical field and more precise dissection of the splenic vessels even in difficult situations [4].

L. Casciola, M.D. • A. Patriti, M.D., Ph.D. (✉)
G. Ceccarelli, M.D.
Division of General, Minimally Invasive and Robotic Surgery, Department of Surgery, San Matteo degli Infermi Hospital, Via Loreto, 3, Spoleto 06049, Italy
e-mail: albertopatriti@gmail.com

Indications to Minimally Invasive Splenectomy: When a Robot-Assisted Approach?

LS can be considered a well-accepted approach for the differential diagnosis and staging of lymphoproliferative diseases; for restaging after chemotherapy or radiotherapy in abdominal lymphoma, as well as when diseases recurrence is suspected; for the treatment of cystic or solid splenic lesions; and for the surgical treatment of blood disorders. The most accepted indications to LS for hematological diseases are idiopathic thrombocytopenic purpura not responsive to conventional treatments, autoimmune hemolytic anemia, spherocytosis, beta-thalassemia, hairy-cell leukemia, chronic idiopathic myelofibrosis, and splenic lymphoma. To date, studies conducted to investigate the role of robot-assisted splenectomy (RS) did not show any significant advantage over LS [4]. Nevertheless, the endo-wristed movements and three-dimensional view may result advantageous in case of difficult splenectomies in order to reduce the complication and conversion rate. Whether a LS is considered demanding can be ascribed to four factors. Anatomy of the pancreatic tail can make demanding spleen pedicle dissection when a bulky or "intrasplenic" pancreatic tail is present. Anatomy of the splenic vessels is another factor. Splenic artery and vein branching off in multiple, short vessels can hamper their identification and ligation. Spleen volume and consistency is the most common factor determining

K.C. Kim (ed.), *Robotics in General Surgery*, DOI 10.1007/978-1-4614-8739-5_26,

conversion of LS and the only one that can be easily determined in the preoperative setting. The last condition impairing the good outcome of LS is iatrogenic conditions, such as previous radiotherapy [5]. With the exception of splenomegaly, it is not easy to predict preoperatively the difficulties encountered during LS. Therefore, indications to RS should be accurately evaluated during laparoscopic exploration, restricting the robot use to cases not suitable for LS. On the other hand, RS remains a good teaching model due to the absence of a reconstructive phase and could be used to train naïve robotic surgeons in order to deal with more difficult situations.

Technical Aspects

Essential Operating Room Equipment

The Laparoscopic Operating Room

- All laparoscopic equipment must be state of the art and in good working order
- An adjustable, remote controlled electric split-leg table
- The four-arm da Vinci robot is prepared over the patient head
- One monitor for the on-table assistant is placed on the patient left side
- CO_2 insufflators maintaining a pneumoperitoneum of 12 mmHg
- Energy vessel sealing device (Harmonic Ace—Ethicon Endo-Surgery, Cincinnati, OH)
- A set of conventional open instruments should be readily available

Necessary Laparoscopic and Robotic Instruments

- 10-mm 30° robotic laparoscope
- Robotic Cadiere forceps, precise bipolar forceps, monopolar scissors, permanent cautery hook, and Harmonic Ace
- Atraumatic bowel graspers
- Laparoscopic scissors
- Articulated vascular linear stapler (30-mm and 45-mm vascular cartridges)
- Suction-irrigator system
- Titanium clip applier, small and medium
- Plastic locking clip applier, medium and large
- Endoscopic bag

The Procedure

Stage 1

Patient Positioning and Robot Docking

The patient is placed in the supine position. The right arm is padded and tucked at the side. The on-table surgeon stands on the right side. The scrub nurse and instruments are positioned lateral to the right leg (Fig. 26.1). A Mayo stand positioned over the right leg holds the most commonly utilized instruments. Reverse *Trendelenburg and tilting the* table on the right as necessary to take advantage of gravity and the weight of the stomach and transverse colon to improve exposure. The robot is docked over the patient left shoulder.

Port Placement

Five trocars are placed after induction of 12-mmHg pneumoperitoneum by the Veress needle inserted in the left flank (Fig. 26.2):

- 1 × 10–12-mm placed supra-umbilically for the assistant
- 3 × 8-mm intuitive robotic trocars placed in the right upper quadrant, in the epigastrium, and in the left flank are the working ports
- 1 × 10-mm port inserted in the middle point between the left costal margin and the umbilicus is used for the robotic camera
- 1 × 5-mm accessory trocar can be inserted in the epigastrium, between the umbilical port and trocar number 1

Inspection of the Peritoneal Cavity

A thorough inspection of the peritoneal cavity for gross pathology and accessory spleens is performed. If identified, the accessory spleen should be removed before splenectomy.

Stage 2

Approach

RS can be performed from an anterior approach (i.e., vessel division without posterior mobilization

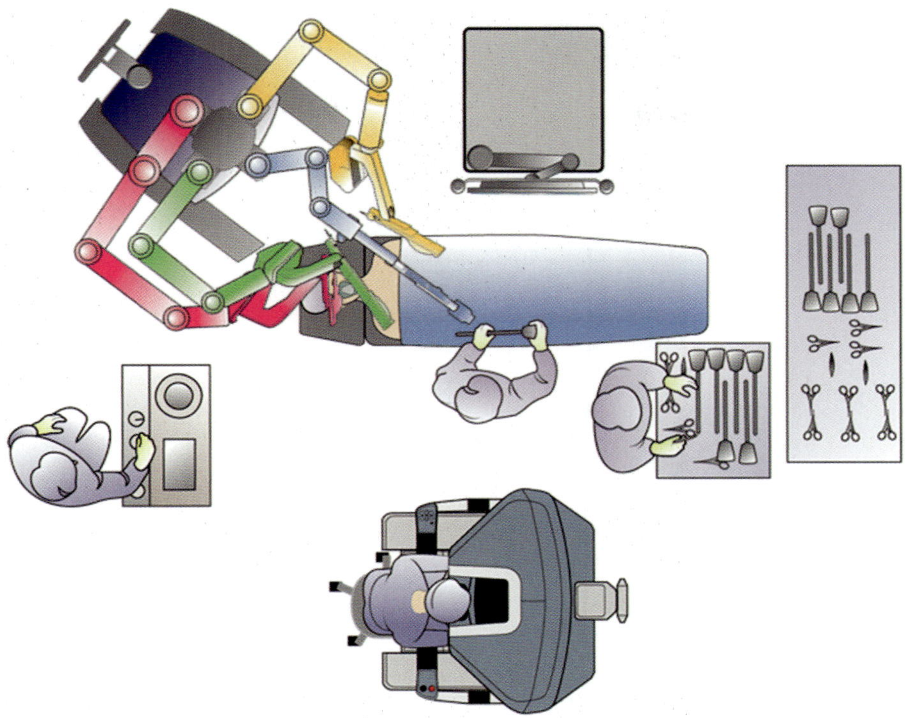

Fig. 26.1 Operating room setup

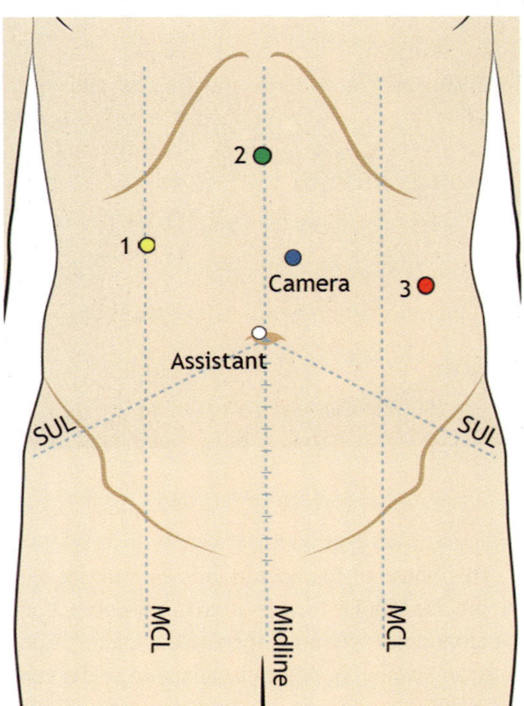

Fig. 26.2 Trocar position

of the spleen). The stomach is retracted to the right with the Cadiere forceps inserted through trocar number 1. The precise bipolar forceps is introduced through port number 2. Port number 3 is used to introduce alternatively the monopolar and the Harmonic scissors. Splenic flexure is mobilized only if necessary in order to expose and divide the splenocolic ligament and the left gastroepiploic vessels. Splenic flexure mobilization can be useful as well to dissect the pancreatic tail and identify the splenic vessels in obese patients.

Short Gastric Vessels

The short gastric vessels are divided using the Harmonic scissors till full exposition of the pancreatic tail and splenic vessels. Alternatively, the short gastric vessels can be clipped and divided with the monopolar scissors (Fig. 26.3).

Pedicle Dissection

The pancreatic tail is exposed using the fourth robotic arm in trocar 1 to completely retract the

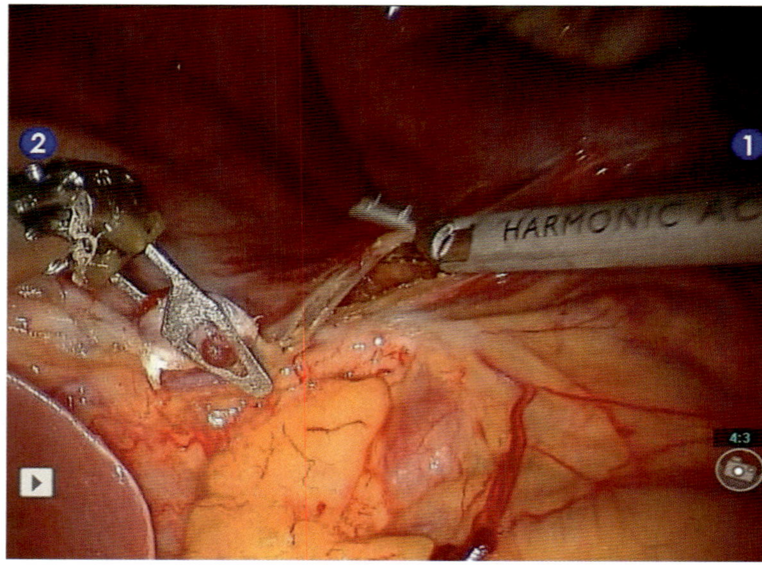

Fig. 26.3 Section of the short gastric vessels with the Harmonic Ace

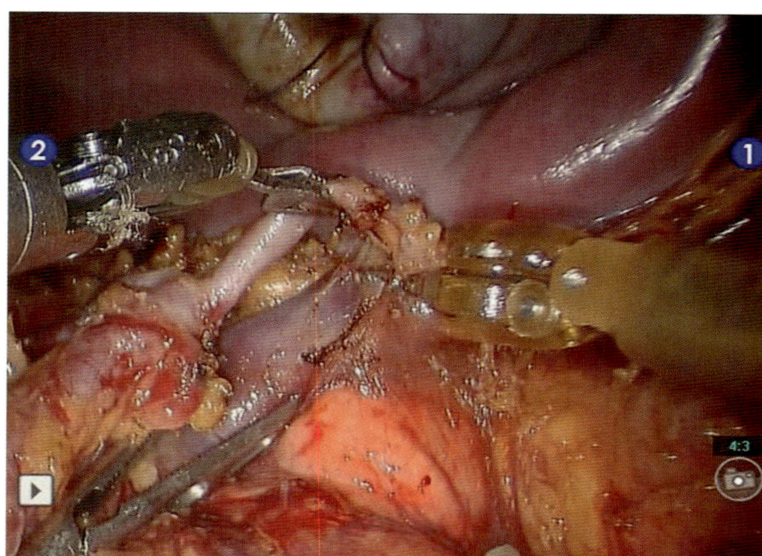

Fig. 26.4 Dissection of the branch of the splenic artery for the inferior splenic pole

stomach on the right side and atraumatic bowel grasper to retract caudally the transverse colon. The splenic artery is circumferentially dissected for a distance of 2–3 cm at the level of the distal portion of the pancreas. If the artery gives off long branches, they can be dissected separately (Fig. 26.4).

This phase of the operation is carried out with the precise bipolar forceps in trocar number 2 and the monopolar scissors or permanent cautery hook in trocar number 3. After visualization of the vein, the splenic artery or its branches are divided between plastic locking clips inserted by the assistant from the umbilical port. The vein is finally

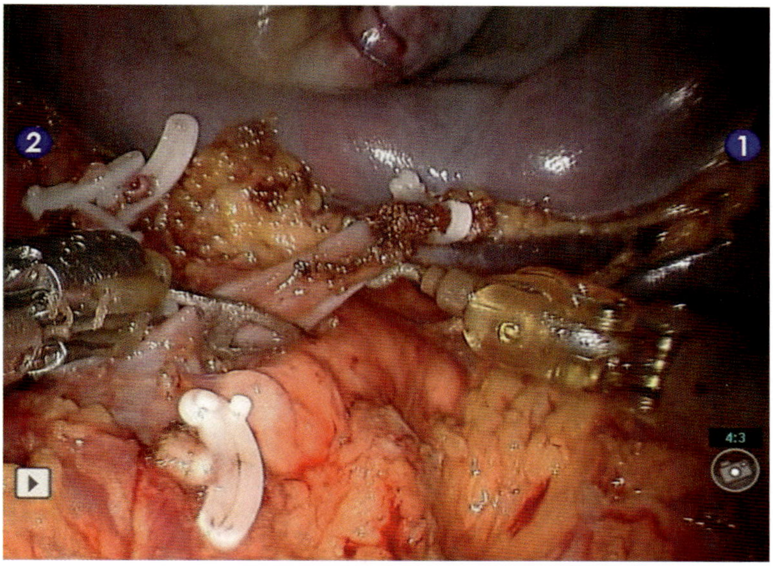

Fig. 26.5 After arterial branches were selectively clipped and divided, the vein is fully dissected and divided

dissected. In order to fully encircle even the larger splenic veins, the vein can be gently grasped by the precise forceps allowing a complete circumferential dissection using the monopolar scissor or permanent cautery hook (Fig. 26.5).

The vein is finally transected between two large plastic locking clips. Main advantage of the robot over traditional laparoscopy is the possibility also to ligate and suture splenic vessels in this phase of the operation (Fig. 26.3).

Stage 3

Spleen Mobilization

The assistant stretches the Gerota fascia caudally using the suction-irrigator and maintains the field clean. The robotic arm in trocar number 2 is used to lift up the spleen by gentle pressure, and by the monopolar scissor in trocar number 3, the splenic ligament are dissected in a caudal-to-cephalad direction (Fig. 26.6).

Stage 4

Specimen Extraction

A 10-mm endoscopic bag is inserted through the umbilical trocar and the robot undocked. Once the specimen is accommodated into the bag, the abdomen is deflated. The umbilical incision can be extended along the left circumference of the umbilicus. When the subcutaneous connective tissue is stretched apart, the linea alba becomes evident. A 3-cm incision is made in a cranial-to-caudal direction. With dilation and a slight traction on the bag, the removal is carried out aseptically without the risk of neoplastic seeding. The bag is opened and the spleen removed for morcellation. The closure is performed by layers

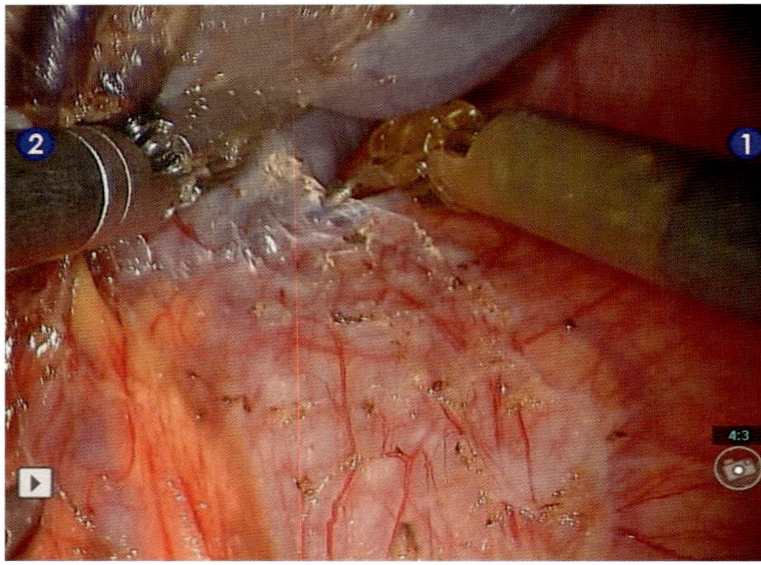

Fig. 26.6 The spleen is lifted up and the posterior ligaments dissected

with an interrupted suture. Generally, the skin incision is hidden by the umbilical scar with a good long-term esthetical result [6].

Drains

A Jackson-Pratt drain is routinely inserted through port number 3 and left in place.

References

1. Delaitre B, Maignien B. Splenectomy by the laparoscopic approach. Report of a case. Presse Med. 1991;20:2263.
2. Casaccia M, Torelli P, Squarcia S, et al. The Italian Registry of Laparoscopic Surgery of the Spleen (IRLSS). A retrospective review of 379 patients undergoing laparoscopic splenectomy. Chir Ital. 2006;58:697–707.
3. Winslow ER, Brunt LM. Perioperative outcomes of laparoscopic versus open splenectomy: a meta-analysis with an emphasis on complications. Surgery. 2003;134:647–53. discussion 54–5.
4. Gelmini R, Franzoni C, Spaziani A, Patriti A, Casciola L, Saviano M. Laparoscopic splenectomy: conventional versus robotic approach – a comparative study. J Laparoendosc Adv Surg Tech A. 2011;21:393–8.
5. Giulianotti PC, Buchs NC, Addeo P, Ayloo S, Bianco FM. Robot-assisted partial and total splenectomy. Int J Med Robot. 2011;7:482–8.
6. Casciola L, Codacci-Pisanelli M, Ceccarelli G, Bartoli A, Di Zitti L, Patriti A. A modified umbilical incision for specimen extraction after laparoscopic abdominal surgery. Surg Endosc. 2008;22:784–6.

Robotic Donor Nephrectomy and Robotic Kidney Transplant

27

Ivo G. Tzvetanov, Lorena Bejarano-Pineda, and José Oberholzer

Minimally Invasive Robotic-Assisted Kidney Transplantation

Living Donor Nephrectomy

Kidney transplantation is the best treatment for patients with chronic renal failure. In 2010, a total of 116,946 patients began renal replacement therapy, but only 2.4 % received a preemptive transplantation as their first treatment modality (2012 USRDS Annual Data Report, http://www.usrds.org). The outcomes of transplanted patients in terms of life expectancy, quality of life, and rate of hospital readmissions per year are more favorable compared to patients treated with dialysis. However, there is a continuously widening gap between demand and availability of kidney grafts due to notorious donor shortage. To address this problem, living kidney donation is the most practical approach [1]. The elective nature of living donor transplantation offers the opportunity to have kidney grafts of excellent quality and the option to perform the procedure when the recipient is in optimal condition, reducing the likelihood of complications associated with uncontrolled comorbidities. In addition, wait time until transplantation and time on dialysis can be minimized. These factors allow better graft and patient survival rates as compared to deceased donor transplantation. The main obstacle of living donation is the exposure of healthy individual to the inherent risk of surgical intervention without a direct health benefit, besides the personal satisfaction for an altruistic action. Therefore, reducing postoperative pain, achieving faster recovery, and minimizing the surgical incisions have become significant factors to increase kidney donation rates. The availability of minimally invasive, laparoscopic surgical technique greatly enhanced living donation rates. The US Food and Drug Administration (FDA) approved the da Vinci Surgical System (Intuitive Surgical, Inc.) in 2000, and its use in living donor nephrectomies was a logical extension of the widely adapted minimally invasive approach. After acquiring extensive experience with the technique in general surgery, the first worldwide transabdominal hand-assisted robotic donor nephrectomy was performed successfully at the University of Illinois at Chicago Hospital within the same year [2]. Since then, our institution has performed over 700 robotic donor nephrectomies with excellent outcomes [3, 4].

Donor Selection and Preoperative Evaluation

Candidates for living donation can be related to the patient as a first- or second-degree relative or an unrelated donor as spouse or a close friend.

I.G. Tzvetanov, M.D. • L. Bejarano-Pineda, M.D.
J. Oberholzer, M.D. (✉)
Division of Transplantation, Department of Surgery, University of Illinois at Chicago, College of Medicine, 840 South Wood Street, CSB Rm 502, Chicago, IL 60612, USA
e-mail: jober@uic.edu

K.C. Kim (ed.), *Robotics in General Surgery*, DOI 10.1007/978-1-4614-8739-5_27,

In the USA, any potential donor should be at least 18 years of age. The workup for living kidney donors has the following purposes:

- Assessment and confirmation of ABO and human leukocyte antigen (HLA) compatibility between donor and recipient. Nowadays, ABO incompatibility or pre-sensitization to a given donor does not necessarily preclude successful transplantation. Preoperative desensitization protocols for cross-match positive or ABO incompatible pairs are increasingly successful (add paper by Thielke J as first and me as last author).
- Medical evaluation of the candidate assessing the current medical status and determining the medical and surgical risks to the donor. Every medical condition should be discussed and clarified.
- Anatomy and functional assessment of the kidneys.
- Psychological evaluation to uncover any psychiatric disorders and psychological or social problems that may disqualify the candidate and resolve doubts or misinformation related to the procedure and its implication.

A multidisciplinary team makes final approval of the potential donor. The decision regarding which kidney to be harvested is based on the function and anatomy. Usually the left kidney is procured, due to its anatomy (longer left renal vein) and the lower complexity of the left nephrectomy.

Surgical Procedure

Patient Preparation and Positioning

The donor is admitted the day of the procedure. Administration of bowel preparation the night before the surgery is used in some centers, but does not offer much advantage and even delays postoperative recovery. During the induction of general anesthesia, Foley catheter and oral gastric tube are regularly placed. Prophylactic antibiotics are administrated. Pneumatic compression stockings are mandatory. For a left nephrectomy, the patient is rolled into the right lateral decubitus position with a cushioned beanbag and axillary roll. The abdomen is prepped and draped in a standard sterile fashion. An adequate fixation of the patient to the operative table is important, because any instability after docking the robotic system could jeopardize the safety of the procedure.

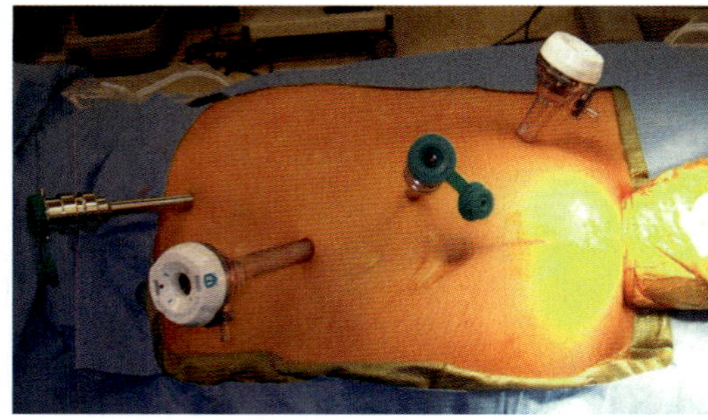

Fig. 27.1 Port placement in the donor

Incision and Port Placement (Fig. 27.1)

The herein described robotic-assisted donor nephrectomy is a transabdominal procedure, which is usually done through four laparoscopic ports and one 7-cm infraumbilical incision. A longitudinal or transverse abdominal incision can be made, based on the patient's preference. The most commonly performed incision even in male donors, is a 7-cm transverse suprapubic Pfannenstiel incision. This incision provides better cosmetic appearance and is the optimal approach for hand assistance. In very tall, male donors, a lower midline incision will provide more optimal distance between the incision and the hilum of the kidney. The incision should not be made excessively close to the laparoscopic operative field, because it would limit the range of motion of the assisting hand. Utilization of hand port is not mandatory. In our practice, the assistant's hand, previously wrapped with protective, sterile foil around the wrist and forearm, is inserted directly through the incision. This maneuver does not cause any problems with the maintenance of pneumoperitoneum and, according

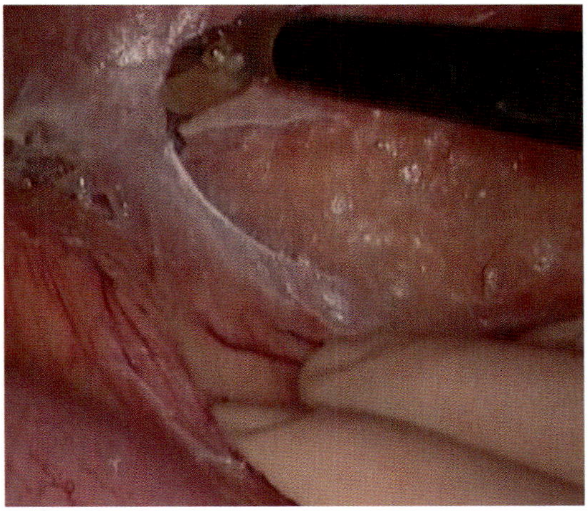

Fig. 27.2 Mobilization of the left colon

to our observations, significantly decreases the incidence of wound infections.

Once the assistant's hand is inserted in the abdomen, the kidney to be harvested is palpated to identify the position of the hilum. This maneuver allows precise robotic port placement. Under hand control from inside the abdomen, a 12-mm laparoscopic port is placed above the umbilicus, close to the midline, at the level of the renal hilum. This port is required for the 30° robotic camera system. To achieve good triangulations, the two 8-mm robotic working ports are placed along the left midclavicular line. They are located proximal and distal, 10–12 cm apart from the camera port. Lastly, the 12-mm port is placed in the left lower quadrant to assist with suction, clipping, stapling, and cutting. At this point, the robotic system is docked and integrated to the ports, and pneumoperitoneum is achieved with 12–14-mmHg CO_2 insufflation. To obtain additional working space, the robotic arms are used to give additional lift on the ports.

Mobilization of the Left Colon (Fig. 27.2)

The assisting surgeon's right hand is introduced into the abdominal cavity, and the descending colon is retracted medially and freed from lateral peritoneal attachments exposing the left paracolic gutter. The operating surgeon controls the electrocautery hook with his right hand and bipolar pickups with the left hand. The descending and the sigmoid colon are then fully mobilized. The splenocolic ligament is also transected and additionally cauterized with bipolar pickups. Following the exact plain between the mesentery of the left colon and the Gerota's fascia allows bloodless exposure of the anterior surface of the left kidney even in cases with significant intra-abdominal adiposity. Occasionally, if the lower pole of the spleen overlays the upper pole of the kidney, the posterior splenic attachments are transected and the spleen is partially mobilized. The operating surgeon has to be very cautions to avoid injury of the body and tail of the pancreas, which may also be overlaying the upper pole of the kidney.

Identification of the Ureter (Fig. 27.3)

The mobilized left colon is retracted medially by the assisting surgeon, and the retroperitoneal space is exposed. The dissection is carried along the anterior surface of the left psoas muscle, starting from lateral towards medial until the left ureter is identified. The three-dimensional (3D) view offered by the robotic system allows a quick and safe identification of the left ureter. The ureter is circumferentially dissected and mobilized distally to the point where it crosses the iliac vessels. A generous amount of adipose tissue should be conserved around the ureter in order to preserve its blood supply. A short Penrose drain is introduced, placed around the mobilized ureter, and clipped to itself to hold the ureter. This technique allows atraumatic lateral retraction of the ureter by the assisting surgeon using a locking grasper. This maneuver keeps the ureter in view and prevents injury during the dissection around the lower pole of the kidney. If a lower polar artery, originating from distal abdominal aorta is present, this vessel needs to be identified and exposed carefully because its unintentional injury would deprive the ureter of blood supply.

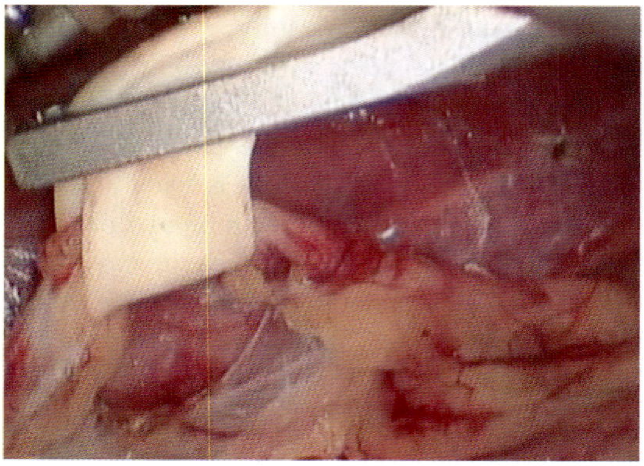

Fig. 27.3 Mobilization of the ureter

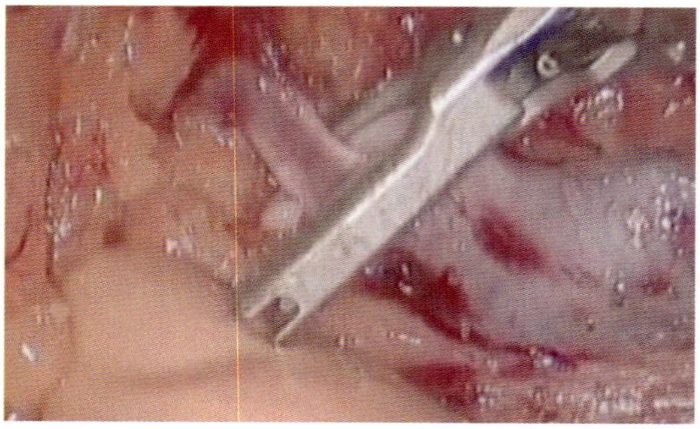

Fig. 27.4 Dissection of the left adrenal vein

Identification of the Renal Vein

The gonadal vein is identified medial to the ureter and dissected off superiorly until its junction with the left renal vein. This maneuver allows safe identification of the renal vein at the proper distance from its bifurcation within the renal hilum. The tissue in front of the vein is transected and the vein exposed medially to its junction with the inferior vena cava (IVC). In rare cases, with retroaortic left renal vein, the dissection is carried as medial as possible. The gonadal vein is transected between two robotically placed hem-o-lock clips. Along the upper border of the renal vein, the left adrenal vein is identified. It is circumferentially dissected, double clipped, and transected (Fig. 27.4).

In most of the cases, at least one lumbar vein will be joining the left renal vein. We have identified up to five lumbar veins, forming a venous network and draining into the lower and posterior surface of the renal vein. The precision during the isolation and transaction of these veins cannot be overemphasized. In these cases, the articulating skills of the robotic system and the 3D vision give significant advantage over conventional laparoscopic instruments.

Dissection Around the Upper Pole and Adrenal Gland

The adrenal gland is identified proximal to the left renal vein. The plain between the gland and upper pole of the kidney is followed, and the adrenal is left intact. The adrenal artery, which originates from the left renal artery, should be divided between clips whenever it presents. The upper pole of the kidney is then fully mobilized; this maneuver can be facilitated by the assisting surgeon exercising gentle distal hand retraction of the kidney. If a sizable upper polar artery is present, extra care should be taken to preserve this vessel, since it could supply 20–30 % of the kidney mass. Small upper polar arteries give <5 % of the parenchyma blood supply, and they are not involved in the vascularization of the pelvis, therefore, can be safely sacrificed.

Transection of the Ureter and Posterior Mobilization

The previously mobilized ureter is clipped with two robotic hem-o-lock clips where it crosses iliac vessels and sharply transects right proximal to the clips. Bleeding from the transected surface is a desirable sign, and the small amount of free urine flow in the retroperitoneal space has no consequences. The posterior attachments of the kidney are divided with the assistance of the assisting surgeon's hand, as well as the articulated robotic instruments. During this maneuver, surgeons have to be cautious to avoid much tension on the hilar vessels or to unintentionally rotate the kidney to 180°, which would lead to strangulation and vascular injury.

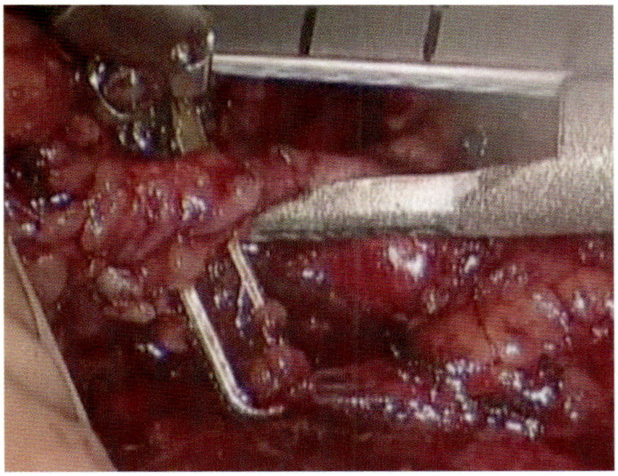

Fig. 27.5 Transection of the renal artery

Identification of the Renal Artery

After completed posterior mobilization, the kidney is gently retracted medially. This allows an easier identification of the renal artery. The ganglionic and lymphatic tissues surrounding the renal artery need to be transected, allowing exposure of the artery. The vessel needs to be circumferentially dissected at the level of its origin from the aorta. Be very careful to not injure possible early arterial branches. If multiple arteries are present, every vessel has to be dissected freely as described. After completion of the dissection, the only connection of the kidney is the renal artery and vein. The precision during this part of the operation cannot be overemphasized, and the advantages of the robotic system are evident.

Division of the Hilar Vessels and Kidney Graft Extraction (Figs. 27.5 and 27.6)

After the kidney is completely mobilized and the vascular dissection completed, 5,000 U of heparin is given intravenously to the donor and left circulating for 2–3 min. The kidney is supported medially by the assistant's hand. The left robotic arm retracts the artery gently, while the right arm holds the robotic hem-o-lock clip ready. The assistant surgeon advances the Endo TA stapler, with vascular load, through the 12-mm left lower quadrant port. Utilization of the Endo TA stapler allows additional length of the artery to facilitate the implantation of the graft. The renal artery is stapled as close as possible to its origin from the aorta. After checking the proper deployment of the stapling line, the robotic clip is placed to enhance hemostasis. The artery is sharply divided with robotic scissors at least 3–4 mm distal from the stapler line. If multiple arteries are present, they are sequentially stapled and transected in a similar fashion. After completing the artery division, 50 mg of protamine is given intravenously to the donor to counteract the effect of heparin. Of note: It is not safe to only use a hem-o-lock clip for securing the arterial stump. The use of a stapler device is mandatory. We only use a hem-o-lock to avoid minimal bleeding at times observed from the staple line.

The kidney is now placed in a lateral (natural) position and the renal vein exposed. The operating surgeon exercises gentle lift and traction to the hilum, straitening the vein. The vessel is divided as medial as possible with an Endo GIA vascular stapler and, subsequently, inserted by the assisting surgeon through the left lower quadrant assisting port. Care should be taken to avoid engaging previously placed plastic clips into the stapler line. Using angulations of the shaft of the stapler is helpful.

The kidney graft is rapidly removed from the abdominal cavity and placed in a container with cold solution with the temperature below 4 °C and flushed with cold preservation solution.

Field Inspection and Closure

Once the kidney graft is removed, the cavity is inspected for bleeding. The arterial and venous stumps are visualized, and the condition of the stapler line verified. If any doubt about the reliability, it should be over sawn with 5-0 Prolene suture, which is relatively easy with the articulated robotic arms. Some bleeding from left over adipose capsule is controlled with electrocautery. Be cautious to the presence of chylous and lymphatic leak. If any of these situations are identified, it should be controlled with suture ligation.

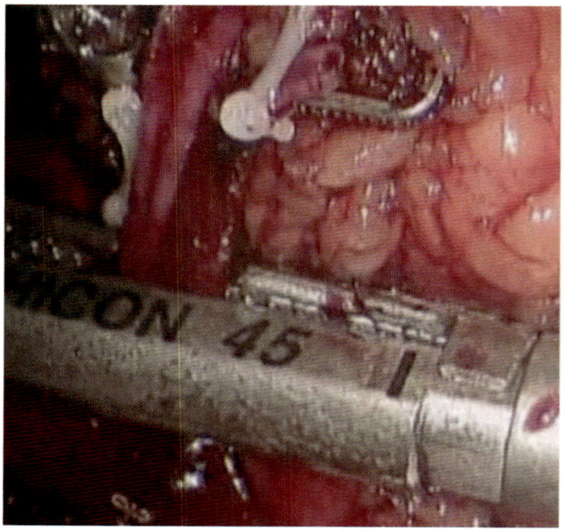

Fig. 27.6 Transection of the renal vein

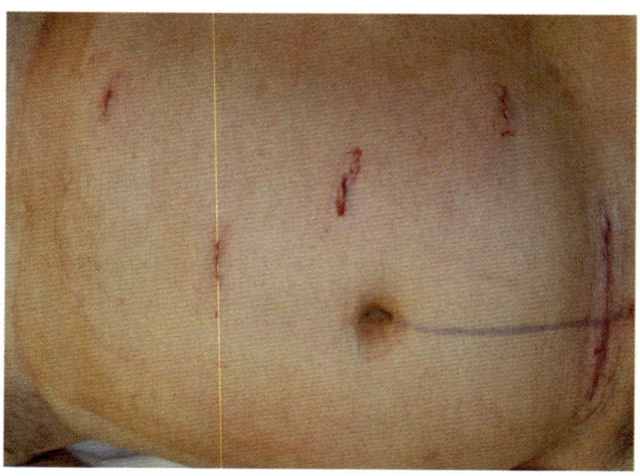

Fig. 27.7 Port positioning in the donor after closure

The robotic system is disengaged and ports removed. Closure of the 12-mm port sides is not mandatory, but is recommended. The 7-cm incision is closed anatomically by layers. Skin incisions are closed cosmetically (Fig. 27.7).

Graft Backbench Preparation

After the kidney is removed and placed in cold storage, the stapler line from the vein is excised and the artery cannulated. The graft is flushed with cold infusion using University of Wisconsin solution until clear fluid is seen coming out from the vein. The surface of the kidney should be inspected, and if the flash is not uniform, the hilum needs to be examined for an unintentionally transected arterial branch. The residual adipose capsule is excised and ligated around the hilum in order to prevent accumulation of lymphoceles, which mostly originate from the graft (in our center, we have essentially eliminated the incidence of lymphoceles by careful backbench preparation). Part of the adipose capsule around the lower pole, in proximity to the ureter, is left to preserve the blood supply. If multiple arteries are present, decision regarding vascular reconstruction or separate implantation depends on the actual position of the vessels.

Right Donor Nephrectomy

The anatomical features of the right kidney make it less preferred for harvesting, mostly due to the shorter length and greater fragility of the right renal vein. The transplant team at our institution prefers to remove the left kidney, even in the presence of multiple arteries. The main indication for harvesting the right kidney is the presence of anatomical defects compatible with transplantation in the right kidney (e.g., small unique renal stone, a large cyst) or a significant difference in function between both kidneys. In this case, the rule is to harvest the kidney with inferior function but with a glomerular filtration rate within normal range. For robotic-assisted right donor nephrectomy, the patient is placed in left decubitus position. The 7-cm incision is performed the same way as described for left nephrectomy, while the port sites are placed in mirror image location. Occasionally, one additional port is placed in the left upper quadrant for liver retraction, which may be necessary during the mobilization of the upper pole. After medial mobilization of the right colon, the ureter is identified and IVC is exposed. Occasionally, Kocher maneuver may be necessary. Following the IVC proximally, the right renal vein is identified and circumferentially dissected free. The renal artery is localized after posterior mobilization and medial retraction of the kidney. The articulated arms of the robot and 3D vision are extremely useful for the renal artery dissection when located posterior to the IVC. The rest of the procedure follows the same steps as described for left nephrectomy.

Postoperative Donor Care

After completion of the operation, the patient is relocated in supine decubitus position and extubated. Pain control is achieved preferentially with opioids. Under appropriate hydration, it is safe to use short term with i.v. NSAIDS. The patient is encouraged to ambulate the same day, and a liquid diet is started 4–5 h after the operation. The morning after surgery, a complete blood cell count and basic metabolic panel are performed. Foley catheter is also removed. General diet is given, and if no complications are experienced, the donor is discharged home on the second or third postoperative day.

Discussion

Currently, according to widely accepted consensus, every transplant center, which performs living donor kidney transplantation, must offer the donors some of the available minimally invasive modalities for donor nephrectomy. Considering the experience in our institution, with over 700 cases performed in the last 11 years, we conclude that robotic donor nephrectomy is a safe procedure with a minimal number of complications. The majority of observed complications have occurred at the beginning of our learning curve. The most significant complications, requiring conversion to open procedure, include (1) three intraoperative renal artery stump bleeding and a (2) single case of intraoperative renal vein laceration (all occurred at the beginning of our experience, last event was in late 2001). Other early postoperative complications include one symptomatic chyloperitoneum and one intra-abdominal hematoma without an identifiable source, both treated laparoscopically. We also encountered three cases of bowel obstruction due to adhesions, also treated laparoscopically. The superficial wound infection rate has been, overall, <2 %.

Major vascular complications during laparoscopic donor nephrectomy, although uncommon, can be potentially fatal [5]. To avoid major postoperative bleeding, we embraced the concept and reiterate it again that vascular clips alone are inadequate for safe hemostasis after transection of the main renal artery. Therefore, we recommend using vascular staplers for transfixion in every vascular transaction involving the renal artery and vein, in order to minimize the risk of early postoperative bleeding from the stumps of the renal vessels. Other limitations, such as prolonged setup time and difficult instrument exchange, addressed to the robotic system, mainly occur during the initial experience, and with appropriate mentoring, are rapidly overcome [6].

Recipient

While we use robotic technology for all donor nephrectomies, the use in the recipient operation is limited to overweight patients, otherwise denied access to conventional kidney transplantation by most transplant centers. Obesity is a common comorbidity among potential kidney transplant recipients in the USA [7], causing a longer time on the waiting list for kidney transplantation as compared to nonobese recipients. Decreased graft and patient survival have been demonstrated in obese renal transplant recipients experiencing wound infections [8]. Considering the negative impact of obesity in outcomes and increased risk of complications, many centers are skeptic to list morbidly obese patients for renal transplantation.

Recent studies suggest that body mass index (BMI) >30 kg/m^2 is an independent risk factor for surgical site infection (SSI), which is directly correlated to decreased graft survival. However, obese recipients who avoid SSI have similar outcomes to nonobese recipients [9]. These results show the need to implement new surgical techniques in obese kidney transplant recipients that prevent complications such as SSI.

Minimally invasive surgical technologies have shown benefits that include reduced recovery period, fewer wound complications, and reduced surgical scars. However, complex procedures such as kidney transplantation have been considered technically demanding by conventional laparoscopy [10]. The introduction of precise surgical robotic systems, such as the da Vinci Surgical System (Intuitive Surgical, Inc.), expanded the possibilities for more difficult surgeries and became promising in kidney transplantation.

Based on our extensive experience applying the robotic system for different procedures such as pancreatectomies, donor nephrectomies, and liver resections, we developed the robotic-assisted kidney transplant procedure. One of the goals with this new surgical approach was to minimize the difficulties in providing kidney transplantation for obese patients with ESRD [11]. Over the last three and a half years at the University of Illinois at Chicago Hospital, we performed 70 kidney transplants on obese patients using the da Vinci robotic surgical system. Initial results showed the advantages and feasibility of the robotic-assisted procedure [12].

Surgical Technique

Backbench Preparation of the Graft

Regardless of the origin of the kidney graft, living or deceased donor, backbench preparation for robotic implantation has some specific steps. The purpose is to facilitate orientation of the organ and minimize bleeding after the implantation. The adipose capsule is meticulously ligated with 3-0 silk during excision. The renal vein and artery are dissected towards the hilum and marked with a marking pen, depending on the site of implantation, right or left. Lastly, the ureter is appropriately shortened and spatulated.

Patient Positioning and Port Placement (Fig. 27.8)

After induction of general anesthesia, a three-way Foley catheter is placed to allow irrigation of the bladder. The patient is positioned supine with parted and flexed legs; shoulder block and tape were used to avoid sliding of the patient during the operation. After the patient is prepped in the sterile fashion, a 7-cm midline incision, approximately 5 cm below the xiphoid process, is made for the placement of the hand access device (Lap Disc, Ethicon, Cincinnati, OH, or Gelfoam or similar). Depending on the body habitus of the recipient, the location of this midline incision could be closer to the umbilicus in order to allow easier access to the surgical field for the bedside hand-assisting co-surgeon.

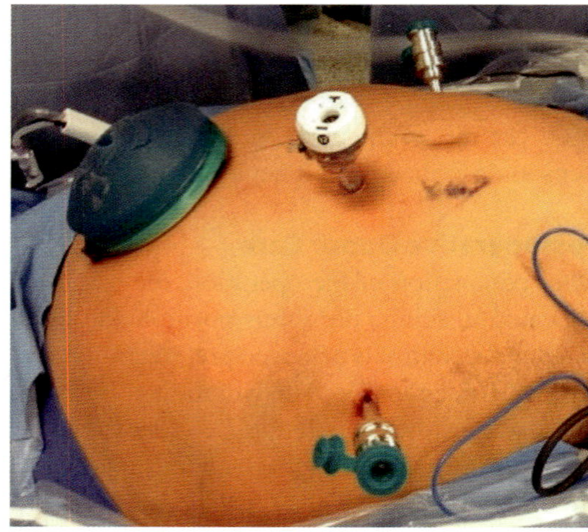

Fig. 27.8 Port placement in the recipient

Pneumoperitoneum is achieved at 15-mmHg CO_2 insufflation. Laparoscopic ports are positioned in the following manner: (1) one 12-mm port for the 30° robotic scope is inserted in the right side of the umbilicus; (2) two 7-mm robotic ports are inserted, one is placed in the right flank and the other in the left lower quadrant; and (3) a 12-mm assistant port is then placed on the left side of the umbilicus between the camera and the left lower quadrant robotic port. If it is needed, an additional 5-mm port could be placed in the right flank between the camera and the robotic port.

Once the ports are located, the patient is placed in 30° Trendelenburg position with the right side elevated (for implantation to the right external iliac vessels). The robot system is docked into position from the patient right leg site parallel and slightly diagonal to the body.

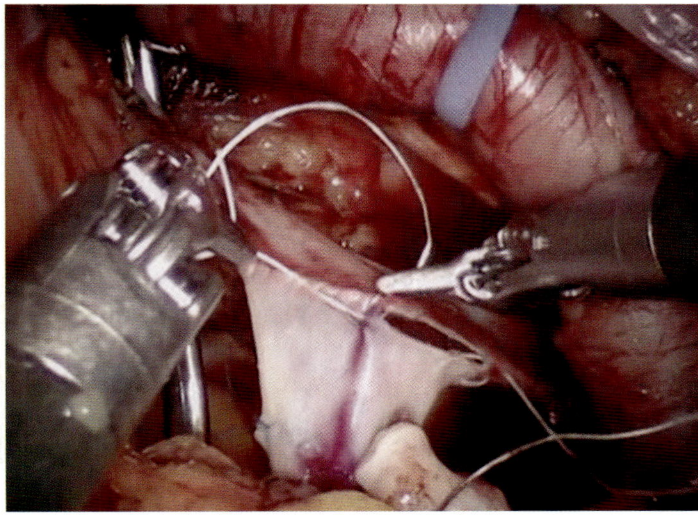

Fig. 27.9 Anastomosis of the renal vein

Vascular Exposure

The operation begins with minimal mobilization of the right colon and exposure of the right external iliac artery and vein. The iliac vessels are dissected freely using bipolar forceps and a hook electrocautery. In order to facilitate the exposure and the dissection around the external iliac vein, a vessel loop is used to retract the artery upwards. Another vessel loop is placed around the iliac vein to allow the dissection on the posterior surface of the vein. Since the iliac vessels need to be completely mobilized at least 5 cm in length, any collateral vessels found need to be suture ligated with Prolene 5-0 and transected.

Graft Implantation and Reperfusion

Once the external iliac vessels are completely dissected free, two robotic bulldog clamps are used to clamp the external iliac vein. Robotic Potts scissors are used to create a venotomy to about 15 mm in length. Twelve-centimeter, double-needle, 5-0 Gore-Tex suture with a knot in the middle is placed at the corner of the venotomy. The kidney graft is inserted in the abdominal cavity by the assisting surgeon and positioned parallel to the dissected iliac vessels. Venovenous anastomosis is completed in an end-to-side fashion with running suture (Fig. 27.9).

If needed, interrupted stitches of 5-0 Prolene are used to reinforce the anastomosis. The external iliac artery is then clamped between robotic bulldogs and an oval-shaped window; proportional to the size of the renal artery of the graft is made in the anterior wall of the artery using robotic scissors. To facilitate this maneuver, a 5-0 Prolene stitch is placed through the anterior wall of the artery, and gentle pulling is applied. The arterial anastomosis is completed in an end-to-side fashion with 12-cm double-needle 6-0 Gore-Tex suture with a knot in the middle (Fig. 27.10).

Once the reconstruction is completed, venous clamps are removed first, followed by immediate removal of the arterial clamps. The reperfusion of the organ and hemostasis are additionally verified, and bleeding points secured with 6-0 Prolene suture. We routinely use robotic fluorescence camera and IV injection of 3 ml of indocyanine green. This allows confirmation of the complete and homogenous reperfusion of the renal graft. At this point, the pressure of the pneumoperitoneum is decreased to 8–10 mmHg to minimize possible negative effect of high intra-abdominal pressure on the graft perfusion.

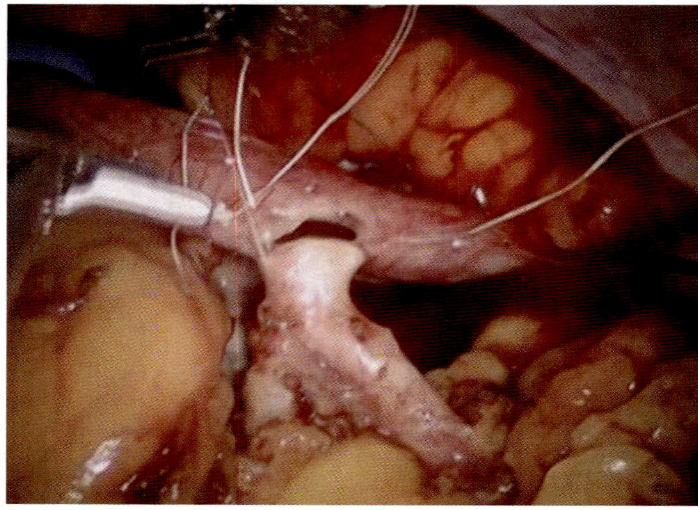

Fig. 27.10 Anastomosis of the renal artery

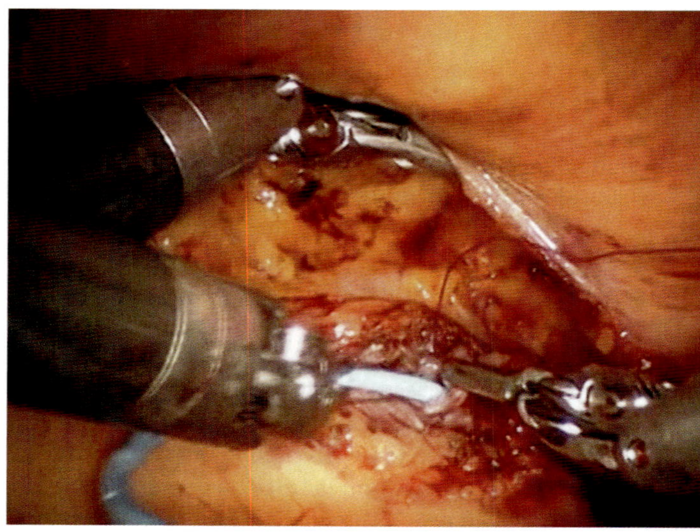

Fig. 27.11 Ureteroneocystostomy

Ureteroneocystostomy

The bladder is distended with diluted methylene blue solution in order to facilitate its identification. The muscular layers are incised, the bladder mucosa is prepared, and the muscular layers are detached laterally to facilitate the subsequent creation of an antireflux mechanism. The ureter is anastomosed to the bladder with running 5-0 Monocryl suture using typical antireflux technique suturing full thickness of the ureteral wall with the mucosal layer of the bladder. Utilization of ureteral stent is optional (Fig. 27.11). Upon completion of the anastomosis, the seromuscular layer is closed over the ureteroneocystostomy with 3-0 Vicryl to create an antireflux mechanism.

At the end of the procedure, the minilaparotomy is closed with running 0 PDS, and the two 12-mm port sites are closed with an endoclosure device and 0 Vicryl suture (Fig. 27.12).

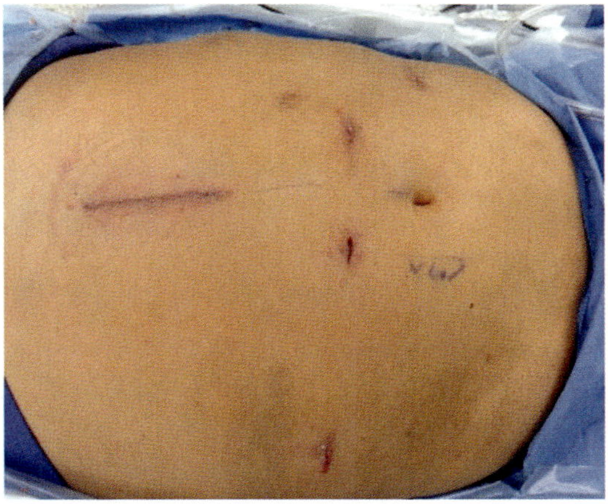

Fig. 27.12 Port positioning in the recipient after closure

Discussion

Applying this standardized technique, within the last three and a half years, we performed more than 70 robotic-assisted kidney transplants in obese recipients. The only selection criterion is BMI >30 kg/m^2, without an upper limit. The highest BMI of transplanted patient was 58 kg/m^2, and the mean BMI of the group was 45 kg/m^2. High immunologic risk or multiple previous surgeries were not considered a contraindication to perform a robotic-assisted procedure. The only exclusion criteria were severe atherosclerosis of the iliac vessels in the recipient and the graft vessels (in case the graft is from a deceased donor). We performed a case–control study where we compared our first 28 robotic-assisted kidney transplants to a frequency-matched retrospective cohort of obese recipients who underwent kidney transplantation by open technique. We observed one wound complication in this robotic group, which was a hematoma in a patient on anticoagulation. No SSI was observed in this sample of robotic-assisted kidney-transplanted obese recipients as compared to 28 % in the control group and up to 40 % in previous studies [9]. Besides the advantages of minimally invasive surgery as early mobilization and high patient satisfaction, we have observed excellent graft function [12].

Based on the experience in our institution, we can state that robotic-assisted kidney transplantation for obese recipients is a safe and effective operation. By achieving excellent kidney graft function and minimizing surgical complications, this surgical technique gives the opportunity to the disadvantaged group of obese patients with ESRD to have more realistic access to transplantation. Of note: This is a very advanced application of robotic surgery and requires extensive experience in robotic surgery. Surgeons attempting this procedure require the full armamentarium of robotic surgical skills, including advanced vascular suture techniques.

Acknowledgments To Dr. Enrico Benedetti and Dr. Pier Giulianotti for their expertise and great efforts in supervising and leading us to accomplish this program. Without your contribution, it would not have been possible.

References

1. Levey AS, Danovitch G, Hou S. Living donor kidney transplantation in the United States–looking back, looking forward. Am J Kidney Dis. 2011;58(3):343–8. PubMed PMID: 21783290.
2. Horgan S, Vanuno D, Sileri P, Cicalese L, Benedetti E. Robotic-assisted laparoscopic donor nephrectomy for kidney transplantation. Transplantation. 2002; 73(9):1474–9. PubMed PMID: 12023627.
3. Gorodner V, Horgan S, Galvani C, Manzelli A, Oberholzer J, Sankary H, et al. Routine left robotic-assisted laparoscopic donor nephrectomy is safe and effective regardless of the presence of vascular anomalies. Transpl Int. 2006;19(8):636–40. PubMed PMID: 16827680.
4. Horgan S, Galvani C, Gorodner MV, Jacobsen GR, Moser F, Manzelli A, et al. Effect of robotic assistance on the "learning curve" for laparoscopic hand-assisted donor nephrectomy. Surg Endosc. 2007;21(9):1512–7. PubMed PMID: WOS:000249555400008. English.
5. Friedman AL, Peters TG, Jones KW, Boulware LE, Ratner LE. Fatal and nonfatal hemorrhagic complications of living kidney donation. Ann Surg. 2006;243(1):126–30. PubMed PMID: WOS: 000234311800020. English.
6. Galvani CA, Garza U, Leeds M, Kaul A, Echeverria A, Desai CS, et al. Single-incision robotic-assisted living donor nephrectomy: case report and description of surgical technique. Transpl Int. 2012;25(8):e89–92. PubMed PMID: WOS:000306273400001. English.
7. Friedman AN, Miskulin DC, Rosenberg IH, Levey AS. Demographics and trends in overweight and

obesity in patients at time of kidney transplantation. Am J Kidney Dis. 2003;41(2):480–7. PubMed PMID: 12552513.

8. Aalten J, Christiaans MH, de Fijter H, Hene R, van der Heijde JH, Roodnat J, et al. The influence of obesity on short- and long-term graft and patient survival after renal transplantation. Transpl Int. 2006;19(11): 901–7. PubMed PMID: 17018125.
9. Lynch RJ, Ranney DN, Shijie C, Lee DS, Samala N, Englesbe MJ. Obesity, surgical site infection, and outcome following renal transplantation. Ann Surg. 2009;250(6):1014–20. PubMed PMID: 19779327.
10. Rosales A, Salvador JT, Urdaneta G, Patino D, Montlleo M, Esquena S, et al. Laparoscopic kidney transplantation. Eur Urol. 2010;57(1):164–7. PubMed PMID: 19592155.
11. Segev DL, Simpkins CE, Thompson RE, Locke JE, Warren DS, Montgomery RA. Obesity impacts access to kidney transplantation. J Am Soc Nephrol. 2008;19(2):349–55. PubMed PMID: 18094366. Pubmed Central PMCID: 2396750.
12. Oberholzer J, Giulianotti P, Danielson K, et al. Minimally invasive robotic kidney transplantation for obese patients previously denied access to transplantation. Am J Transplant. 2013;13(3):721–8.

Part X

Surgical Techniques: *Hernias*

Robot-Assisted Ventral and Incisional Hernia Repair

28

Brad Snyder

General Overview

When the abdominal contents are able to eviscerate through a fascial defect, an hernia is defined. This may lead to loss of domain, visceral disproportion, bowel obstruction, and/or chronic pain. The umbilical hernias (a congenital defect) and epigastric hernias (acquired fascial decussation) make up what is known in general as ventral abdominal wall hernias. Incisional hernias, on the other hand, are secondary to a surgical procedure. Most practicing surgeons will find themselves evaluating these hernias for repair.

Ventral abdominal hernia (primary or incisional) repair is a common surgical procedure. About 90,000–100,000 repairs are performed every year in the USA. There is a reported incidence of 3–20 % in the 5-year period post-laparotomy [1, 2].

The principle idea for repair is to approximate the fascial edges of the hernia and prevent recurrence. There are several techniques for repairing these ventral hernias. The traditional ventral hernia repair, using an open technique with a simple suture closure, was associated with a high rate of wound complication secondary to large flaps in the abdominal wall layers, as well as recurrence rates between 25 % and 63 % [3, 4]. The open ventral hernia repair with prosthetic mesh using a tension-free technique has lowered the recurrence rate to 10–40 % [5, 6], but it also increased the incidence of significant wound complications including mesh infections [5–7]. Laparoscopic repair of incisional hernias was introduced in 1992 [8, 9], leading to improvements in recovery time, hospital stay, complication rates, and cost. Published recurrence rates have been reduced to 0–9 % [10–13]. These recurrences have been attributed primarily to improper positioning of the mesh (with <3 cm overlap of mesh and fascia) and to the use of tacking or stapling devices for fixation rather than abdominal wall suturing using suture passers [13, 14].

The primary complications of laparoscopic ventral hernia repair are seroma formation, wound infection, ileus, and hematoma [10–13]. Although laparoscopic repair has been associated with faster recovery, fewer complications, and a lower recurrence rate compared to open technique, there continues to be a significant incidence of postoperative pain associated with the transabdominal wall sutures. Several authors [2, 12, 15–17] have reported a 2 % incidence of significant postoperative pain lasting more than 2–8 weeks after repair. Significant postoperative pain has also been described in association with helicoids staples and tackers. Three exploratory laparotomies were required in such cases [2, 18]. Additionally, a randomized controlled

B. Snyder, M.D. (✉)
Department of Surgery, Memorial Hermann Texas Medical Center, Houston, TX, USA
e-mail: Brad.Snyder@uth.tmc.edu

K.C. Kim (ed.), *Robotics in General Surgery*, DOI 10.1007/978-1-4614-8739-5_28,

study showed a significantly higher pain level in suture placement compared to tackers for mesh fixation [19]. The pain is described by patients as a single point of constant, sharp burning in a dermatome pattern at the points of transabdominal sutures or tackers; this pain has been attributed to tissue and nerve entrapment. These suture sites require prolonged hospital stay, local injections, and the occasional readmission for pain control.

The da Vinci Robot (Intuitive Surgical, Sunnyvale, CA, USA) offers numerous advantages over the open and traditional laparoscopic approach. These include six degrees of motion, three-dimensional (3D) imaging, and superior ergonomics, to name a few, that enable easy and precise intracorporeal suturing [2]. This can serve as a means to eliminate transabdominal fixation sutures and tacks all together.

In addition, the da Vinci Robot can be used to primarily suture the fascial defect closed followed by circumferential fixation of the mesh. Two reports of robotic ventral hernia repair did not close the ventral hernia primarily nor did they employ a continuous running suture; instead, they used interrupted sutures to secure the mesh [20, 21]. However, closing the defect primarily will significantly increase the overlap of the mesh, and continuously running the suture increases surface area of suture to the fascia. Together, these changes eliminate the need for transabdominal sutures or helicoid tackers that can cause significant postoperative pain while maintaining, if not improving, the strength of the repair.

Procedure Overview

Patient Positioning

Patients are placed in the supine position with both arms tucked at their sides and the entire abdominal wall exposed and prepped. In all cases, the bladder and stomach should be decompressed. An adhesive drape is used to cover the patient's abdomen; this also facilitates marking the size, shape, and location of the fascial defect (see Fig. 28.1).

Trocar Placement

The abdominal cavity is accessed right or left upper abdomen via a 5 mm subcostal incision and is later exchanged for a robotic 5 mm trocar. A 12 mm trocar is placed for the camera, and a final 5 or 8 mm robotic trocar is placed in the lower abdomen. These are placed in the lateral abdomen under direct visualization as far lateral as possible to maximize distance away from the fascial defect.

Robot Positioning and Docking

The robot is docked to the patient immediately if there are no adhesions or there is a sufficient distance from the adhesions to safely visualize and move within the peritoneal cavity. A 10 mm Intuitive robotic camera positioned 30° up is used. The lysis of adhesions is performed with sharp and blunt dissection using limited electrocautery or ultrasonic devices. Robotic instrumentation used for the adhesiolysis is typically the 8 mm monopolar shears. After reduction of the hernia contents, the peritoneal sac is generally left in place. The hernia defect is measured, and an appropriately sized prosthetic mesh designed for intra-abdominal use is prepared to overlap all margins of the defect or defects by 5 cm prior to primary closure of the fascial defect.

If the defect is midline, the robot can be docked at 90° to the bed from the opposite side of the trocar placement. If the defect favors a particular side, the robot is docked from that side with trocars placed on the opposite side as the defect. It is important to be familiar with the setup of the da Vinci Robot and to approximate the ideal placement of the trocars so as to obtain the optimal range of motion for repair of larger ventral hernias. Depending on the location of the ventral hernia, all efforts should be made to position the robotic camera and trocars as far away from the fascial defect as possible. Considerations for port placement must be made to accommodate the 3–5 cm overlap of mesh and fascia. In general, a 10–15 cm circumferential circle can be drawn around the edge of the fascial defect. The robotic

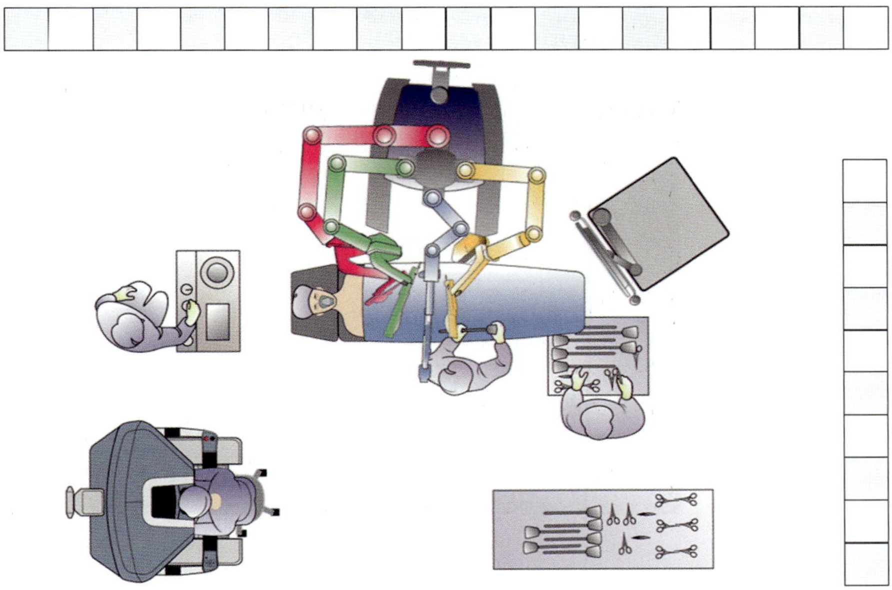

Fig. 28.1 Patient positioning and room setup for robotic ventral hernia repair

trocars can then be placed anywhere along the semicircle outline as long as they are 8 cm apart from one another along a perpendicular line to the axis of the robot and the hernia (see Fig. 28.2).

As the external arms of the robot typically articulate down with this repair, a docking approach over the head or pelvis will be inadequate for arm movement. Optimally, one should keep the side of the bed elevated where the trocars insert to insure proper movement of the robotic arms. The cart comes in directly in line with the defect and the camera port. Also, a utility port should be placed at the start of the operation for delivering the mesh into the abdomen; however, a utility port is not necessary for most patients. The location of the robot cart must also accommodate the bed, anesthesiologist, and bony prominences, such as the shoulder and anterior superior iliac spine, which may limit the range of motion. In addition, the trocars should be placed at the most extreme lateral, cranial, and caudal positions that will still allow anterior work without interfering with the bed, anesthesiologist, and bony prominences. The most lateral possible position of the

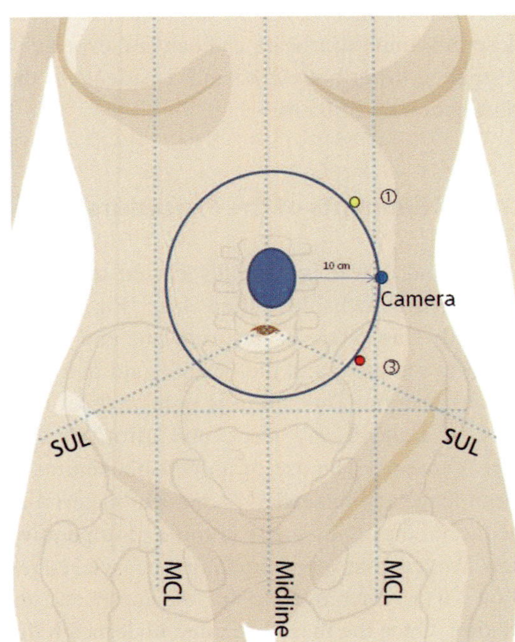

Fig. 28.2 Typical port placement along a 10 cm circumferential circle drawn around the primary ventral abdominal wall defect

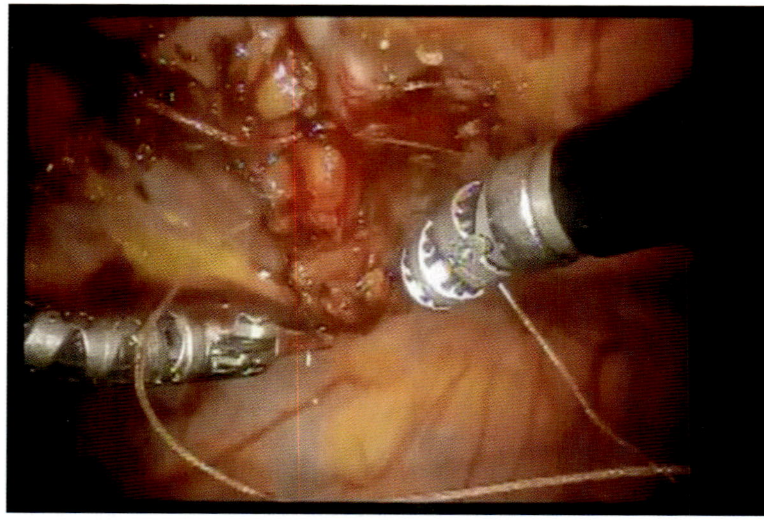

Fig. 28.3 The primary defect is closed primarily

two instrument arms will allow the most range of motion and anterior abdominal wall suturing. The extremes for instrument length must also be considered prior to trocar placement. The current da Vinci instruments have a 34 cm reach; however, close proximity to trocars and camera, especially in smaller, lower body mass index patients, is the most common difficulty.

Critical Elements of the Procedure

The fascial defect is typically closed using the running 0-absorbable suture (see Fig. 28.3). Typically this suture is run from one end of the defect to the other and then back again in a continuous fashion. The suture is tightened periodically to remove any slack and afford fascial approximation. The use of absorbable sutures is to not leave any unneeded permanent material in the fascial that could cause chronic postoperative pain. We feel that approximating the fascial edges allows us greater overlap for the mesh and its fixation. Once the mesh is fixated underneath the defect, there is little to no tension on the primary repair; therefore, there is less concern about tension on this repair than if this would be a primary repair alone. Nonetheless, it is not our main concern if the primary closure does not hold completely or not since there will be an underlay of mesh to prevent the hernia recurrence. Simply put, the primary repair is to allow greater overlap and additional security to the repair.

Once the fascial defect is closed, the mesh is positioned superiorly and inferiorly as it was outside the abdomen, and a spinal needle is inserted at each marked point through the abdominal wall for verification of correct placement. A strong, permanent suture already fixated at the 12 o'clock and 6 o'clock positions of the mesh is then used to circumferentially suture the mesh to the abdominal wall taking care to take bites of the posterior fascia with each pass (see Fig. 28.4). These bites are full thickness through the posterior fascia and into the abdominal wall musculature. While the musculature does not add to the overall strength of the fixation, it is important to know that full-thickness purchases of the fascial are being obtained. Care must be taken not to acquire too big of a bite through the muscle because this may cause undue pain with little gain in repair strength. If the defect is below the arcuate line, one must obtain transversalis fascia with each bite. The suturing is started at the 12 o'clock position on the mesh, run to the 6 o'clock position, and then back to the 12 o'clock (see Fig. 28.5). It is easiest to

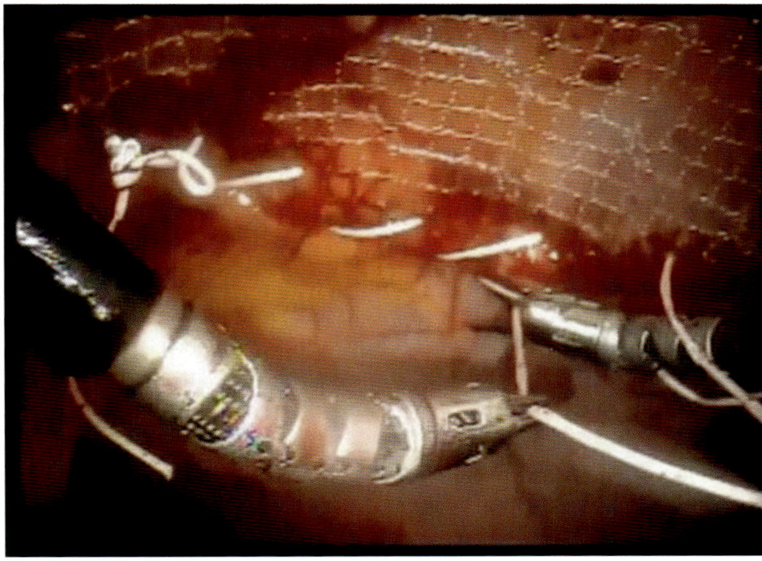

Fig. 28.4 The mesh is sewn in place with a continuous, running, nonabsorbable suture using "baseball" stitch conformity

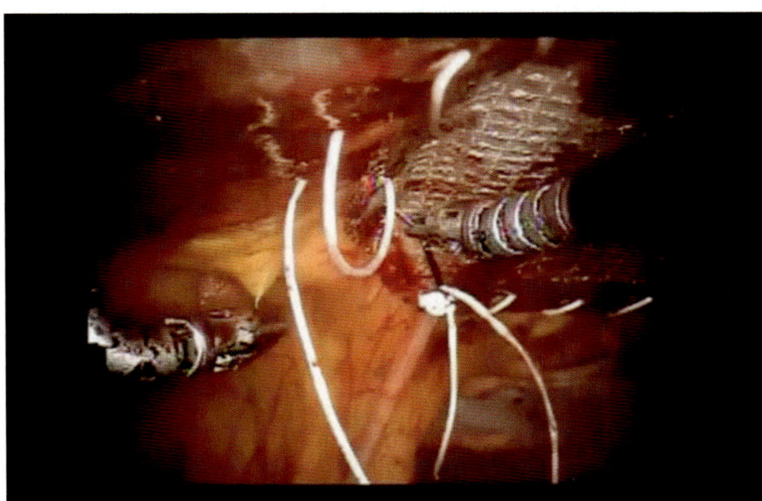

Fig. 28.5 The suture is run to each corner of the next suture and tied to its tail to secure the running suture and mesh

start on the side of the mesh that is furthest away from the camera. That is, if your ports are on the patient's left side, the entire right side of the mesh is sewn first. Once the suture from the 12 o'clock position is run to the 6 o'clock position and tied to the next suture, the left side of the mesh, closest to the camera, is run back up to the 12 o'clock position and tied to itself. The suture is kept loose so as not to tighten the mesh closely against the abdominal wall until the opposite suture is again started in a similar manner.

No trans-fascial or transabdominal sutures are placed. No drain is used. The 12 mm trocar site is then closed with absorbable suture using a suture passer, pneumoperitoneum is released, and the skin is closed.

Hybrid Versus Totally Robotic Approach

The robotic assisted ventral hernia repair should be considered a hybrid technique unless the hernia is a primary defect with no adhesions or contents to reduce. In this case, all sutures and mesh can be placed before docking and the case can be completed with one dock. It may be necessary at times, however, to perform lysis of adhesions laparoscopically or robotically and close the defect, at which time the robot is undocked to assess the size and shape of mesh to be used on the defect. In these particular cases, the arms are simply lifted off the trocars for measurement and placement of the mesh. The robot does not need to be moved away from the bedside.

Discussion of Advantages, Limitations, and Relative Contraindications

Laparoscopic ventral hernia repair was introduced in the 1990s and since has gained wide acceptance [8, 9]. With published data showing recurrence rates equal or less than the open mesh repair, fewer complications, shorter operative times, and decreased lengths of stay [16, 22, 23], it has become a readily used tool in the general surgeon's arsenal. In the robotic technique for ventral hernia repair, the surgeon must adopt standard robotic port placement to safely and successfully perform intracorporeal suturing of the fascial defect and mesh fixation with circumferential fascial fixation. The da Vinci Robot has been shown to have advantages over standard laparoscopy for suturing because of its instrument's six degrees of freedom with the EndoWrist that utilizes intra-abdominal articulations and true 3D imaging. This makes this device the ideal tool for intracorporeal suturing of mesh to the posterior layer of the anterior abdominal wall for ventral hernia repair. In addition, there is less abdominal wall trauma and postoperative pain at the working trocar ports as the fulcrum is not entirely at the abdominal wall but at the EndoWrist instruments.

The robot-assisted intracorporeal suturing technique adds numerous advantages to the standard technique for laparoscopic ventral hernia repair. While previous reports have confirmed the need to suture the mesh at 2–5 cm intervals [12–14] as a means of reducing the recurrence rates associated with laparoscopic hernia repairs, we feel that continuous circumferential suturing applies those principles while evenly distributing the tension throughout the mesh. Mesh fixation with tacking alone has been associated with higher recurrence rates [14, 24]. Transabdominal sutures and tackers are often placed using measurements and fascial defect approximation without direct visualization of the edge of the fascial defect. This method can result in incorrect placement and increases the risk of recurrences. The robotic technique places the approximated fascial defect edges in the middle of the mesh, thus maximizing the overlap of the mesh.

The transabdominal sutures and tackers have been directly related to severe postoperative pain that lasts for months [11–13, 18, 25]. The pain is attributed to direct trauma, nerve impingement, and soft tissue entrapment. Patients may require repeated local injections and occasionally readmission for pain control [12, 13]. In our experience, the major source of pain has not been tackers as much as transabdominal sutures. This has lead to multiple patients requiring prolonged pain medication, frequent injections, and even a surgery to remove the suture. Complications associated with tackers usually result from them being misplaced or incompletely placed. They may dislodge, increasing the formation of adhesions directly to the tack and under surface of the mesh. Exposed mesh has also been associated with bowel erosion. This technique has a potential risk for future small bowel obstruction and septic complications in the presence of a prosthetic mesh. Our technique for the robot-assisted laparoscopic repair of ventral hernia using intracorporeal suturing allows for stable suture fixation under direct visualization and eliminates the need for tackers because a running suture is used for circumferential fixation. The entire repair is performed under direct visualization, with precise placement and confirmation of depth into the posterior fascia for all sutures placed. The fascial sutures encompass 1 cm bites of fascia, minimizing trauma to the abdominal wall.

Intracorporeal suturing of the fascia allows the midline to be re-approximated allowing for possible primary repair, more physiologic abdominal wall movement, and greater overlap of the mesh to the defect fascial edges. Slick, nonabsorbable sutures were used to minimize adhesion formation and provide adequate strength for a lasting repair without slippage of the mesh. In addition, this suture is easy to handle in the abdomen and slides through the mesh allowing ease of tightening the suture along the circumference of the mesh. Robot-assisted laparoscopic ventral hernia repair offers yet another advantage by providing the suturing option under excellent visualization for the repair of difficult hernias with bony or muscular margins, such as lumbar, suprapubic, and subcostal hernias. Several of our patients had hernias on or near lateral borders of the abdomen making mesh fixation with tackers difficult. This allows the surgeon to take very precise bites of tissue to anchor the mesh repair.

Limitations of this robot-assisted technique are obvious for large ventral hernias as they approach the working ports and camera, making this technique technically challenging. In addition, obese patients pose a challenge preoperatively because it may be difficult to determine the ideal trocar placement.

Outcomes Review

Between 2009 and 2011, these authors had a person experience with this procedure, and we performed a retrospective review of 15 patients who underwent robotic-assisted ventral hernia repair with intracorporeal, primary closure of fascial defects with a running 0-absorbable suture, followed by underlay mesh fixation using a continuous running, circumferential, nonabsorbable suture. Standard laparoscopic ventral hernias were also performed during this time, but were not directly compared in a prospective fashion. Data for age, gender, body mass index, American Society of Anesthesiologists (ASA) score, previous abdominal operations, size and number of defects, ability to close defect primarily and type of suture used, size and type of prosthetic mesh implanted including suture used for circumferential suturing, operative time, laparoscopic time, robotic docking time, robotic console time, anesthesia time, estimated blood loss, number of trocars required to complete surgery, length of hospital stay, operative and postoperative complications, hernia recurrences, and duration of follow-up were collected. American Society of Anesthesiologists (ASA) score over 3 and/or fascial defects larger than 15 cm in any one dimension assessed by clinical, radiology, or diagnostic laparoscopy were not repaired using robotic technique and therefore are not reported here.

Of the 15 patients, all had robotic-assisted ventral hernia repair and were available for follow-up. All the fascial defects were closed primarily before the mesh repair. Median follow-up time was 23 months (range 2–33 months). Five had a BMI greater than 30 kg/m^2, mean 31.53 (range 27–41.65). The mean ASA score was 2.4. All but two patients (86 %) had previous surgery; however, no one had previous attempts at hernia repair. Most hernias were in or near the midline. Multiple defects were found in five of the patients (33 %). The mean fascial defect size was 37.39 cm^2 (range 6.28–117.75 cm^2). The mean operative time was 114±21 min and console time was 74±16 min (range 42–143). The mean length of hospital stay was 2.4±1.1 days (range 0.25–10). None of the patients required conversion to open or traditional handheld laparoscopic technique after the initial trocar insertion. There were no mortalities.

One patient required a prolonged hospital stay (6 days) for pain control, and one patient had both prolonged hospital stay (10 days) for pain control and postoperative urinary retention. Since there was no comparative laparoscopic arm, subjective patient pain scales or narcotic usage was not measured specifically within the retrospectively reviewed group. There were no seromas, prolonged ileus, or infections of the mesh or wound reported in this series. There was one recurrence diagnosed by physical exam. This recurrence was from the patient with a lumbar hernia that presented many difficult challenges with regard to port placement, patient positioning, mesh placement, and fascial closure.

The average time for robot-assisted laparoscopic ventral hernia repair using intracorporeal sutures (114 min) seems to be comparable to the times reported in the literature for standard laparoscopic ventral hernia repair and previous robotic ventral hernia repair in pig models [2, 12–14]. Our series included lysis of adhesions of the anterior abdominal wall while maintaining a comparable time to a previous report of robotic ventral hernia in pigs without adhesions. The sizes of the defects in this study (6–118 cm^2) were comparable to those reported for standard laparoscopic repair [12, 13, 25].

Conclusion

The robotic-assisted ventral hernia technique is feasible and may reduce postoperative pain by eliminating trans-fascial sutures. Further evaluation is needed and long-term data is lacking to assess the benefit to the patient, but future studies are investigating this very thing. Randomized prospective trials to compare robotic versus laparoscopic ventral hernia repair where operative time, hospital stays, objective measurements of postoperative pain, chronic pain, and hernia recurrence are measured. A study like this would be more appropriately poised to answer the question: is a robotic ventral hernia repair better than a laparoscopic repair? What is certain at this time is that robotic ventral hernia is feasible and safe and appears to be highly effective.

References

1. Mudge M, Hughes LE. Incisional hernia: a 10-year prospective study of incidence and attitudes. Br J Surg. 1985;72:70–1.
2. Schluender S, Conrad J, Divino CM, et al. Robot-assisted laparoscopic repair of ventral hernia with intracorporeal suturing. Surg Endosc. 2003;17: 1391–5.
3. LeBlanc KA, Heniford BT, Voeller GR. Innovations in ventral hernia repair. Contemp Surg. 2006: 1–8
4. Van der Linden FT, Van Vroonhoven TJ. Long-term results after surgical correction of incisional hernia. Neth J Surg. 1988;40:127–9.
5. Stoppa RE. The treatment of complicated groin and incisional hernia. World J Surg. 1989;13:545–54.
6. Laber GE, Garb JL, Alexander AI, et al. Long-term complications associated with prosthetic repair of ventral hernias. Arch Surg. 1998;133:378–82.
7. White TJ, Santos MC, Thompson JS. Factors affecting wound complications in repair of ventral hernias. Am Surg. 1998;64:276–80.
8. Heniford BT, Park A, Ramshaw BJ, et al. Laparoscopic repair of ventral hernias: nine years' experience with 850 consecutive hernias. Ann Surg. 2003;238:391–400.
9. Perrone JM, Soper NJ, Eagon JC, et al. Perioperative outcomes and complications of laparoscopic ventral hernia repair. Surgery. 2005;138:708–15.
10. Carbajo MA, Martin del Olmo JC, Blanco JI, et al. Laparoscopic treatment vs open surgery in the solution of major incisional and abdominal wall hernias with mesh. Surg Endosc. 1999;13:250–2.
11. Franklin ME, Dorman JP, Glass JL, et al. Laparoscopic ventral and incisional hernia repair. Surg Laparosc Endosc. 1998;8:294–9.
12. Heniford BT, Ramshaw BJ. Laparoscopic ventral hernia repair: a report of 100 consecutive cases. Surg Endosc. 2000;14:419–23.
13. Heniford BT, Park A, Ramshaw BJ, et al. Laparoscopic ventral and incisional hernia repair in 407 patients. J Am Coll Surg. 2000;190:645–50.
14. Sanders LM, Flint LM, Ferrara JJ. Initial experience with laparoscopic repair of incisional hernias. Am J Surg. 1999;177:227–31.
15. Earle D, Seymour N, Fellinger E, et al. Laparoscopic versus open incisional hernia repair: a single-institution analysis of hospital resource utilization for 884 consecutive cases. Surg Endosc. 2006;20:71–5.
16. Harrell AG, Novitsky YW, Peindl RD, et al. Prospective evaluation of adhesion formation and shrinkage of intra-abdominal prosthetics in a rabbit model. Am Surg. 2006;72:808–13.
17. McKinlay RD, Park A. Laparoscopic ventral incisional hernia repair: a more effective alternative to conventional repair of recurrent incisional hernia. J Gastrointest Surg. 2004;8:670–4.
18. Berger D, Bientzle M, Muller A. Postoperative complications after laparoscopic incisional hernia repair. Surg Endosc. 2002;16:1720–3.
19. Bansal VK, Misra MC, et al. A prospective randomized study comparing suture mesh fixation versus tacker mesh fixation for laparoscopic repair of incisional and ventral hernias. Surg Endosc. 2011;25(5):1431–8.
20. Tayar C, Karoui M, Cherqui D, et al. Robot-assisted laparoscopic mesh repair of incisional hernias with exclusive intracorporeal suturing: a pilot study. Surg Endosc. 2007;21(10):1786–9.

21. Ballantyne GH, Hourmont K, Wasielewski A. Telerobotic laparoscopic repair of incisional ventral hernias using intraperitoneal prosthetic mesh. JSLS. 2003;7(1):7–14.
22. Dubay DA, Wang X, Kirk S, et al. Fascial fibroblast kinetic activity is increased during abdominal wall repair compared to dermal fibroblasts. Wound Repair Regen. 2004;12:539–45.
23. Giulianotti PC, Coratti A, Angelini M, Sbrana F, et al. Robotics in general surgery: personal experience in a large community hospital. Arch Surg. 2003;138:777–8.
24. LeBlanc KA, Booth WV. Laparoscopic repair of incisional abdominal hernias using expanded polytetrafluoroethylene: preliminary findings. Surg Laparosc Endosc. 1993;3:39–41.
25. LeBlanc KA. The critical technical aspects of laparoscopic repair of ventral and incisional hernias. Am Surg. 2001;67:809–12.

Part XI

Surgical Techniques: *Pediatric*

Pediatric Robotic Surgery

29

John J. Meehan

General Considerations

Most surgical equipment is designed for adults. Pediatric surgeons need to find ways of making the adult equipment and instrumentation fit in the world of pediatric surgery. The da Vinci robotics was no exception and was never designed with children in mind. Since the start of the robotic era, very little has been done to redesign or add technology for kids. Pediatric surgeons are forced to find unique ways to make this technology work in children. Despite the daunting size of this 500 kg robot next to a 5 kg infant, many simple adjustments can be made in order to accommodate the da Vinci system for minimally invasive procedures in children.

The first step in determining whether a pediatric procedure is possible with the da Vinci is to consider the diagnosis and anatomy in relation to the potential working region. Procedures, which concentrate in a focused location have the highest probability of success. Procedures that may need to sweep from one quadrant of a cavity to an opposite quadrant may need further consideration. Utilizing a hybrid approach incorporating laparoscopy or even an open segment of an operation may be appropriate for some procedures. Careful planning also must include ideal patient positioning, trocar placement, and trocar depth. Discussing the envisioned progress of the case with all team members including anesthesia ahead of time can help avoid difficulties later in the procedure.

Positioning

With a height of about 6 ft, the current robot appears enormous hovering over a small child. Access to patients becomes limited. The robotic arms must have adequate clearance in regard not only to the patient but also to the OR table and in relation to the other robotic arms. In order to avoid instrument arm to OR table collisions, we recommend elevating the smaller patients using foam padding (Fig. 29.1).

This allows the robot arms a greater range of motion external to the patient as the arms of the robot are less likely to collide with the OR table. Raising the patient off the main OR table with a compressible pad also affords better access to the patient for the bedside assistant and anesthesiologist. We routinely place children 10 kg or less on two foam eggcrate style pads and one foam pad for children between 10 and 20 kg in size. Larger children are usually fine without additional elevation. An important additional consideration is assuring adequate clearance of the external robot arms over the patient. Serious injury could occur if the robotic arms torque down onto a patient unchecked. We prefer placing a solid barrier securely mounted to the OR table to help protect the patient. An example is shown in Fig. 29.2.

J.J. Meehan, M.D., F.A.C.S. (✉)
University of Washington School of Medicine, Seattle Children's Hospital, 4800 Sand Point Way NE, Seattle, WA 98105, USA
e-mail: John.meehan@seattlechildrens.org

K.C. Kim (ed.), *Robotics in General Surgery*, DOI 10.1007/978-1-4614-8739-5_29,

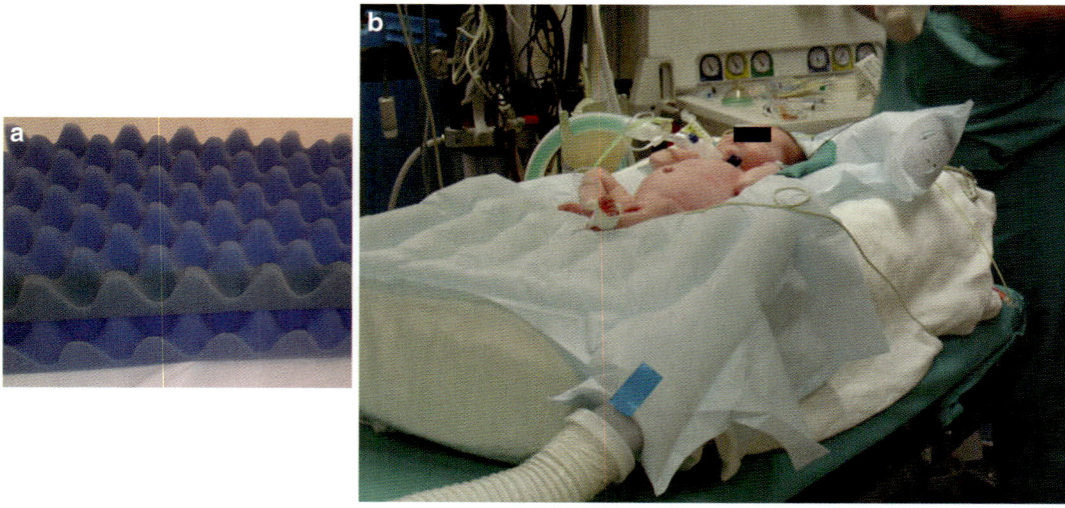

Fig. 29.1 Foam padding (**a**) helps elevate the small patients off of the table which aids in gaining adequate access to the child during a robotic procedure (**b**)

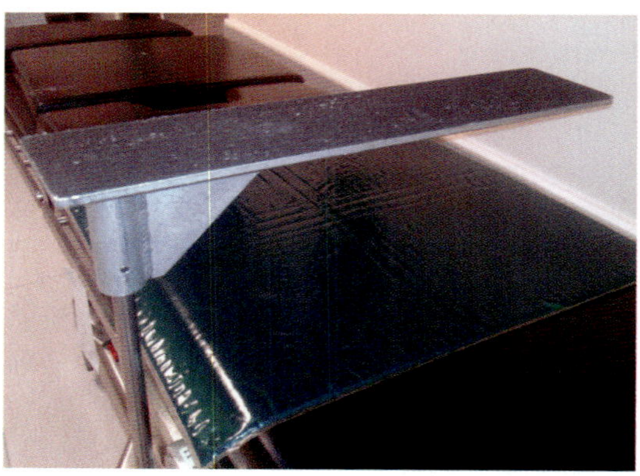

Fig. 29.2 A table-mounted barrier is helpful to prevent the large robotic arms from making contact with the patient

Trocar Location

Trocar placement in robotic procedures may not be the same as trocar placement in standard MIS procedures. In standard MIS, ergonomic issues influence how far apart the surgeon may place the trocars. Sites that are too lateral will cause shoulder and neck discomfort for the operating surgeon and can make an otherwise easy case somewhat tedious and physically taxing. However, the ergonomic concerns are eliminated in robotic surgery. Trocars placed too close together create a new problem, namely, robotic arm collisions. In fact, making the robot trocars further apart can reduce robot arm external collisions. But this benefit is only good up to a certain point; if the trocars are too far apart, they may be approaching the target at too shallow of an angle and the external arm could make contact with the patient or the OR table.

Trocar Depth

Available working space for the da Vinci robotic instruments is limited by the minimum requirements that are needed for instrument articulation. While this is almost never a problem in adult surgery, this can be an enormous issue in the abdomen of a small child. The remote center of the robotic trocar is the point in three-dimensional space in which the robot arm will pivot around. This location is represented on the da Vinci robotic trocar with a thick black line (Fig. 29.3).

The distance from remote center to end of trocar is a set length at a distance of 2.90 cm. The manufacturer recommends that the robotic trocar is inserted inside the patient such that the remote center is placed just at the inside edge of the body cavity. Therefore, 2.90 cm of trocar length should

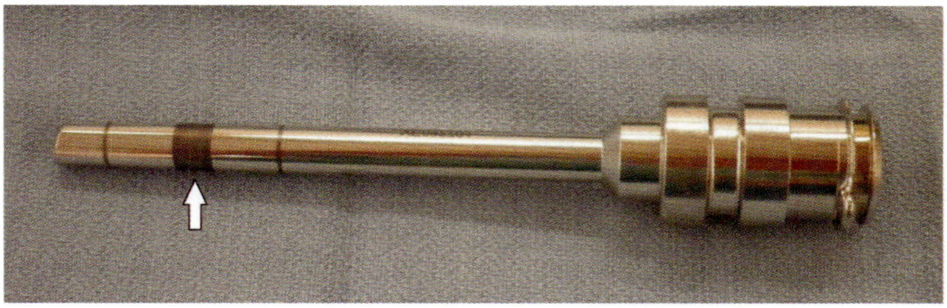

Fig. 29.3 The da Vinci 5 mm robotic trocar demonstrating the remote center (*arrow*)

be inside the patient. Next, we must consider the articulating instrument. The shortest 5 mm da Vinci instrument is the needle driver. Measuring the needle driver from the tip of the instrument to the most proximal articulating joint is a distance of 2.71 cm. Adding this distance to the articulating length yields a minimum distance of 5.61 cm. In other words, the target organ must be a minimum of 5.61 cm away from the abdominal or chest wall. Other instruments are even longer. In small children, this distance is considerable and the amount of usable working space beyond this minimum distance can disappear quickly.

However, there is a potential adjustment which may allow for a little additional room in selected patients. Although the remote center marking on the da Vinci trocar was originally intended to be visible just inside the patient, we can adjust the trocar so it is just outside the patient instead. The entire abdominal or thoracic wall of small children may only be 1 cm. Therefore, by routinely extracting the trocar back such that the remote center is positioned just outside the patient instead of just inside the patient, we can effectively increase our workable domain and potentially improve instrument maneuverability. We have found that this simple adjustment can have tremendous impact on our ability to perform a procedure.

Scope

While the optics of the 3D system has been a huge advantage for robotic surgery, it has also uncovered some limitations due to the diameter. The 12 mm 3D da Vinci scope is essentially two 5 mm scopes down the shaft of a single scope. But this 12 mm 3D scope simply will not fit in the intercostal space of smaller children and is huge for abdominal procedures in neonates. In 2005, Intuitive released a 5 mm 2D scope for use with the da Vinci Standard robot. This 5 mm scope was a key improvement even though it was only a 2D system. The 5 mm camera paved the initial wave of neonatal cases and allowed robotic neonatal surgery to flourish for a few years. Numerous neonatal congenital anomalies were repaired robotically for the first time in both the abdomen and the chest. These procedures included duodenal atresia repairs in children as young as one day of age and a CDH repair in a 2.2 kg 6-day-old baby [1, 2]. Pulmonary lobectomies for congenital cystic adenomatoid malformation (CCAM) and pulmonary sequestration were also now possible [3]. We also performed the first EA-TEF repair with da Vinci system in 2007 although this was unpublished. Neonatal robotic surgery was off to a flying start.

There is no question that the 5 mm 2D scope opened up a tremendous variety of potential robotic cases. Eventually, the 8.5 mm 3D scope came available and is now available in HD. However, the 8.5 mm can be a bit too large for the intercostal space in some neonates. The 5 mm 2D scope still had a significant place in the pediatric robotic theater. Unfortunately, this 5 mm scope was only made for the Standard and S systems. Once the Si system was unveiled, Intuitive Surgical announced that they would not make a compatible scope with the Si new platform. Shortly thereafter, the company discontinued support of the 5 mm 2D scope entirely (Fig. 29.4).

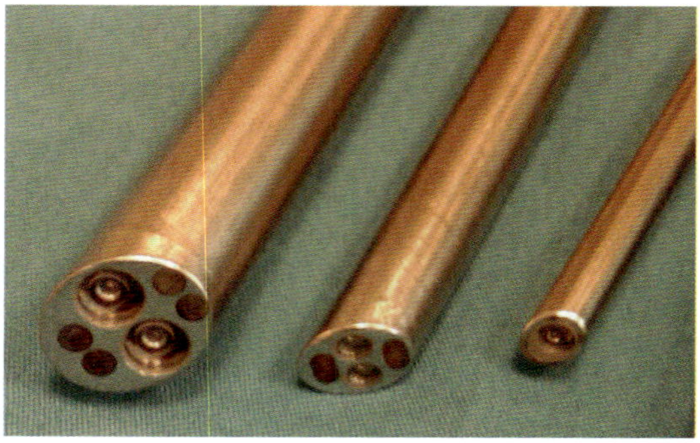

Fig. 29.4 A comparison between the original robotic scopes for the Standard da Vinci camera. (*left*, 12 mm 3D; *middle*, 8.5 mm 3D; *right*, 5 mm 2D). The 5 mm 2D scope is no longer manufactured

Instruments

The 8 mm platform was launched in 2001. Smaller diameter instruments were made available in 2005 with the release of the 5 mm instruments. The smaller diameter was welcomed by pediatric surgeons who had already become accustomed to using 5 and 3 mm laparoscopic instruments. The 5 mm robotic instrument is a reasonable instrument diameter for small children. But these 5 mm instruments are not without a new limitation: the articulating length is longer than the 8 mm counterpart. As discussed in the preceding sections, trocar depth can be adjusted to offset this problem. Another disadvantage of the 5 mm instruments is that selection is exceedingly limited with only a few types of 5 mm instruments being made. As of the beginning of 2013, the 5 mm instrument product line has gone essentially unchanged with almost no new instrument choices or improvements.

The 4th Arm

The da Vinci system has an option for an additional instrument arm. While potentially useful in adults or larger children, the neighboring space external to a small child or neonate is already limited and the additional arm may add additional constraints. Although we occasionally use the 4th arm for a handful of procedures, the robot's current large size limits its usefulness in children. We consider using the 4th arm if the child is greater than 20 kg. The one exception is the choledochal cyst resection with Roux-en-Y reconstruction. We will describe that case later in this chapter.

Specific Pediatric Procedures

Table 29.1 lists all of the robotic procedures we have performed in children.

The list is quite extensive which demonstrates the diversity of the surgical problems in pediatric patients. Many of these procedures such as cholecystectomy, Heller myotomy, adrenalectomy, splenectomy, and colon resections are similar to adult procedures and are discussed in detail elsewhere in this text. Pediatric urology is covered elsewhere as well. Describing the details of all of the procedures in this list is a book in itself so we will concentrate on selected cases that are ideal robotic pediatric operations or deserve special mention. Following the pediatric principles and adjustments outlined in the preceding sections can help a surgeon adequately plan for nearly any pediatric robotic procedure.

Fundoplication

The fundoplication is a key procedure in the training of a pediatric surgeon new to robotics. Along with the cholecystectomy, the fundoplication is a familiar laparoscopic procedure and is one of the most common operations in pediatric general surgery. Therefore, we must emphasize that the fundoplication is an important procedure in understanding the subtle differences between robotic surgery and laparoscopic surgery and will help a new robotic surgeon learn the basics before moving on to more complex procedures.

Most pediatric fundoplications are performed via the transabdominal approach, and the Nissen fundoplication is the most common fundoplication [4]. Other less common fundoplications are the Toupet and Thal partial wraps. The choice for the type of fundoplication is the surgeon's preference, but all have been shown to be effective [5].

Table 29.1 Pediatric robotic procedures: a comprehensive list of procedures we have performed using the da Vinci surgical robot

- Abdomen
  - Cholecystectomy
  - Fundoplication
  - Heller myotomy
  - Pyloroplasty
  - Adrenalectomy
  - Neuroblastoma
  - Splenectomy
  - Small bowel resection
    - Crohn's
    - Enteric duplication
    - Meckel's diverticulum
  - Partial colon
    - Left colectomy
    - Ileocecectomy
    - Right colectomy
    - Sigmoid colectomy
  - Total proctocolectomy with pull-through
  - Kasai portoenterostomy
  - Choledochal cyst
  - Duodenal anomalies
    - Duodenal atresia
    - Duodenal web
    - Annular pancreas
  - Ladd's procedure
  - Jejunal or ileal atresia
  - Puestow
  - Gastrotomy with foreign body retrieval
  - Congenital diaphragmatic hernia (Morgagni)
  - Nephrectomy
  - Ovarian cystectomy
  - Ovarian teratoma
  - Urachal remnant
  - Utricle
- Chest
  - Pulmonary resections
    - CCAM
    - Pulmonary sequestration
  - Thymectomy
  - Cystic hygroma
  - Mediastinal masses
    - Congenital anomalies
      - Bronchogenic cyst
      - Esophageal duplication
    - Tumors
      - Ganglioneuroma
      - Neuroblastoma
      - Ganglioneuroblastoma
      - Germ cell tumor
      - Teratoma
- Esophageal atresia with tracheoesophageal fistula
- Congenital diaphragmatic hernia (Bochdalek)
- Eventration of the diaphragm

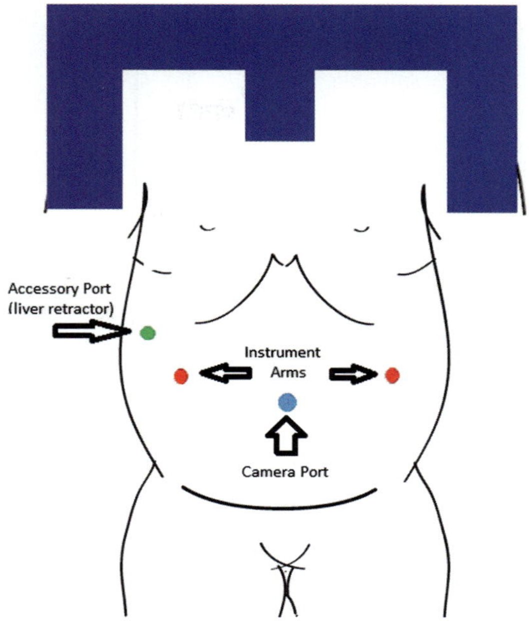

Fig. 29.5 The robotic trocar for a fundoplication. Notice the lateral placement of the working ports, which are more lateral than the standard laparoscopic locations. A 3 or 5 mm retractor port for the liver is placed in the *right upper quadrant*

Laparoscopically, the fundoplication procedure has been performed regularly since the mid-1990s with good results [6]. The learning curve for the laparoscopic approach has been estimated somewhere between 25 and 30 cases [7]. Although many well-trained laparoscopic surgeons will argue about the futility of the robot for this procedure, we have found that it is an excellent training case. More importantly, the learning curve is much shorter, perhaps as short as five cases [8].

Trocar locations are slightly modified from the laparoscopic approach (Fig. 29.5).

While the camera location is still at the umbilicus, the left and right working ports are slightly more lateral in comparison to the laparoscopically placed trocars. The more lateral placement avoids robotic arm collisions between the instrument arms and the camera arm external to the patient. The retracting port for the liver is in the same location as is customarily placed along the patient's right flank. The robot cart is positioned

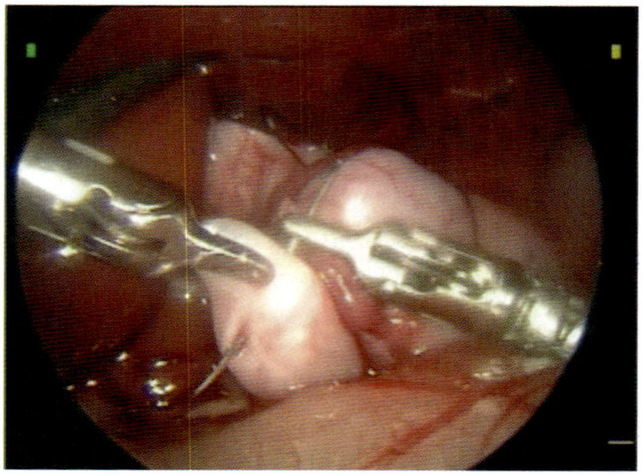

Fig. 29.6 The fundoplication is constructed using interrupted nonabsorbable sutures

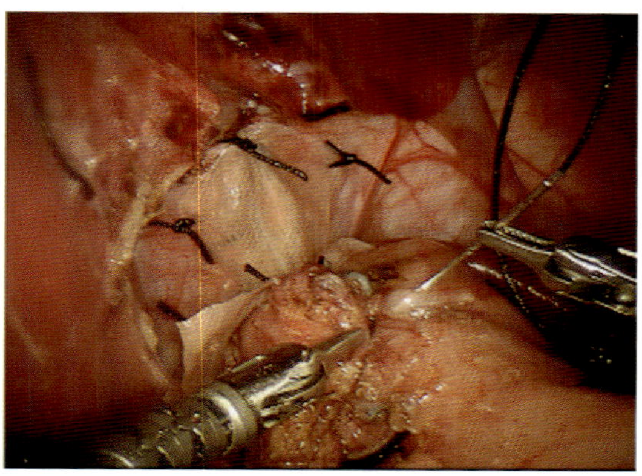

Fig. 29.7 Unable to close the hiatus primarily, patch closure of the large congenital hiatal defect was required prior to this fundoplication

directly over the patient's head. Dissection begins by exposing the hiatus and taking down the short gastric vessels. We prefer both a minimal hiatal dissection as well as a minimizing the number of short gastric we sacrifice. The wrap is constructed with nonabsorbable suture and generally should be at least 3 cm in length (Fig. 29.6).

Suturing the completed wrap to the underside of the diaphragm is optional and we recommend this additional step if the patient had a large hiatal defect that required repair. Occasionally, a patch for a congenital diaphragmatic hiatal hernia may be needed (Fig. 29.7). Results are similar to the laparoscopic approach.

Ladd's Procedure

Malrotation results from a failure of the intestine to return to the abdomen in the proper orientation during embryology. In normal embryogenesis, the bowel has two rotational axes that result in the proper orientation of the bowel. The rotations occur outside the abdominal cavity early in gestation. As the bowel reenters the abdomen, the small bowel becomes fixed along its most proximal segment to form the C-loop of the duodenum, which terminates with the ligament of Treitz. Meanwhile, the large bowel becomes fixed to the retroperitoneum by attachments along the right gutter. Most importantly, the mesentery to the small and large bowel lies in a long fan of mesenteric attachments that extend from the right lower quadrant all the way to the left upper abdomen and the ligament of Treitz. This fixed long fan of mesentery is why normally rotated bowel usually does not twist. However, in malrotation, the mesentery is very narrow. Upon return of the bowel to the abdomen, the small bowel that did not rotate properly usually has the majority of the small bowel off to the right of the abdomen. The duodenal loop never properly forms and the duodenum can often go straight inferiorly instead of making the proper C-loop. The ascending colon is often to the left of the small bowel and duodenum so the retroperitoneal attachments that were supposed to tether the ascending colon to the right gutter now grab onto anything in the right abdomen, usually the small bowel but in a random fashion. These attachment bands are called Ladd's bands in reference to the pediatric surgeon William Ladd who first described the operation that also bears his name [9]. Ultimately, a patient can present with either partial or complete obstruction from these bands, and a chronic condition that is hard to diagnose may exist for years without an upper GI study. The biggest worry, however, is the development of a volvulus. This occurs as a result of the narrow vascular pedicle, and rapid operative intervention is critical before the bowel is lost from ischemia.

The Ladd's procedure has four steps: (1) Detorse the bowel. The volvulus always occurs in a clockwise fashion, and the bowel must be

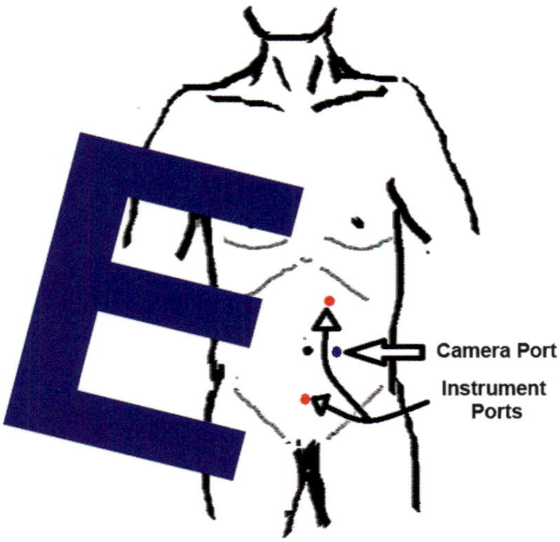

Fig. 29.8 Port locations for the robotic Ladd's procedure

turned counterclockwise until the mesentery is straight (remember the phrase "turn back time"). (2) After the torsion has been reduced, the Ladd's bands are taken down freeing all adhesions. (3) The most important step in reducing the risk of a recurrence is widening the mesentery. The peritoneal surface of narrow pedicle between the duodenum and the ascending colon is incised on one side and the mesentery splayed out in order to widen it. (4) Finally, the appendix in a malrotated patient is never in the right lower quadrant, so an appendectomy is part of the procedure to reduce the possibility of diagnostic confusion if appendicitis ever developed in such a patient.

Malrotation can present with or without volvulus. The patient with malrotation and midgut volvulus is a true surgical emergency, and we do not advocate attempting a minimally invasive procedure in these patients. However, the patient who has chronic abdominal pain or partially obstructive symptoms who is found to have malrotation on upper GI but no evidence of volvulus or acute obstruction may be a good candidate for an elective minimally invasive procedure. Besides children, these patients could also be adults who have a long history of abdominal pain or emesis and have gone through a multitude of doctor visits over the years. The diagnosis is confirmed by an upper GI as stated previously. The robotic trocar locations for a Ladd's procedure are shown in Fig. 29.8.

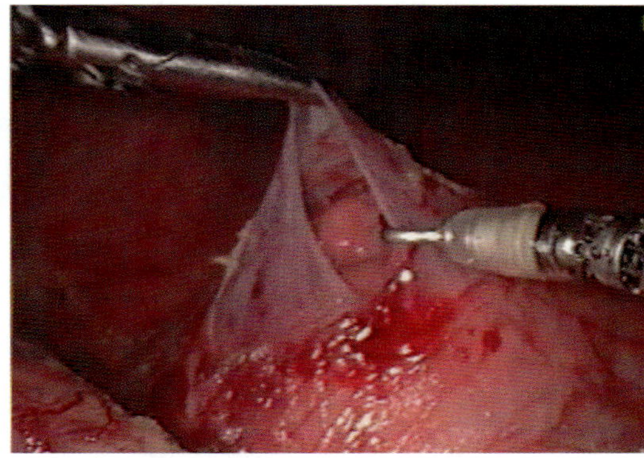

Fig. 29.9 Intraoperative photo of a Ladd's procedure showing the numerous Ladd's bands

The key area of work is the right upper quadrant. Begin by taking down all Ladd's bands, usually starting laterally and working medially (Fig. 29.9). The entire course of the duodenum should be freed along its lateral aspect. On the medial aspect of the duodenum, the anterior sleeve of mesentery is incised longitudinally and blunt dissection is used to widen the mesentery. Finally, the appendix is taken at the conclusion of the procedure.

Kasai Portoenterostomy

Patients with biliary atresia require a Kasai procedure for biliary drainage where a Roux limb of intestine is brought up to the portal plate to facilitate drainage of the bile. The key step in the open Kasai operation is the precise dissection of the portal plate for the best chance of obtaining adequate biliary drainage. This procedure was done laparoscopically for several years, but the results were less than optimal [10]. A voluntary moratorium was placed on the MIS Kasai procedures by the International Pediatric Endoscopic Group (IPEG) at their annual scientific meeting in Buenos Aries in September of 2007 [11]. The lack of precision in the technique was suspected, although some data suggested that CO_2 insufflation may have also played a role [12]. This failure suggests that the Kasai procedure has no margin for error and exposes the deficiencies in standard laparoscopy for a procedure that

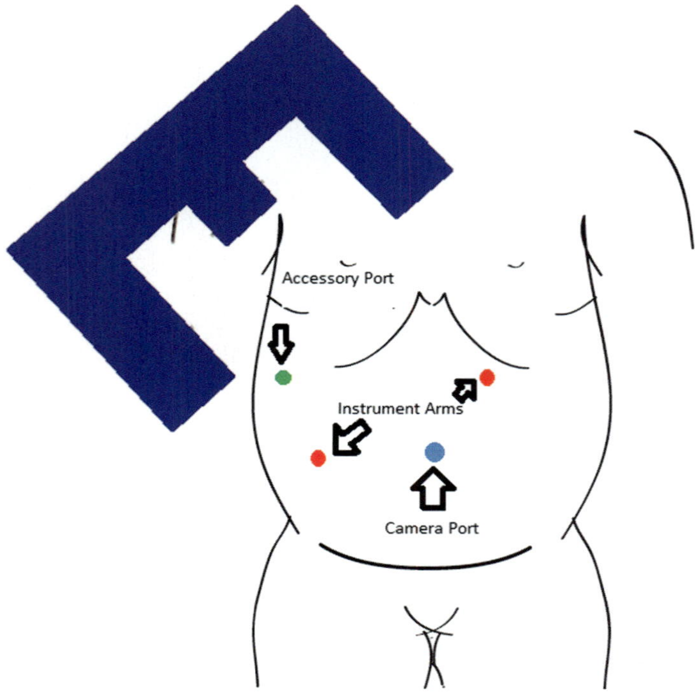

Fig. 29.10 Port locations for the robotic Kasai portoenterostomy. Note that a 12 mm scope is preferred for the Kasai to take advantage of an extracorporeally Roux limb construction. *Note*: This port placement scheme is also used for the duodenal atresia repair except an 8.5 mm scope is preferred for the umbilical camera port

requires precision like the Kasai for biliary atresia. Robotic surgery offers a level of precision and improved optics that may be the solution. The robotic approach allows the surgeon to dissect the portal plate at the appropriate angle and with absolute precision. The port placement for the robotic Kasai is shown in Fig. (29.10).

Despite the small size of these children at 4–8 weeks and usually only about 4 kg, we recommend using the 12 mm scope for the robotic Kasai. This camera size is selected because the neonatal bowel can easily be extruded through a 12 mm umbilical incision to create an extracorporeal Roux-en-Y limb, whereas trying to construct one intracorporeally in such a small child is difficult. The patient is supine in a slight reverse Trendelenburg position and rotated slightly to the left. After gaining access to the abdomen, a cholangiogram should be attempted before the robot is docked to confirm the diagnosis. The rudimentary gallbladder is retracted cephalad to expose the porta hepatis. The remnants of the cystic duct are dissected back to the fibrosed common hepatic and bile ducts. We recommend leaving a portion of the gallbladder attached to the liver bed and to use this as a handle for liver retraction through the remainder of the case. The atretic extrahepatic biliary system is then dissected up to the bifurcation of the portal vein (Fig. 29.11).

It is very important to avoid cauterization at the portal plate as this may inadvertently damage critical biliary drainage channels. The portal plate should be separated from the atretic extrahepatic biliary tissue using the scissors at a precise angle such that potential biliary channels have the highest probability to drain (Fig. 29.12).

After the portal plate has been precisely dissected, the Roux-en-Y jejunojejunostomy is created extracorporeally. The small bowel is marked about 15–20 cm distal to the ligament of Treitz. The robot is then undocked from the trocars and the 12 mm umbilical trocar removed.

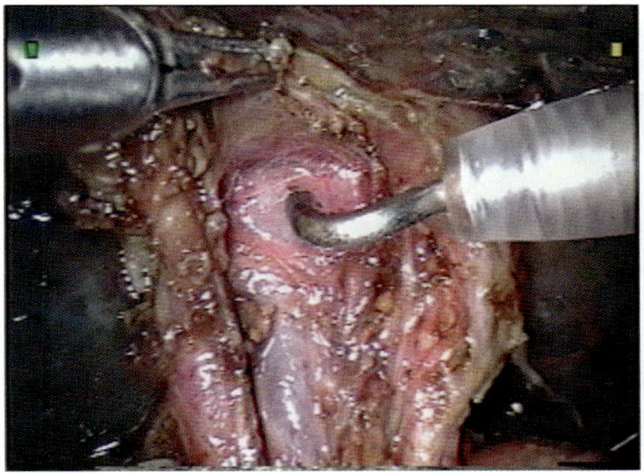

Fig. 29.11 Robotic dissection at the bifurcation of the portal vein and exposure of the portal plate

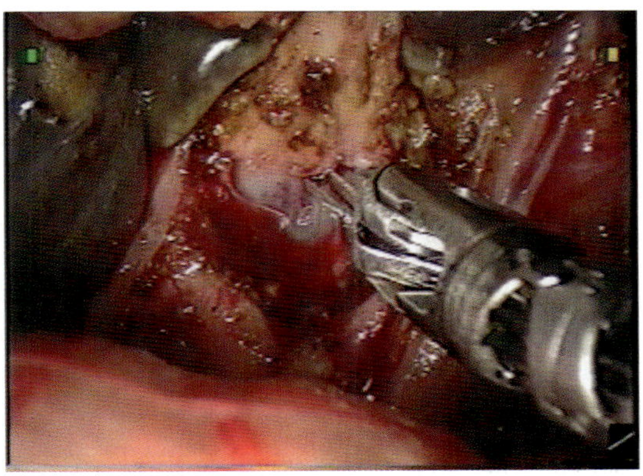

Fig. 29.12 Dissection of the portal plate

The neonatal bowel easily comes through the 12 mm umbilical port with no need to extend the incision. The marked bowel is then brought up through the umbilical wound, and a 30 cm Roux limb is constructed using interrupted absorbable sutures extracorporeally. The Roux limb is then dropped back into the abdomen and the trocar reintroduced and the pneumoperitoneum reestablished. The robot is re-docked to the same trocars and a retrocolic portoenterostomy is created (Fig. 29.13).

We use 4-0 absorbable suture to anchor the anastomosis on each side of the portoenterostomy followed by interrupted 5-0 or 6-0 PDS sutures to complete the anastomosis. Next, the gap in the colonic mesentery where the Roux limb passes is closed to prevent an internal hernia. Finally, the last portions of the rudimentary gallbladder are removed from the liver bed concluding the operation. Initial results are encouraging [13, 14]. A multi-institutional study is needed to investigate if a robotic Kasai procedure is the answer to the MIS approach in neonates with biliary atresia.

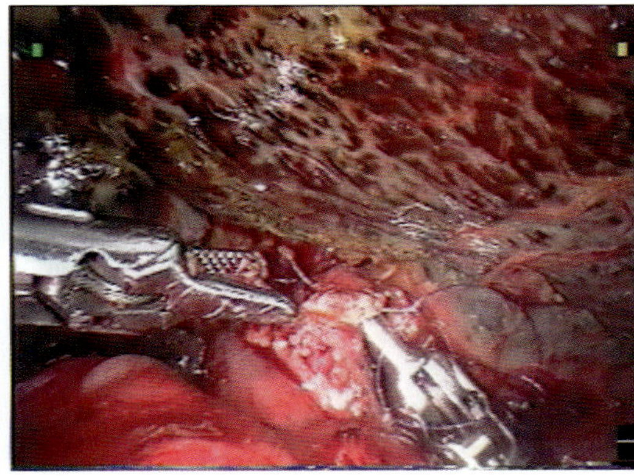

Fig. 29.13 Constructing the hepaticojejunostomy

Choledochal Cyst

The choledochal cyst resection with reconstruction is a complex procedure that is very challenging with standard laparoscopic instruments. The challenging dissection and significant suturing required in the reconstruction make this an ideal robotic case. Choledochal cysts are more prevalent in females and Asian populations [15]. Patients can present with right upper quadrant pain, fever, and jaundice. Ultrasound often demonstrates the cyst, and a CT scan will demonstrate a more detailed anatomical picture for surgical planning. Alternative radiographic images can be obtained from ERCP or MRCP. The age of presentation can be as young as just a few months of age up through young adults. Similar to the Kasai, smaller children may be candidates to have their Roux limb constructed extracorporeally through the 12 mm umbilical port incision if their abdominal wall is thin enough. Larger children may have an abdominal wall that is too thick to allow a Roux limb construction extracorporeally. Intracorporeal Roux limb construction is a better option for these

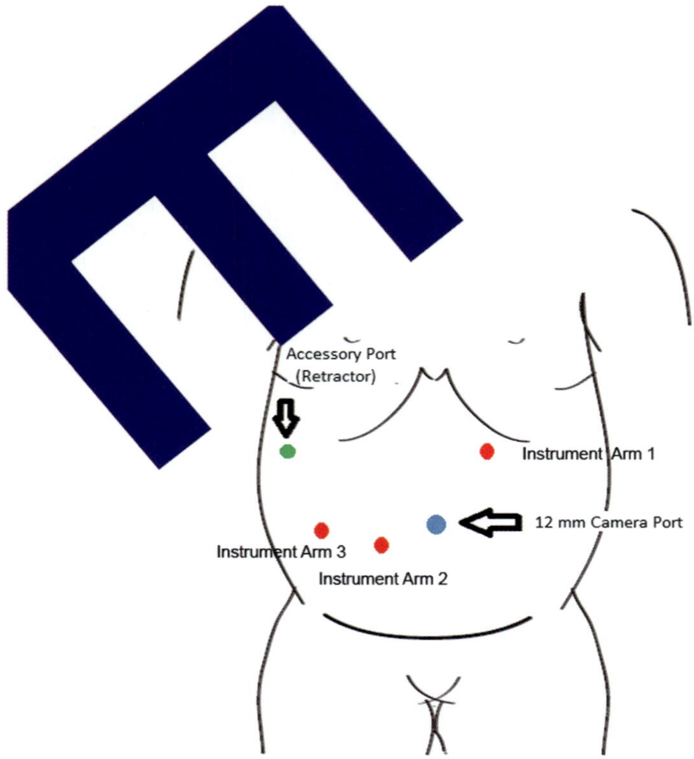

Fig. 29.14 Port locations for the robotic choledochal cyst resection and Roux-en-Y choledochojejunostomy reconstruction

patients, and the robot helps to facilitate this step. Trocar placement is shown in Fig. (29.14).

A cholangiogram can be done at the onset of the procedure prior to robot docking and is generally recommended. If the child is more than 20 kg, we opt for using the 4th arm of the robot to retract the gallbladder upwards to expose the porta hepatis. In smaller children, we find the 4th arm too cumbersome due to the small size of the patient. Retraction of the gallbladder and dissection of the cystic duct is the first task. The cystic duct is identified, ligated, and divided and the dissection carried towards the common bile duct, leaving the gallbladder attached to the liver bed. The gallbladder is used through the remainder of the case as a grasping handle to retract the liver. Once the junction from the cystic duct to common bile duct has been identified, the extrahepatic biliary dissection is performed to fully expose the choledochal cyst (Fig. 29.15).

We sometimes elect to open the cyst on the anterior surface in order to see the back wall better as these cysts are often densely adherent to the portal vein. The biliary tree is dissected proximally to the duodenum as close as possible and ligated. The cyst is then dissected towards the liver until the entire cyst has been isolated. Transection of the common duct cephalad to the cyst completes the resection and reconstruction begins. A Roux-en-Y limb is created as described in the Kasai procedure, and the choledochojejunostomy anastomosis is accomplished with PDS suture (Fig. 29.16).

Preliminary laparoscopic data suggests that reconstruction can be done via a choledochoduodenostomy without the need of a Roux limb [16]. This type of reconstruction significantly shortens the length of time of the case, but long-term data regarding potential complications is lacking.

Duodenal Atresia

The repair of the newborn with duodenal atresia (DA) is a very difficult laparoscopic procedure. Only a few pediatric surgeons routinely

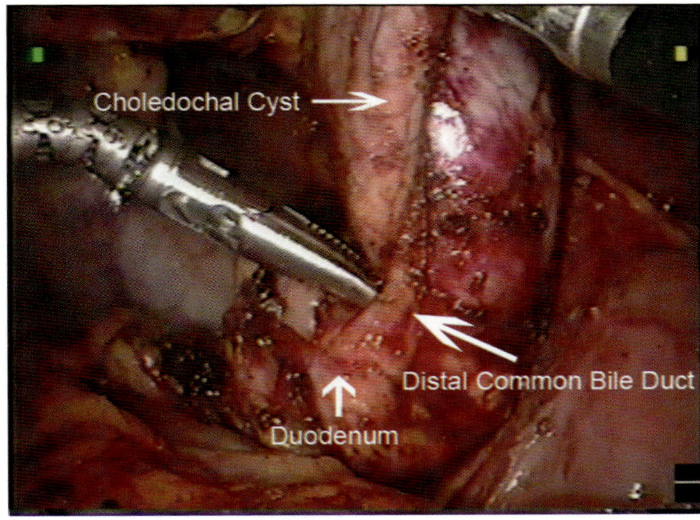

Fig. 29.15 Robotic dissection of the choledochal cyst

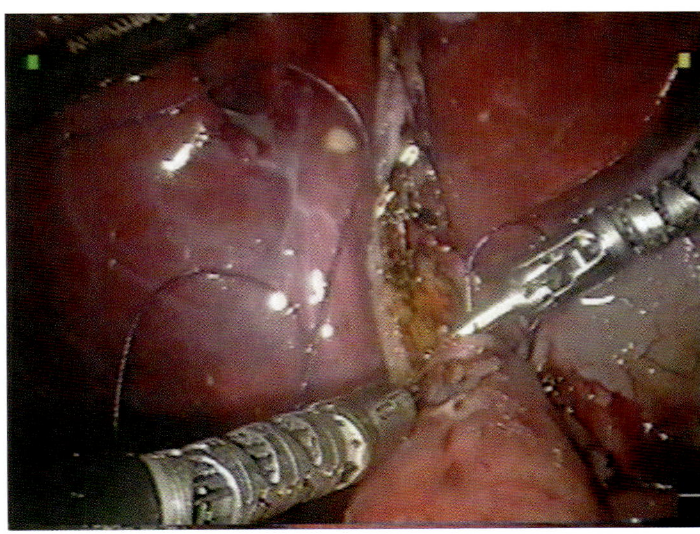

Fig. 29.16 Robotic construction of the Roux-en-Y choledochojejunostomy

perform this procedure using laparoscopic instrumentation simply because the technique is too challenging to suture the small diameter bowel in such a tight space. A novel approach using permanent material has been performed laparoscopically using nitinol U-clips (Medtronic Surgical, Minneapolis, MN, USA), but is not in widespread use [17]. The robot offers the significant suturing advantages. The youngest patient to have robotic surgery was the first duodenal atresia ever performed with the da Vinci robot, a 1-day-old newborn that weighed only 2.4 kg.

With the baby supine in reverse Trendelenburg position and rotated slightly to the left, the trocars are identical as the Kasai arrangement already shown in Fig. (29.10). However, there is no need to use the large 12 mm scope in the duodenal atresia case and we opt for the 8.5 mm scope instead. A 5 mm accessory port is placed on the right flank just above the liver edge and about 1 cm below the costal margin. This port is used to retract the liver with the aid of a fan retractor as necessary or could also be used for a suction device by the bedside assistant once the proximal and distal bowel segments are opened.

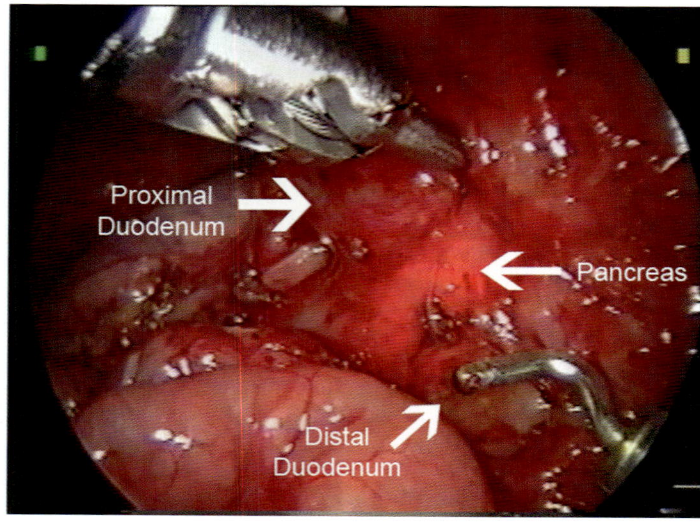

Fig. 29.17 Dissection demonstrating the proximal and distal duodenum in a baby with duodenal atresia. The pancreas is also visible as well as the separation between the two segments of bowel

The 5 mm robotic instrument ports must be strategically placed to allow for adequate internal movement as the patients are often only about 3 kg or less. The robot is brought in over the patient's right shoulder at about a 45° angle. A needle driver or Maryland is used in the surgeon's left hand and the hook cautery in the right hand. The procedure begins by taking down the hepatic flexure of the colon in the right upper quadrant, thereby exposing the duodenum. The dilated proximal duodenum is usually easy to locate, but finding the small distal duodenum may take some time during dissection (Fig. 29.17).

Care should be taken during the dissection to avoid the common bile and pancreatic ducts as they enter the duodenum. This junction could be in either the proximal or distal segment. Once the proximal and distal extents of the duodenum are exposed, the proximal segment is opened transversely and the distal longitudinally. We recommend constructing the duodenal anastomosis in a diamond configuration whenever possible, as described in the open procedure by Kimura [18]. If desired, the anesthesiologist can help pass a small NGT tube into the stomach, which can be fed into the distal bowel and flushed with saline, looking for possible downstream webs or atresias. Interrupted suturing is preferable, but a running locked configuration in short runs is acceptable on the back row. A running suture for the entire length should be avoided as this may encourage a stricture. The front row should be constructed in an interrupted fashion (Fig. 29.18).

Mediastinal Mass

This is a broad category of diagnoses and includes both benign and malignant tumors as well as congenital anomalies. The congenital anomalies include bronchogenic cyst and esophageal duplication. Bronchogenic cysts are often located at the carina but can be in other locations as well. Esophageal duplications can occur anywhere along the tract of the esophagus and may present with dysphagia or reflux. Resection may require reconstruction of the esophageal wall or even a protecting fundoplication if they are located low in the chest. Mediastinal tumors can occur in a number of locations depending on their cell line of origin. The location in either the anterior or posterior mediastinum often helps predict the diagnosis.

The differential diagnosis of a posterior mass includes ganglioneuroma, ganglioneuroblastoma, and neuroblastoma. These tumors arise from the sympathetic chain and may even traverse the diaphragm. Ganglioneuromas are benign tumors that are slow growing or may have arrested in growth completely (Fig. 29.19).

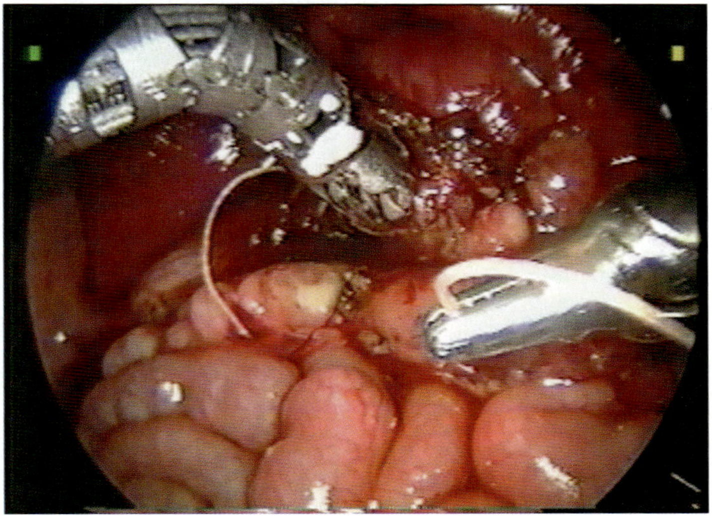

Fig. 29.18 Nearing the end of the diamond duodenoduodenostomy in duodenal atresia. The 5 mm robotic instrument is placed down the narrow distal limb to prevent back-walling the anastomosis

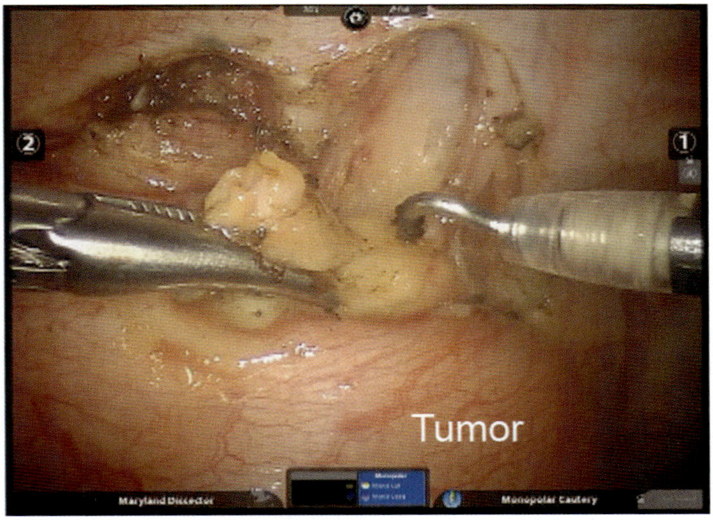

Fig. 29.19 Resection of a ganglioneuroma. The 3D vision of the da Vinci system helps to see how these tumors dive in between the ribs

Primary resection is the only therapy required for these tumors. Neuroblastomas are malignant and can be quite large on initial presentation. Confirming the diagnosis with a biopsy followed by chemotherapy is the best option for large lesions, while smaller lesions may be amenable to a primary resection. Proper staging will include bone marrow aspiration and biopsy, and chemotherapy is tailored based on tumor biology. Ganglioneuroblastomas carry an intermediate classification due to their occasional propensity to recur locally but require primary resection only.

The anterior masses include teratomas, germ cell tumors, and thymomas. Teratomas are more commonly benign and may be asymptomatic for years (Fig. 29.20). However, they can also be malignant, and it is important to draw serum values for alpha fetoprotein (AFP) and beta human chorionic gonadotropin (beta-HCG) levels prior to resection. Elevation of these serum markers is highly suggestive a malignant tumor. Subsequent measurements after resection are helpful to monitor for potential recurrence in patients with malignant teratomas [19]. If the serum levels are normal, the teratomas are almost certainly mature

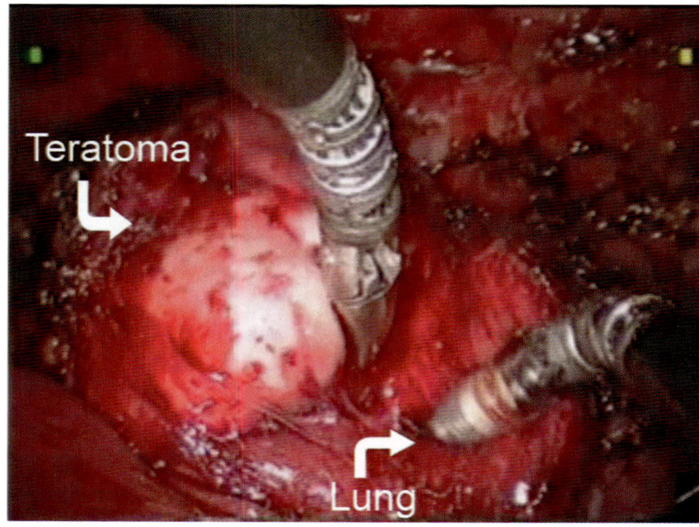

Fig. 29.20 A mediastinal teratoma

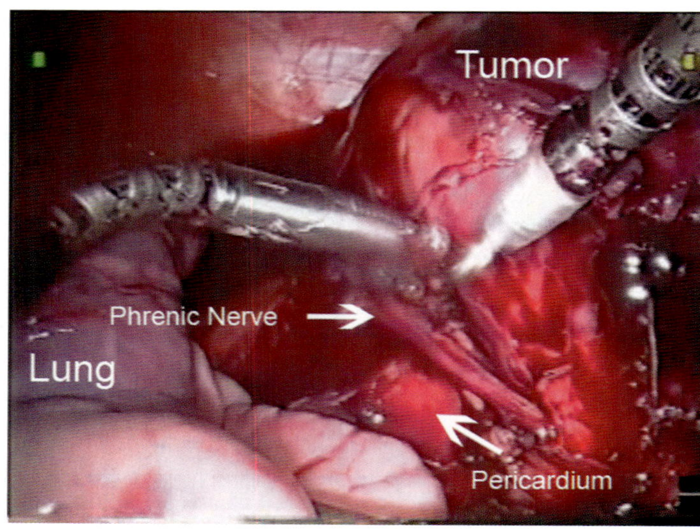

Fig. 29.21 A large 10 × 11 cm germ cell tumor adherent to the pericardium. Note the proximity of the phrenic nerve (*arrow*)

teratomas and benign. Finally, the tumors of thymic origin include thymomas and germ cell tumors. Germ cell tumors may also have increased beta-HCG and AFP, often originate in thymic tissue, and can grow to an enormous size (Fig. 29.21).

The robotic articulations are particularly useful for navigating around mediastinal masses reducing the need for additional trocars. We often can accomplish the entire resection of just about any mediastinal mass with only 3 trocars; one camera port and 2 instrument ports. The simple rule for setting up the case can be remembered by placing the robot cart wherever the tumor is situated. For example, if the mass is anterior and superior, the robot will come in from an anterior and superior angle. Likewise, if the mass is posterior and inferior, the robot will be bought in from a posterior and inferior angle (Fig. 29.22).

Congenital Diaphragmatic Hernia: Bochdalek Hernia

The posterolateral Bochdalek CDH occurs due to the failure of the diaphragm to close properly in

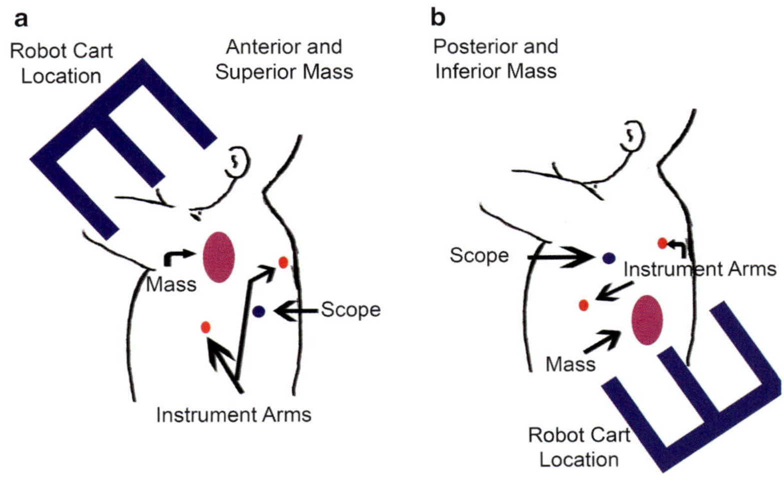

Fig. 29.22 Example trocar locations and robot cart positioning for mediastinal masses: (**a**) anterior and superior mass and (**b**) posterior and inferior mass

embryology. The defect is always posterior and lateral, but the size of the defect can be quite variable. The most posterolateral rim may have no diaphragm at all making it difficult to find adequate tissue to complete the repair. Moreover, this anatomic location is hard to reach in standard thoracoscopy as it is deep in the sulcus of where the diaphragm should be and the suturing angles thoracoscopically are less than ideal. The abdominal approach is even more challenging but not because the region is hard to reach, in fact it is fairly easy to reach. But these children have a scaphoid abdomen with a lack of domain because the viscera developed inside the chest. Moreover, bringing the viscera back into the abdomen crowds the very tight abdominal compartment even further adding to the problem regarding lack of domain. Therefore, most pediatric surgeons agree that the thoracoscopic approach is preferred. It should be noted, however, that we have occasionally done the abdominal approach robotically for very small patients when the articulating instruments are too long from the chest [1]. Regardless, the thoracoscopic approach to the Bochdalek CDH remains our preferred approach.

Non-robotic thoracoscopic failure rates have been alarmingly high in some series [20, 21]. The articulating instrumentation used in robotics may solve this problem [22]. But not all aspects of the procedure need the robot. Viscera reduction is better accomplished using standard thoracoscopic instruments. Large sweeping movements from one section of the chest to another are necessary for reducing the viscera, and the da Vinci is not very adept at moving in this manner. Therefore we reduce the viscera thoracoscopically before docking the robot. Defects that are too large for a primary repair will require a patch closure. The material is brought in through a 5 mm trocar rolled up like a carpet. Once inside, it can be easily unrolled and sewn in place. In patients with a tight primary closure, the patch material can be used as a reinforcement sewing it directly over the repair.

The patient is placed in a lateral decubitus position. The robot will come in from the patient's feet, at a slight angle towards the patients back (Fig. 29.23). This means that the robot arms will be maneuvering over the patient's head during the case. It is critically important to place a protective solid barrier over the baby's head to prevent the robot arms making inadvertent contact with the patient. We prefer a table-mounted laryngoscopy holder commonly used in head and neck procedures (Fig. 29.24).

The robotic trocars need to be placed perfectly in a neonatal repair as the small neonatal chest has very little additional room for the articulations. Cheating

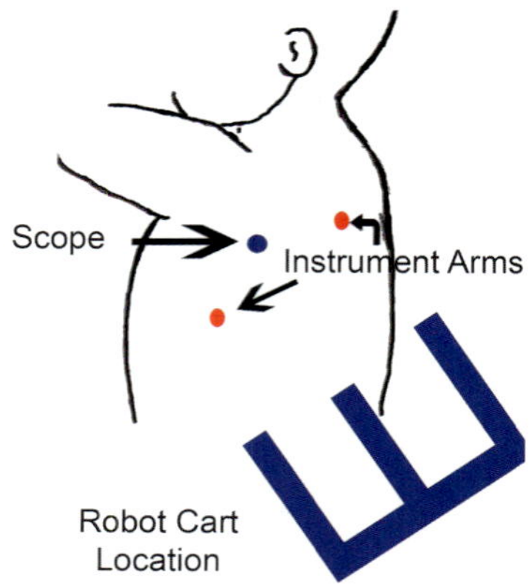

Fig. 29.23 Trocar placement for the robotic Bochdalek CDH repair

the remote center to the outside of the chest helps gain important additional articulating length.

The procedure begins by first reducing the viscera by using laparoscopic peanuts and gentle traction. Once the viscera are reduced, the robot can then be docked. Mobilize the diaphragmatic edge of the defect as it fuses with the posterolateral chest wall as best as possible (Fig. 29.25).

This mobilized rim of tissue can help attain a primary closure, which is preferred over patch closure. Close the defect using interrupted horizontal mattress sutures (Fig. 29.26).

We prefer to work from lateral to medial but either direction is acceptable. Pledgets help distribute the tension on the diaphragm and may reduce tearing of the muscle. Occasionally, closing the most posterolateral aspect can be particularly difficult because no rim of tissue is available for mobilization. In these patients, consider passing the suture out of the chest and around a rib, making a small external skin incision to assist with this maneuver. Usually only one or two sutures around the rib are required. We have not needed this rib stitch very often using the robot because we can often get adequate mobilization and proper suturing angles without it. Once the posterolateral section is closed, the repair proceeds medially. Patch closure, if necessary, is accomplished by suturing the lateral aspect first and proceeding medially. A chest tube is usually not necessary following closure.

Congenital Diaphragmatic Hernia: Morgagni Hernia

Repair of the Morgagni CDH is another ideal robotic case and relatively easy. The foramen of Morgagni is anterior and essentially midline on the diaphragm although it is often skewed slightly to the right side. The defect occurs as a result of failure of the fusion of the pleuroperitoneal surface of the diaphragm at the costosternal trigone. Unlike the Bochdalek CDH, which often presents at birth with respiratory compromise, these patients may go years or even decades without the diagnosis suspected. The defect may be found incidentally during a chest X-ray for unrelated issues. Occasionally, a patient may present with a bowel obstruction from viscera trapped in the hernia. More commonly, patients complain of mild substernal chest pain or indigestion. Because of its anterior location, the angles for suture repair of this defect using the standard laparoscopic instrumentation are challenging. Primary repair is preferred although a patch closure may be necessary for larger defects. Port placement is shown in Fig. (29.27).

Typically, only one camera port and two instrument ports are required without the need for an accessory port. The viscera reduction is performed first followed by resection of the hernia sac, which is usually, but not always, present. A rim of tissue on the anterior abdominal wall is mobilized with the hook cautery, and repair is performed using horizontal mattress sutures (Fig. 29.28).

Pledgets can be used if desired. Prosthetic material can be rolled up like a carpet and brought in through one of the instrument trocars for larger defects if a patch closure is needed.

Thymectomy

Myasthenia gravis (MG) is a poorly understood autoimmune disorder where the body produces antibodies that block muscle cells from receiving neurotransmitters from the nerve cell. This leads to muscle weakness of voluntary muscles. Patients can present with fatigue, generalized

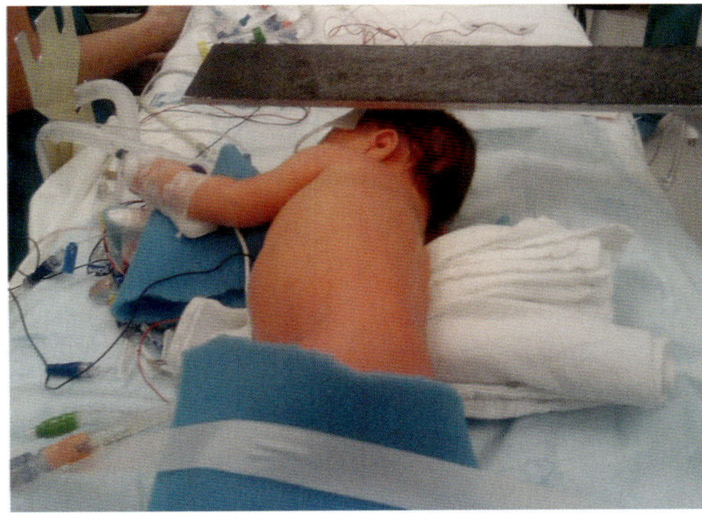

Fig. 29.24 A protective barrier is positioned over the baby's head. This is a critically safety precaution in the CDH repair as the robot arms will maneuver over the patient's head during the operation

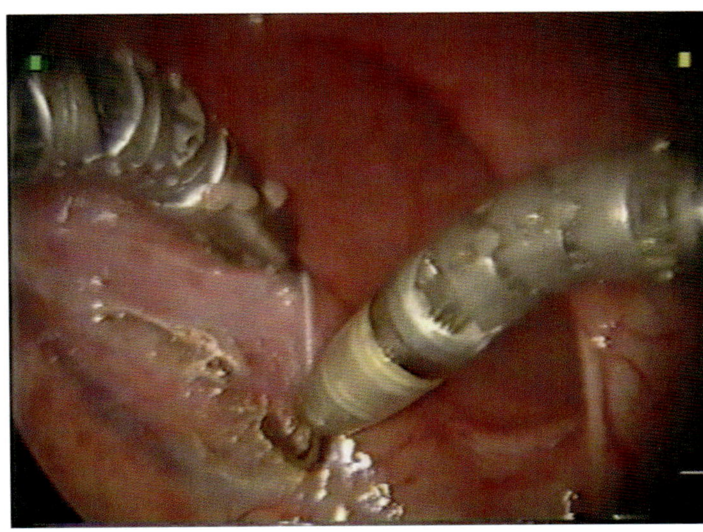

Fig. 29.25 Mobilizing tissue to create a suitable diaphragm rim for suturing

weakness, facial paralysis, or even breathing difficulties from weakness of the chest wall muscles. The muscles around the eye are often affected first leading to the classic eyelid droop or even double vision. While the weakness may be noticed on physical exam, reflexes are often normal. The diagnosis is confirmed by nerve conduction studies and detection of acetylcholine receptor antibodies. Steroids that can help reduce the immune response and pyridostigmine, which may improve the communication between nerves and muscles, are the mainstay of medical therapy. Respiratory compromise often results in hospitalization during acute exacerbations. Patients with refractory symptoms are candidates for thymectomy as this may alleviate the need for medications.

The robotic thymectomy is an ideal approach to the thymus which often extends beyond the mediastinum and up into the neck. Preliminary studies are already in print and the initial robotic results are encouraging [23]. We prefer a left thoracic approach. A dual lumen endotracheal tube is preferable and will assist with collapse of the left lung. The patient is placed in a supine position rolled slightly to the right with a small bump

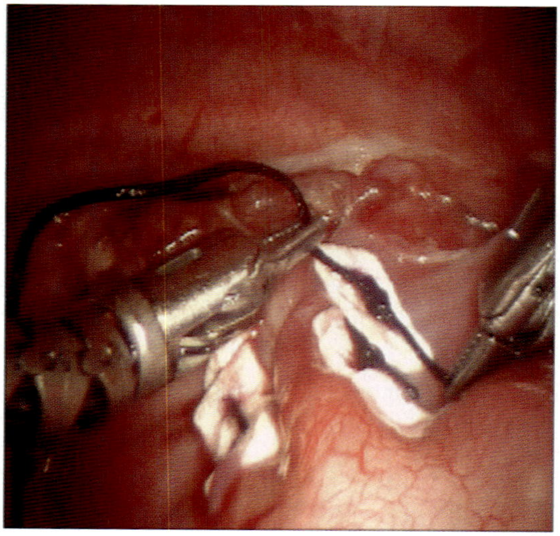

Fig. 29.26 Closure of the Bochdalek CDH using interrupted horizontal mattress sutures and pledgets

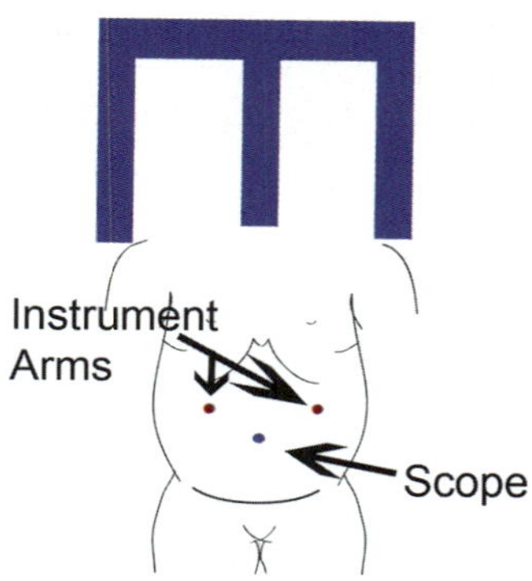

Fig. 29.27 Port placement for the Morgagni CDH repair

under the left scapula. The left arm is positioned over the face and trocars are placed as shown in Fig. (29.29).

The entire procedure can be accomplished with only three ports although an assistant port can be added for lung retraction if necessary. The scope selection is a 30° scope and alternating between an upward and downward look is helpful throughout the case. The phrenic nerve is identified early in the procedure, and care should be employed when dissecting near this sensitive structure (Fig. 29.30).

Dissection is followed cephalad and then medially. A significant portion of the gland may reside in the right chest or the right neck but is all easily accessible from the left chest using the robotic instruments. The innominate vein is identified and care taken to fully dissect the entire gland out of the neck holding adequate retraction to pull the cephalad tail of the thymus down into the mediastinum (Fig. 29.31).

A complete resection is critical for the best chance for resolution of symptoms. A postoperative chest tube is rarely necessary. At the completion of the operation, we automatically send all patients to the pediatric ICU as a precaution because of their baseline weakness but have never had any postoperative respiratory issues. Most patients are discharged in 24–48 h following surgery.

Esophageal Atresia with Tracheoesophageal Fistula

Repair of the neonate with a TEF is considered the Holy Grail in pediatric surgery, and absolute precision is required for the esophageal anastomosis. Using a minimally invasive approach is slowly gaining popularity but has not gained wide acceptance. The first MIS TEF repair was reported in 2001 [24]. Several series have been reported since then, but the procedure is still being done by only a small subset of pediatric surgeons. One of the problems is the rarity of this condition in relation to a problematic learning curve in order to become familiar with the procedure. Initial stricture and leak rates are relatively high but eventually approach those of open surgery [25]. Despite this shortcoming, advantages such as avoiding of a thoracotomy are of great benefit as profound scoliosis is a major concern for neonates that undergo a thoracotomy [26].

Theoretically, the robot could solve the problem of the precision with 3D vision and more accurate placement of the sutures. Unfortunately, this is a procedure, which is still a bit difficult for the current robotic da Vinci system because of the size of the instrumentation in relation to the patient. Most newborns with TEF are quite small, often under 3 kg in size. The robotic 8.5 mm

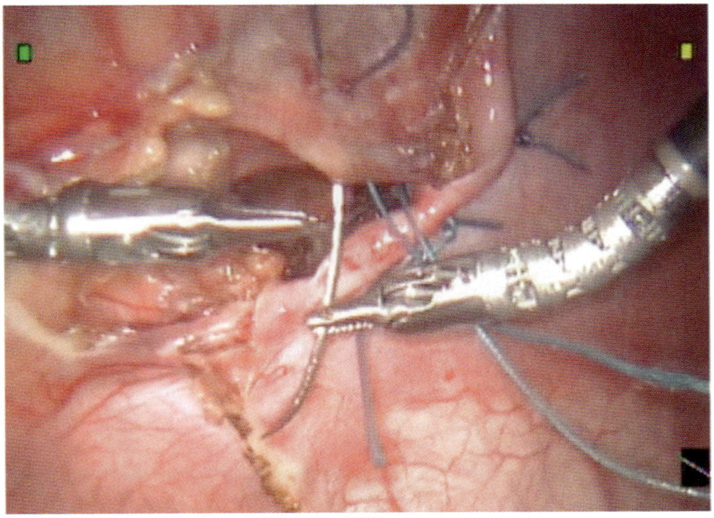

Fig. 29.28 Repair of the Morgagni CDH

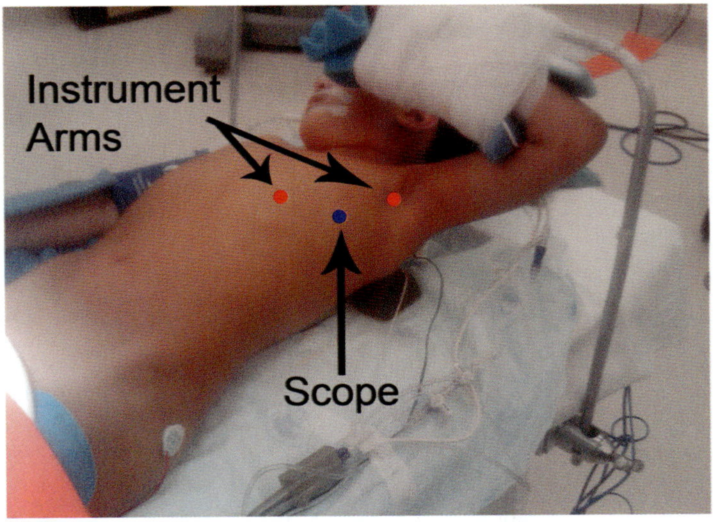

Fig. 29.29 Positioning and trocar placement for the robotic thymectomy. The da Vinci robot will come in over the patient's right shoulder

scope is a very tight fit between the rib space of such a small baby, and the lack of workable space for the articulating instruments makes this operation extremely challenging. These constraints are potentially compounded if the newborn has any one or more of the numerous others associated anomalies often seen with TEF as part of the VACTERL association (V, vertebral; A, anorectal malformation; C, cardiac; TE, tracheoesophageal fistula; R, renal; L, limb). Therefore, the robotic TEF repair is unlikely to be a common procedure with the current da Vinci robot unless significant improvements are made. As a guideline, The TEF baby generally needs to be above 3 kg and very few TEF babies are that large. We did our first TEF repair in 2007 with a da Vinci Standard system and the 2D 5 mm scope which is no longer available. This procedure can also be accomplished with the 8.5 mm scope but the rib space is very tight. However, in the hopes that this technology will eventually improve with diameter equipment and shorter articulating lengths, we will go on to describe the steps to robotic repair of the TEF. Although there are five different

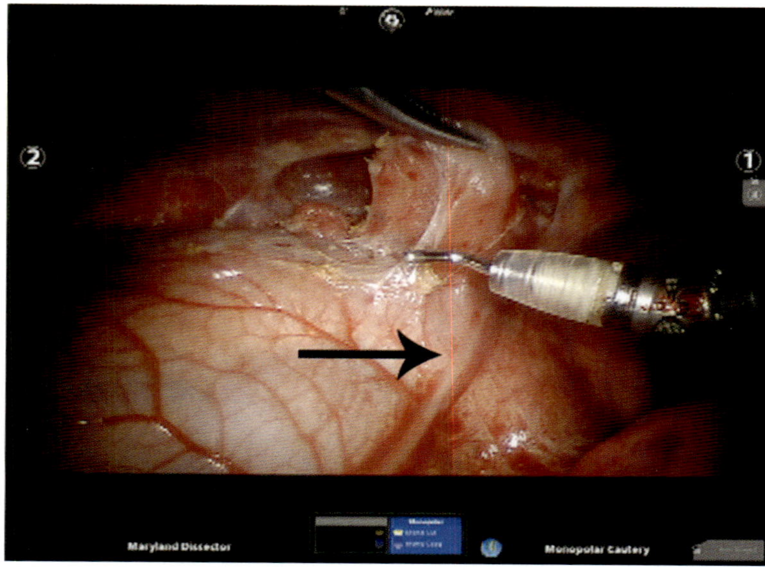

Fig. 29.30 Identification of the phrenic nerve (*arrow*) is the first task in the robotic thymectomy

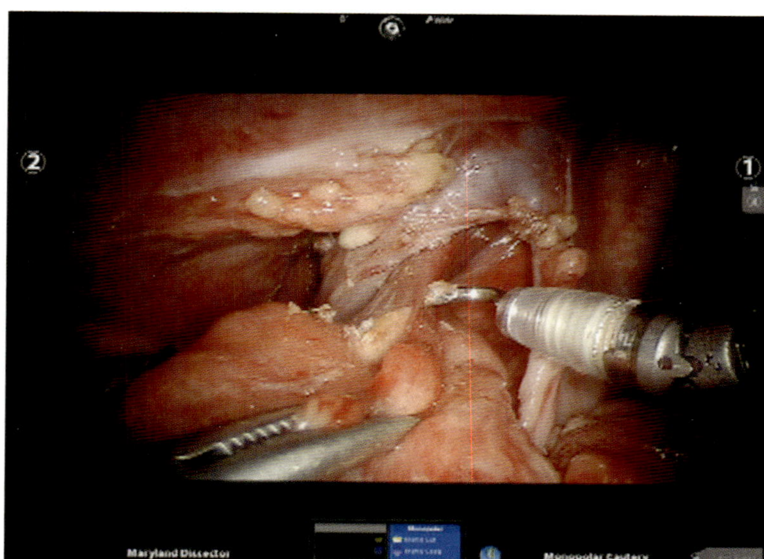

Fig. 29.31 Dissection of the thymus around the innominate

types of TEF, we will describe repair of the most common variant, the proximal esophageal atresia with distal tracheoesophageal fistula.

Bronchoscopy is strongly recommended at the beginning of the procedure to confirm the suspected anatomy. The trocar placement is shown in Fig. 29.32 and a transpleural approach is required.

The first step is identification and division of the azygos vein. The vessel can be taken down and divided using a thermal sealing device such as the LigaSure. Alternatively, clips can be used to ligate the vessel and scissors brought in for division. Dissection then begins in the mediastinum with identification

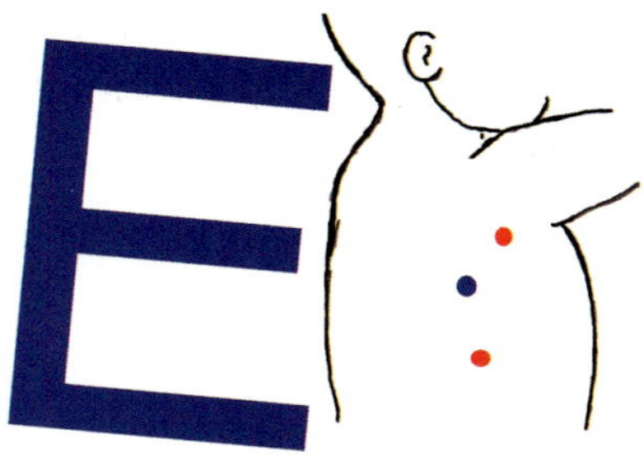

Fig. 29.32 Trocar placement for the robotic esophageal and TEF repair

of the proximal esophagus, the distal esophagus, the trachea, and the fistula connecting the trachea to the distal esophagus. The anesthesiologist can assist the surgeon by manipulating a nasogastric (NG) tube to help demonstrate the upper pouch. The fistula is often just a couple of tracheal rings inferior to the upper pouch and usually attaches just 1 or 2 mm proximal to the carina (Fig. 29.33).

The fistula takedown is the next important step that can be done in a variety of ways. One recently advocated method is to simply clip the fistula close to the origin at the trachea using an endoscopic clip applier [27]. Alternatively, the fistula can be divided in a piecemeal fashion to minimize the leak from the trachea and closed sequentially with interrupted absorbable sutures. Another choice would be to come across the fistula all at once with the scissors, but this may cause significant airway pressure loss until the open trachea is closed. We prefer the piecemeal approach, suturing the trachea as the fistula is divided. Once control of the fistula has been established, attention is turned at bringing the two ends of the esophagus together with mobilization of the esophagus. Mobilization needs to be adequate to bring the two ends together without undue tension, but this needs to be balanced with avoiding overdissection and potential esophageal ischemia. Grasping the friable neonatal esophagus with robotic instrumentation poses another challenge and should be done with a minimum of trauma. Once again, it is often helpful to utilize the assistance of the anesthesiologist by manipulating the NG tube to aid in the proximal pouch mobilization. The anastomosis is performed using interrupted anastomosis 4-0 or 5-0 suture. The first suture may not bring the two ends together all the way but can be regarded as a traction suture lining up the repair for the remainder of the anastomosis. Subsequent sutures can be used to pull the two ends completely together. We recommend placing the knots on the inside of the lumen for the back row and on the outside for the front row. Have the anesthesiologist gently slide a NG tube past the completed back row and down into the distal esophagus before completing the front row (Fig. 29.34).

The surgeon may have to help guide the tube with a grasper or needle driver. The NG tube then serves as a stent or sizer for the repair. Although some surgeons prefer to leave it in place, it can be removed at the completion of the procedure. Complete the front row of sutures over the NG tube with the knots on the outside of the esophagus. A chest tube is left in place following the repair and should stay in place until a swallowing study is performed about 7 days postoperatively. The chest tube can be removed and feeds initiated once there is no evidence of a leak.

The Future

The wide range of procedures that can be done robotically in children is huge as the combination of acquired and congenital anomalies creates an enormous variety of surgical pathology. The da Vinci has gained tremendous popularity in adult urology, gynecology, and more recently in adult general surgery. Enthusiasm is now also growing in pediatric general surgery. However, improvements in the technology are needed in order to gain widespread acceptance. Downsizing the diameter is an important step as the 5 and 8 mm robotic instruments are competing against 3 mm laparoscopic instrumentation. The articulating length is also an issue, as space becomes a significant issue in smaller patients. This can be accomplished either in the instrument itself or by shortening the length of the robotic port from remote center to the end of the cannula. The tissues of newborns and premature babies are very fragile, and instrumentation with delicate but fine

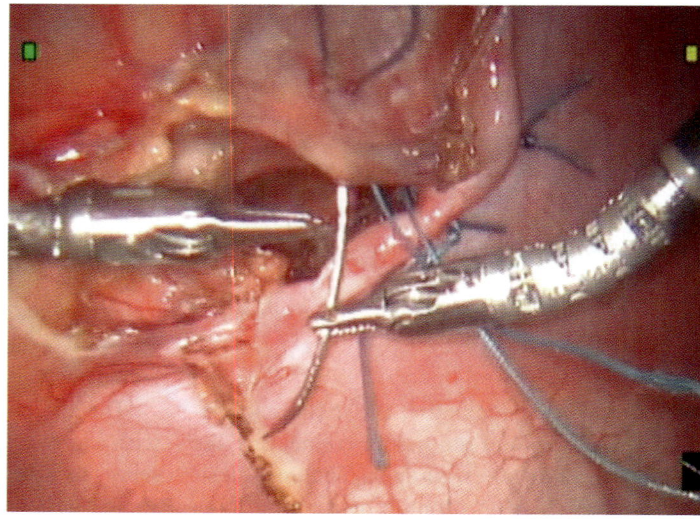

Fig. 29.33 Exposure of the tracheoesophageal fistula (*arrow*). The proximal esophagus (PE), distal esophagus (DE), and trachea (T) are also visible

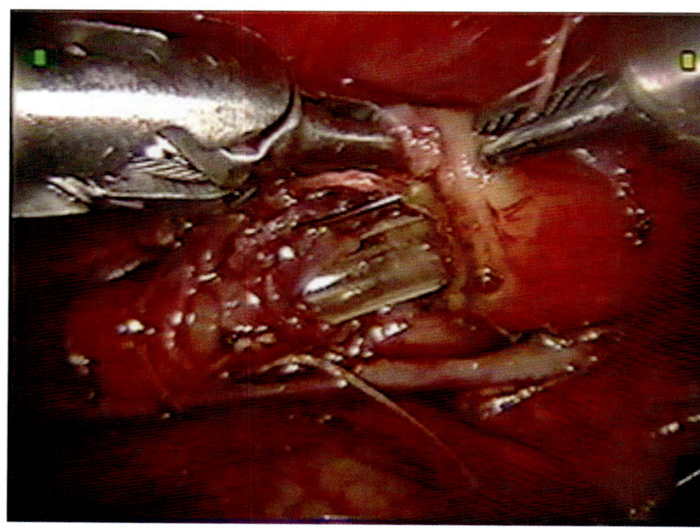

Fig. 29.34 The NG tube is passed distally to assist with the anastomosis in the repair of the esophageal atresia

tips is another item for the future as we expand this technology to smaller and smaller babies.

There are many laparoscopic procedures that are often too challenging for the standard handheld instruments, and the robotic approach has the potential to overcome the deficiencies of laparoscopy in children. Cholecystectomies and fundoplication are excellent training cases, and surgeons new to robotic surgery should start their experience with these simple cases before moving on to more challenging procedures. There are many operations where we feel the current robot is already superior to laparoscopy including duodenal atresia, choledochal cysts, Ladd's procedure, the Kasai portoenterostomy, thymectomy, mediastinal masses, and all forms of congenital diaphragmatic hernia. The introduction of the Tissue Sealer in 2012 may prove to be a major game changer as this device has the potential to be useful for pulmonary lobectomies in children with pulmonary sequestrations and CCAMs. Animal testing for this application is still needed but could lead to a revolution in the way pediatric surgeons view the robotic technology. Additionally, development of pediatric specific instrumentation with finer grasping qualities could help expand the realm of procedures for neonates and perhaps even premature kids. Finding ways to utilize the Firefly technology for neuroblastoma, rhabdomyosarcoma, and other pediatric tumors could help pave the way for a whole new perspective for pediatric oncological surgery. The possibilities are endless and there is plenty of room to grow as pediatric robotic surgery is literally in its infancy.

References

1. Meehan JJ, Francis P, Sandler A. Robotic repair of duodenal atresia. J Pediatr Surg. 2007;42(7):E31–3.
2. Meehan JJ, Sandler A. Robotic repair of a Bochdalek congenital diaphragmatic hernia in a small neonate: robotic advantages and limitations. J Pediatr Surg. 2007;42(10):1757–60.
3. Meehan JJ, Phearman L, Sandler A. Robotic pulmonary resections in children: series report and introduction of a new robotic instrument. J Laparoendosc Adv Surg Tech A. 2008;18(2):293–5.
4. Mattioli G, Esposito C, Lima M, Garzi A, Montinaro L, Cobellis G, Mastoianni L, Aceti MG, Falchetti D, Repetto P, Pini Prato A, Leggio S, Torri F, Ruggeri G, Settimi A, Messina M, Martino A, Amici G, Riccipetitoni G, Jasonni V. Italian multicenter survey on laparoscopic treatment of gastro-esophageal reflux disease in children. Surg Endosc. 2002;16(12):1666–8.
5. Esposito C, Montupet P, van Der Zee D, Settimi A, Paye-Jaouen A, Centonze A, Bax NK. Long-term outcome of laparoscopic Nissen, Toupet, and Thal antireflux procedures for neurologically normal children with gastroesophageal reflux disease. Surg Endosc. 2006;20(6):855–8.
6. Meehan JJ, Georgeson KE. Laparoscopic fundoplication in infants and children. Surg Endosc. 1996;10:1154–7.
7. Meehan JJ, Georgeson KE. The learning curve associated with laparoscopic antireflux surgery in infants and children. J Pediatr Surg. 1997;32(3):426–9.
8. Meehan JJ, Meehan TD, Sandler A. Robotic fundoplication in children: resident teaching and a single institutional review of our first 50 patients. J Pediatr Surg. 2007;42(12):2022–5.
9. Ladd WE. Surgical diseases of the alimentary tract in infants. N Engl J Med. 1936;215:705–8.
10. Wong KK, Chung PH, Chan KL, Fan ST, Tam PK. Should open Kasai portoenterostomy be performed for biliary atresia in the era of laparoscopy? Pediatr Surg Int. 2008;24(8):931–3.
11. Gundeti MS. Pediatric robotic and reconstructive urology: a comprehensive guide. Oxford: Wiley-Blackwell; 2012.
12. Laje P, Clark FH, Friedman JR, Flake AW. Increased susceptibility to liver damage from pneumoperitoneum in a murine model of biliary atresia. J Pediatr Surg. 2010;45(9):1791–6.
13. Dutta S, Woo R, Albanese CT. Minimal access portoenterostomy: advantages and disadvantages of standard laparoscopic and robotic techniques. J Laparoendosc Adv Surg Tech A. 2007;17(2):258–64.
14. Meehan JJ, Elliott S, Sandler A. The robotic approach to complex hepatobiliary anomalies in children: preliminary report. J Pediatr Surg. 2007; 42(12):2110–4.
15. Huang CS, Huang CC, Chen DF. Choledochal cysts: differences between pediatric and adult patients. J Gastrointest Surg. 2010;14(7):1105–10.
16. Liem NT, Pham HD, le Dung A, Son TN, Vu HM. Early and intermediate outcomes of laparoscopic surgery for choledochal cysts with 400 patients. J Laparoendosc Adv Surg Tech A. 2012;22(6): 599–603.
17. Spilde TL, St Peter SD, Keckler SJ, Holcomb 3rd GW, Snyder CL, Ostlie DJ. Open vs. laparoscopic repair of congenital duodenal obstructions: a concurrent series. J Pediatr Surg. 2008;43(6):1002–5.
18. Kimura K, Tsugawa C, Ogawa K, Matsumoto Y, Yamamoto T, Asada S. Diamond-shaped anastomosis for congenital duodenal obstruction. Arch Surg. 1977;112(10):1262–3.
19. Billmire DF, Grosfeld JL. Teratomas in childhood: analysis of 142 cases. J Pediatr Surg. 1986;21(6): 548–51.
20. Lansdale N, Alam S, Losty PD, Jesudason EC. Neonatal endosurgical congenital diaphragmatic hernia repair: a systematic review and meta-analysis. Ann Surg. 2010;252(1):20–6.
21. Arca MJ, Barnhart DC, Lelli Jr JL, Greenfeld J, Harmon CM, Hirschl RB, Teitelbaum DH. Early experience with minimally invasive repair of congenital diaphragmatic hernias: results and lessons learned. J Pediatr Surg. 2003;38(11):1563–8. Review.
22. Slater BJ, Meehan JJ. Robotic repair of congenital diaphragmatic anomalies. J Laparoendosc Adv Surg Tech A. 2009;19(s1):s123–7.
23. Hartwich J, Tyagi S, Margaron F, Oitcica C, Teasley J, Lanning D. Robot-assisted thoracoscopic thymectomy for treating myasthenia gravis in children. J Laparoendosc Adv Surg Tech A. 2012;22(9):925–9.
24. Lobe TE, Rothenberg SS, Waldschmidt J, Stroeder L. Thoracoscopic repair of esophageal atresia in an infant, A surgical first. Pediatr Endosurg Innova Tech. 1999;3:141–8.
25. Szavay PO, Zundel S, Blumenstock G, Kirschner HJ, Luithle T, Girisch M, Luenig H, Fuchs J. Perioperative outcome of patients with esophageal atresia and tracheo-esophageal fistula undergoing open versus thoracoscopic surgery. J Laparoendosc Adv Surg Tech A. 2011;21(5):439–43.
26. Sistonen SJ, Helenius I, Peltonen J, Sarna S, Rintala RJ, Pakarinen MP. Natural history of spinal anomalies and scoliosis associated with esophageal atresia. Pediatrics. 2009;124(6):e1198–204.
27. Rothenberg SS. Thoracoscopic repair of esophageal atresia and tracheo-esophageal fistula in neonates: evolution of a technique. J Laparoendosc Adv Surg Tech A. 2012;22(2):195–9.

Part XII

Surgical Techniques: *Microsurgery*

Robotic-Assisted Microsurgery for Male Infertility and Chronic Orchialgia

30

Jamin V. Brahmbhatt, Ahmet Gudeloglu, and Sijo J. Parekattil

General Overview of Current Applications

The introduction of the operative microscope in the 1920s revolutionized surgery of microscopic structures. Today another revolution is upon us with the incorporation of robotic technology into microsurgery. The advantages of robotic assistance include high-resolution three-dimensional optics, enhanced precision with elimination of tremor and 5:1 motion scaling, improved surgeon ergonomics, and ability to control multiple instruments without need for a skilled assistant. These benefits have led to its utilization for treatment of male infertility and chronic orchialgia through vasectomy reversal, subinguinal varicocelectomy, testicular sperm extraction, and targeted denervation of the spermatic cord.

In 2004 Kuang et al. performed the first robotic-assisted andrological procedure with an ex vivo vasovasostomy [1]. The first randomized prospective study comparing the robotic-assisted vasovasostomy (RAVV) and pure microsurgical vasovasostomy (MVV) showed advantages in terms of decreased operative time and decreased sperm granuloma at the anastomosis [2]. Also in 2004, Fleming et al. reported excellent patency on two patients that underwent the first bilateral robotic-assisted vasovasostomy (RAVV) [3]. The first robotic-assisted subinguinal varicocelectomy (RAVx) was described in 2008 [4, 5]. Since then the techniques and outcomes have improved significantly with robotic assistance for male infertility [6, 7].

Chronic orchialgia (CO) is a common clinical condition that is often under diagnosed. The condition may affect over 100,000 men annually [8, 9]. CO is defined as intermittent or constant, unilateral or bilateral testicular pain lasting more than 3 months [10]. The pain can be idiopathic or caused by nerve irritation or hyposensitivity through vasectomy, hernia repair, sports injury, abdominal surgery, or any intervention that can irritate the genitofemoral or ilioinguinal nerves. Although the exact mechanism for CO is not well understood, one common theme is a two-hit theory (Fig. 30.1). There is a baseline inflammatory or genetic process that leads to Wallerian degeneration (Fig. 30.2) of the peripheral nerves. This leads to hypersensitivity of the ilioinguinal and genitofemoral nerves. A second inciting event, trauma, surgery, or irritation of these nerves then leads to chronic neuropathic pain in this area.

Prevalence can range up to 33 % of men after vasectomy [11] and 63 % after inguinal hernia repair [12–14]. After hernia repair the pain can be neuropathic or non-neuropathic secondary to mesh. Even with such a high prevalence after hernia repair, only 1 % of patients who suffer from

J.V. Brahmbhatt, M.D. • A. Gudeloglu, M.D.
S.J. Parekattil, M.D. (✉)
Department of Urology, Winter Haven Hospital and University of Florida, 199 Avenue B NW, Suite 310, Winter Haven, FL, USA
e-mail: jamin.brahmbhatt@winterhavenhospital.org; ahmet.gudeloglu@winterhavenhospital.org; sijo.parekattil@winterhavenhospital.org

K.C. Kim (ed.), *Robotics in General Surgery*, DOI 10.1007/978-1-4614-8739-5_30,

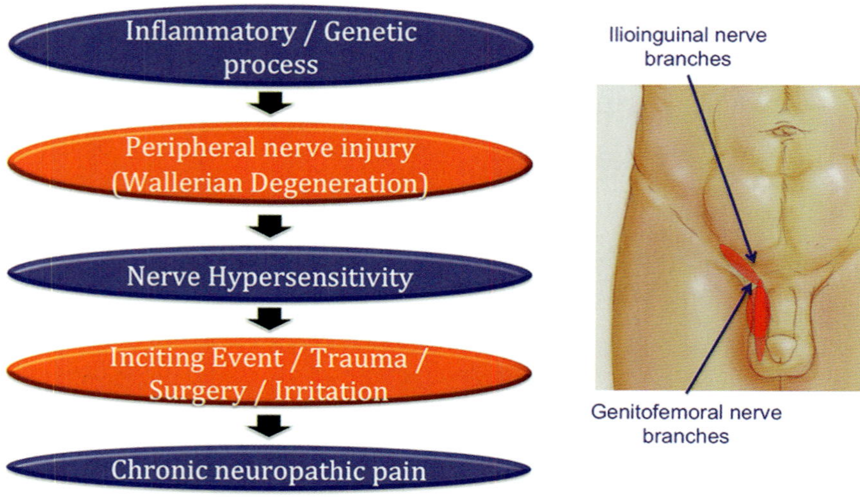

Fig. 30.1 Two-hit theory on cause of chronic orchialgia

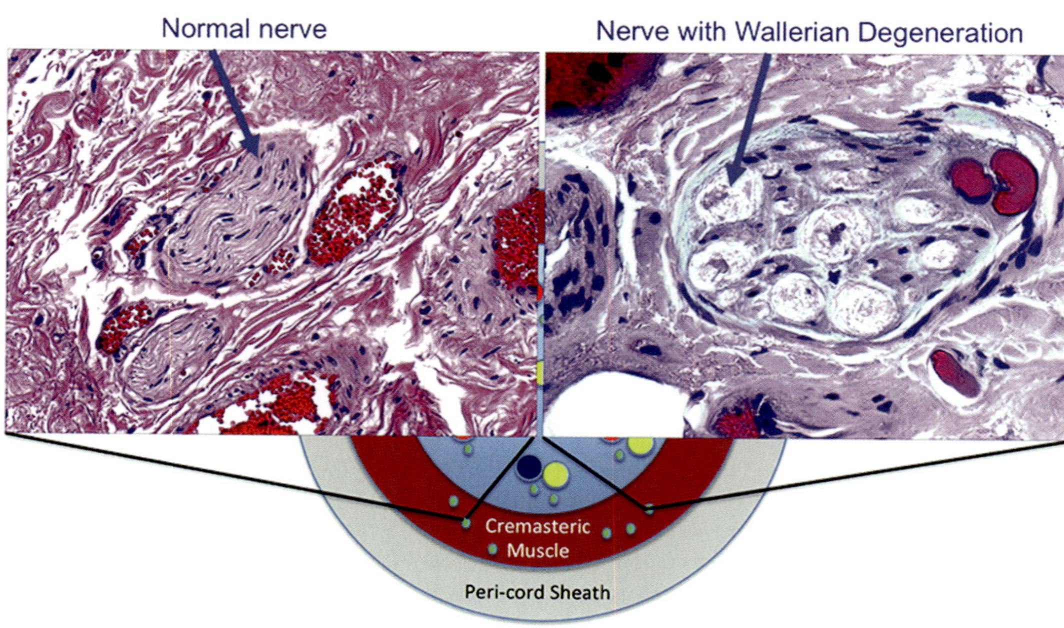

Fig. 30.2 Nerve fiber with and without Wallerian degeneration on H&E staining

CO may be referred for further evaluation [15]. Parekattil et al. in 2008 reported on the advantages of robotic-assisted targeted microsurgical denervation of the spermatic cord (RMDSC) for chronic groin and testicular pain [7, 8]. The technique targets denervation at specific nerves found to have abnormal fibers (Wallerian degeneration) within the spermatic cord [16]. The three primary locations for abnormal nerves (highest to lowest) are cremasteric nerve fibers, perivasal tissue and vasal sheath, and posterior lipomatous/posterior-arterial tissue.

In this chapter we will highlight specific procedures for the management of male infertility and chronic orchialgia: robotic-assisted microsurgical vasovasostomy, vasoepididymostomy, subinguinal varicocelectomy, and targeted denervation of the spermatic cord.

Preoperative Preparation

Anticoagulant medications or supplements are generally held 5–7 days prior to the procedure. A broad-spectrum antibiotic is administered at least 30 min prior to skin incision. Mechanical lower extremity compression stockings are used for deep venous thrombosis prophylaxis.

Operative Setup and Patient Positioning

The patient is placed in a supine position and prepped and draped in a standard surgical fashion. Skin incisions are made and appropriate operative tissues are exposed. The robot is brought in from the right side of the patient for the microsurgical portion of the case (Fig. 30.3). Figure 30.4 illustrates the trocar robotic arm placement. Trocars are loaded to allow the instruments to function and to stabilize their movements outside the patient's body. Instruments are advanced 4–5 cm beyond the tip of the trocar to optimize range of motion. A 0° camera lens is used to optimize the visual field during procedures.

Figure 30.5 illustrates our utilization of the VITOM (Karl Storz Inc., Tuttlingen, Germany) camera system for enhanced 16–18× magnification with a nitrogen powered fifth arm (Point setter arm, Karl Storz Inc., Tuttlingen, Germany). The real-time video images from VITOM are transported to the surgeon console utilizing the TilePro (Intuitive Surgical, Sunnyvale, CA) robotic surgical console software system to provide simultaneous real-time images to the microsurgeon. Figure 30.6 illustrates the cockpit view of the surgeon console (1) the da Vinci Si 3D HD camera view, (2) the VITOM optical 16–18× camera lens system view, and (3) a 40–100× optical microscopic view from the intra-op andrology laboratory microscope (Nikon Inc., Tokyo, Japan).

Robotic-Assisted Microsurgical Vasovasostomy

Technique

The proximal and distal vas deferens (beyond the previous vasectomy site) is palpated through the scrotal skin. Through the skin the distal vas is fixed into place with a towel clip (Fig. 30.7). Local anesthetic is infiltrated into this area. A 1–2 cm vertical incision is made over the vas starting inferiorly from the previously placed towel clip (Fig. 30.8). Using fine electrocautery and sharp dissection, the distal and proximal ends of the vas are dissected free. The distal vas is dissected to allow a tension-free anastomosis to the proximal vas. The proximal vas is carefully transected with a #11 blade. Microscopic examination of the proximal vas fluid is performed. If no sperm is present in this proximal fluid, robotic-assisted microsurgical vasoepididymostomy (RAVE) is performed. If sperm is found, then RAVV is performed. The adventitia from either end of the vasa is now secured together with a 3-0 prolene suture to allow a tension-free anastomosis.

The robot is now positioned from the right of the patient to perform the microsurgical vasovasostomy. Black diamond micro-forceps are inserted on the right and left robotic arms. The micro Potts scissors are inserted onto the fourth robot arm. The 0° camera lens is inserted onto the robot camera arm. The two ends of the vas are placed over a 1/4 in. Penrose drain. The assistant passes the 9-0 nylon suture that is kept in its inner packaging to the surgical field. The suture is grasped using the black diamond right-hand grasper and cut to about 2 in. length using the micro Potts scissors. The 9-0 nylon suture is held and manipulated using the black diamond forceps in both left and right arms as needle drivers. The posterior muscularis layer of the two ends of the vas is now approximated (Fig. 30.9). Two or three double-armed 10-0 nylon sutures are now placed inside out to reanastomose the posterior mucosal lumen of the vas (Fig. 30.10). Three double-armed 10-0 nylon sutures are used to close the anterior mucosal lumen of the vas

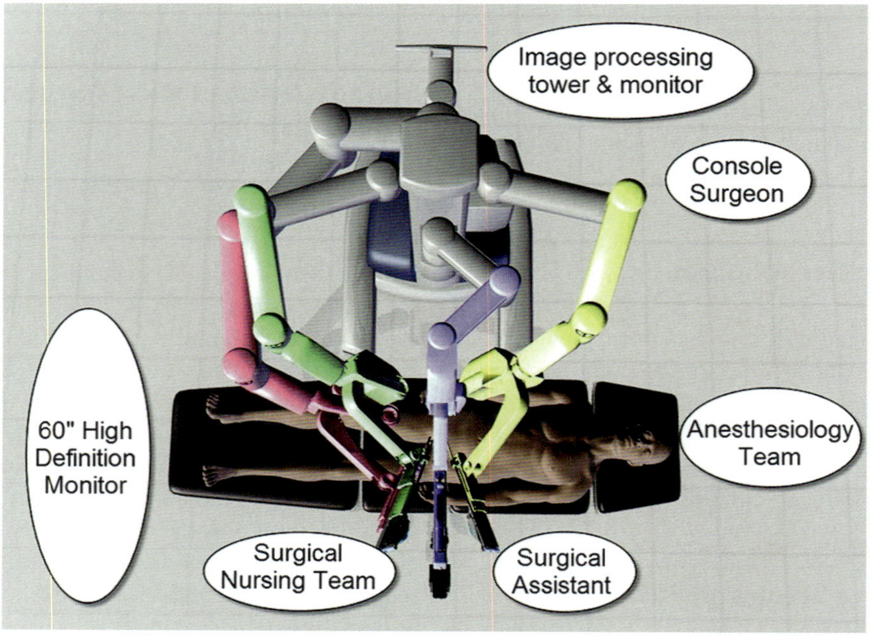

Fig. 30.3 General robotic position and setup for microsurgery cases

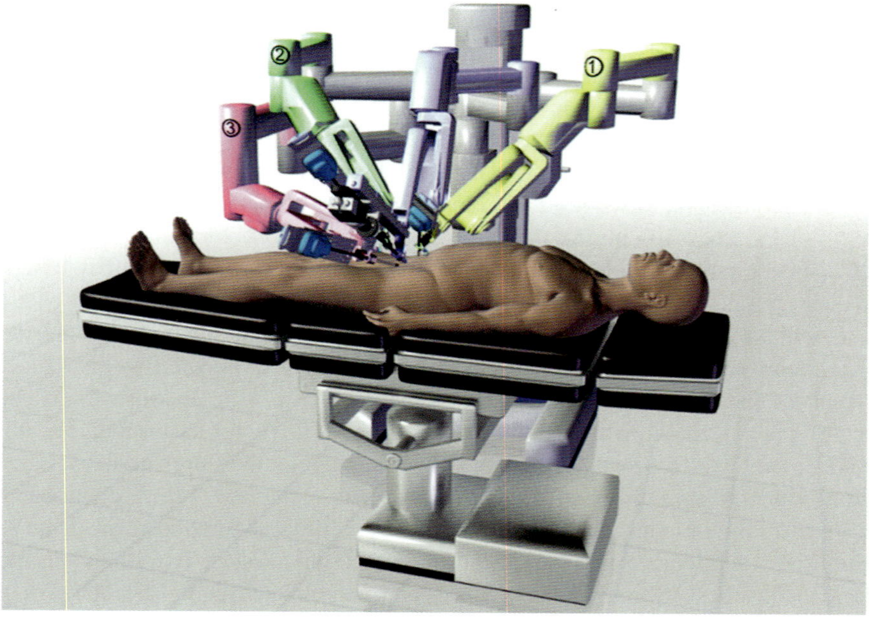

Fig. 30.4 Robotic arm and trocar placement for microsurgery cases

(Fig. 30.11). Five to six 9-0 nylon sutures are used to approximate the anterior muscularis layer of the vas (Fig. 30.12). The same procedure is now performed on the contralateral side by repositioning the robotic arms. The Penrose drain is gently removed from under the repair. The vas is placed back into the scrotal cavity and the tissue and skin are closed with absorbable suture.

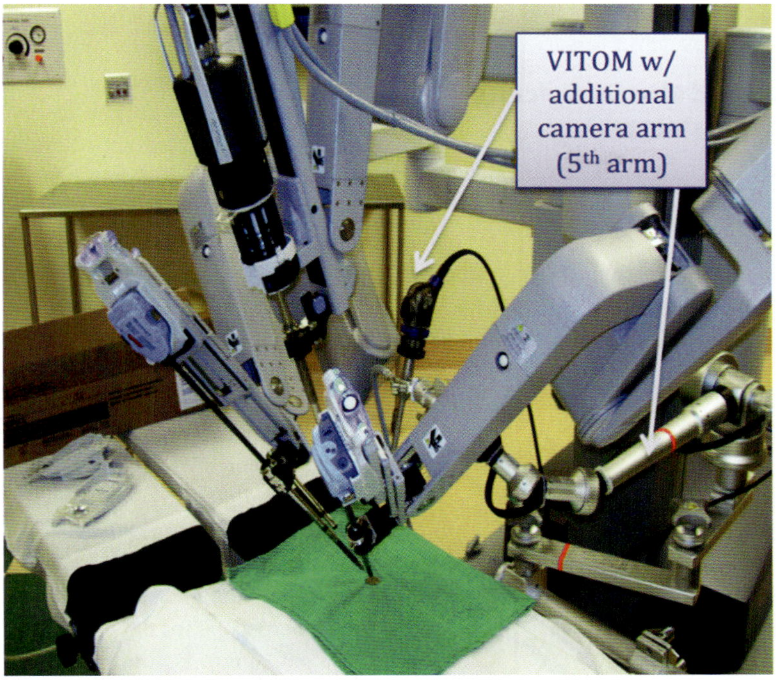

Fig. 30.5 Positioning of VITOM on nitrogen powered fifth robotic arm

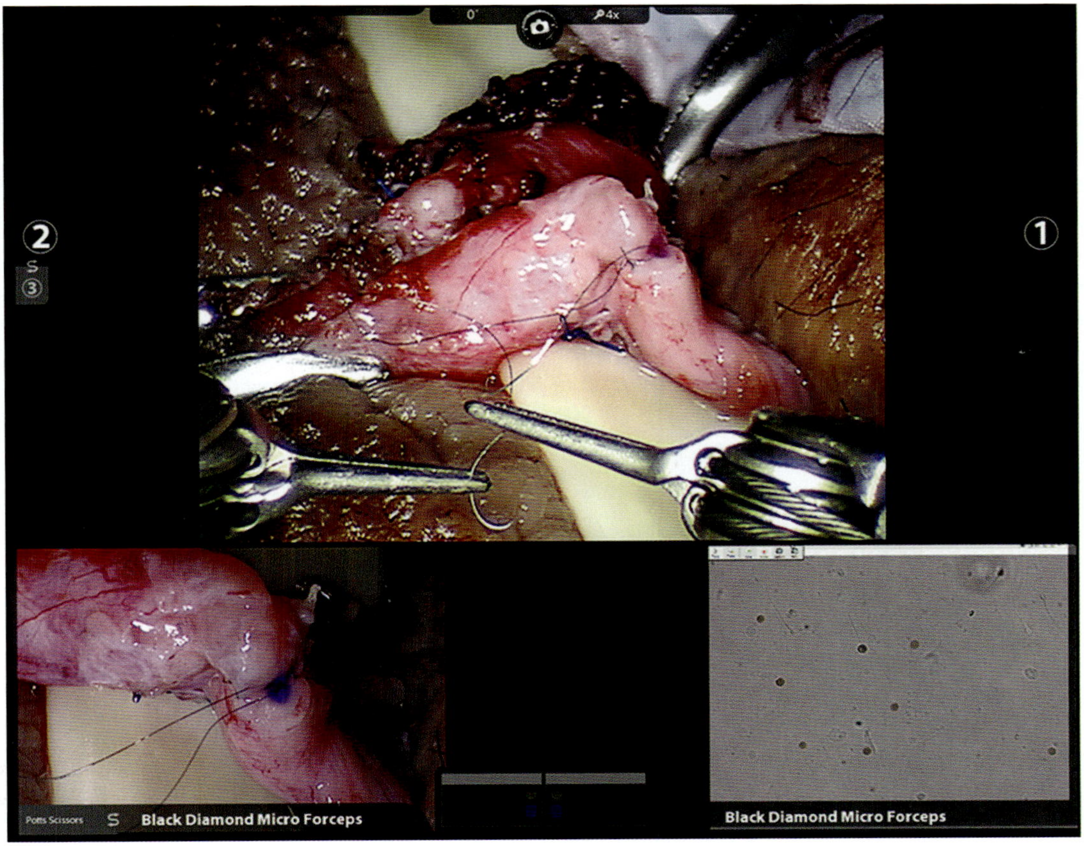

Fig. 30.6 Cockpit view of surgeon console with TilePro software

Robotic-Assisted Microsurgical Vasoepididymostomy

Technique

The RAVE procedure starts from above when there is no sperm in the fluid from the proximal vas. The scrotal incision is enlarged by 1–2 cm inferiorly. The testicle is delivered and the tunica is incised to expose the epididymis. The adventitial layer of the epididymis is incised above the level of epididymal obstruction (blue/gray zone with dilated epididymal tubules above this area). A 3-0 prolene suture is used to attach the testicle to the adventitia of the vas to prevent tension between the anastomosis. The vas is stripped off the adventitia and flipped towards the epididymal tubules. The robot is now positioned similar to above. Two 10-0 nylon double-armed suture needles are placed longitudinally through a single epididymal tubule to expose the tubule (Fig. 30.13). This tubule is then incised longitudinally using the micro Potts scissors between the two suture needles to create a lumen in the tubule (Fig. 30.14). The fluid is then aspirated and examined under a separate phase contrast microscope for the presence of sperm.

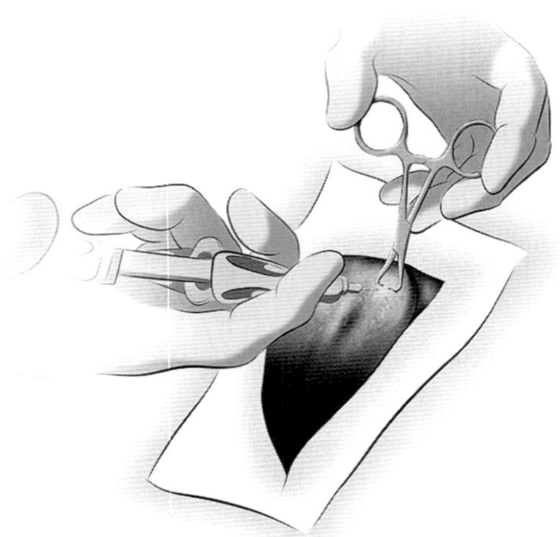

Fig. 30.7 Skin and vas under towel clip for robotic vasectomy reversal

When sperm is confirmed, two double-armed 10-0 nylon needles in the epididymal tubule are advanced through and then all four of the needles are brought inside out on the vas mucosal lumen to involute the epididymal tubule lumen into the vas lumen (Fig. 30.15). Five to six 9-0 nylon sutures are placed circumferentially to approximate the muscularis of the vas to the adventitia of the epididymal tubule (Fig. 30.16). The testicle and anastomosis are carefully delivered back into the scrotum. The dartos layer and skin are closed.

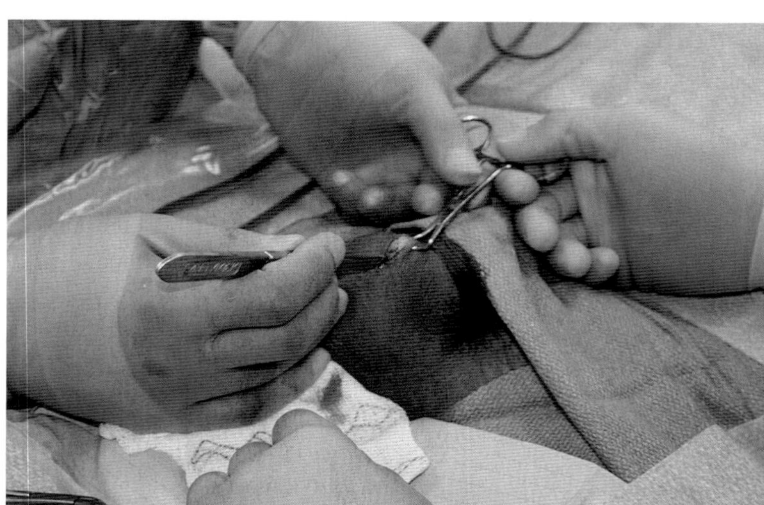

Fig. 30.8 Midline skin incision for robotic vasectomy reversal

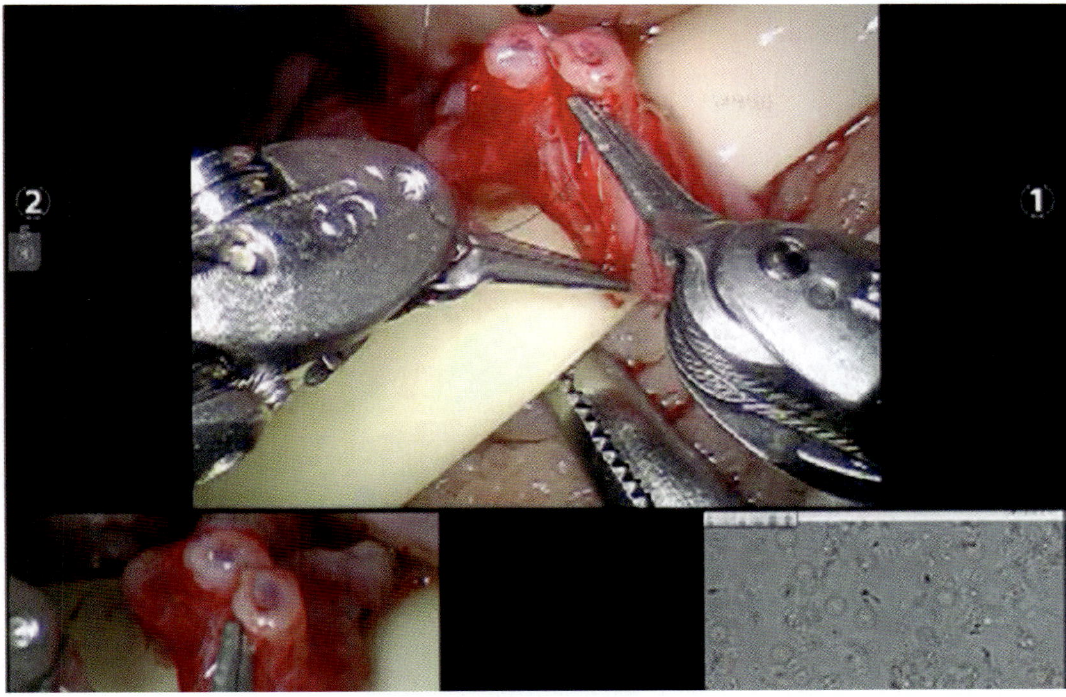

Fig. 30.9 RAVV posterior muscular anastomosis

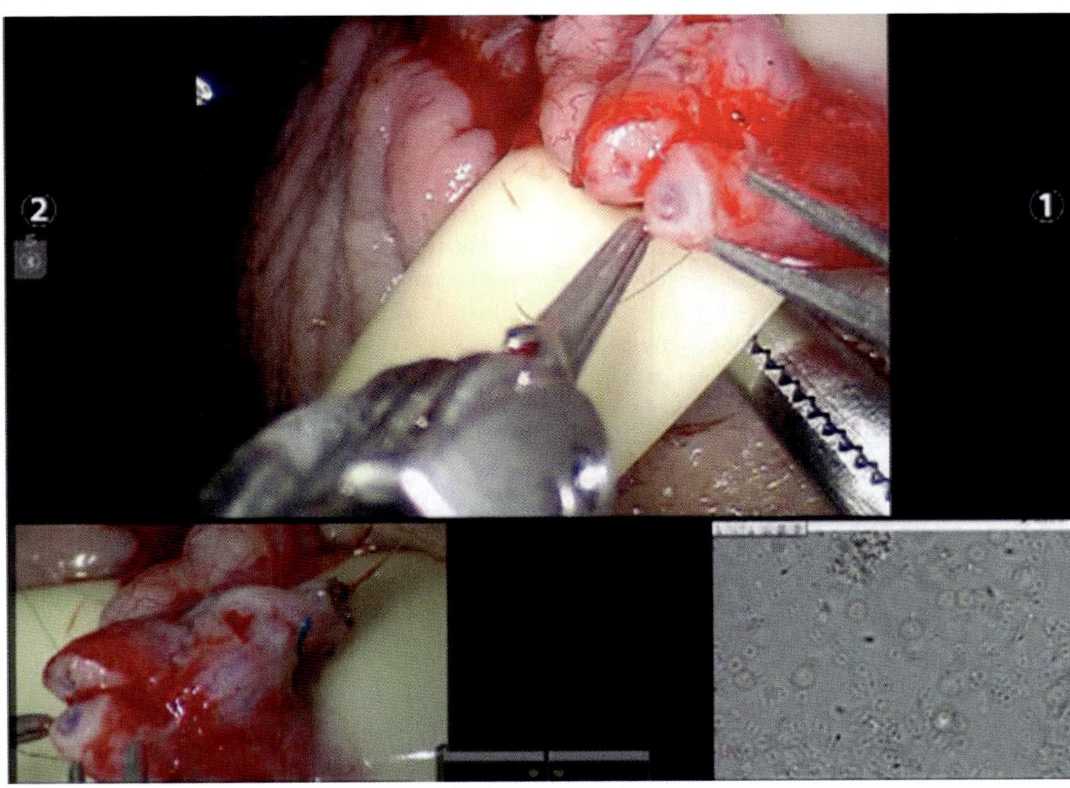

Fig. 30.10 RAVV posterior luminal anastomosis

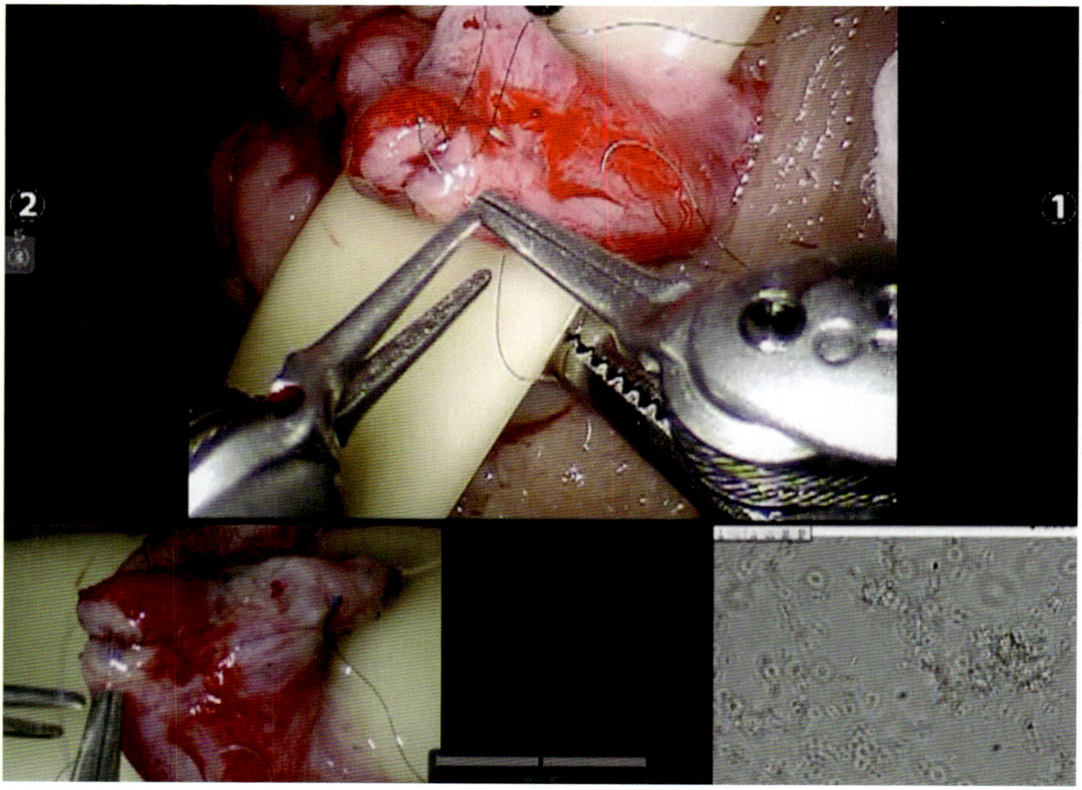

Fig. 30.11 RAVV anterior luminal anastomosis

RAVV/RAVE Outcomes Review

Between July 2007 and March 2013, 147 robotic-assisted vasectomy reversals (90 bilateral RAVV, 57 RAVE) were performed by a single fellowship-trained microsurgeon. Twenty of these patients had chronic scrotal pain after vasectomy and the rest wished to regain fertility. Median patient age was 42 years and median duration from vasectomy 7 years for RAVV and 11 years for RAVE. Median OR setup duration was 30 min and median robotic OR duration was 120 min and 150 min for RAVV and RAVE, respectively. After 23 months median follow-up, patency rates (more than one million sperm per ejaculate) were 97 % in the RAVV group and 60 % in the RAVE group. Pain relief occurred in 88 % of the patients who underwent RAVV or RAVE for chronic scrotal pain related to vasectomy.

To our knowledge this is the world's largest robotic-assisted microsurgical vasectomy reversal serial and appears to be safe and feasible. The advantages such as a stable microsurgical platform, ergonomic surgeon instrument controls, elimination of tremor, magnified immersive 3D vision, and simultaneous tri-view ability all contribute to reach comparable patency rates with experienced standard microsurgery centers. Further evaluation and longer follow-up is needed to assess its clinical potential and the true cost-benefit ratio.

Robotic-Assisted Microsurgical Varicocelectomy

Technique

A 1–2 cm subinguinal incision is made over the external inguinal ring. A tongue depressor is placed underneath the cord to keep the cord elevated. The robot is positioned from the right of the patient.

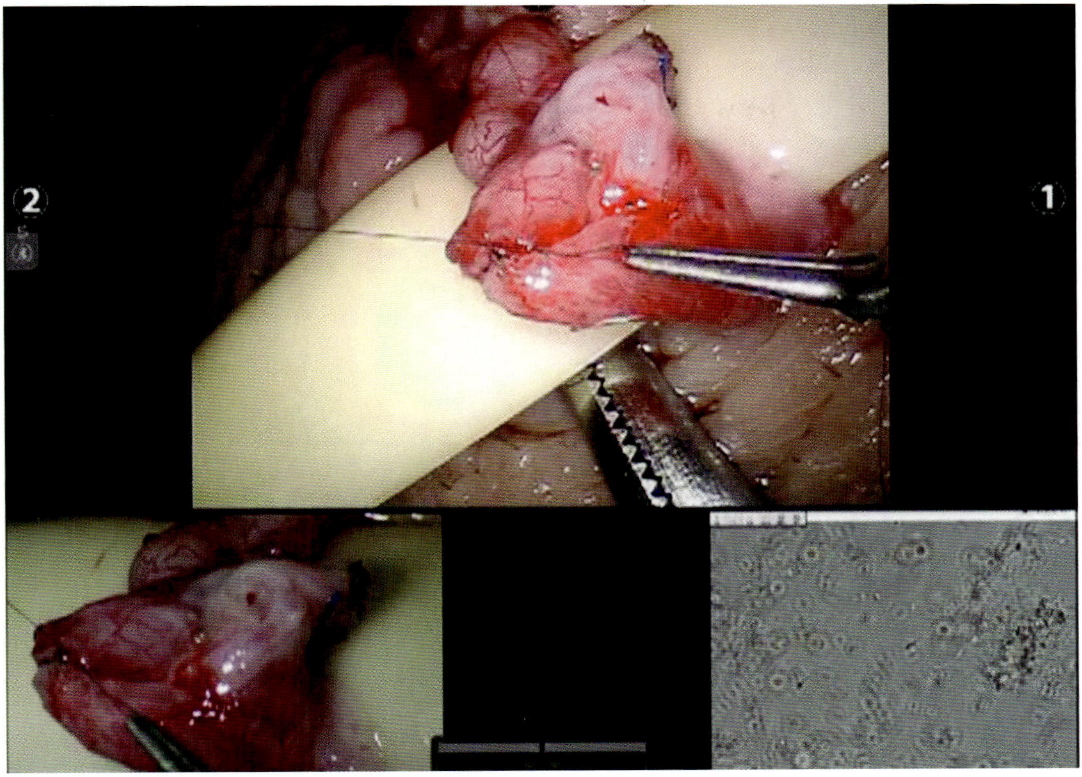

Fig. 30.12 RAVV anterior muscular anastomosis

A zero degree camera lens is utilized. The black diamond micro-forceps are used in the right robotic arm, the micro bipolar forceps in the left arm, and the curved monopolar scissors in the fourth arm. The anterior cremasteric sheath of the spermatic cord is now incised to separate the cord structures.

The artery(ies) is identified using real-time micro-Doppler (Vascular Technology Inc, Nashua, NH). All dilated veins are isolated and tied using 3-0 silk (Fig. 30.17). Vein mapper may be used to help enhance identification of veins (Fig. 30.18). Vessels are cut with curved monopolar scissors. The cord is placed back into the incision and the deep tissue and skin are now closed.

RAVx Outcomes Review

From June 2008 to March 2013, 211 RAVx cases were performed in 180 patients. Indications for the procedure were the presence of a grade two or three varicocele and the following conditions: azoospermia in 18 patients, oligospermia in 53 patients, and chronic orchialgia with or without oligospermia in 109 patients. The median duration per side was 20 min (10–80). Median follow-up was 34 months (1–57). Seventy-eight percentage with oligospermia had a significant improvement in sperm count or motility, 28 % (five patients) with azoospermia converted to oligospermia, and 92 % of the testicular pain patients had a significant reduction in pain (84 % of these patients had targeted denervation of the spermatic cord in addition to varicocelectomy). Two recurrences or persistence of varicocele occurred, one patient developed a small postoperative hydrocele, and two patients had postoperative scrotal hematomas (treated conservatively). The fourth robotic arm allowed the surgeon to control one additional instrument during the cases decreasing reliance on the microsurgical assistant. The fourth arm also enabled the surgeon to perform real-time

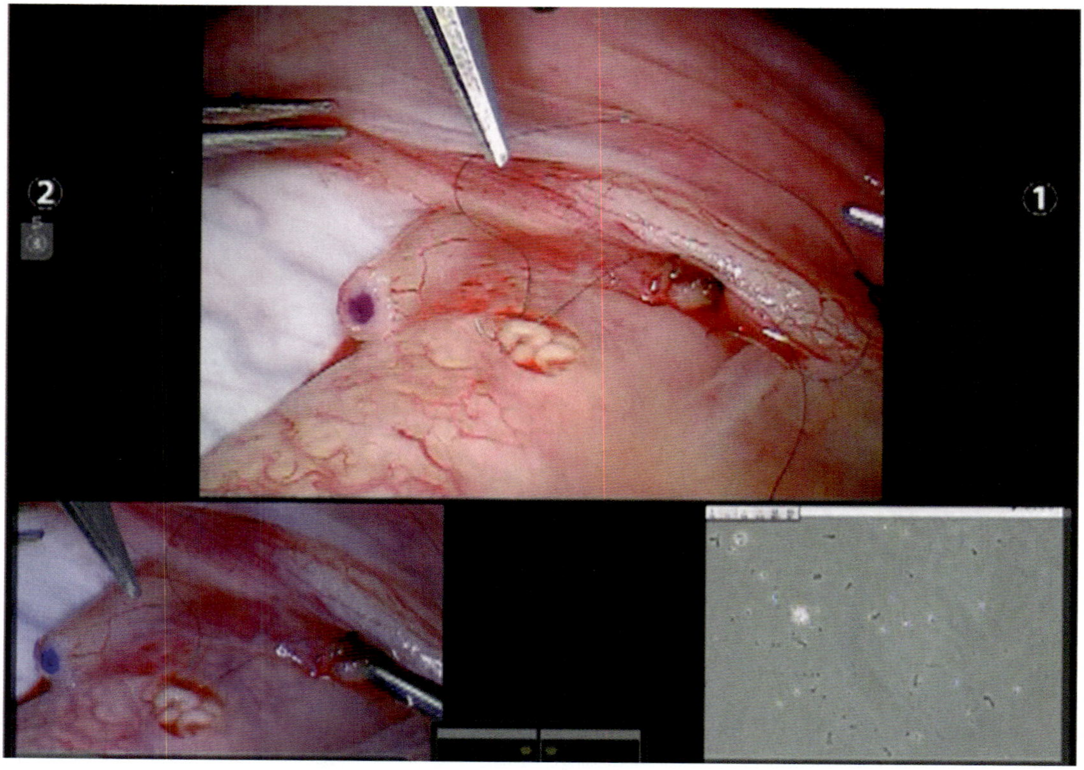

Fig. 30.13 RAVE exposed epididymal tubule

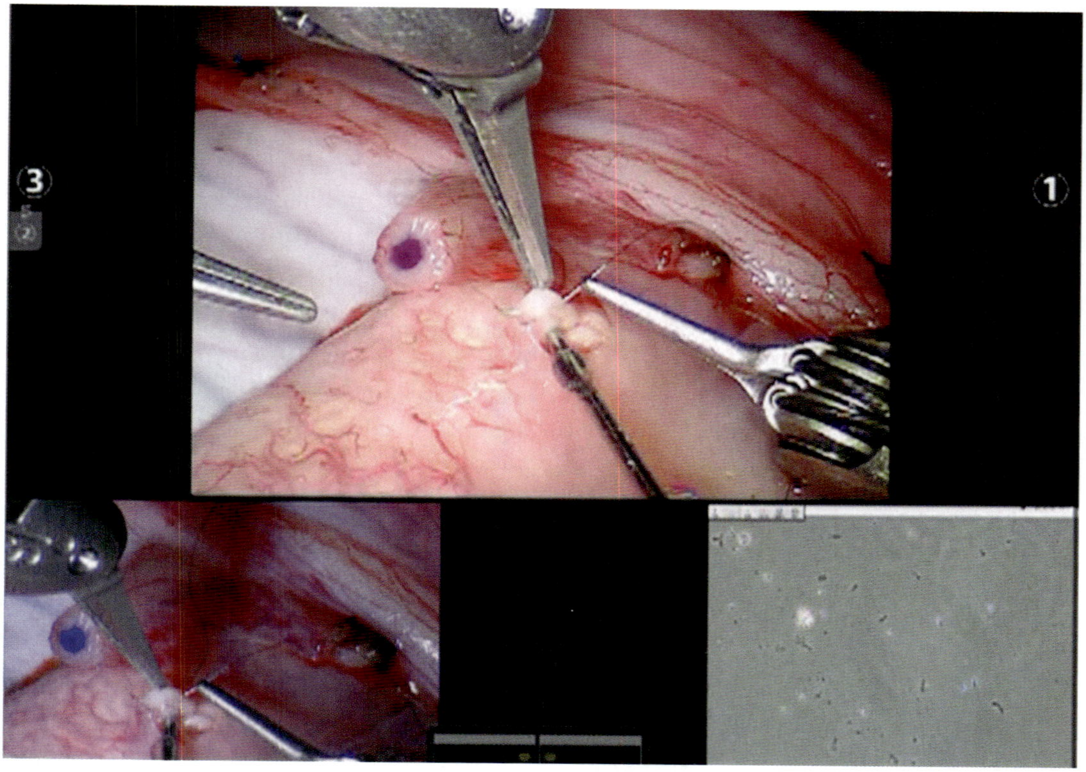

Fig. 30.14 RAVE incision of epididymal tubule

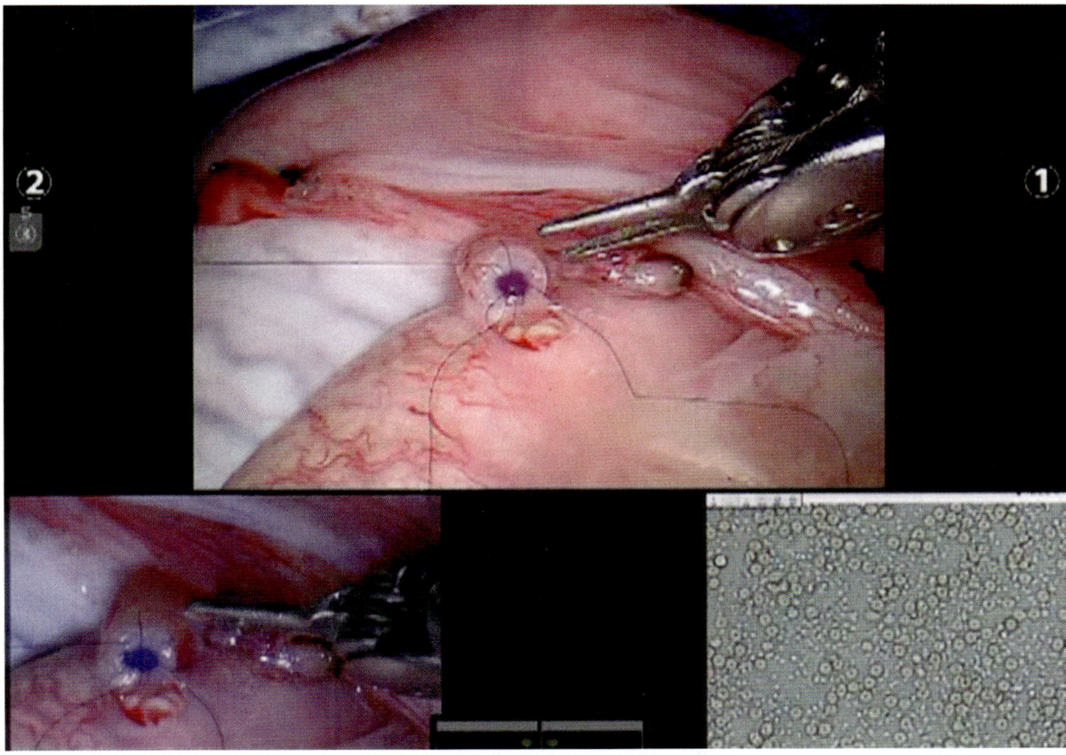

Fig. 30.15 RAVE involution vasoepididymostomy

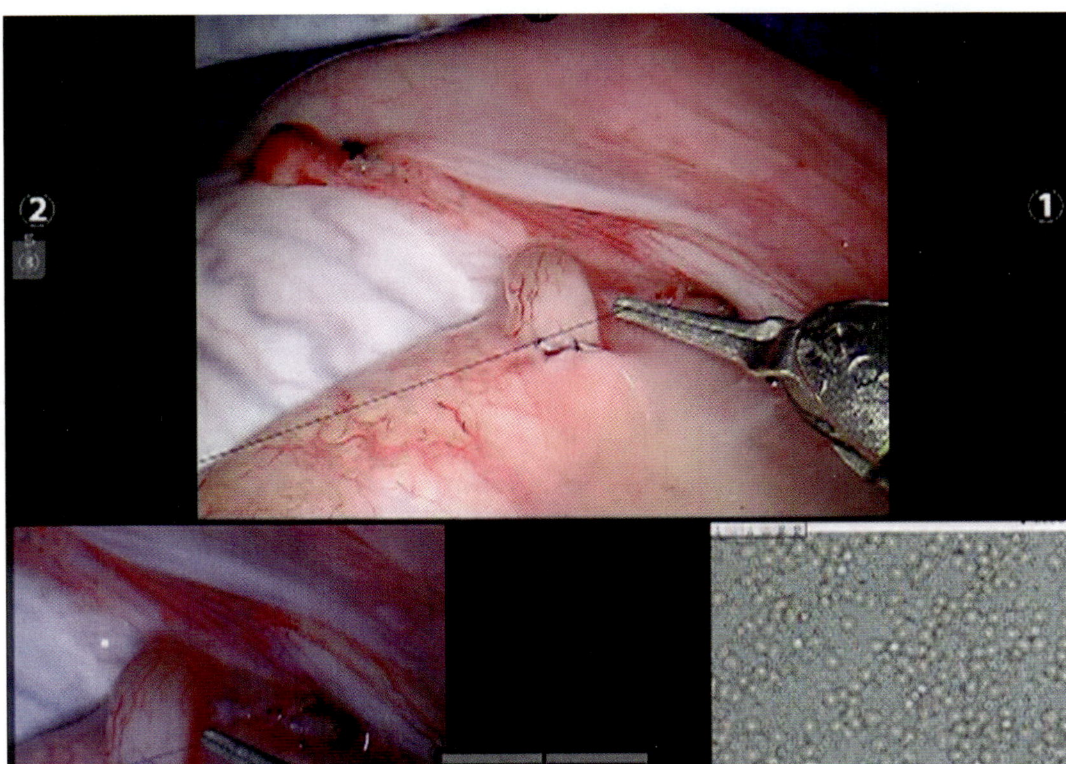

Fig. 30.16 RAVE vas muscularis to epididymal adventitia approximation

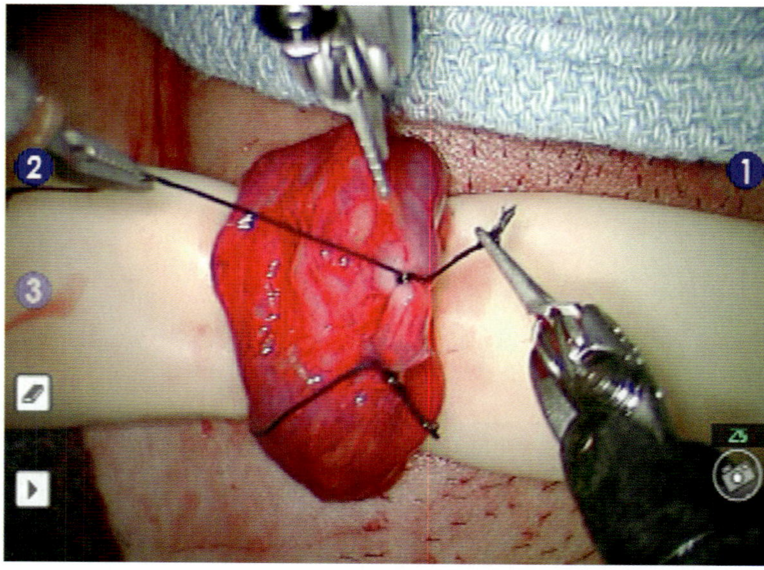

Fig. 30.17 Isolation and ligation of dilated vein

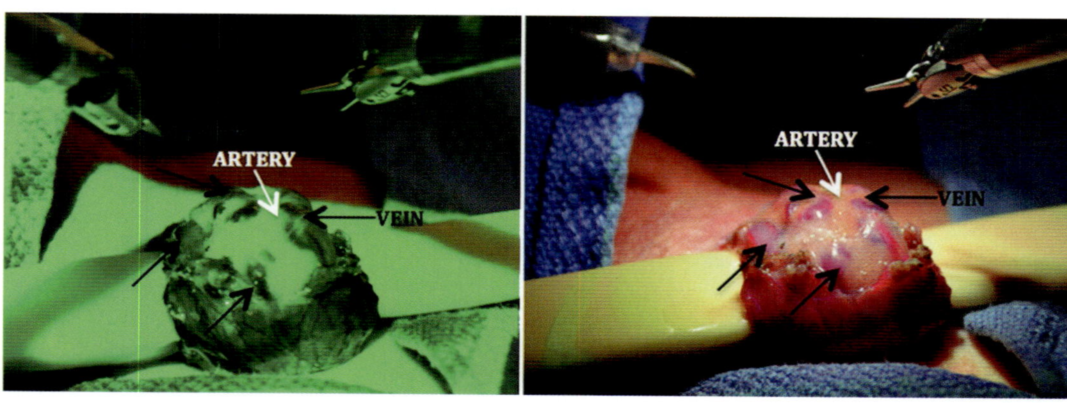

Fig. 30.18 Vein mapper assistance during robotic varicocelectomy

intraoperative Doppler mapping of the testicular arteries while dissecting the veins with the other arms if needed.

RAVx appears to be a safe, feasible, and efficient alternative to pure microsurgical varicocelectomy. The preliminary human results appear promising. Further evaluation and comparative effectiveness studies are warranted.

Robotic-Assisted Microsurgical Testicular Sperm Extraction

Technique

A vertical 4–5 cm incision is made in the scrotal median raphe. The incision is carried down to the tunica vaginalis that is incised to allow

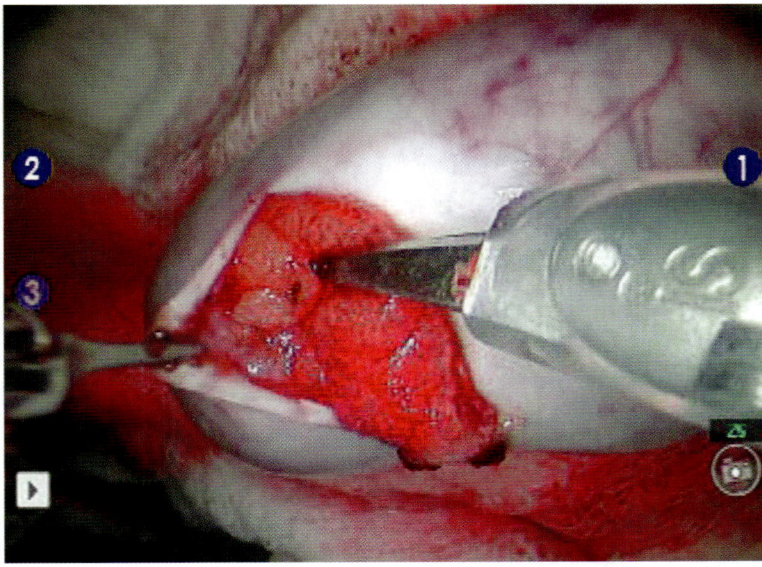

Fig. 30.19 Exposure of larger seminiferous tubules

delivery of the scrotum. The robot is now positioned from the patient's right side as described earlier. Black diamond micro-forceps are placed in the right and fourth robotic arms. Curved monopolar scissors are placed in the left robotic arm. Once the testicle is isolated, a 2–3 cm transverse incision over the tunica exposes the seminiferous tubules. The tunica of the testicle is everted to fully expose all the tubules in the testicle. The testicular lobules are carefully dissected through to find areas that appear to have larger seminiferous tubules (Fig. 30.19). These areas are sampled and the specimens are examined immediately with phase contrast microscopy by a trained embryologist. Sampling is performed until sperm sufficient for multiple-assisted reproductive technique cycles are collected.

In cases where no sperm are readily found, the testicle is thoroughly evaluated. Dissection through the deeper lobules of the testicle is performed and sampling is performed. The additional black diamond micro-forceps in the fourth robotic arm can be very helpful in deep dissection to help retract the superficial lobules out of the way as the surgeon is evaluating the deeper lobules. Once adequate sperm has been retrieved or adequate sampling has been performed, the tunical incisions in the testicle are closed with 6-0 prolene running suture. The testicle in placed back into the tunica vaginalis cavity within the scrotum and closed in layers.

Robotic-Assisted Targeted Denervation of Spermatic Cord

Technique

A 1–2 cm transverse subinguinal incision is made. The incision is carried down until the spermatic cord is reached. Spermatic cord is brought up to the surface. Posterior medial and lateral dissection and cauterization are performed to ligate branches of the ilioinguinal and genitofemoral nerves in this area.

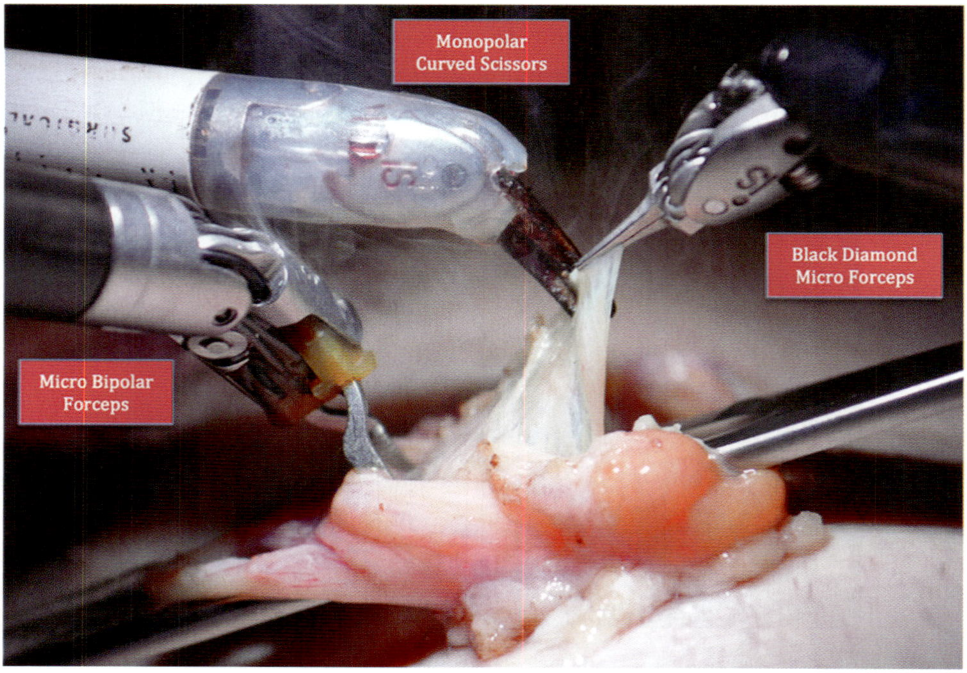

Fig. 30.20 Standard robotic instrumentation for targeted denervation

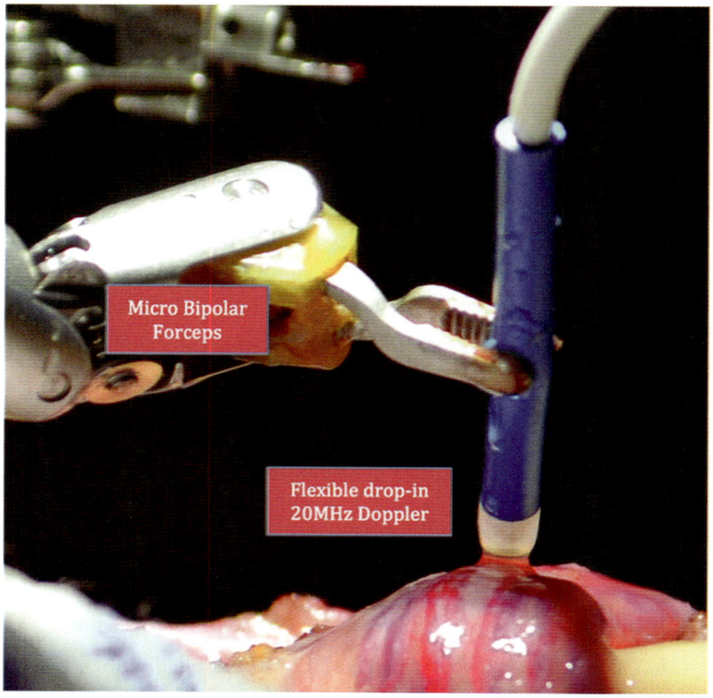

Fig. 30.21 Flexible CO_2 laser instrumentation during targeted denervation

The robot is positioned from the right of the patient. A 0° camera lens is utilized. The right, left, and the fourth robot arms are loaded with black diamond micro-forceps, Maryland bipolar grasper, and monopolar curved scissors, respectively (Fig. 30.20). If a flexible CO_2 laser fiber (Omniguide, Cambridge, MA) dissection is used, then the fourth arm is replaced with a black diamond micro-forceps to hold the Flexguide laser holder (Fig. 30.21).

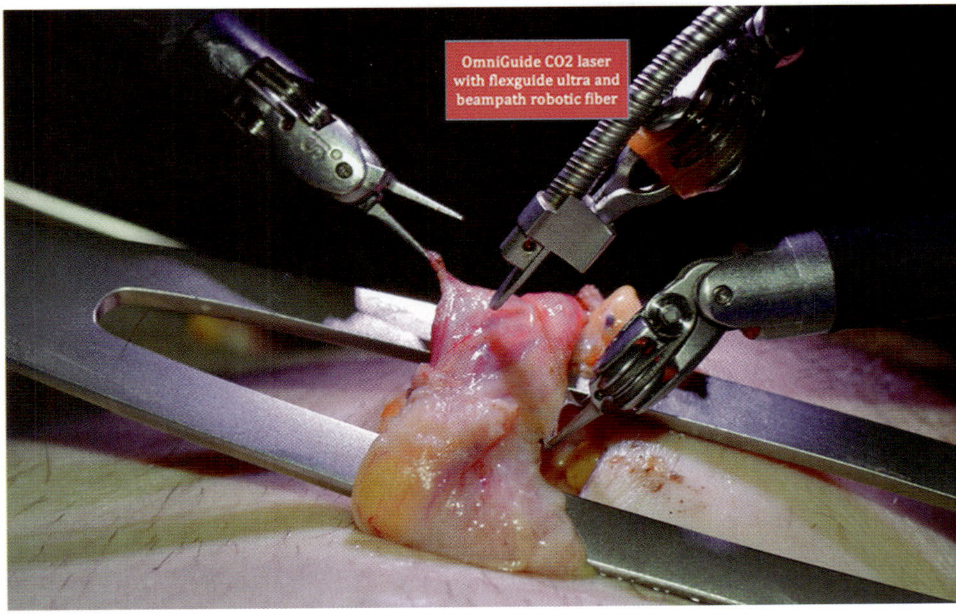

Fig. 30.22 Confirmation of testicular artery using micro-Doppler

Fig. 30.23 Hydrodissection of residual nerve fibers on perivasal tissue

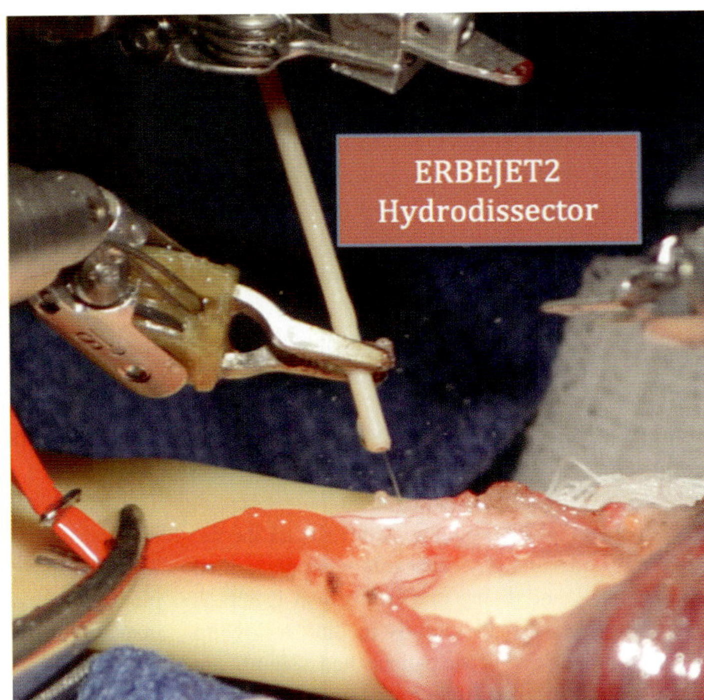

The anterior cremasteric muscle is divided. The presence of a testicular artery is confirmed (Fig. 30.22) with real-time intraoperative micro-Doppler (Vascular Technology Inc, Nashua, NH). The posterior cremasteric fibers and posterior fat component are ablated. The vas is isolated and generally the artery and vein to the vas are dissected away from the vas. The perivasal tissue is now ablated. Hydrodissection of the perivasal tissue is now performed (Fig. 30.23) using the

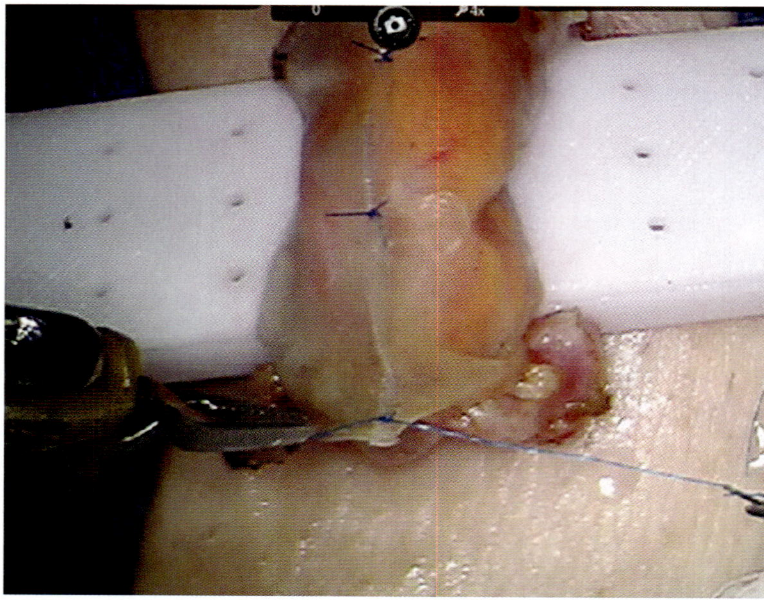

Fig. 30.24 Secured axoguard around spermatic cord

ERBEJET2 hydrodissector (ERBE Inc., Atlanta, GA) to ablate residual nerve fibers.

The cord is now wrapped with axoguard (Axogen Inc., Gainesville, FL) bio-inert wrap to prevent neuroma formation and irritation of ligated nerve ends. The wrap is loosely secured using 6-0 prolene interrupted sutures (Fig. 30.24). The robot is now undocked. The cord is placed back into the incision and the deep tissue and skin are now closed.

RMDSC Outcomes Review

Between October 2008 and March 2013, 496 RMDSC procedures have been performed. The pain was assessed utilizing a standardized validated pain assessment tool: PIQ-6 (QualityMetric Inc., Lincoln, RI). Pain scores and physical exam were performed preoperatively and then postoperatively at 1, 3, 6, 9, and 12 months. At 28 months median follow-up (1–54 months), 86 % of the patients had a significant decrease in their pain (70 % complete response and additional 16 % greater than 50 % reduction in their pain score) by 6 months post-op. The procedure failed to provide pain relief in 55 patients. Median operative duration was 15 min (10–150). Complications included one testicular ischemia, nine hematomas, and two seromas. Two testicular arteries and one vasal injury were all repaired intraoperatively with robotic-assisted microsurgical techniques without any further sequel.

The fourth robotic arm allowed the surgeon to control one additional instrument (micro-Doppler or hydrodissector) leading to less reliance on the microsurgical assistant. Targeted robotic-assisted microsurgical denervation of the spermatic cord seems safe and feasible, and the preliminary results appear promising. Further follow-up and further evaluation is warranted.

Conclusion

The use of robotic assistance is rapidly expanding in many fields that perform microsurgery. The advantages include a stable microsurgical platform, ergonomic control of microsurgical instruments, elimination of tremor and magnified 3D vision with cockpit view, and less reliance on a surgical assistant. As techniques evolve robotic-assisted microsurgery can provide endless opportunities for more efficient and less morbid procedures. The use of these technologies needs to be assessed for its true cost–benefit ratio. Hopefully, this technology will only further provide benefits for our patients.

References

1. Kuang W, Shin PR, Matin S, Thomas Jr AJ. Initial evaluation of robotic technology for microsurgical vasovasostomy. J Urol. 2004;171(1):300–3. Epub 2003/12/11.
2. Schiff J, Li PS, Goldstein M. Robotic microsurgical vasovasostomy and vasoepididymostomy: a prospective randomized study in a rat model. J Urol. 2004; 171(4):1720–5. Epub 2004/03/17.
3. Fleming C. Robot-assisted vasovasostomy. Urol Clin North Am. 2004;31(4):769–72. Epub 2004/10/12.
4. Corcione F, Esposito C, Cuccurullo D, Settembre A, Miranda N, Amato F, et al. Advantages and limits of robot-assisted laparoscopic surgery: preliminary experience. Surg Endosc. 2005;19(1):117–9. Epub 2004/11/19.
5. Shu T, Taghechian S, Wang R. Initial experience with robot-assisted varicocelectomy. Asian J Androl. 2008; 10(1):146–8. Epub 2007/12/19.
6. Parekattil SJ, Gudeloglu A. Robotic assisted andrological surgery. Asian J Androl. 2013;15(1):67–74. Epub 2012/12/18.
7. Parekattil SJ, Brahmbhatt JV. Robotic approaches for male infertility and chronic orchialgia microsurgery. Curr Opin Urol. 2011;21(6):493–9. Epub 2011/09/22.
8. Parekattil SJ, Cohen MS. Robotic surgery in male infertility and chronic orchialgia. Curr Opin Urol. 2010;20(1):75–9. Epub 2009/11/06.
9. Levine LA. Microsurgical denervation of the spermatic cord. J Sex Med. 2008;5(3):526–9. Epub 2008/02/29.
10. Costabile RA, Hahn M, McLeod DG. Chronic orchialgia in the pain prone patient: the clinical perspective. J Urol. 1991;146(6):1571–4. Epub 1991/12/01.
11. McMahon AJ, Buckley J, Taylor A, Lloyd SN, Deane RF, Kirk D. Chronic testicular pain following vasectomy. Br J Urol. 1992;69(2):188–91. Epub 1992/02/01.
12. Alfieri S, Amid PK, Campanelli G, Izard G, Kehlet H, Wijsmuller AR, et al. International guidelines for prevention and management of post-operative chronic pain following inguinal hernia surgery. Hernia. 2011;15(3):239–49. Epub 2011/03/03.
13. Hakeem A, Shanmugam V. Current trends in the diagnosis and management of post-herniorraphy chronic groin pain. World J Gastrointest Surg. 2011;3(6): 73–81. Epub 2011/07/19.
14. Poobalan AS, Bruce J, King PM, Chambers WA, Krukowski ZH, Smith WC. Chronic pain and quality of life following open inguinal hernia repair. Br J Surg. 2001;88(8):1122–6. Epub 2001/08/08.
15. Hindmarsh AC, Cheong E, Lewis MP, Rhodes M. Attendance at a pain clinic with severe chronic pain after open and laparoscopic inguinal hernia repairs. Br J Surg. 2003;90(9):1152–4. Epub 2003/08/29.
16. Parekattil SJ, Gudeloglu A, Brahmbhatt JV, Priola KB, Vieweg J, Allan RW. Trifecta nerve complex – potential anatomic basis for microsurgical denervation of the spermatic cord for chronic orchialgia. J Urol. 2013;190(1):265–70.

Part XIII

Education and Training

Developing a Curriculum for Residents and Fellows

31

Brian Dunkin and Victor Wilcox

Introduction

This chapter is designed as a resource for anyone seeking to develop a curriculum for surgical residents and fellows in robotic surgery. It is organized in the same fashion as a curriculum is developed covering the topics of needs assessment, goals and objectives, didactic and skills educational methods, outcome measures, and evaluation and feedback. The chapter outlines the currently available resources to provide cognitive and technical skills training, highlighting the advantages to each and the barriers to their implementation. It also provides examples of current best practices for each part of the curriculum identified either in the literature or through personal communication with experts in the field. The chapter focuses on training for use of the da Vinci® Surgical System (Intuitive Surgical Inc., Sunnyvale, California, USA), the only FDA-approved surgical robot available in the USA, but the principles for training are the same for any robotic platform.

B. Dunkin, M.D., F.A.C.S. (✉)
Department of Surgery, Houston Methodist Hospital
6550 Fannin Street, Suite 1661A, Houston,
TX 77030, USA

V. Wilcox, M.D
Research Fellow, Department of Surgery, Houston
Methodist Hospital, 6550 Fannin Street, Suite 1661A,
Houston, TX 77030, USA

Needs Assessment

The first step in curriculum design is to perform a thorough needs assessment. This requires determining the learning needs of the target audience, identifying gaps in their current learning, and setting priorities. In 2005, there were 25,000 robotic cases reported; that number grew to 355,000 in 2011 and is on pace to surpass 400,000 cases in 2012 (Fig. 31.1) [1]. Over 1,000 hospitals now boast a robotic surgery platform, and the robot is becoming commonplace in gynecological, urological, thoracic, and general surgery procedures. The robot holds particular importance to certain subspecialties such as urology where the public knowledge of and demand for robotically performed radical prostatectomies have led to an increasing centralization of cases in hospitals equipped with robots where 85 % of all of these procedures are currently performed in the USA [2]. As the use of the robot in surgery becomes ever more prominent, the need for residents and fellows to be trained on the system becomes greater. Adding to this clinical demand are the unique aspects of robotic surgery in regard to patient safety and team communication that are not part of other surgical procedures. These factors and the complexity of the robotic system indicate that robotic surgery training is ideally introduced during residency and fellowship to allow for a longitudinal training experience over a significant period of time. Despite this need, a minority of training programs offers a structured curriculum for robotic surgery. Additionally, a

K.C. Kim (ed.), *Robotics in General Surgery*, DOI 10.1007/978-1-4614-8739-5_31,

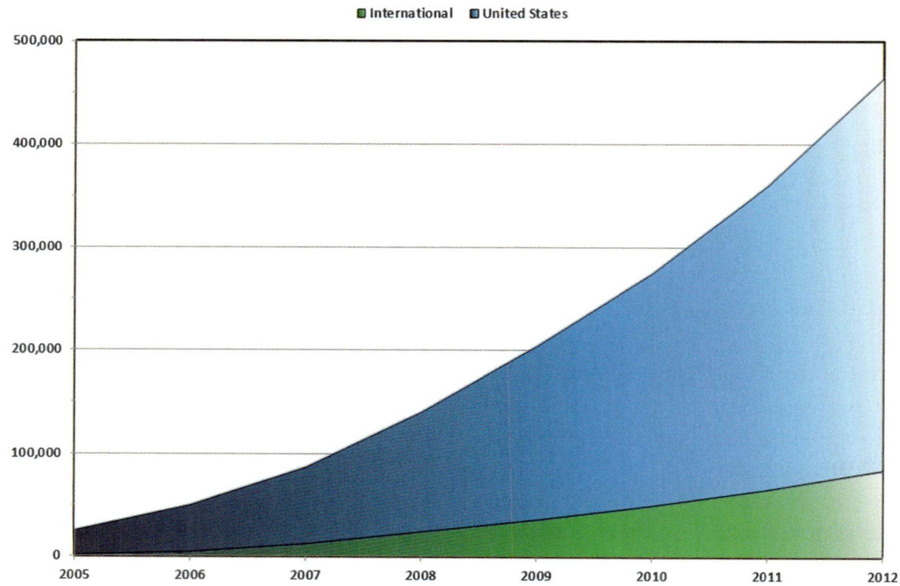

Fig. 31.1 Rapid rise in robotic surgical procedures with extrapolated estimates through 2012

lack of accepted clinical measures of competency in robotic surgery has led to great variability in credentialing requirements for use of the robot at different hospitals. The end result is a failure to guarantee that any particular training curriculum will provide all the evidence of competency that an institution requires for the graduating resident or fellow to practice [3]. Clearly, the increasing volume of robotic surgery across multiple specialties, coupled with the unique aspects of robotic procedures, complexity of the platform, and variability in training opportunities is strong evidence that there is a need for more structured curricula introduced as early as possible into surgical residency and fellowships.

Goals and Objectives

Once a formal needs analysis is performed, the next step in curriculum development is to determine the goals and objectives of the curriculum. Goals are general ideas of what the curriculum needs to accomplish such as "provide residents and fellows with a comprehensive robotic education to make them more proficient in robotic surgery." Objectives are more specific action items often worded as "After completing this curriculum the learner will be able to…" Goals are determined based on the needs analysis and objectives created for each goal that are specific actionable items. For example, one goal is to teach residents and fellows to be proficient in robotic surgery. An objective to meet this goal might be that after completion of the curriculum, the resident will be able to describe the components of the da Vinci Si robotic system.

Expertise in a surgical domain requires both knowledge and technical skill. Interestingly, of all the curricula reviewed for this chapter, many had written overall goals and specific objectives for what was to be achieved technically, but few had specific cognitive objectives. In developing a meaningful curriculum with measurable outcomes, it is essential to pay particular attention to well-developed goals and objectives.

Knowledge

All medical device manufacturers are committed to the safe use of their products and take measured steps to achieve this by their users. Intuitive Surgical Inc., the manufacturer of the da Vinci Surgical System (dVSS) is no different. As a result, the company has developed the da Vinci Surgery Training Pathway and the da Vinci Residency/Fellowship Training Program. The

Surgical Training Pathway is focused on practicing physicians who want to learn to perform robotic surgery, while the Residency/Fellowship program is focused on "senior" level residents (those in the last 2 years of training) and fellows across multiple specialties. Both programs utilize online modules and assessments developed specifically for each da Vinci platform (Si, Si-e, S, and Standard) coupled with live in-person hands-on training using the actual robotic system and either inanimate or animate models. The online modules for both are available for free through the da Vinci Surgery Online Community accessed through Intuitive's website (http://www.intuitivesurgical.com) [4].

The da Vinci Residency/Fellowship Training Program is arranged into three steps: Step 1—preclinical phase, Step 2—clinical preparation phase, and Step 3—online modules and assessments. Step 1 is focused on residents and fellows who are not yet prepared to operate the dVSS clinically—either as a patient-side assistant or as a console surgeon. There are four components to this step (1) online dVSS courses and exams for each system, (2) hands-on dVSS overview, (3) procedure observation, and (4) literature review. The first component consists of professionally developed on-line video modules with a self-assessment quiz to be completed after viewing. There are four goals for this component (1) describe the features and benefits of the dVSS, (2) review the surgeon console components, (3) review the patient cart components, and (4) review the vision cart components. No objectives are listed to achieve these goals. It is anticipated to take approximately 2 h to review the material, and residents/fellows who complete the module and take the self-assessment quizzes will receive an online certificate of completion. There is no description of what is entailed in the second component of Step 1—hands-on dVSS overview. For the third component, procedure observation, it is suggested that this can be accomplished by viewing live cases or recorded cases from the da Vinci online video library. No goals or objectives are described for this component and no suggested cases. The fourth and final component of Step 1 is a literature review. Multiple robotic surgery articles are available through the Intuitive website, but no suggested articles, structure of review, or goals and objectives for this component are available.

Step 2 of the da Vinci Residency/Fellowship Training Program is focused on residents and fellows who are beginning their participation in dVSS surgery. It has six components (1) energy control lab for da Vinci Si users, (2) da Vinci port placement philosophy, (3) dVSS docking practicum, (4) dVSS skills training, (5) procedure observation, and (6) literature review. Components 1–4 are all done with an instructor using the real dVSS platform in an inanimate lab, and while instructions for how to set-up and conduct the labs are provided, there are no goals and objectives described. Components 5 and 6 are identical to that describe for components 3 and 4 in Step 1.

Step 3 of the da Vinci Residency/Fellowship Training Program entails online modules and assessments for each of the available dVSS models on the market. The components of each module and the goals of each component are shown in Table 31.1. There are extremely comprehensive descriptions of the dVSS system with professionally edited videos and images coupled with self-assessment quizzes within each module and a final comprehensive "Staff Assessment" test at the end. As a result, this material is frequently incorporated into curricula developed by individual training programs to satisfy the cognitive component.

The most comprehensive industry agnostic curriculum is the Fundamentals of Robotic Surgery (FRS) Curriculum being developed under the direction of three co-principle investigators (Satava, Smith, and Patel) with funding from industry and government [5]. The FRS program has brought together experts from multiple surgical societies and in the fields of education and performance metrics to build a basic curriculum in robotically assisted surgery that could be adopted by multiple specialties. Since 2011 there have been four FRS conferences focused on identifying the essential components of knowledge and skill required to perform robotic surgery. The vision is to create didactic content coupled with hands-on skills practice and team training that lead to measurable competence. A high stakes written examination and hands-on skills test are also planned to serve as validated measures of knowledge and

Table 31.1 Components and goals for da Vinci online modules

Intuitive da Vinci online training modules	
Module	Training goals
da Vinci Si (or Si-e, S, Standard) system	
Overview	• Provide an overview of the features and benefits of the dVSS • Review the surgeon console components • Review the patient cart components • Review the vision cart components
OR setup and system connections	
OR configuration	• Demonstrate how to arrange the system components into a basic OR configuration
System connections	• Review the steps for properly connecting all the system cables
Start-up	• Demonstrate the start-up process
Shutdown	• Demonstrate the shutdown process
Vision system	
Components	• Introduce the components of the vision system – CORE – Camera assembly – CCU – Illuminator – Touch screen monitor
Vision system controls	• Review vision system controls available on the touch screen monitor and camera head
White balance	• Explain the white balancing procedure
Endoscope calibration	• Review the steps for endoscope and camera calibration
Draping	
Patient cart	• Review the patient cart components that require draping • Demonstrate the steps required to drape the patient cart
Camera assembly	• Provide an overview of the camera assembly components • Demonstrate the steps required to drape the camera
Touch screen monitor	• Demonstrate the steps required to drape the touch screen monitor
Docking	
Port placement	• Review the basic da Vinci port placement philosophy • Discuss the accessories needed for port placement • Explain remote center technology
Camera arm positioning	• Summarize the steps for setting up and aligning the camera arm to maximize range of motion
Instrument arm positioning	• Summarize the steps for setting up and aligning the instrument arms to maximize range of motion
Docking	• Review the steps for docking the patient cart • Explain the guidelines for minimizing trauma to the incision site • Provide tips for retaining correct position of the camera and instrument arms during the docking process
Endoscope insertion and removal	• Review the correct procedure for inserting and removing the endoscope and camera assembly
Instrument insertion and removal	• Review the procedure for inserting and removing the *EndoWrist* instruments manually • Demonstrate the correct procedure for removing and inserting the *EndoWrist* instruments using the guided tool exchange (GTE)
Safety features	
Fault modes and error handling	• Review recoverable and non-recoverable fault modes • Discuss basic safety features and error handling procedures • Explain the battery back-up feature • Discuss the process for contacting customer service • Review the process for accessing the events logs

(continued)

Table 31.1 (continued)

Intuitive da Vinci online training modules	
Module	Training goals
Emergency switches	• Review the function and purpose of the emergency stop button • Review the function and purpose of the emergency power off switches
Energy control	• Review the system energy and control features
Procedure conversions	• Review the procedure steps for converting to an open or laparoscopic procedure in an emergency situation
Final OR staff assessment	
Da Vinci Si OR staff assessment	• Quiz covering the material in all of the modules

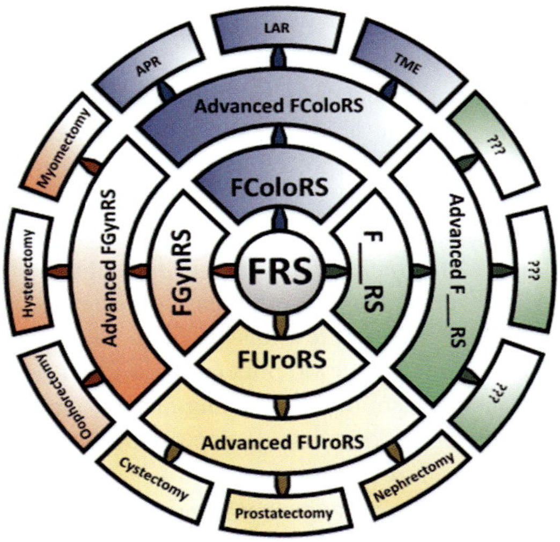

Fig. 31.2 The Sweet tree of curriculum templates

skill at the completion of the curriculum. The program is arranged into three phases—preoperative, intraoperative, and postoperative—and the goals and objectives of this curriculum are evolving. FRS is meant to serve as the core knowledge and skills required by any specialty to perform robotic surgery, with more advanced modules left to be developed by specific specialties (Fig. 31.2).

Another example of a curriculum with clear goals and objectives in the knowledge domain has been created at the Lehigh Valley Health Network under the direction of Dr. Mario Martino. This curriculum is available through the "The Medicine Network" website which serves as a central repository for curricula and resources for robotic training for medical students, residents, and fellows [6]. The goal of the Lehigh Valley Health Network robotic surgical training curriculum for residents is to train all OB-GYN and general surgery residents to be competent bedside assistants in complex robotic surgery. The curriculum has two phases—bedside training and console training. Within bedside training, there are five competencies with clearly identified goals and objectives in both knowledge and skill.

Technical Skill

Most curricula focus on the technical skills required to perform robotic surgery. For the da Vinci Residency/Fellowship Training Program, technical skills are rehearsed using the actual dVSS in either an inanimate or animate laboratory setting and under the guidance of a trained proctor. While the Program provides suggested "scripts" of what should be done in the lab and what measures should be recorded, there are no specific goals or objectives outlined.

The FRS Curriculum sought to develop a deconstructed task list essential for all specialties. Participating expert surgeons engaged in a 2-day workshop using the Delphi method where ideas from each institution's curriculum were evaluated and then ranked by anonymous vote. The guiding principles in selecting tasks were that they be oriented around three dimensions, incorporate as many elements of real surgical skills as possible, be cost effective, easy to administer and reliably evaluate, utilize physical models that could be placed under any robotic platform, and preferably already have validating evidence supporting their use. After the first selection round, tasks were organized into a matrix and then another round of voting performed to assign importance. Tasks falling two standard deviations below the mean task score were eliminated. The resulting task list (Table 31.2) serves as a basis for training objectives for a core global curriculum.

The Lehigh Valley Health Network curriculum requires skills practice using the Fundamentals of Laparoscopic Surgery (FLS—http://www.flsprogram.org) as well as inanimate and simulator training on the robotic platform but does not provide details of this practice or outline goals and objectives.

Dulan et al. from the University of Texas Southwestern Medical Center have developed and published a comprehensive, proficiency-based curriculum [7]. While this curriculum uses the da Vinci Residency/Fellowship Training Program for its didactic content, it systematically created goals and objectives for developing technical skills. This process brought together six experienced experts from various disciplines to identify the skills necessary to perform robotic surgical procedures for any specialty. From this discussion, they developed a deconstructed task list that served as the basis for their objectives in the skills curriculum (Table 31.3).

Lyons et al. from the Methodist Institute for Technology, Innovation, and Education (MITIE^{SM}) have used a similar consensus conference of experts to deconstruct robotic surgery skills into a somewhat shorter list of tasks which then served as a basis for developing a proficiency-based skills curriculum using the da Vinci Skills Simulator (Table 31.4) [8].

Didactic and Skills Educational Methods

After deciding on the objectives that will best achieve the learning goals of the curriculum, the next step is to identify available content and educational methods and select those that will maximize the impact of the curriculum on the target learners. In the case of robotic surgery, training objectives require both didactic and skills training. For didactic content, training can be in the form of computer-based modules, reading of the literature, or traditional classroom training. For skills training, the choices include working with inanimate models, participating in animal or cadaver surgeries, and working with virtual reality simulators.

Didactic Educational Methods

As described in the section "Goals and Objectives," many training programs currently leverage the online content provided by Intuitive Surgical Inc. through their da Vinci Residency/Fellowship Training Program to serve as the didactic portion of their curriculum. These modules include high-quality multimedia presentations, and the trainee can select training specific to the robot model available to them (Standard, S, Si, or Si-e). Each of the six modules takes approximately 2 h to complete and includes self-assessment questions. There are certificates of completion for each individual module and for completing a comprehensive written exam at the end of the entire online program. Many curricula require trainees to print out these certificates and submit them to their training director prior to embarking on skills training or working as a bedside assistant. Directors may want to require each trainee to complete more than one or even all of the model-specific modules depending on the generation of robot(s) in use at their institution. Intuitive also has a large library of procedure videos that can serve as a source of training material during the didactic phase of training. Although this library is comprehensive in scope, the value of the videos for helping residents and fellows to independently learn about robotic procedures may be limited as they are highly edited; usually do not review patient selection, room setup, or port placement; and often are without audio.

While the intuitive online modules are well designed and freely available, some feel that the didactic portion of a curriculum should be developed and validated independent of a vendor. This not only allows content to be directly targeted at the curriculum's learning objectives but also allows for ongoing evolution and refinement of the content to meet evolving needs and improvement of the program based on feedback and outcomes evaluations. The Lehigh Valley Health

Table 31.2 FRS task list in order of decreasing importance

Task	Description
Situation awareness	Aware of status of team, equipment essential to the procedure, and patient status; maintains effective communication
Eye–hand instrument coordination	Learn to accurately and efficiently manipulate the bedside instruments with economy of motion; pass objects between instruments
Needle driving	Accurately and efficiently pass needle through targeted tissue without tearing, damaging adjacent structures, or dropping the needle
Atraumatic handling	Manipulating tissue with graspers without causing avulsion or crush injuries; understanding of haptics
Safety of operative field	Appropriate placement and positioning of instruments so as to avoid injury to tissues from instrument collision outside of the field of view
Camera	Effectively maneuver the camera in a controlled manner maintaining focus, proper orientation and angle, and avoiding tissue contact
Clutching	Maintaining full range of motion in an efficient, ergonomic manner without collision of console controls; efficient, accurate use of pedals
Dissection, fine and blunt	Accurately utilizes instruments to bluntly or precisely dissect tissue in correct plains maintaining traction and countertraction and adequate exposure without injuring surrounding structures
Closed loop communication	Maintain effective communication with team members using names, clear requests, and using callbacks as per TeamSTEPPS®
Docking	Guides team in docking the robot efficiently with proper positioning and alignment, attaches arms to trocars, avoids moving OR table
Knot tying	Accurately and efficiently ties secure knots with economy of motion and without causing tissue damage or ischemia
Instrument exchange	Efficiently, accurately, and safely removes
Cutting	Efficiently and accurately cuts the right structure without collateral damage or going past-point
Energy sources	Applies energy appropriately without collateral damage
Foreign body management	Safely removes all foreign bodies from the patient with the appropriate instruments, confirming removal and instrument counts
Robotic Trocars	Safely inserts trocars with correct orientation and spatial orientation relative to the target; uses direct visualization after first trocar
Suture handling	Efficiently, accurately, and safely places running and interrupted sutures to adequate appose tissues avoiding suture breakage or tissue damage
Wrist articulation	Efficiently uses all degrees of freedom in full range of motion
Ergonomic positioning	Maintains good posture with comfortable position of body and limbs during the entire procedure
System settings	Can properly configure console settings for scope angle, magnification, and motion speed and scaling
Multiple arm control	Can efficiently activate and employ the fourth arm in the procedure without collisions
OR setup	Properly arranges bedside cart where most accessible and safe while maintaining sterile field
Robot system errors	Understands and troubleshoots system errors to correct them when possible avoiding unnecessary conversion
Undocking	Efficiently and safely removes robotic equipment and trocars and inspects port sites
Transition to bedside assist	Safely and efficiently removes instruments and ports performing port site inspections

Network created such content that is freely available online [9]. It incorporates multimedia- and computer-based training with live video and animations. Trainees learn about the history of robotic surgery as well as the future expectations for the field. They also learn the benefits, indications for, and recent advancements in the robotic platforms. The program teaches about the surgeon

Table 31.3 Deconstructed robotic surgery curriculum tasks list from UT southwestern

Task	Description
Cognitive skills	
Console setup	Setting up and adjusting console settings as needed during surgery
Docking	Surgeon guides OR nurse in positioning bedside robot and attaches arms to trocars
Robotic trocars	Appropriate port location strategies and placement technique
Robotic positioning	Placing the bedside cart in the location where the operative field is most accessible
Communication	Closed loop communication between console surgeon, bedside assistants and OR team
Robot component names	Knowledge of robotic component terminology
Instrument names	Knowledge of instrument terminology
Technical skills	
Energy sources	Activation and control of cautery or other energy sources
Camera	Maneuvering the camera to obtain a suitable view
Clutching	Maintaining comfortable range of motion for manual controls
Instrument exchange	Changing out instruments used in the operation
Fourth arm control	Activating the fourth arm through clutching and using it in the operation
Basic eye–hand coordination	Using manual controls to accurately manipulate bedside instruments and perform tasks
Wrist articulation	Understanding and using the full range of motion of the *EndoWrist* (Intuitive Surgical)
Depth perception	Appreciating spatial relationships of instruments and tissue
Instrument to instrument transfer	Passing objects between the instruments
Atraumatic handling	Using graspers to hold tissue or surgical material without crushing or tearing
Blunt dissection	Using instruments to separate tissues bluntly
Fine dissection	Using instruments to perform precise dissection of delicate structures
Retraction	Holding tension on an object to facilitate surgical manipulation
Cutting	Using the scissors to cut at a precise location
Interrupted suturing	Suturing single stitches with the robot
Running suturing	Suturing continuous stitches with the robot

Table 31.4 MITIE deconstructed task list for robotic surgery

	Task	Description
1	Pick and place	Pick up an object and set it down in a specific location
2	Two-handed transfer	Transfer an object from one hand to another in space
3	Wrist manipulation	Use wristed instruments to advantage
4	Camera control	Manipulate camera for optimal view
5	Clutching	Use clutch control to optimize position of hands at surgeons console and minimize working space
6	Third arm	Use of third arm for retraction and manipulation
7	Suturing	Suturing efficiently and accurately
8	Energy	Use of energy—monopolar and bipolar

console, vision cart, bedside cart, and instrumentation. In addition, trainees learn safety measures and what to consider when selecting patients for robotic versus laparoscopic surgery. There is a self-assessment test at the end of the program which requires passage at a rate of 80 % in order to receive a completion certificate. While this material was developed with medical students as the target audience, it is well done and clearly applicable to residents and fellows as well.

After successful completion of the Lehigh Valley online modules, the trainee is prescribed mentored learning time in the laboratory to learn more about port placement, docking, and working as a first assistant. Patient management skills are also mentored both in the clinic and on the hospital wards as trainees learn to identify good candidates for robotic surgery and manage patients postoperatively. Trainees are also mentored on systems-based practice in which they review robotic cases to identify variation in quality and areas for improvement. In addition, mentors teach professionalism and demonstrate effective communication between the trainee and members of the robotic surgery team and the Lehigh program has developed in-house evaluation tools for measuring performance in these areas.

The FRS Curriculum has also developed an outline to create vendor agnostic didactic content matched to the deconstructed educational tasks identified through expert consensus conferences. It is planned for this material to be developed with input from multiple specialty societies and made available through an online host.

Skills Educational Methods

In addition to the online didactic training module, the da Vinci Residency/Fellowship Training Program outlines technical skills rehearsal using the actual dVSS and is meant to be administered by trained Intuitive proctors at approved training sites. Currently this program is not readily available and residents or fellows who want this type of experience must go through the da Vinci Surgery Training Pathway at an approved animate lab for a fee.

A number of institutions have published robotic skills curricula, including the departments of Obstetrics and Gynecology at the University of Alabama, the University of North Carolina at Chapel Hill, and the Lehigh Valley Health Network. Each teaches the same set of skills using in-house robots and inanimate models either home grown or acquired from a third party vendor [10, 11]. Practice begins with learning to dock the robot safely. It then progresses to skills rehearsal using inanimate models. The Chamberlain Group (Great Barrington, MA) offers a number of inanimate surgical skills models that are commonly used for this purpose (see Table 31.5) (Figs. 31.3, 31.4, 31.5, and 31.6) [12]. They also offer kits with multiple models that may prove more economical (see Figs. 31.7 and 31.8). Unfortunately, there are no validated metrics of performance on these tasks that can be used for formative or summative feedback.

In contrast, Genevieve et al. from the University of Texas Southwestern (UTSW) have developed the most comprehensive and validated series of inexpensive, inanimate exercises in a fashion similar to the Fundamentals of Laparoscopic Surgery (FLS) [13]. Using the deconstructed task list in Table 31.3, these investigators set out to develop tasks on physical models that would incorporate these desired skills. Care was taken to minimize cost and use durable materials that could standup to repetitive practice. Through this development process, nine exercises (Table 31.6) (Figs. 31.9, 31.10, 31.11, 31.12, 31.13, 31.14, 31.15, 31.16, and 31.17) were chosen to be used in a box trainer utilizing standardized templates, the Standard da Vinci system, a zero degree camera, and various 8 mm articulating robotic instruments. The tasks were ordered according to increasing level of complexity. Prior to the performance of each exercise, the manual controls of the console unit were placed in an optimal neutral position by the proctor; for tasks 1, 3, and 4, no clutching or camera adjustments were allowed, whereas clutching and camera adjustments were encouraged for the other tasks. Tasks 1, 4, 5, 8, and 9 used FLS models (http://www.flsprogram.org), including a pegboard, suture block, slitted Penrose drains, and premarked gauze. Modifications of the FLS models included creation of a hexagonal pegboard for task 5 and extension of the Penrose drain slit to 2 cm with placement of 5 target pairs for task 9. Commercially available models (Manipulation Skill Drill Pod, The Chamberlin Group, http://www.thecgroup.com) were used for tasks 3 and 6 and modified by placing them on standardized

Table 31.5 Inanimate models used in intuitive skills training

Chamberlain group model	Skill session instructions
Item 4068 (Fig. 31.3)	*Manipulation* Trainees take a ring from the center, transfer it to the other hand, and place it on the corresponding outer peg. After moving all four rings, they then reverse the process *Instruments* Two large needle drivers *Evaluation* Trainees are timed and suffer time penalties of 5 s for dropping rings and 5 s for omitting any hand-offs
Item 4072 (Fig. 31.4)	*Dissection* Trainees use blunt or sharp dissection to dissect through the superficial layer of the model and dissect out the embedded vessel, mobilizing it across a specified length (should be marked) *Instruments* Two Maryland bipolar forceps *Evaluation* Trainees are timed and suffer time penalties of 5 s for injuries to vessels and 10 s for avulsions of the vessels from the proximal or distal attachments
Item 4075 (Fig. 31.5)	*Transection* Trainees take grasp the model with the ProGrasp™ forceps at the indicated spot, then transect the tissue beginning at the lowest numbered area 1 and proceeding one at a time to area 6 *Instruments* Large needle driver, curved scissors, and ProGrasp™ forceps (with third arm) *Evaluation* Trainees are timed on each wave transected and suffer time penalties of 5 s for transecting outside of the marked boundaries
Item 4073 (Fig. 31.6)	*Suturing* Trainees use the 20cm length suture to close the "I" using running suture and 4 knots; they then repair the "S" defect using the three 10cm lengths of suture with figures of eight through marked areas on the model and tied with four knots each *Instruments* Two Large Needle Drivers w/ 3 × 10cm lengths and 1 × 20cm length of 3-0 Vicryl™ RB-1 *Evaluation* Trainees are timed and suffer time penalties of 5 s for dropping a suture, 10 s for breaking a suture, 5 s for driving needle outside of the marked zone, and 5 s for incomplete tissue approximation

templates. Tasks 2 and 7 were created de novo. Task 2 used freehand drawings of polygons and error markings such that when targets were appropriately acquired by the camera, a uniform rectangular shape was visible on the monitor as witnessed by the proctor. Task 7 used a rubber band with inked targets placed at 1 cm intervals. A video illustrating the appropriate technique as well as pitfalls to avoid was created for use as a standardized tutorial.

Objective scoring based on the previously validated FLS approach [14–16] was used and included time and carefully defined errors (Table 31.6); for example, accuracy was measured in mm (tasks 4, 7, and 9), and surface area of cuts outside of the circular line was measured graphically (task 8). Based on observation of expert and novice performance, cutoff times (maximal allowable task duration) were assigned for each task. The following formula was used: Score = (cutoff time) − (completion time) − (weighting factor × sum of errors); to heavily penalize suboptimal performance, errors were weighted by a factor of 10 (tasks 1–7, 9) or 50 (task 8, Pattern Cut, requiring all cuts to be within the marked line). A higher score indicated superior performance. A score of zero was assigned if a negative value was derived. Similarly, if a protocol violation occurred, such as using the wrong technique, as witnessed under direct observation by the proctor during testing, a score of zero was assigned.

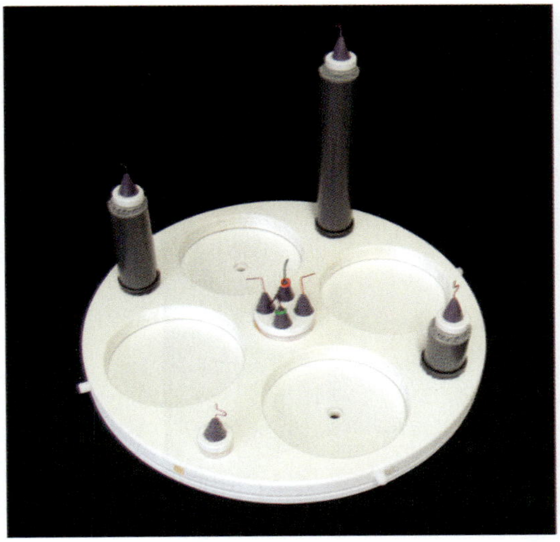

Fig. 31.3 Chamberlain Group Item 4068

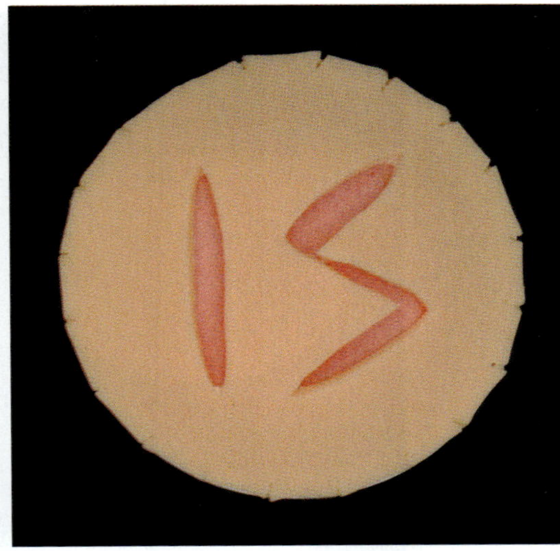

Fig. 31.5 Chamberlain Group Item 4075

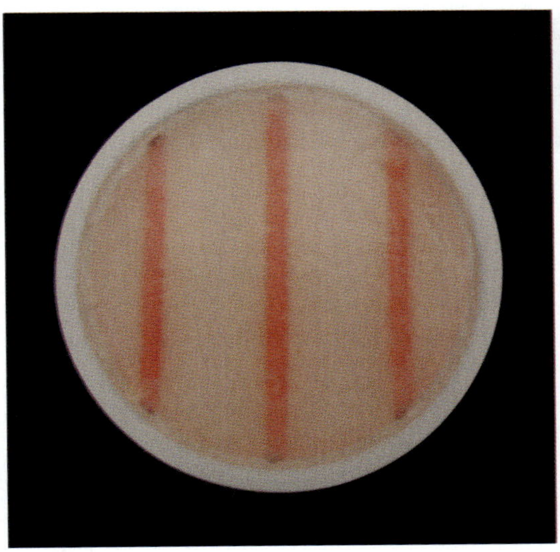

Fig. 31.4 Chamberlain Group Item 4072

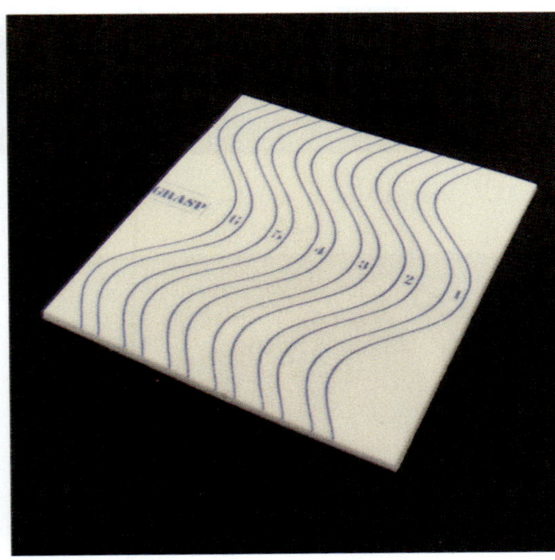

Fig. 31.6 Chamberlain Group Item 4073

A robotic expert (extensive prior clinical experience) performed five consecutive repetitions of each task and the mean −2 s.d. values were chosen as preliminary proficiency levels; data were suitably homogeneous and there were no outliers (>2 s.d.). A normalized score was defined as the task score divided by the proficiency score; a composite score was defined as the sum of all nine normalized task scores. A robotic novice (no prior robotic and minimal laparoscopic exposure) performed all components of the curriculum, including three consecutive repetitions of tasks 1–9 as a measure of baseline performance; the baseline novice and expert scores were compared to evaluate construct validity, defined as the ability of a test to measure the trait that it purports to measure. The novice then practiced the nine tasks until proficiency was reached on two consecutive repetitions for each task and underwent proctored post-testing (one repetition per task).

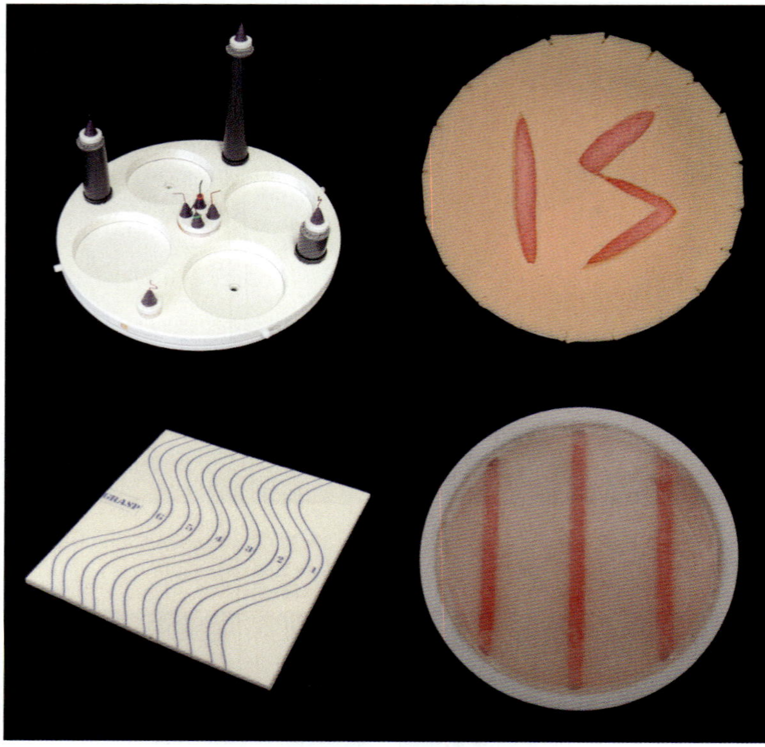

Fig. 31.7 Robotic system skills kit from the Chamberlain Group

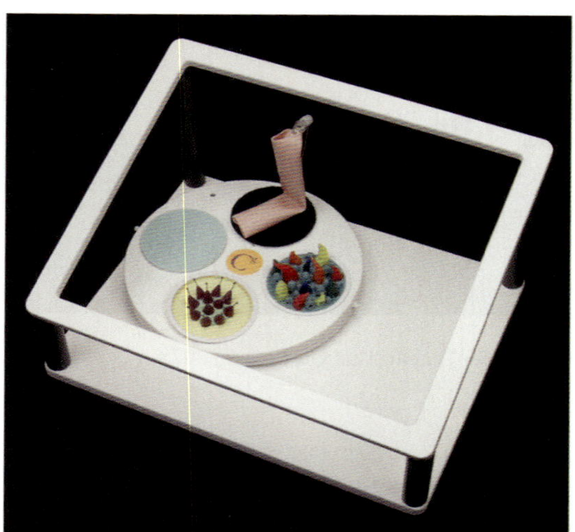

Fig. 31.8 Robotic skills kit from the Chamberlain Group

The novice completed inanimate training in 7 h. Baseline novice and expert performance were significantly different according to composite scores (546 ± 26 vs. 923 ± 60, $p < 0.001$), thus supporting overall construct validity. For the individual tasks, novice and expert performance was significantly different for tasks 1, 3–7, and 9 but not for tasks 2 and 8.

The novice reached proficiency on all 9 tasks after performing 111 practice repetitions. Significant pretest to posttest improvement was noted according to the composite scores (500.8 vs. 839.2, $p = 0.004$), thus supporting overall curricular effectiveness in terms of skill acquisition. From a resource standpoint, curriculum development materials (models, supplies, and box trainer) cost $2,227 excluding the cost of the robotic system and instruments and suture. Incremental cost for training the novice was minimal (<$10), since the only consumable materials included Penrose drains, rubber bands, and pattern cut gauze.

Hung et al. developed a more simplified set of physical models (Fig. 31.18) and established both construct validity (i.e., experts performed better on the models than novices) and superior training benefit when compared to a virtual reality

Table 31.6 UTSW data w/prelim construct data

Task	Model		Instructions
I	Peg transfer (Fig. 31.9)	Model	FLS peg board
		Instruments	Two large needle drivers (left and right)
		Description	The six pegs are picked up in turn by a large needle driver from a pegboard on the surgeon's left, transferred in space to a needle driver in the right hand instrument, and then placed on the corresponding right side of the pegboard. After all pegs are transferred to the right, the process is reversed
		Errors	Dropping peg out of the field of view
		Cutoff time	300 s
		Proficiency score	234 (66 s with no errors)
II	Clutch and camera movement (Fig. 31.10)	Model	Flat template with geometric shapes
		Instruments	None
		Description	Using the camera, follow the path from shape A to B and continue on clockwise from shape to shape until arriving back at shape A. At each shape, the camera must freeze and the trainee must verbalize that they have their final image. Error dots and lost corners will be counted and the trainee will continue on to the next shape
		Errors	Visualization of the red error dots or lack of visualization of the corners of the geometric shape
		Cutoff time	300 s
		Proficiency score	248 (52 s with no errors)
III	Rubber band transfer (Fig. 31.11)	Model	Curved wire posts on custom template
		Instruments	Two large needle drivers (left and right)
		Description	Two rubber bands are picked up in turn by a large needle driver from the curved wires on the surgeon's left, transferred in space to a needle driver in the right hand and then placed on the curved wire on the corresponding right-hand side. After the two rubber bands are transferred from left to right, the process is reversed
		Errors	Dropping rubber band out of the field of view or avulsion of wire hooks
		Cut-off Time	300 s
		Proficiency Score	229 (71 s with no errors)
IV	Simple suture (Fig. 31.12)	Model	FLS suture block with penrose drain
		Instruments	Two large needle drivers (left and right) and one curved scissors (fourth arm)
		Description	Use the 12 cm 2-0 silk suture to suture through the two targets on the Penrose drain, tie one surgeon's knot and two square knots, and then cut the tails to approximately 1 cm
		Errors	Inaccuracy, suture breakage, knot slippage, air knot, incorrect tail length, frayed suture, model avulsion, bunny ears
		Cutoff time	600 s
		Proficiency score	509 (91 s with no errors)
V	Clutch and camera peg transfer (Fig. 31.13)	Model	Hexagon peg board (6.5 cm between posts)
		Instruments	Two large needle drivers (left and right)
		Description	The peg starts at post A and is moved by the left hand to post B. At post B, pick up the peg with the right hand, position the camera to view post C, and then move the peg to post C. Continue in like fashion until returning to post A
		Errors	Dropping peg out of the field of view
		Cutoff time	300 s
		Proficiency score	251 (49 s with no errors)

(continued)

Table 31.6 (continued)

Task	Model		Instructions
VI	Stair rubber band transfer (Fig. 31.14)	Model	Curved wire post on pedestals and custom template
		Instruments	Two large needle drivers (left and right)
		Description	With the left hand instrument, pick up the rubber band on post A and place it on post B. The right hand picks up the rubber band on post B and places it on post C. Then, with the left hand, transfer it back to post A. The camera should follow the movement of the instruments from post to post
		Errors	Dropping a rubber band outside the field of view, avulsion of the wire hooks
		Cutoff time	300 s
		Proficiency score	242 (58 s with no errors)
VII	Run and cut rubber band (Fig. 31.15)	Model	10 cm rubber band with 1-cm inked targets
		Instruments	Two large needle drivers (left and right), one curved scissors (fourth arm)
		Description	Grasp the rubber band at every other black mark and cut the intervening black mark. Repeat this until every black target is cut
		Errors	Cutting outside of the black marks
		Cutoff time	300 s
		Proficiency score	202 (98 s with no errors)
VIII	Pattern cut (Fig. 31.16)	Model	FLS pattern cut testing gauze
		Instruments	One Maryland forces (left), one curved scissors (right), and one cadiere forceps (fourth arm)
		Description	Activate the fourth arm to hold the free inferior portion of the gauze. Activate the third arm and cut the circle making sure to have black lines on both sides of the cut gauze showing that all cuts were made on the black line and not outside of it
		Errors	Cuts outside of the black line
		Cutoff time	300 s
		Proficiency score	147 (153 s with no errors)
IX	Running suture (Fig. 31.17)	Model	FLS suture block with penrose drain with five black targets on each side of the 2-cm slit
		Instruments	Two large needle drivers (left and right), one curved scissors (fourth arm)
		Description	Using a 16-cm 2-0 silk suture, suture through the first set of targets and tie one surgeon's knot and two square knots. Place running sutures through the next three pairs of inked targets and tie one surgeon's knot and two square knots on the last pair of targets. Cut the tails to approximately 1 cm
		Errors	Inaccuracy, breakage of suture, slippage of knot, air knot, incorrect tail lengths, frayed suture, avulsion of the model, and bunny ears
		Cutoff time	600 s
		Proficiency score	340 (260 s with no errors)

simulator as measured in an animate lab setting [17].

The Fundamentals of Robotic Surgery Curriculum is in the process of developing the tasks and metrics it will require for skills rehearsal and testing. A modified Delphi process is being utilized for this process with a goal of goal of creating three-dimensional tasks than incorporate all of the deconstructed FRS skill sets (Table 31.2), be cost effective, have high fidelity at least for testing purposes, be easy to administer with good inter-rater reliability, use physical models, and focus on tasks that have prior validation when possible. The committee is also considering tasks to practice docking and trocar insertion.

Virtual Reality Skills Training

There are a number of simulator platforms that provide training options for robotic surgery with virtual reality environments (Table 31.7). These platforms offer another way to provide a longitudinal training experience for residents and fellows. Mimic Technologies Inc. (Seattle, Washington, USA) founded in 2001 with department of defense funding has developed two simulators, one with a stand-alone simulated console, and another that docks and works with the dVSS surgeon console. The simulated console, called the Mimic dV-Trainer™, uses a relatively small booth and cable-suspended controls to provide practicing surgeons with the hands-on feel of a real robotic platform (Fig. 31.19). The system incorporates a comprehensive set of validated exercises to take aspiring robot surgeons from novice to intermediate skill level. Trainees on the console learn basic arm control, then use of three arms, camera control, energy usage, suturing, and knot tying. Multiple validation studies have confirmed its face, content, and construct validity. It also has validated orientation and skills training modules (see Figs. 31.20 and 31.21) as well as a validated performance analysis and scoring system called MScore™ (see Fig. 31.22). The system costs in the ballpark of $100,000 with an additional annual service fee. It is fairly compact, fitting on a table or desk with a set of pedals for the floor. It also requires an attached

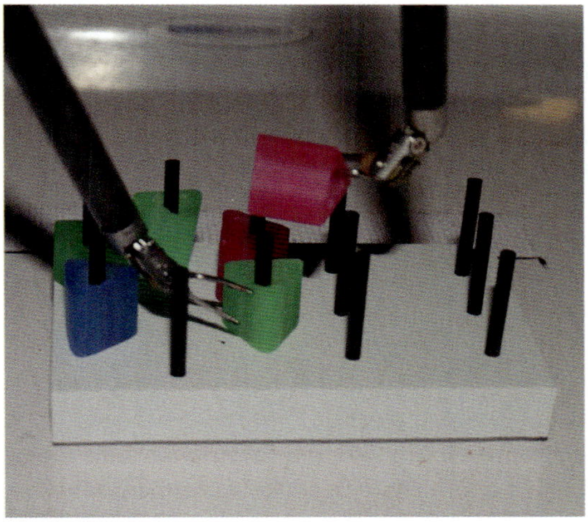

Fig. 31.9 UTSW task 1—peg transfer

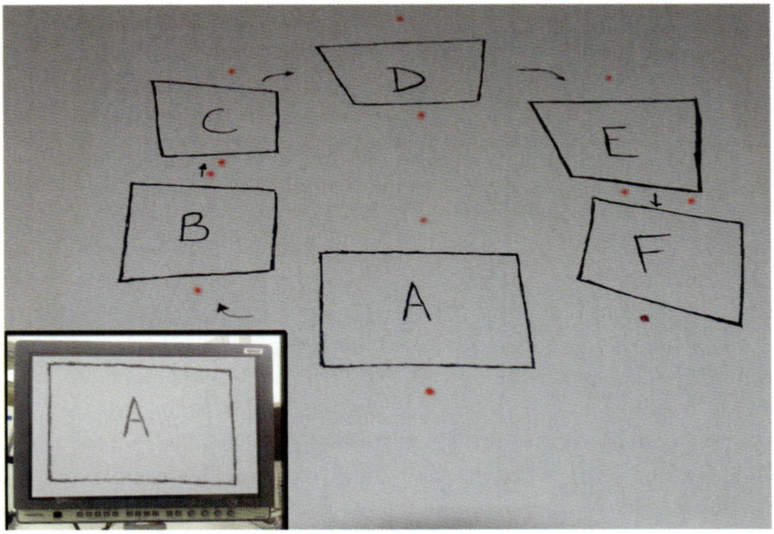

Fig. 31.10 UTSW task 2—Clutch and Camera MOvement

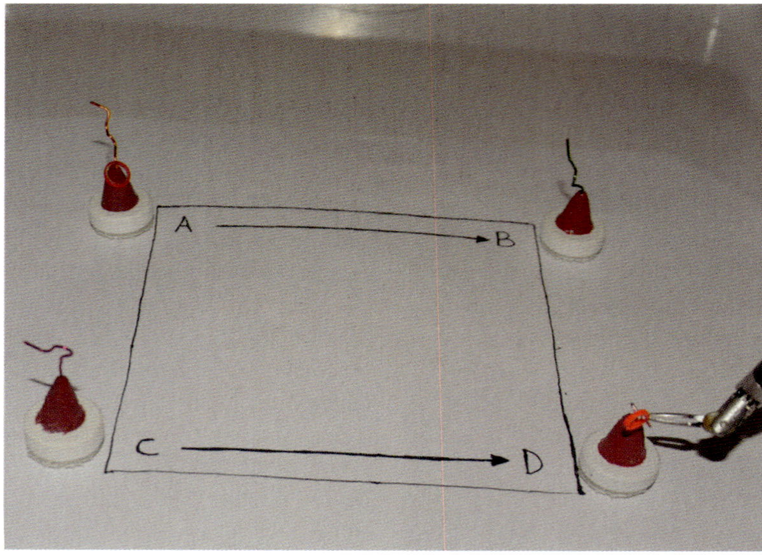

Fig. 31.11 UTSW task 3—rubber band transfer

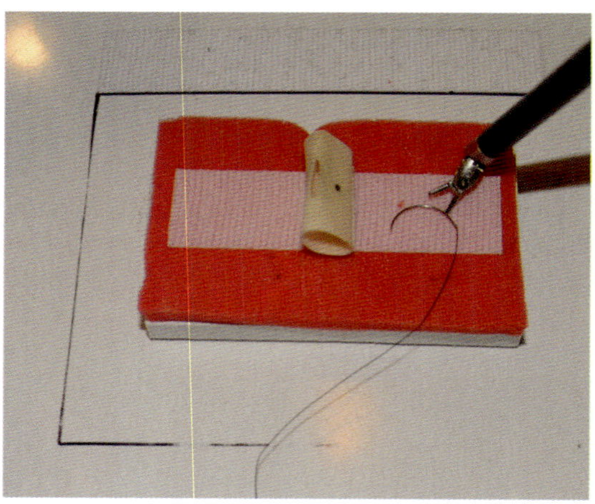

Fig. 31.12 UTSW task 4—simple suture

desktop computer. MIMIC has sought to aid the development of curriculum by adding an "MShare" section to their website where curriculum developers can share their work with other Mimic users to foster collaboration among various institutions [18].

Intuitive has collaborated with Mimic since 2003, and in 2011, licensed some of the software of the Mimic simulator to be incorporated into a stylized computer module that connects to the back of the da Vinci Si platform and is called the da Vinci Skills Simulator (Fig. 31.23). This "backpack" utilizes the real da Vinci surgeon console with a computer-generated environment. Its cost is comparable to the MIMIC simulator, and multiple studies have been published establishing a difference in performance between novices and experts on this simulator. Because the dVSS is often packaged as part of the sale of a new da Vinci Si platform, there are now over 400 "backpack" simulators in institutions around the world. Despite this unprecedented availability, however, a well-defined and validated proficiency-based skills curriculum on this platform has yet to be developed.

The HOST™ (Hands-on Surgical Training) is a haptic enabled augmented reality system available on the RoSS (Robot Surgical Simulator, Simulated Surgical Systems, LLC, Williamsville, NY) and is another option for simulated robot training (Fig. 31.24). It comes with basic skill modules for camera control, arm movement, clutch, three-arm control, suturing, tying, clipping, and suture cutting. There have been limited studies to show face and content validity, and the training modules are currently being assessed for validity. Its size is comparable to a da Vinci surgeon console, and its cost ranges from $100,000 to $125,000. HOST features a

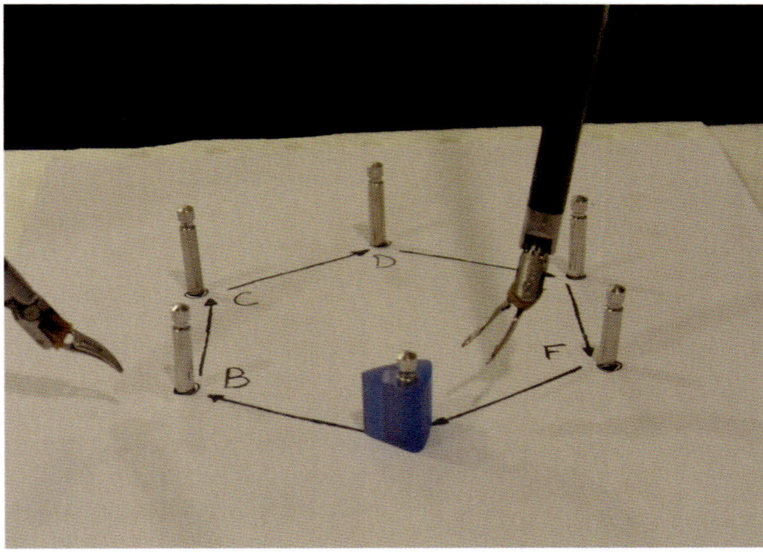

Fig. 31.13 UTSW task 5—clutch and camera peg transfer

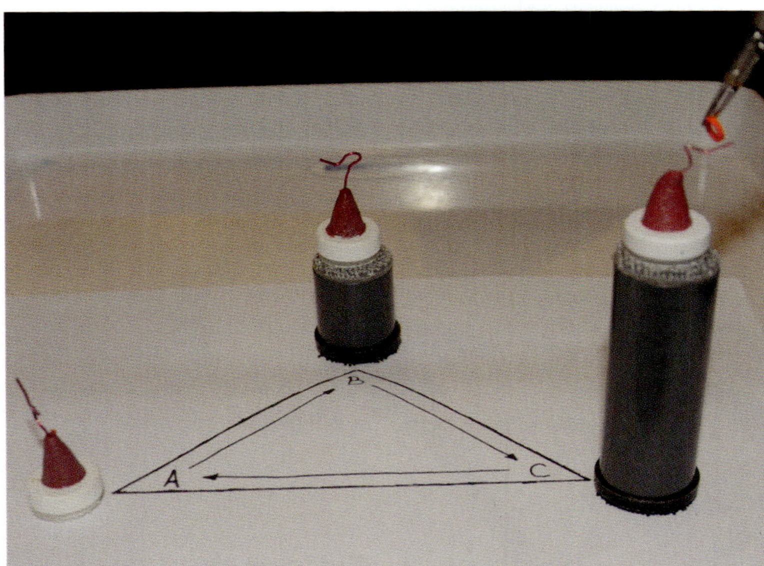

Fig. 31.14 UTSW task 6—stair rubber band transfer

mode that uses a novel reversal of the master–slave relationship where the trainee watches a surgery taking place, and the trainee's hands are moved by the simulator so that he or she can feel himself performing the same surgery. The system includes modules mostly suited to training urologists and gynecologists but also includes a few modules that would benefit general surgeons such as adrenalectomy and nephrectomy.

The least expensive option currently available for virtual reality robotic surgery is the SEP-Robot simulator from SimSurgery (Boston, MA; Fig. 31.25). Priced between $40,000 and $45,000 plus an annual service plan, this system has no

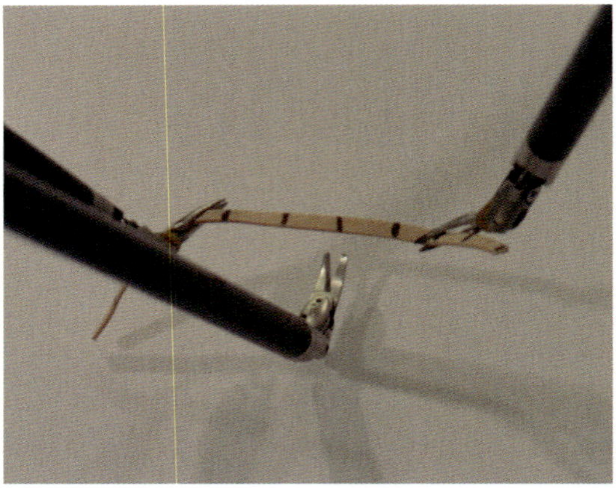

Fig. 31.15 UTSW task 7—run and cut rubber band

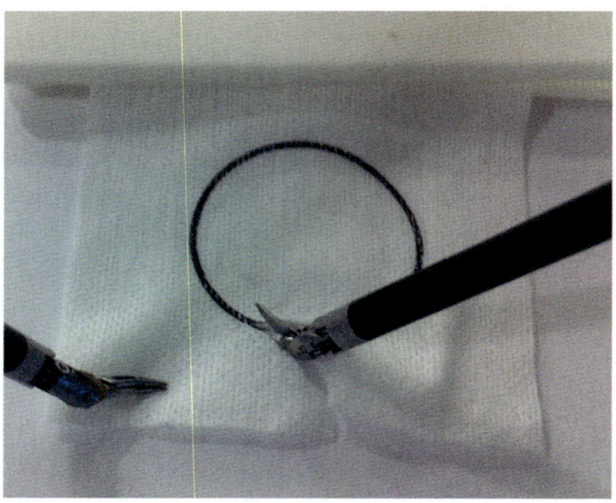

Fig. 31.16 UTSW task 8—pattern cut

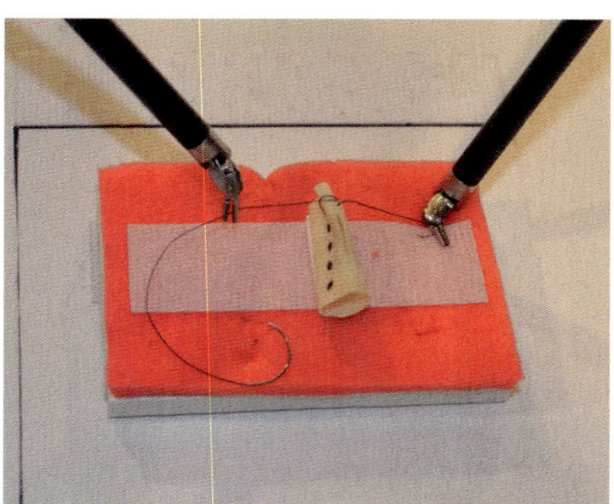

Fig. 31.17 UTSW task 9—running suture

console and rather depends on arm boards, a monitor, and a turnkey computer. This simulator provides modules to simulate a cholecystectomy and other minimally invasive procedures. It is currently, the cheapest, most mobile simulator option in use.

Team Training

All surgery requires a team to work together in a coordinated fashion, but robotic surgery is unique in that the surgeon is not "scrubbed" into the surgical field and is immersed in a visualization environment that limits his or her situation awareness. In addition, if an intraoperative crisis should occur that requires converting from robotic surgery to an open approach, the robotic instruments and platform must be removed and "undocked" in a coordinated fashion. As a result, precise communication within a well-coordinated team is paramount to a successful robotic surgery program. At the Methodist Institute for Technology, Innovation, and Education (MITIE, Houston, Texas), intraoperative robotic surgery crisis scenarios have been developed which require the operating surgeon and circulating nurse to work in a coordinated fashion to convert from robotic to open surgery. Studies are being conducted to validate the metrics of these performances with plans to incorporate this type of experience into not only resident and fellow training but also into hospital quality initiatives.

Outcome Measures

The ultimate measure of a curriculum is to determine if it has enabled trainees to achieve the outlined goals and objectives. For robotic surgery, the ultimate goal is for a resident or fellow who successfully completes the curriculum to have the knowledge and skills required to safely and effectively perform robotic surgery. Ideally, this outcome would be measured in the clinical domain during real surgical procedures.

Traditionally, validated measures of clinical performance have been difficult to come by in surgery. More recently, however, one such tool has been developed in the laparoscopic domain called GOALS (the Global Operative Assessment of Laparoscopic Skills) [19]. This simple tool can be used to reliably differentiate between novice and expert surgeons performing laparoscopic surgery. Using GOALS as a template, Goh et al. developed a similar clinical assessment tool for robotic surgery called GEARS (the Global Evaluative Assessment of Robotic Surgery) (Fig. 31.26) [20]. This validated global assessment form uses a 5-point Likert scale with descriptive anchors at 1, 3, and 5 to evaluate performance in six domains—depth perception, bimanual dexterity, efficiency, autonomy, force sensitivity, and robotic control. This clinical assessment tool has been shown to reliably differentiate the performance of novice, intermediate, and experts during robotic surgery with excellent consistency and inter-rater reliability. Such a powerful clinical assessment tool can be used to validate robotic training curricula and prove their effectiveness.

Another measure of clinical performance is the ability for a trainee to independently complete a step of a surgical procedure. The Lehigh Valley Health Network curriculum breaks down robotically assisted hysterectomy into ten steps with time limits assigned to each (Table 31.8) [21]. The trainee is allowed to progress as far as possible within the time limit for each step and scored on a 3-point Likert scale with a minimum total score established for proficiency. While this tool may not have been tested for high-stakes validity, it is practical and appears powerful in giving residents formative feedback on their performance.

Finally, the da Vinci Si dual-console robotic platform may be an additional aid for training. It allows for two surgeons (i.e., expert and trainee) to sit at their own surgeon console connected to the patient-side robotic platform. Both participants can view the surgery in three dimensions, and control of the instruments can be "passed" back and forth between the two consoles. This may allow an attending surgeon to perform a surgery while a resident or fellow observes and to selectively allow the trainee to perform parts of the procedure. There is very limited data on the efficacy of the dual-console system. Smith et al. recently published a series of 50 cases done on the dual console in which they used the second console for observation and verbal assistance [22]. They found no compromise in patient outcomes or operative times and felt the platform provided a feasible way to train residents with varying levels of experience.

Evaluation and Feedback

In order to facilitate ongoing improvement of the curriculum and to ensure it evolves to meet the changing needs of trainees, a mechanism to garner evaluation and feedback about curriculum performance is crucial. This is usually done by having trainees complete a survey about their experience. It is important to gain feedback from curriculum moderators and technicians as well. As an example, in their curriculum development, Dulan et al. used a 5-point Likert scale to ask trainees how well they felt the curriculum trained them in each of the deconstructed tasks they identified [7]. This feedback cycle can be further improved by surveying trainees after they have completed residency or fellowship and moved into practice. In this way it can be determined how well the curriculum prepared graduates to meet the credentialing requirements of their new institutions and how prepared they felt for independently performing robotic surgery in practice.

Conclusion

The resources and examples described in this chapter describe a number of options for program directors wishing to provide robotic surgery training to their residents or fellows. The right approach for any program will be dictated by their own needs assessment and goals

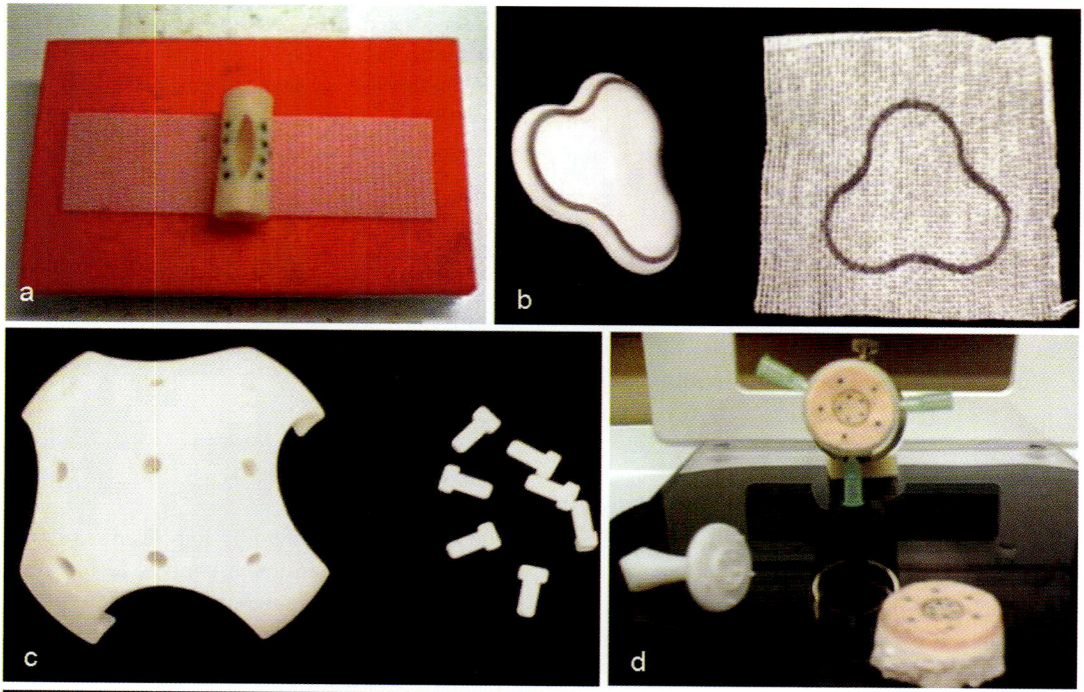

	Exercise	Task and Skills tested
A	Horizontal Mattress Suture	Perform running horizontal mattress targeting each marked point on penrose tube. Start by anchoring stitch at point furthest away. Errors counted for loose knots, broken suture, and missing pre-marked targets.
B	Clover Pattern Cut	Sharply cut marked pattern on gauze while staying within black boundary. Errors counted for each deviation outside black boundary using a 1x1 cm grid.
C	3-D Dome and Peg Transfer	Pick up 9 plastic pegs from remote location and transfer them into semi-spherical dome. Errors are counted for dropped or misplaced pegs.
D	Circular Target	Place suture needle through 10 marked points arranged in a concentric pattern, going from inside to outside points and progressing in running fashion. Errors counted for broken suture and missing pre-marked targets.

Fig. 31.18 Hung et al. inanimate exercises for fundamentals of robotic surgery

as well as the availability of robotic platforms for training and financial and personnel resources (Fig. 31.27). Ideally, after implementing a curriculum, trainees would be objectively measured in their clinical performance using validated tools such as GEARS. Implementing well-constructed curricula coupled with validated measures of knowledge and skill is the best way to assure that graduating residents and fellows will be well equipped to become credentialed to perform robotic surgery and provide optimal care to their patients.

Table 31.7 Virtual reality robotic surgery simulators

Simulator	Advantages	Disadvantages	Price estimate
Mimic	• Fits on table top • Feels like the console • No need for robot console • Validated MScore™ system	• Proprietary surgeon console interface	\$100,000 + annual maintenance fee
da Vinci skills simulator	• Fits on back of robotic console • Uses actual console	• Requires use of robot for non-operative purposes • Less validation available of scoring system	\$100,000 + annual maintenance fee
RoSS HOST	• Includes video of many surgeries • No need for robot console	• Requires space equivalent to a da Vinci console • Limited training material for general surgeons • Limited validation studies available	\$100,000–\$125,000
SEP robot	• Low cost • Compact and mobile • No need for robot console	• Limited validation studies available • Uses disconnected *EndoWrist* without similar haptic feedback	\$40,000–\$45,000

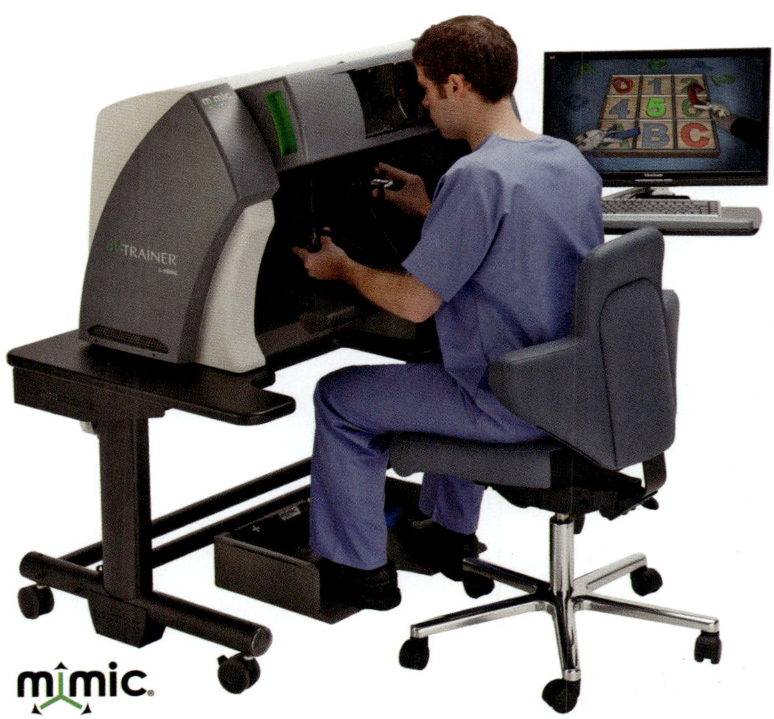

Fig. 31.19 MIMIC console

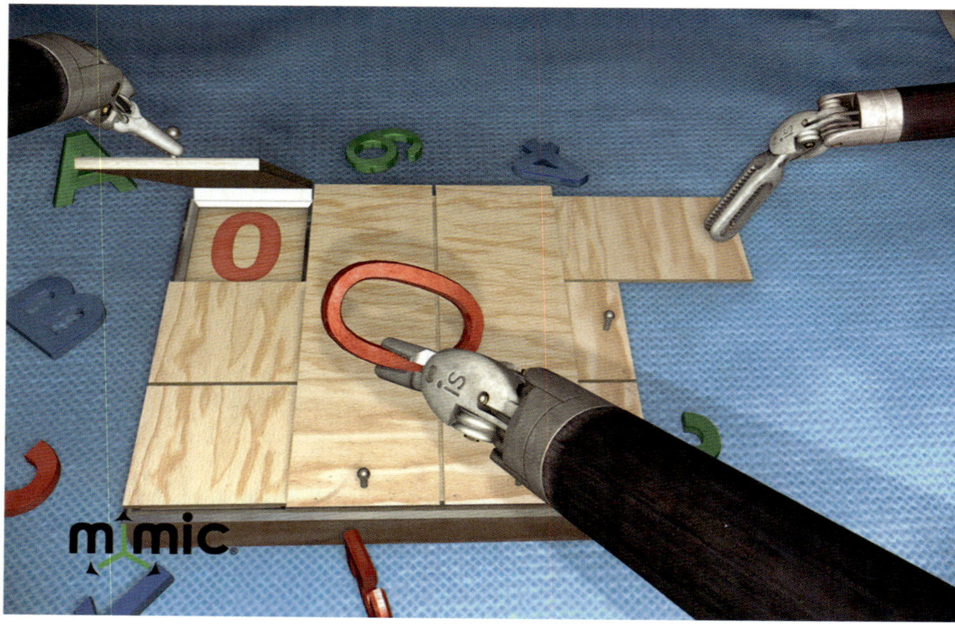

Fig. 31.20 MIMIC advanced arm manipulation

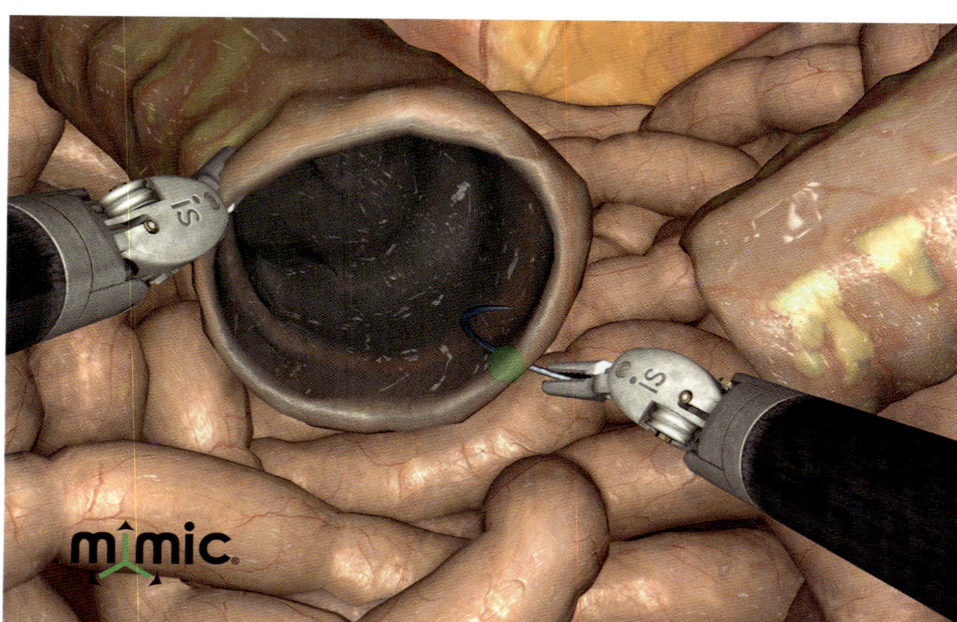

Fig. 31.21 MIMIC needle driving

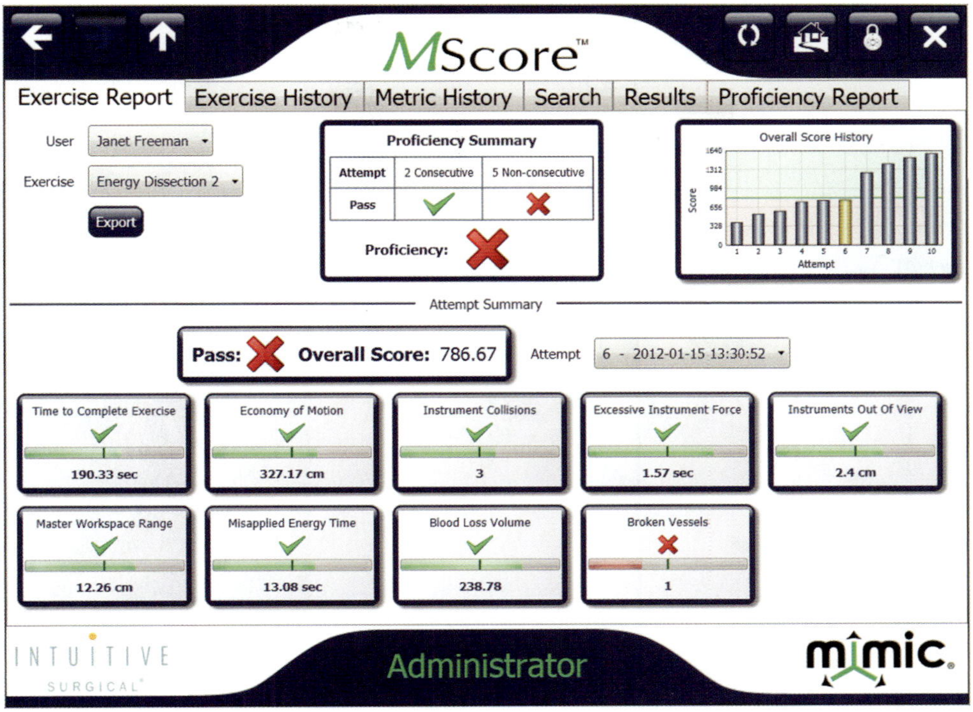

Fig. 31.22 MIMIC MScore display

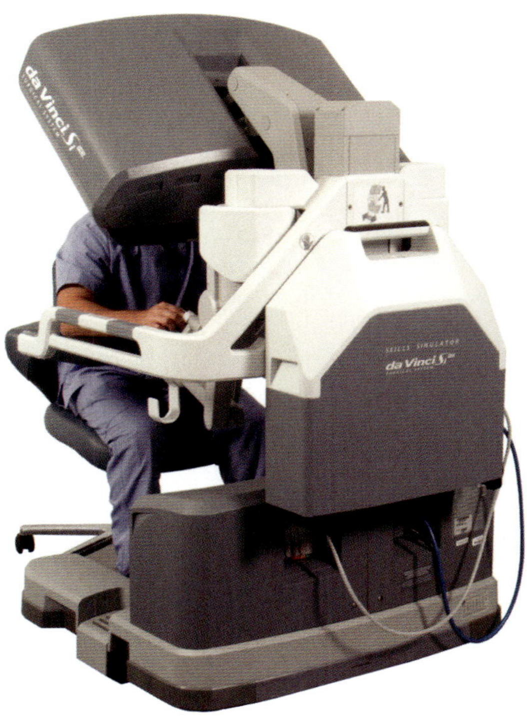

Fig. 31.23 da Vinci Si skills simulator backpack on robot console

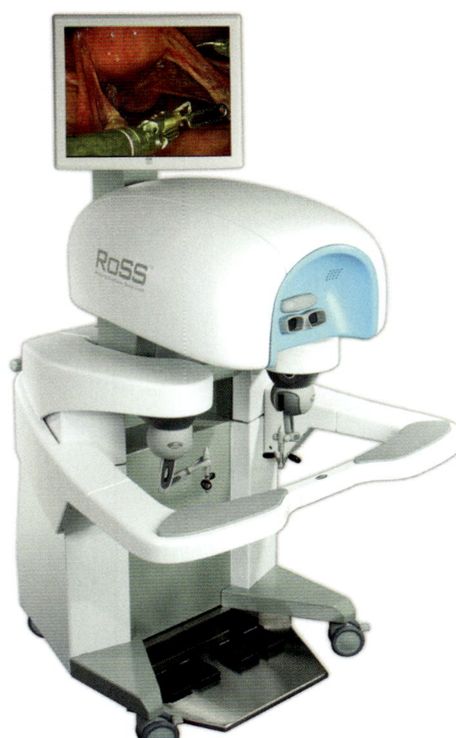

Fig. 31.24 RoSS HOST robotic simulator system

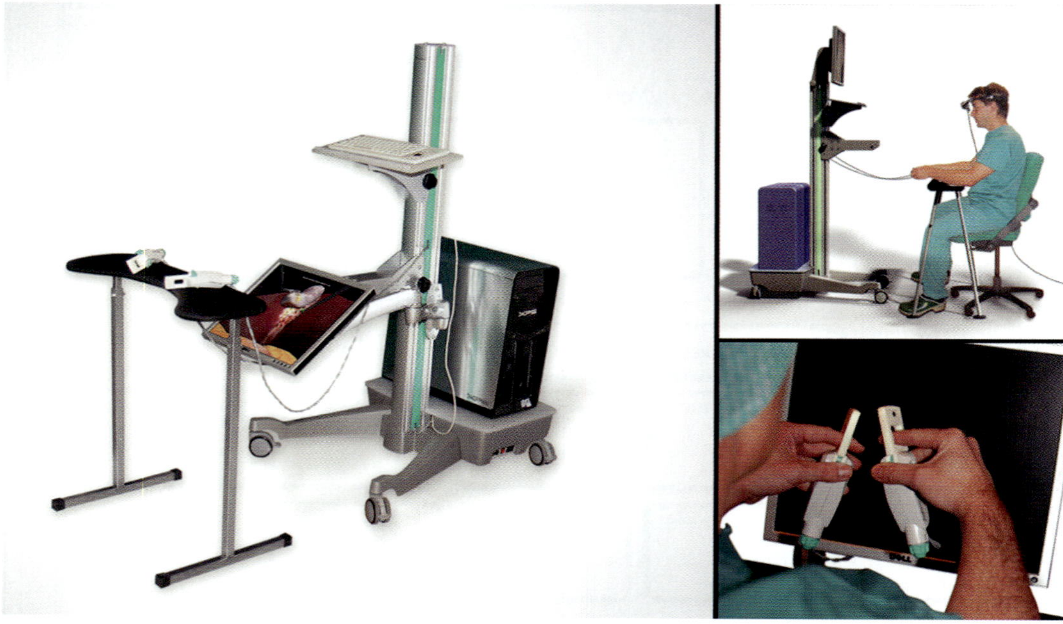

Fig. 31.25 SEP robotic simulator system

Depth perception

1	2	3	4	5
Constantly overshoots target, wide swings, slow to correct		Some overshooting or missing of target, but quick to correct		Accurately directs instruments in the correct plane to target

Bimanual dexterity

1	2	3	4	5
Uses only one hand, ignores nondominant hand, poor coordination		Uses both hands, but does not optimize interaction between hands		Expertly uses both hands in a complementary way to provide best exposure

Efficiency

1	2	3	4	5
Inefficient efforts; many uncertain movements; constantly changing focus or persisting without progress		Slow, but planned movements are reasonably organized		Confident, efficient and safe conduct, maintains focus on task, fluid progression

Force sensitivity

1	2	3	4	5
Rough movements, tears tissue, injures nearby structures, poor force control		Handles tissues reasonably well, minor trauma to adjacent tissue, rare suture breakage		Applies appropriate tension, negligible injury to adjacent structures

Autonomy

1	2	3	4	5
Unable to complete entire task, even with verbal guidance		Able to complete task safely with moderate guidance		Able to complete task independently without prompting

Robotic control

1	2	3	4	5
Consistently does not optimize view, hand position, or repeated collisions even with guidance		View is sometimes not optimal. Occasionally needs to relocate arms. Occasional collisions and obstruction of assistant.		Controls camera and hand position optimally and independently. Minimal collisions or obstruction of assistant

Case Difficulty

1	2	3	4	5
Ideal anatomy		Moderate difficulty		Very challenging, unusual anatomy

Fig. 31.26 GEARS evaluation form

Table 31.8 Lehigh valley health network clinical assessment of robotic hysterectomy

Task	Needs improvement 1	Good 2	Excellent 3
Procedure preparation (50 min)			
Patient positioning	Patient required repositioning > 3 times	Patient required repositioning 2–3 times	Patient properly positioned the first time
Equipment setup, port placement, and docking	Required considerable assistance (> 50%)	Required assistance	Accurately performed with little or no assistance
Incision	Does not use landmarks, poor incision placement, or poor handling of scalpel	Appropriate incision in terms of location and size, comfortable handling of scalpel	Handled scalpel expertly
Anatomic landmarks and boundaries	Did not accurately identify required landmarks and boundaries	Identified required landmarks and boundaries	Identified all known structures, landmarks, and boundaries
Procedure (10 min)			
Transect round ligaments and open broad ligament	Does not use surface landmarks to transect accurately, inappropriate incision placement, and poor instrument handling	Appropriate incision in terms of location and size for accurate transection, at ease with the instruments	Expert handling of instruments to transect ligaments
Identify pararectal and paravesical spaces	Did not identify spaces accurately	Identified the spaces with minimal assistance	Identified the space without assistance
Procedure (10 min)			
Isolate, seal, and transect the infundibulopelvic ligaments	Did not identify the ligament or failed to properly transect or seal it	Identified the ligament, transected the ligament, and appropriately sealed it	Identified all known structures and accurately transected and sealed the ligament
Identify the ureters	Unable to accurately identify required landmarks and boundaries	Required assistance to identify required landmarks and boundaries	Accurately identified all required landmarks and boundaries
Bladder procedure (10 min)			
Dissection of the bladder	Appears unsure and excessively hesitant while dissecting	Controlled and safe dissection using correct anatomical plane; minimal trauma to tissues	Superior atraumatic dissection using correct anatomical planes while handling instruments confidently during the dissection
Procedure (20 min)			
Isolate uterine artery, cardinal ligaments, and uterosacral ligaments	Did not accurately identify required structures, landmarks, and boundaries	Identified required structures, landmarks, and boundaries	Identified all known structures, landmarks, and boundaries
Transect ligaments	Does not use surface landmarks to transect accurately, inappropriate placement of incision, or poor handling of instruments	Appropriate incision in terms of location and size to transect accurately; looked at ease with instruments	Handled instruments expertly to transect ligaments

Procedure (20 min)			
Perform vaginal colpotomy	Does not use surface landmarks; inappropriate incision placement	Appropriate incision in terms of location and size; purposeful movements with delivery of specimen if applicable	Performed without hesitation, limited cautery with ease of specimen delivery if applicable
Procedure (10 min)			
Closure of cuff	Poor quality closure, insecure ends, air knots identified, poor handling of suture instruments, and suture cut during tying	Incisions reapproximated without visualization of air knots, ends of cuff closed, and safe maneuvering of instruments	Cuff closed securely, purposeful suture placement, superior closure with hemostasis, and no suture breakage
Procedure (20 min)			
Undocking, removal of ports, and cystoscopy	Unsafe practices such as undocking before removing instruments, pneumoperitoneum, or overdistention of the bladder	Safely undocks and removes ports with minimal guidance; safe performance of cystoscopy	Efficiently undocks without guidance; skilled and purposeful manipulation of cystoscope
Procedure (20 min)			
Incision closed to out of room time	Poor quality of knot tying, knots the slip frequently, or excessive trauma to tissues or vessels	Competent knot tying, minimal trauma to tissue and vessels, and minimal blood loss	Superior knot tying, atraumatic tissue and vessel handling, and secure knots without slippage
Postoperative procedure (20 min)			
Assist with room turnover	No assistance with room turnover	Assists anesthesia with waking and transferring	Assists with all aspects of room turnover
Resident performance			
Equipment handling	Looks awkward	Confident handling of the scope	Skilled, competent handling of the scope
Movement of hands-on controls	Many unnecessary movements	Some unnecessary movements	All purposeful movements
Flow of procedure	Hesitated often unsure of what to do	Usually confident with occasional hesitation	Confident and sure of what to do at all times
Score			
Overall performance rating	*Needs improvement (8–18)*	*Pass (20–36)*	*Competent (39–54)*

Fig. 31.27 Robotic surgery curriculum development flowchart

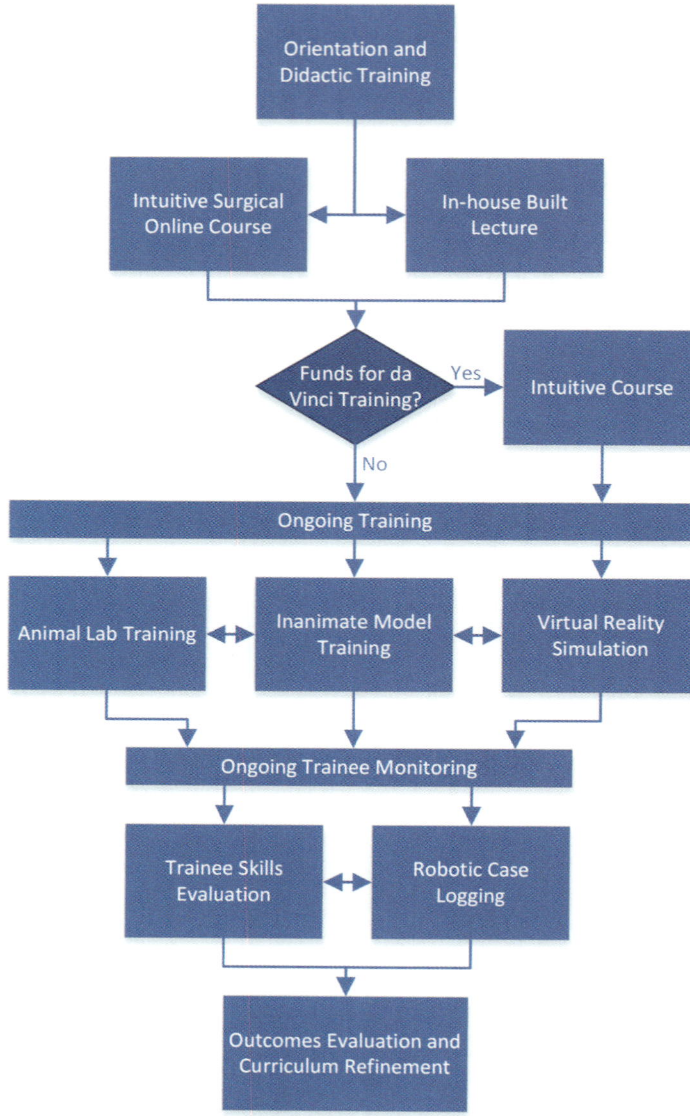

References

1. Satava RM, Smith RP, Patel VM. Fundamentals of robotic surgery: outcomes measures and curriculum development. Bostom, MA: Society of Laparoscopic Surgeons; 2012. p. 1–5. http://www.simulationfirst.com/frs/FRS%20White%20Paper%20for%20Boston%20SLS.pdf.
2. Stitzenberg KB, Wong YN, Nielsen ME, Egleston BL, Uzzo RG. Trends in radical prostatectomy: centralization, robotics, and access to urologic cancer care. Cancer. 2012;118(1):54–62.
3. Erickson BK, Gleason JL, Huh WK, Richter HE. Survey of robotic surgery credentialing requirements for physicians completing OB/GYN residency. J Minim Invasive Gynecol. 2012;19(5):589–92.
4. Intuitive Surgical da Vinci Surgery Online Community. http://www.davincisurgerycommunity.com/. Accessed 14 Oct 2012.
5. Satava RM, Smith RP, Patel VM. Public Form Fundamentals of Robotic Surgery Curriculum Development in Celebration, Florida (Interim Progress Report); 2011. http://www.modelbenders.com/papers/FRS_Outcomes_Conference_Report.pdf. Accessed 21 Oct 2012.

6. Robotics Surgery Training Network. A network dedicated to robotic surgery. http://www.robotictraining.org. Accessed 11 Dec 2012.
7. Dulan G, Rege RV, Hogg DC, Gilberg-Fisher KM, Arain NA, Tesfay ST, et al. Developing a comprehensive, proficiency-based training program for robotic surgery. Surgery. 2012;152(3):477–88.
8. Lyons C, Goldfarb D, Miles B, Joseph R, Link R, Bass B, Dunkin BJ. Which skills really matter? Proving face, content, and construct validity for a commercial robotic simulator. Surg Endosc. 2013;27(6):2020–30.
9. Learn About Robotic Surgery. http://www.selectroboticsurgery.org/. Accessed 25 Oct 2012.
10. University of Alabama School of Medicine Obstretrics and Gynecology Residency Program Robotics Curriculum. http://www.obgyn.uab.edu/residency/edrobotics. htm. Accessed 4 Nov 2012.
11. Geller EJ, Schuler KM, Boggess JF. Robotic surgical training program in gynecology: How to train residents and fellows. J Minim Invasive Gynecol. 2011; 18(2):224–9.
12. Products of the Chamberlain Group "Bringing Practice to the Practice of Medicine". http://www.thecgroup.com/products. Accessed 24 Oct 2012.
13. Dulan G, Rege RV, Hogg DC, Gilberg-Fisher KM, Arain NA, Tesfay ST, et al. Proficiency-based training for robotic surgery: construct validity, workload, and expert levels for nine inanimate exercises. Surg Endosc. 2012;26(6):1516–21.
14. Fried GM, Feldman LS, Vassiliou MC, Fraser SA, Stanbridge D, Ghitulescu G, et al. Proving the value of simulation in laparoscopic surgery. Ann Surg. 2004;240(3):518–25.
15. Sroka G, Feldman LS, Vassiliou MC, Kaneva PA, Fayez R, Fried GM. Fundamentals of laparoscopic surgery simulator training to proficiency improves laparoscopic performance in the operating room – a randomized controlled trial. Am J Surg. 2010; 199(1):115–20.
16. Fraser SA, Klassen DR, Feldman LS, Ghitulescu GA, Stanbridge D, Fried GM. Evaluating laparoscopic skills: setting the pass/fail score for the MISTELS system. Surg Endosc. 2003;17(6):964–7.
17. Hung AJ, Jayaratna I, Teruya K, Desai MM, Gill IS, Goh AC. Comparative assessment of three standardized robotic training methods. BJU Int. 2013;112(6): 864–71.
18. Mimic Innovation in Simulation. http://www.mimic-simulation.com/. Accessed 15 Dec 2012.
19. Vassiliou MC, Feldman LS, Andrew CG, Bergman S, Leffondré K, Stanbridge D, et al. A global assessment tool for evaluation of intraoperative laparoscopic skills. Am J Surg. 2005;190(1):107–13.
20. Goh AC, Goldfarb DW, Sander JC, Miles BJ, Dunkin BJ. Global evaluative asssessment of robotic skills: validation of a clinical assessment tool to measure robotic surgical skills. J Urol. 2012;187(1):247–52.
21. Martino M. Robotic surgery resident assessment form with rubric. Lehigh Valley Health Network; 2011. https://sites.google.com/site/medicinenetwork/apgo-creog/robotics-curriculum/lehigh-valley-health-network. Accessed 6 Jan 2013.
22. Smith AL, Scott EM, Krivak TC, Olawaiye AB, Chu T, Richard SD. Dual-console robot surgery: a new teaching paradigm. J Robot Surg. 2013;7(2):113–8.

Challenges and Critical Elements of Setting Up a Robotics Program

32

Randy Fagin

Background

There are currently thousands of da Vinci surgical systems at hospitals around the world. They are being used by surgeons on every continent except Africa and Antarctica, and when it comes to setting up, maintaining, and growing a successful daVinci surgery program, I can say with complete confidence that most of these hospitals consider themselves unique in the challenges they face. Most feel quite strongly that the culture and size of their hospital, the resources they have access to, the politics of medicine where they live, the size of their city, the number and personality of the surgeons they work with, and the presence of unions or residents or both all pose unique challenges that are unlike any other program. I've heard it so often that there must be some statistic like "every 8 s a healthcare team member involved in daVinci surgery says…Well that may work for THEM, but you don't understand, things are different here."

However, when you examine successful da Vinci surgery programs across the globe, you find that regardless of the size of the hospital or city, no matter what the politics and competitive forces are at play in their medical community, regardless of whether their surgeons are demanding or supportive, whether their staff has unions or they work with residents, there is a clear and common pathway to success in setting up, maintaining, and growing a da Vinci surgery program. This common pathway contains six elements:

1. A clear noble purpose
2. The right leadership structure
3. Consistent communication pathways
4. Standardization
5. Parallel tasks
6. A continuous improvement cycle

Before we explore these six elements, we must start by acknowledging a few truths:

1. Just because your hospital owns a da Vinci surgical system, and there are surgeons who come to that hospital to use, it does not mean you have a da Vinci surgery program. It is possible that all you have is a surgical tool that surgeons come to use.
2. If your hospital has successfully increased the number and type of da Vinci surgeries it performs, it still does not mean that you have a da Vinci surgery program. It is possible that all you have is a surgical tool that more surgeons are choosing to use as more surgeons and patients see the value in da Vinci surgery.

A daVinci surgery program exists only when elements 1, 2, and 3 exist

1. A clear noble purpose
2. The right leadership structure
3. Consistent communication pathways

and its success is dependent on its ability to apply elements 4, 5, and 6

R. Fagin, M.D. (✉)
Texas Institute for Robotic Surgery, Hospital Corporation of America, Austin, TX, USA

Intuitive Surgical International, Austin, TX, USA

K.C. Kim (ed.), *Robotics in General Surgery*, DOI 10.1007/978-1-4614-8739-5_32,

4. Standardization
5. Parallel tasks
6. A continuous improvement cycle

In the following pages I will detail for you a straightforward and reproducible plan for creating a da Vinci surgery program at your hospital and driving its success using the above six elements and the resources you already have in place.

A Clear Noble Purpose

We are in the business of helping people, treating diseases, and changing lives for the better. We all would like to see our volumes and revenue increase and often, our success is judged by our ability to achieve those goals. However, increases in revenue and surgical volume can be the result of work towards your goal, but they cannot be the goal itself. To create a da Vinci surgery program every team member must come to work with a common, clear, and noble purpose beyond the fulfillment of their job's responsibilities and beyond the achievement of increasing volume and revenue.

To find your program's noble purpose, start by having your surgeons and administrative leadership answer the following questions:

"What do we want our da Vinci surgery program to achieve?"

"How are we going to measure that success?"

Do you want to achieve the best clinical outcomes in your city? Then you need to define what a "best clinical outcome" is for each surgery and specialty, decide how you will measure for these "best clinical outcomes," and determine the path towards achieving that goal. Maybe you want to be at the leading edge of new surgical innovations. Then you need to define what will count as an innovation, decide who your surgeon champions are that will be developing these innovations, determine how you will prioritize which innovations your program will support, and agree on how you will measure the success of using these innovations and how you will share your innovations with others. Is your program centered around a small number of key surgeons or is it structured to accommodate a diverse population of surgeons from practices across your city? You need to define who you are as a program, find your noble purpose, before you can achieve true and lasting success.

This noble purpose must be what is referred to as a S.M.A.R.T. goal. It must be *S*pecific, *M*easurable, *A*ttainable, *R*elevant, and *T*ime-bound.

Specific

Your goal must be clear and unambiguous. It must tell you who will be involved, what you wish to accomplish, and why you are doing it.

Measurable

You need well-defined criteria that you will use to measure your progress towards the goal.

Attainable

The goal you choose should not be easy to achieve but realistic enough that you can attain it.

Relevant

Your goal must be something that matters and will help drive your organization forward.

Time-Bound

You must set a deadline for completing milestones on the way to your goal. Without a deadline, achieving these critical milestones can be overtaken by day-to-day challenges.

The Right Leadership Structure

Once you have determined your noble purpose, you need to put into place a leadership structure that will facilitate your achieving the goals you have set. To develop the right leadership structure you need to first ensure that you are looking

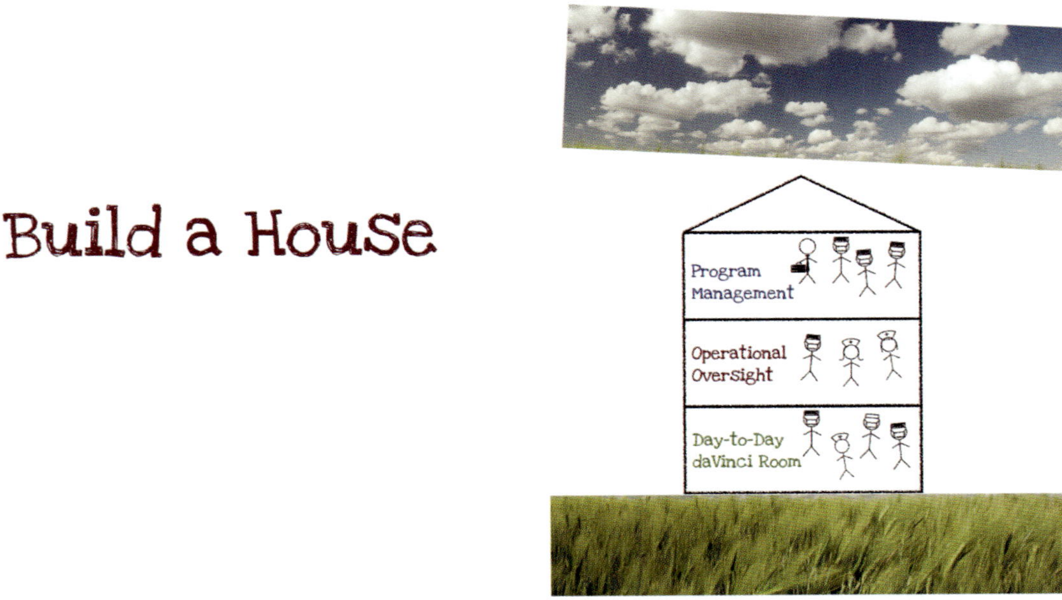

Fig. 32.1 Building a house

beyond the da Vinci surgical system as a tool that your surgeons use and are treating all da Vinci surgery in your hospital as its own service line. This means you cannot think of da Vinci surgery as part of your urology service line, part of your GYN service line, part of your general surgery service line, etc. da Vinci surgery must be its own service line with leaders and leadership that attend to its needs and are accountable to its noble purpose across surgical specialties, as we would traditionally describe them. This is a unique thought for a hospital that is used to creating silos of leadership around surgical specialties that are defined by the residency a surgeon completed (Urology, OB/GYN, General Surgery, etc.). Once we accept that da Vinci surgery is its own service line, and that it is a service line that crosses many surgical specialties, then we are ready to look at the leadership structure that will support it. Think about building the leadership structure for your da Vinci surgery service line like building a house. The house we are going to build has three levels (Fig. 32.1).

The ground floor of the house is literally the ground floor of your da Vinci surgery program. It is the boots on the ground support you depend on in your operating room for *day-to-day* operations. It includes your surgical techs, nurses, anesthesia providers, surgeons, housekeepers, and your da Vinci coordinator. Remember, since we agree that da Vinci surgery is its own service line, we need to ensure that we have a nurse coordinator that is specific to this service line—our da Vinci coordinator.

The second floor of the house is where your *operational oversight* team lives. This is typically a member of your operating room leadership team, your da Vinci coordinator, and one of your surgeon leaders. If the da Vinci service line were a company, the operational oversight team would be the Chief Operating Officer. Their role is focused on the establishment and optimization of day-to-day operations in the program. They advise the program management team (*see next section*) on key planning issues and make recommendations on planning and resource allocation. Based on the noble purpose of your program, they set operational and/or performance goals, establish processes for improvement, ensure quality control, and inform all the other "floors of the house" of their progress and achievements. In short, they look at what happens in every da Vinci surgery, ensure that all team members learn from what happens in every room and not just their room, and use that knowledge to create, implement, and measure improvements that bring the program closer to achieving its noble purpose.

The third floor of the house is the *program management* team. This team consists of an administrative leader (typically someone with a "C" in their title CEO, COO, CAO, CNO, CFO, CMO,…) and surgeon champions representing each of your surgical specialties performing da Vinci surgery. If we go back to our company analogy, the program management team serves as the Chief Executive Officer. Their role is focused on looking to the future, aligning and directing their team members, interfacing between the hospital leadership/board and the program team members, and managing the allocation of financial and physical resources. In short, they are the visionary leader who ensures that the program's human and physical resources are allocated and aligned to work towards achieving their noble purpose.

Consistent Communication Pathways

In order for the leadership structure to function effectively in driving the program towards their noble purpose, consistent communication pathways must be created and enforced. Unfortunately, the typical communication pathways are ineffective at solving problems. Typically, people communicate with those who are either geographically closest to them, or who possess the highest "rank." A surgeon and an anesthesiologist work out how they will position the patient in a way that satisfies both of them only to have a new combination of surgeon and anesthesiologist the next day forcing them each to go through the exercise all over again. Or maybe a surgeon is unhappy with the support he is getting in the operating room so he marches up to the CEO's office to tell him how important he is to the hospital and why the CEO needs to fix "*his*" operating room. If we go back to our house analogy, this means people are trying to solve problems within a single level of the house, or they are skipping a level of the house. This simply does not work. Problems cannot be solved within a level of the house or by skipping a level of the house. To have an effective communication pathway we need to build stairs for our house (see Fig. 32.2).

Notice that the stairs only go up one floor at a time. So the surgeon and anesthesiologist who do not agree on positioning need to bring their concerns to the operational oversight team, one level up. This operational oversight team that lives on the second floor can then perform a review of best practices and literature. They can then bring their findings to the program management team for modification and/or approval (one level up). The program management team's approval then travels one level down to operational oversight, who can then implement safe and standardized patient positioning for ALL the da Vinci operating rooms (one level down). Problem solved. If the surgeon is unhappy with the support in his operating room, skipping a level and going to the CEO does not help. The CEO can't fix the operating room. The surgeon needs to be directed to the operational oversight team (one level up), who will address the concerns and create a solution that will be implemented in ALL da Vinci operating rooms (one level down) so no matter which team member is supporting the surgeon's case, the support will be correct and consistent.

Be prepared, people aren't used to this and will try to circumvent the system on a regular basis. Someone will ask a team member in the room to solve a problem, or someone will call an executive team member to complain. It takes time, but be consistent and direct people one level up to solve their problems and hold each level responsible for making sure that solutions are implemented across team members only one level down.

So now we have successfully created the foundation of our da Vinci surgery program by putting into place elements 1, 2, and 3:

1. A clear noble purpose
2. The right leadership structure
3. Consistent communication pathways

Next we need to create success within our program, so it's time to move on to elements 4, 5, and 6:

4. Standardization
5. Parallel tasks
6. A continuous improvement cycle

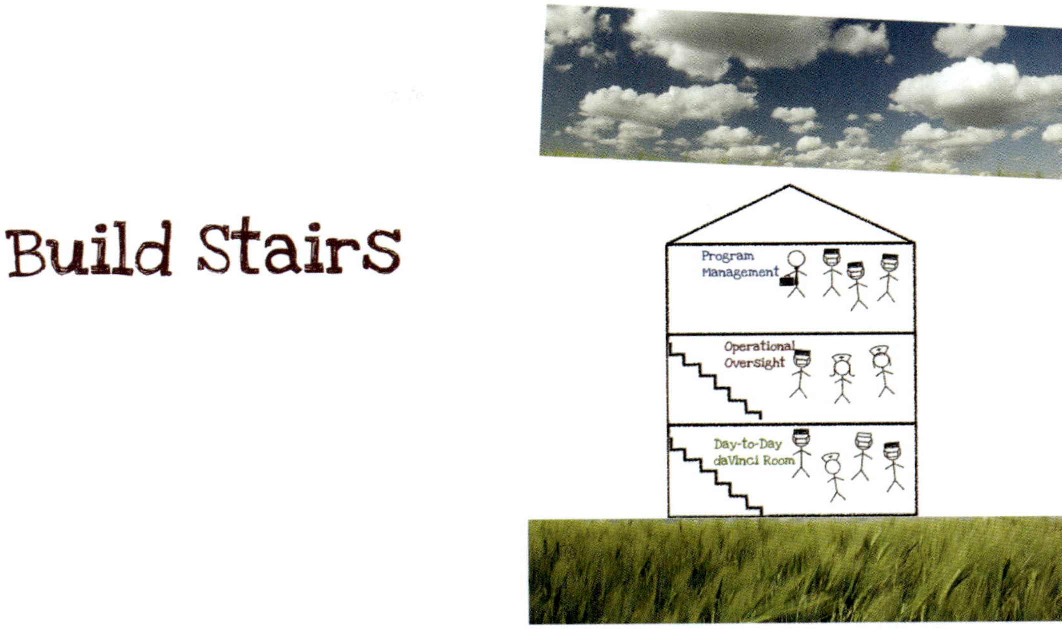

Fig. 32.2 Build stairs

Standardization

There is variability everywhere in our operating rooms, from pick lists and room setup to equipment and personnel. We live in a world where a single surgeon will have a 5–10 page printout that outlines what they want for a particular case. For a medium-sized da Vinci program, that can mean a few dozen surgeons who perform a few dozen different types of operations with the da Vinci surgical system, each with a unique 5–10 page printout. It may seem like a good idea, giving each surgeon what they request, but it's actually very bad for the surgeon, the team, and the patient. Let's do a little math. If there are just 10 da Vinci surgeons, 6 surgical technologists, 8 circulator nurses, and 15 anesthesiologists, there will be a 1 in 7,200 chance that if you were to walk into that operating room twice in 1 year, you would see the same group of 4 people. And that doesn't take into account the differing pick lists for each type of case as preferred by each surgeon. In this environment, how often do you think a team member will miss a detail? Way too often. One of the beauties of da Vinci surgery for the surgeon and the operating room team is its ability to facilitate standardization. With da Vinci surgery we need fewer instruments because da Vinci instruments articulate and can be used for multiple purposes, by almost all surgeons, for almost all cases. The equipment (the patient side cart and console), as well as its setup, breaks down, and sterilization is common to all surgeons and procedures. Our da Vinci programs, however, have not fully taken full advantage of this great opportunity for standardization. In a room where we have the same equipment and instruments, set up in exactly the same way, for all surgeons, and all surgical cases, how often do you think a team member will miss a detail? Not very often. This is good for the team, good for the surgeon, and good for the patient.

There are three simple ways you can take advantage of the opportunity for standardization in daV inci surgery.

1) Room setup
2) Personnel
3) Instrumentation

Room Setup

The da Vinci operating room should have a standard setup that works for as close to 100 % of your da Vinci surgeries as possible. Depending on your OR size, shape, and the types of cases your hospital performs, this setup may vary slightly from hospital to hospital. But whatever setup you choose, you want it to be the standard for nearly all your da Vinci cases. To find your standard setup, start by clearing out any unnecessary items from the room. These unnecessary items are both visual and physical barriers to communication and workflow. Next, using just the items you need every day, work with your team to create a configuration that keeps the sterile field in one area and the non-sterile field in another. Doing this will improve the efficiency and flow of patients and personnel on the non-sterile side and the performance of surgical tasks on the sterile side.

Personnel

As we saw from the example in the opening paragraph, even a small core team can present problems with standardization. Despite these challenges, we must work to standardize our da Vinci team. By designating a core da Vinci team that is highly familiar and proficient in the setup, use, breakdown, and care of the daVinci surgical system, we can improve the quality of patient care, the consistency with which that care is delivered, and the efficiency of the team's performance. When you are looking to reduce the variability in your team you need to be sure you look beyond the surgical tech and circulating nurse and include anesthesia. Anesthesia is the often forgotten, but critical member of the da Vinci team. Their involvement as a core team member is critical to the smooth and safe performance of da Vinci surgery. Designating and utilizing a core team of anesthesia providers that are familiar with the unique needs of da Vinci surgery including things like patient positioning, ventilation requirements, and fluid needs improve patient safety, quality of care, consistency of care delivery, and operational efficiency.

Instrumentation

Because da Vinci surgeries across specialties use the same core open, laparoscopic, and da Vinci instrumentation, we have a great opportunity to minimize and standardize the instruments we use across surgeons, surgeries, and specialties. You can begin by simply looking across the pick lists for all of your da Vinci surgeries and find the items that are common to a single procedure or all procedures. By taking these common instruments and making a single tray that will be used for many or all da Vinci surgeries, the frequency of use of this single tray will improve the efficiency of setup, breakdown, and sterilization and improve the likelihood that you will have 100 % of what you need 100 % of the time.

Standardizing the instruments used by your surgeons also allows you to standardize how you set up the back table. By standardizing back table setup, your team will be able to function more consistently no matter which team member is scrubbed in the room and no matter who is giving relief.

Parallel Tasks

Traditionally, in the operating room tasks are performed in series (Fig. 32.3). First the team works together to set up the back table, then they work together to drape the robot, then the patient is brought back. The reality is tasks like these can and should be performed by one person. With one person performing these tasks they can then be done simultaneously (Fig. 32.4).

For example, one person can set up the back table at the same time that another person drapes the robot. By executing tasks in parallel you will reduce the time it takes to get all these tasks finished. In addition, if you also take elements that are traditionally done while the operating room is "down" (the "red zone" on Figs. 32.3, 32.4, and 32.5) and convert them to tasks done while the patient is still in the room you will reduce the number of tasks that need to be done in the "red zone" and will reduce you room turnover time (Fig. 32.5).

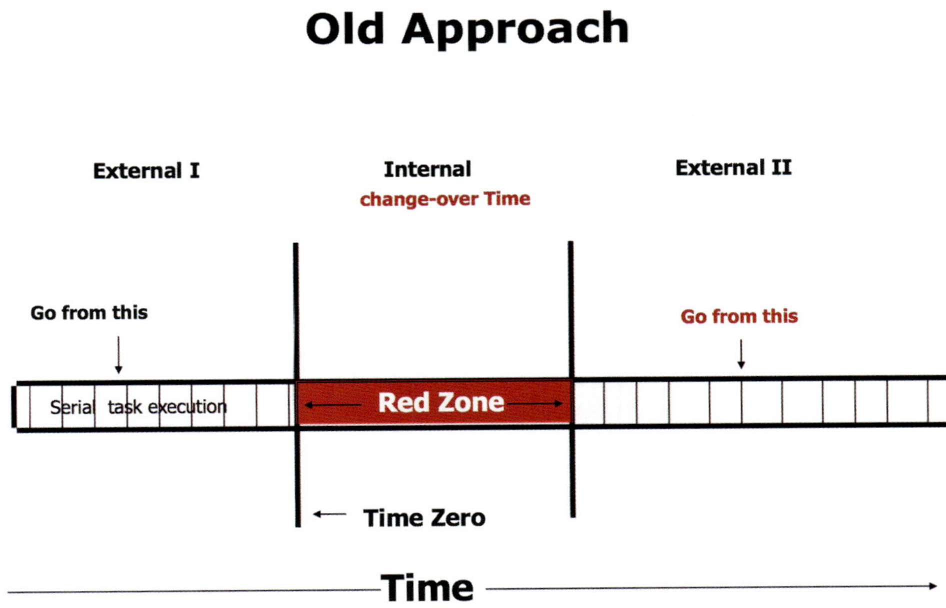

Fig. 32.3 Old approach

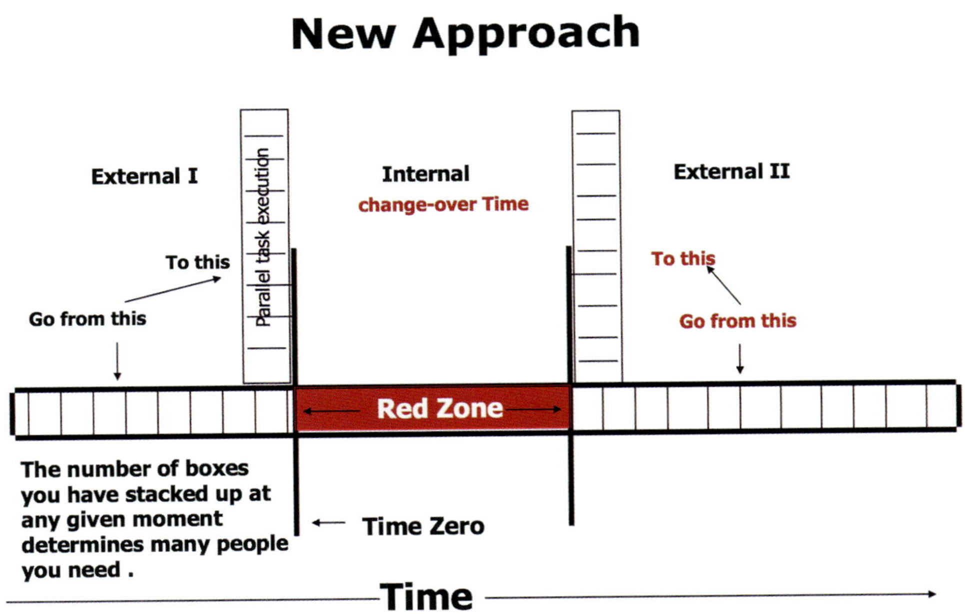

Fig. 32.4 New approach

Operating Room Efficiency: Parallel Task Model

Now that you know the basics lets apply these key concepts in a model that you can implement in the operating room. We are going to go step by step with each figure depicting the roles and parallel tasks for the five critical people in the room: Surgeon, Nurse Circulator, Scrub Tech, Surgical Assistant, and Anesthesia. Under each heading I

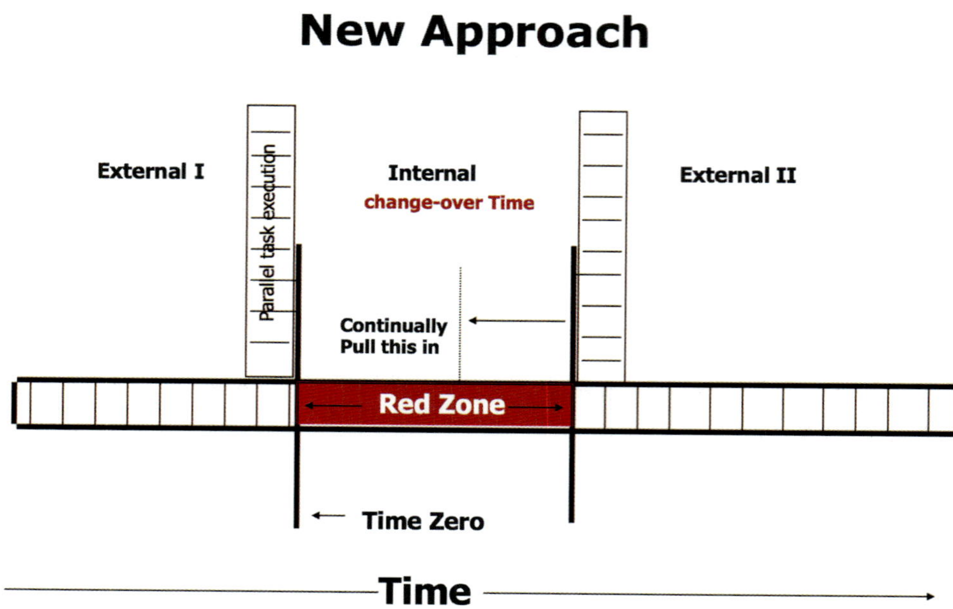

Fig. 32.5 New approach

will list the specific parallel task that is critical for that step in the robotic procedure.

Step 1: Setting Up the Back Table (Fig. 32.6)

Parallel Task: Go Get the Patient Before the Back Table Is Set Up

The key for efficiency at this stage of the procedure is that once the back table is opened the circulator and anesthesia representative go to get the patient. The back table may look like a giant pile at this point but it takes 5–10 min to go to pre-op holding and return with a patient and that is more than enough time for the scrub (and in some places first assistant) to completely set up the back table. There is no need to wait for the back table to be setup to go get the patient. In addition, to make back table set up more efficient, you should work to minimize the instruments you open. You do not need a full open set opened and counted. If you choose, an open set can be in the room left unopened next to the back table and opened only in the case of the rare emergency.

Step 2: Patient Enters the OR (Fig. 32.7)

Parallel Task: Drape the Robot While the Patient Is Being Intubated

When the patient enters the room the surgeon and the circulator should be focused on positioning and prepping the patient while the scrub tech is focused on draping the robot. Remember, anesthesia still needs to intubate the patient then the patient will need to be positioned, prepped, and draped. These activities will take 5–15 min, which gives the scrub more than enough time to drape the robot while the patient is in the room and these other activities are being performed.

Step 3: Patent Draped (Fig. 32.8)

Parallel Task: Team Members Need to Anticipate the Surgeon's Needs not React to Them

Once the patient is draped, the surgeon will make his initial incision, insufflate the abdomen with CO_2 and place the ports. While the surgeon is doing this, the team should be anticipating his/her needs. The circulator should connect the bovie, then the gas in that order since this is the

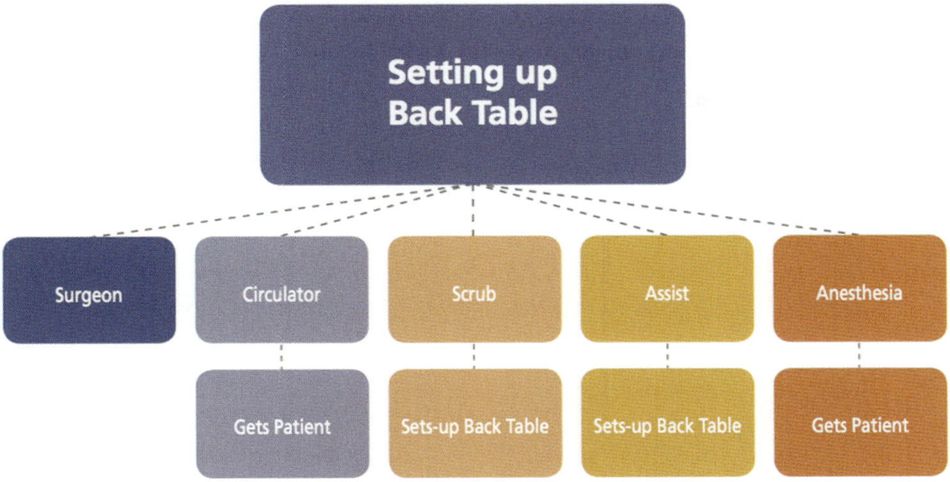

The Key: Create Task Overlap

- **Circulator - Gets patient from pre-op while back table is set up.**
- **Anesthesia - Gets patient from pre-op while back table is set up.**

TASK OVERLAP: NO NEED TO WAIT TO GET PATIENT UNTIL AFTER BACK TABLE SET UP.
Scrub and Assist - Set up back table:
- **Minimize the amount of instruments on the back table. Limit it to *da Vinci* instruments only.**
- **Open surgical tray can remain unopened and placed to the side of back table.**

PRE-SURGERY INSPECTION SHOULD BE CONDUCTED PRIOR TO THE ANESTHETIZATION OF PATIENT

Fig. 32.6 Step 1: Setting up the back table

order in which the surgeon will need it (first incision, then insufflation). The assist's role at this time is to clean and prepare the scope since this is the next item needed. These steps are the same every case so anticipating the needs of the surgeon should be easy and routine. By anticipating surgeon needs instead of reacting to requests efficiency is further improved.

Step 4: Ports Placed (Fig. 32.9)

Parallel Task: Docking Should Be a Team Effort That Includes the Surgeon

The surgeon is the only consistent person in the operating room so he/she needs to be as facile with the docking procedure as the team. Because team members can change from day to day, the ability of the surgeon to complete simple tasks like this will reduce variability and improve efficiency and consistency. Once the robot is docked, the surgeon will move to the console and it is at this point that the circulator should begin his/her paperwork. In many operating rooms the circulator will disrupt the workflow up to this point by trying to complete paperwork or make computer entries. The surgeon's time at the console will provide more than enough opportunity for the circulator to complete the necessary paperwork and make all the required computer entries. By completing charting while the surgeon is at the console, workflow is not disrupted and efficiency is improved.

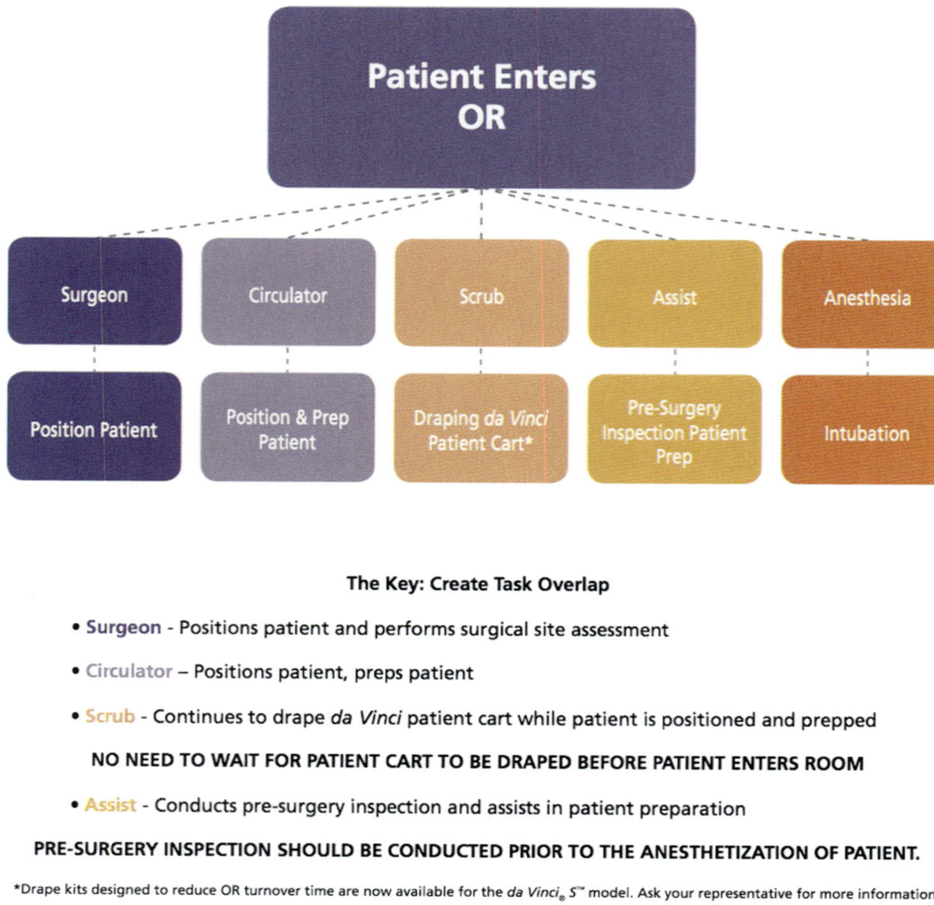

Fig. 32.7 Step 2: Patient enters the OR

Step 5: Surgeon off the Console (Fig. 32.10)

Parallel Task: While the Surgeon Closes the Patient the Robot Should Be Undraped and the Back Table Cleared

When the surgeon stands up from the console, they are telling the room that they are done using the robot and all of the equipment associated with it. This means the robot should not just be rolled back but it should also be undraped and the robotic equipment (reposables, ports, etc.) should be cleaned up and removed from the room. By removing the drapes, cleaning up the robotic equipment and sending it to central sterilization you are performing part of the turnover while the patient is still in the room. The surgeon will take 10–20 min to remove the specimen and close the abdomen, which gives plenty of time for the team to begin stripping the room of unnecessary items.

Step 6: Patient Exits the OR (Fig. 32.11)

Parallel Task: While the Patient Heads to Recovery the Scrub and Assist Complete the Room Cleanup and Begin to Open for the Next Case

With the operation complete, the surgeon heads out to talk the family of the patient he just operated on and the patient who they will be operating on next. While the circulator and anesthesia are bringing the patient to recovery, the scrub and assist should be

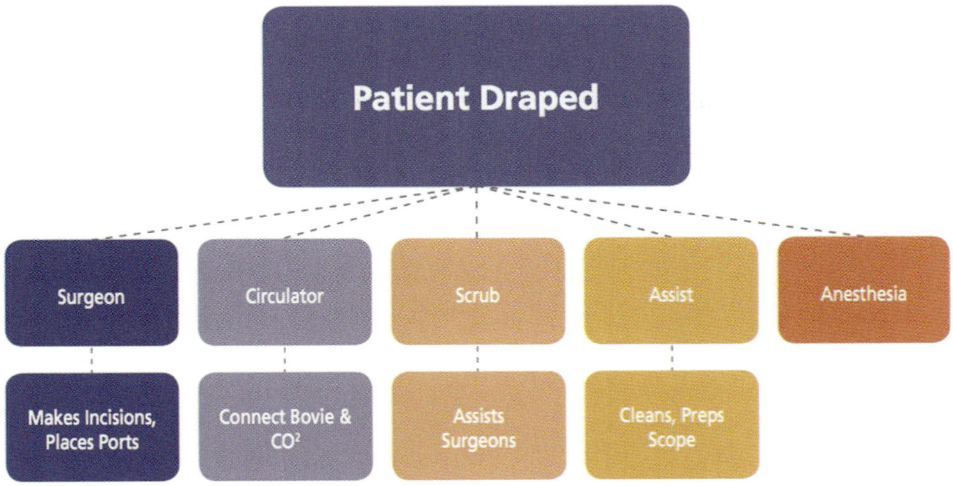

The Key: Create Task Overlap

- **Surgeon** - Insufflates, makes incisions, places camera and instrument ports
- **Scrub** - Assists surgeon with incision, port placement, instrumentation
- **Circulator** - Prepares auxiliary equipment (ESU, gas, etc.)
- **Assist** - Cleans and prepares scope for port placement visualization

TEAM MEMBERS SHOULD ANTICIPATE THE SURGEON'S NEED FOR INSTRUMENTS AND EQUIPMENT.

- Connect Bovie
- Gas tubing connected

Fig. 32.8 Step 3: Patent draped

completing what little is left of room clean up and then should immediately open for the next case. With the back table already cleared and the robot already undraped all that is left to do is take out the garbage, mop, and open for the next case. These few remaining tasks take less than 15 min and should be the only "red zone" items to complete minimizing the time turnover should take.

A Continuous Improvement Cycle

We all recognize that practice makes perfect. Whether you are playing the piano, swinging a golf club, or throwing a football, we recognize that to get better at it, you have to do it, and do it often. When playing the piano you can hear if the notes you are playing are correct. When you swing your golf club you know right away if you sliced it into the woods or hit it straight down the fairway. When you throw a football you know immediately if you connected with or overthrew your receiver. But in the operating room you can find people who have been doing their job for a long time and still aren't very good at it. Why is working in the operating room any different from being a quarterback? Because unlike the quarterback who knows the second he throws the ball if it was a good throw or not, members of the operating room team do not get any feedback on their task performance. How much could a golfer improve if he was only allowed to see where his ball landed 3 months later? How about a basketball player who would be told how many of the

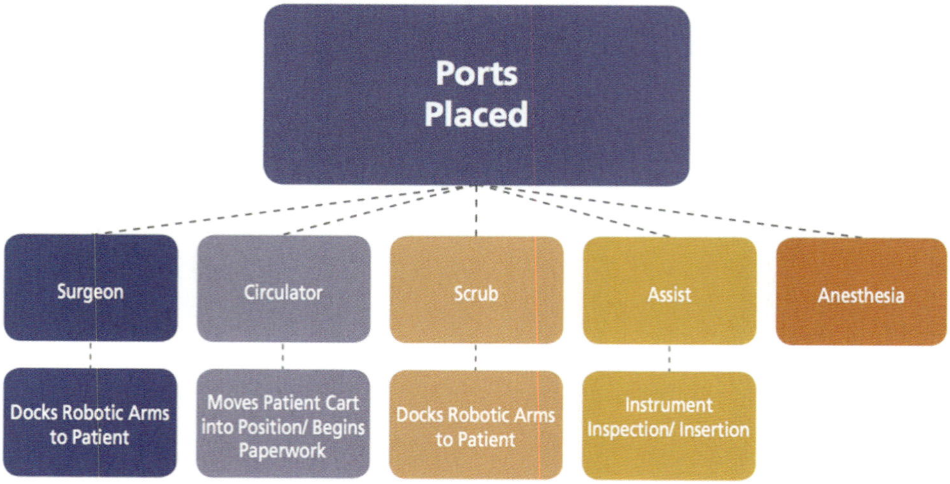

The Key: Create Task Overlap

- Circulator – Moves *da Vinci* patient cart into position. Once locked in place and surgery begins, paperwork can be started.
- **Surgeon** - Docks robotic arms to ports
- Scrub - Assists surgeon in docking of robotic arms to ports
- Assist - Gathers and inspects robotic instrumentation and auxiliary instrumentation and prepares for insertion

DOCKING AND DRIVING THE *DA VINCI* SYSTEM IS A TEAM EVENT THAT SHOULD BE PRACTICED CONTINUALLY. HAVING CONSISTENT TEAM MEMBERS FOR ALL CASES WILL ALSO INCREASE EFFICIENCY.

Fig. 32.9 Step 4: Ports placed

shots he took were baskets only at an annual performance review. Practice only makes perfect when the feedback given is timely, frequent, and relevant and we need to apply this feedback to our operating room teams if we want them to improve. We can provide this feedback to our operating room teams using a five-step process:

1. Standardize an operation and the activities that support it
2. Measure the standardized operation
3. Gauge measurements against requirements
4. Innovate to meet requirements and increase productivity
5. Standardize the new, improved operations

Standardize an Operation and the Activities That Support It

We learned during the section on reducing variability that standardization of simple items like room layout, personnel, and instrumentation can improve team performance and drive quality and efficiency simultaneously. As we look beyond these items and focus on the processes our team members engage in, the same benefits hold true. So it is up to us to give our team members the responsibility of identifying areas of variability and working to create standardized methods for performing activities.

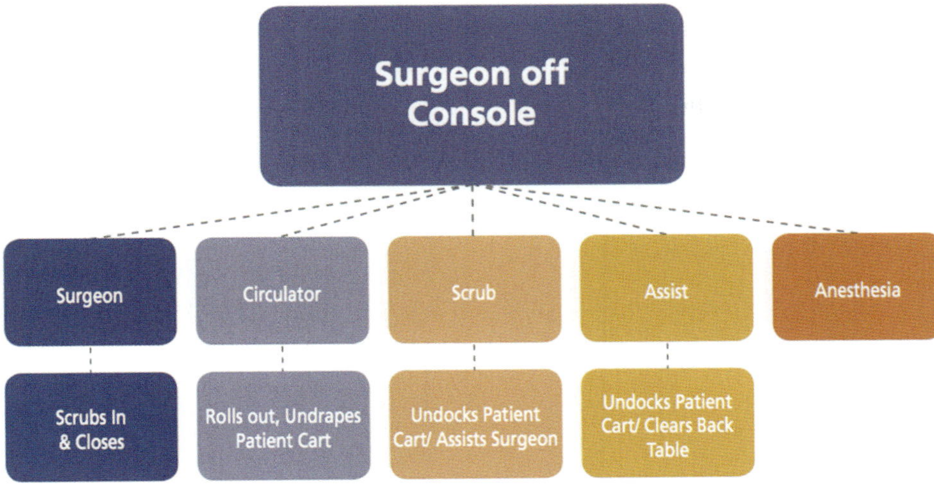

The Key: Create Task Overlap

- **Surgeon** - Scrubs in to close ports
- **Scrub** - Undocks *da Vinci* Patient Cart and assists surgeon in preparation of suture and port-site closure
- **Assist** - Helps in undocking *da Vinci* Patient Cart and begins clearing back table of all *da Vinci* instruments

INSTRUMENTS AND SCOPES SHOULD BE IMMEDIATELY SENT TO CENTRAL PROCESSING FOR CLEANING, STERILIZATION.*

- **Circulator** – Rolls *da Vinci* patient cart out and begins undraping and cleaning the system

ONCE THE SURGEON STANDS UP FROM THE CONSOLE, *DA VINCI* EQUIPMENT IS NO LONGER NEEDED. PATIENT CART SHOULD BE UNDRAPED; ASSISTANT CAN BEGIN TO CLEAR AND CLEAN BACK TABLE.

Fig. 32.10 Step 5: Surgeon off the console

Measure the Standardized Operation

It isn't enough, however, to merely standardize a process. We need to know if all our team members are following the standardized method and we need to be able to gauge how effective this method has been at improving care and efficiency. The only way to do that is to measure what we are doing. So, for any process we currently perform or intend to perform, we must identify a way to measure the performance of the task in an objective way, and implement a way to record those measurements. Because the processes we are measuring are performed by our day-to-day team members on the ground floor of our "house," we must record these measurements on the ground floor. Measurements should be taken at the point closest to where a task being measured is being performed. Doing this will provide you with the most accurate information. This means, to measure performance, you will need to assign the job of collecting these measurements to members of your day-to-day team on the ground floor.

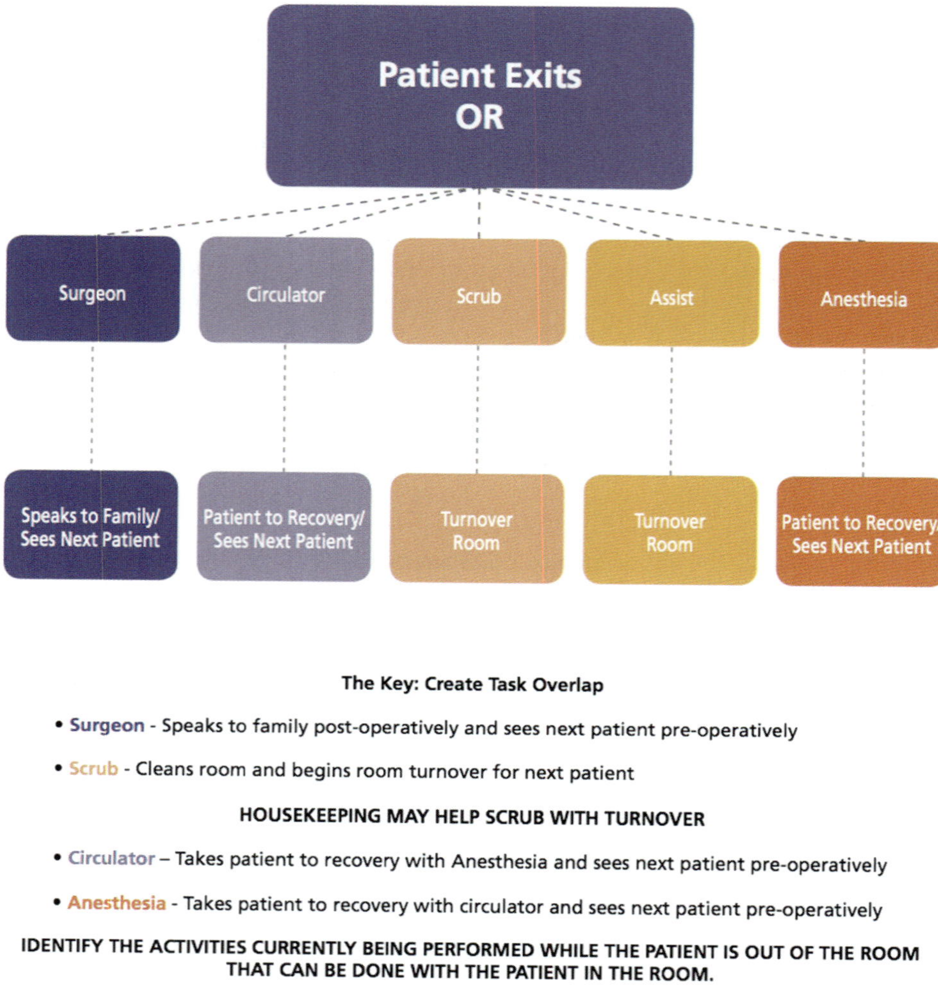

Fig. 32.11 Step 6: Patient exits the OR

Gauge Measurements Against Requirements

Once you have standardized a process and measured the performance of the tasks within that process, you need to know if your results meet your performance goals. To gauge your measurements against your goals, you will need to enlist members of your operational oversight team on the second floor of the house to review the data collected, and compare your current performance to your performance goals.

Innovate to Meet Requirements and Increase Productivity

Although it will be team members on the second floor of your house (operational oversight) that will be responsible for the first three steps, it is the responsibility of your ground floor day-to-day personnel that are charged with step 4; innovating the role they play to improve efficiency and productivity. Because team members, who perform a given role, know that role the best, you need to give them the responsibility of finding innovative ways to work smarter, not harder.

Standardize the New, Improved Operations

So you've standardized tasks, measured performance of that task, met your performance goal for that operation, and improved the efficiency of performing the task. Now you need to standardize this new, optimized task and continue to measure performance to maintain this higher level of functioning.

When you successfully enact a continuous improvement cycle, you will find that the benefits extend beyond improvements in quality, productivity, and revenue. A continuous improvement process, when done correctly, improves engagement of your staff/team, eliminates inefficient work, and teaches people to perform experiments on their work to spot and eliminate waste.

Conclusion

Although there are many challenges in setting up a successful daVinci surgery program, a clear, reproducible path to success is within every program's reach. By defining your clear and noble purpose, building your "house" and setting in place the right leadership structure and communication pathways, working to reduce variability in tasks, focusing on parallel tasks, and engaging in a continuous improvement cycle you can join the hundreds of daVinci surgery programs across the country that have used this model to create growth and success. The results achieved can be dramatic and sustainable and the performance improvements are significant and reproducible. After reading this, if you still believe that your situation is unique, or you cannot implement this entire model because of (insert your reason here) I want you to share with you one more pearl. One of the unique aspects of this model is the ability to implement various fragments of it in part or in total. Regardless of the limitations and challenges your program faces, you can implement those part(s) of this model that you choose, eliminate those part(s) you simply cannot implement due to your unique situation, and still achieve significant benefits in program development and success. So use this model and begin enjoying the improvements in quality, revenue, and success it can bring your program, your practice, and your patients.

Professional Education: Telementoring and Teleproctoring

33

Monika E. Hagen and Myriam J. Curet

Background

The change in modern technique for general surgery from traditional open procedures to minimally invasive techniques has been driven by technological advances, which require effort to master on the part of trainee surgeons [1, 2]. Besides learning the technical aspects of these new technologies for routine standard surgery, new approaches to the anatomy and even entirely new procedures might be necessary when applying minimally invasive techniques. Examples include changing to a medial to lateral dissection during laparoscopic colonic mobilization or the work in new anatomical spaces for procedure such as minimally invasive totally extraperitoneal hernia repair. Therefore, the technical mastering of laparoscopic instruments is often insufficient for the successful performance of procedures that are already mastered with an open approach and each individual laparoscopic procedure requires specific learning.

M.E. Hagen, M.D., M.B.A.
Intuitive Surgical International, Sunnyvale, CA, USA

Department of Digestive Surgery, University Hospital Geneva, 14, rue Gabrielle-Perret-Gentil, Geneva 1211, Switzerland
e-mail: monikahagen@aol.com

M.J. Curet, M.D. (✉)
Intuitive Surgical International, Sunnyvale, CA, USA

Department of Surgery, Stanford University School of Medicine, Stanford, CA, USA
e-mail: mcuret@stanford.edu

While a pool of experienced senior surgeons are usually available in large tertiary hospitals to monitor and mentor their inexperienced colleagues as they learn how to use new technologies or even new procedures, this process can be a bottleneck in the dissemination of new techniques and their availability to the general population. As a result, telementoring or teleproctoring is becoming an increasingly familiar and welcome part of the modern surgical milieu [3, 4].

The goal of telementoring is to provide surgeons with real-time, "over-the-shoulder" guidance from distant, more experienced colleagues as they perform unfamiliar or challenging procedures or use new technology [5]. Using Internet-enabled cameras, microphones, telestration (technology to draw illustrations on the surgeon's monitor), and speakers in the operating theater, telementors are able to observe and guide their mentees as necessary. This approach is particularly well suited to minimally invasive procedures, which already mostly rely on cameras to visualize the operating field; thus, there is less situational awareness to be gained by the physical presence of the mentor. When efficiently scheduled, telementoring might maximize the number of procedures mentors are able to proctor, increasing the overall training rate. This is particularly important for uncommon or newly developed surgical procedures using new tools and techniques such as robotics where the global supply of sufficiently experienced mentors may be limited.

K.C. Kim (ed.), *Robotics in General Surgery*, DOI 10.1007/978-1-4614-8739-5_33,

Value and Limitations of Telementoring

The major advantages of telementoring are in convenience and throughput. A telementor does not need to scrub in or move from one operating room to another; they can remain in their office with all their reference material. Their time is used only when it is needed—thus increasing the efficiency of supervision. Trainee surgeons anywhere around the world with equipment and bandwidth can perform telementored surgery. This can drastically increase the availability of procedures at community and rural hospitals equipped for telementoring and decreases the distances that patients are forced to travel in order to receive the best care. Most importantly, telementoring allows training in and enhances performance of complex surgeries when mentors are not physically present. Telementoring also makes it easier to extend the period of mentoring; a trainee might go from needing a great deal of attention in the beginning to only calling in their telementor for particularly difficult presentations. Because mentors' time is not wasted in transit or scrubbing, their attention costs less and they are able to spend more time with their own patients.

Telementoring does have its disadvantages. A mentor who is physically present is able to step in and complete the procedure if there is a complication; obviously this is not possible in telementoring. This underscores the need for strong preparation of the trainee beforehand. Telementors also must address issues around licensing, credentialing, and privileging ahead of time. Additionally, relying on two-dimensional images can make it difficult to detect or indicate anatomical features. Some or all of these problems may be rendered irrelevant in the future.

Systems and Technical Requirements

There are a variety of telepresence and telementoring systems currently available, among them RP-Vantage (In Touch Health, *Santa Barbara, CA*), Karl Storz OR1 Smartconnect (Karl Storz, *Tuttlingen, Germany*), and Stryker's Video Network Hub (Stryker, *Kalamazoo, MI*). Details of the systems can be reviewed on the webpages of the respective company. The most important prerequisite for operating these systems in a telementoring context is bandwidth, which must be adequate to carry the images and sound in both directions with low latency and high resolution [6]. Generally these systems transmit the laparoscopic camera output from the surgical field, as well as audio and visual feeds from the operating theater to the mentor, while transmitting audio feeds from the mentor's office to the theater. In some systems the mentor is able to draw and make indications on the camera feed view to show the trainee what is being discussed (telestration), and there may be a monitor with a video feed from the mentor's office as well. The telementoring apparatus may be installed in the operating room or on a mobile cart so it may be shared between operating rooms. Patient information confidentiality regulations also require the use of encryption to protect privacy. A minimum setup would utilize a virtual private network (VPN) running on an asymmetrical digital subscriber connection (ADSL) capable of >1 Mbps, encrypted using a 256-bit advanced encryption standard (AES) [4]. As a simplified alternative, Parker et al. reported on ten clinical cholecystectomies during which mentors communicated with trainees over the phone and received short videos of the surgery via Blackberry to comment on the procedure [7]. This or a similar system (e.g., Skype or Google video chat through a laptop) has the potential to provide an effective low-cost backup and allow successful guidance during surgical procedures.

Applications of Telementoring in General Surgery

Reports on telementoring during general surgery procedures as part of advanced laparoscopic training can be found in the literature for a variety of procedures such as colorectal resections [8, 9]. Rosser et al. reported that intraoperative problems were solved successfully by remote guidance for colon resections and fundoplications [10]. Telementoring also may enable care in austere and environments. For example, the US Navy has experimented with a successful implementation of telementoring aboard an aircraft carrier for inguinal hernia surgery when far from port [6]. Telementoring has else been applied to delivery health-care needs in remote areas: Sebajang et al. reported telementoring for 19 laparoscopic general surgery procedures which were performed by surgeons with no formal minimally invasive training [11]. Byrne et al. demonstrated in 34 laparoscopic cholecystectomies that the amount of required telesupport increases with difficulty of the surgical case and physical attendance of the mentor was need in 2 of the 34 cases. Sawyer et al. compared operating times and complications of six age- and sex-matches cases of laparoscopic cholecystectomy with live or telementoring. This group observed no significant differences in operating time and concluded that telementoring is a safe and effective training method for laparoscopic cholecystectomy. In addition, two reports can be found on successful telementoring for laparoscopic adrenalectomy without technical difficulties [12, 13].

Robotic Surgery and Telementoring

While the da Vinci Surgical System (Intuitive Surgical International, Sunnyvale, CA, USA) offers all technical requirements that are needed for "long-distance" telementoring, currently no such application is available on the market (as of July 2012). Teleproctoring and remote case observation for robotic procedures with the da Vinci Surgical System was investigated by Intuitive Surgical International but remains off the market until its value and legal implications are clear (as of July 2012).

Besides classical "long-distance" telementoring, teaching using a dual console setup in the same room or same hospital falls under the definition of telementoring as well. During dual console da Vinci surgery, two surgical consoles are connected to a single patient side cart. Two surgeons can control different functions of the da Vinci Surgical System simultaneously. Console adjustments can be made independently including the image and instrument control mode. Instrument control is individually assigned to either one of the two surgeons, and this setup might be switched at any time during the procedure. Camera control can be performed in the usual way by either surgeon. All instruments lock as usual during camera movements. A virtual pointer—a three-dimensional graphical object that appears overlaid to the video image when activated—can be used by either surgeon when masters are not assigned to instruments.

In the most common scenario, a proctor surgeon, sitting at one of the consoles, controls no, one, or two instrument arms and provides guidance to a surgeon being proctored at the other surgeon console, who controls two, three, or four instrument arms. The four arms are divided between the proctor and the proctee depending on who is performing which tasks. The proctor surgeon would use one or two unassociated masters to activate one or two pointers and then use each pointer to refer to anatomical features or to demonstrate movements of the instruments while speaking with the surgeon being proctored. During this setup, the mentor can demonstrate as well as facilitate the surgery at the same time.

The dual console da Vinci Surgical System is therefore currently a valuable tool for "short-distance" telementoring and its future potential, as a "long-distance" mentoring tool via online data transmission seems evident. In its present version, it appears most valuable in a teaching setting and the second surgical console might serve as a platform for simulation use when not required for clinical cases. Clinical procedures have been performed in the abovementioned setup and described in the literature [14], but its value for surgical education has not yet been scientifically established (as of July 2012).

Conclusion and Future Perspective

Telementoring offers advantages over the physical-presence model of surgical training. As the cost of telementoring equipment decreases and its use as a teaching modality spreads, decentralized surgical training will become more feasible. Additionally, telementoring enhances the capabilities of general surgeons operating in remote locations on patients with complex problems. Once the pool of telementors for a given surgical procedure is adequately large, someone will always be available to provide an emergency consult. It is to be hoped that telementoring receives legislative support, which protects and promotes the availability of qualified telementors.

With the development of telepresence and telerobotics in medicine, the disadvantages of telementoring may be superseded. Telerobotic surgery is ideally suited to telementoring because the telemetry and controls are easily shared between trainee and mentor. If complications arise, a telepresent mentor would be able to complete the surgery, obviating the need for physical presence.

Telementoring is still in its infancy, and evidence-based support for its use to impact learning curves and patient outcome is sparse but promising. The convenience of telemedicine is its great selling point especially as the demands upon the time of physicians increase. As the price of equipment goes down and telementoring's legal status is clarified, expect it to become a common feature of surgical practice, particularly in a robotic setup.

References

1. Abboudi H, Khan MS, Aboumarzouk O, Guru KA, Challacombe B, Dasgupta P, Ahmed K. Current status of validation for robotic surgery simulators – a systematic review. BJU Int. 2013;111:194–205.
2. Rosser Jr JC, Murayama M, Gabriel NH. Minimally invasive surgical training solutions for the twenty-first century. Surg Clin North Am. 2000;80:1607–24.
3. Rosser Jr JC, Gabriel N, Herman B, Murayama M. Telementoring and teleproctoring. World J Surg. 2001;25:1438–48.
4. Antoniou SA, Antoniou GA, Franzen J, Bollmann S, Koch OO, Pointner R, Granderath FA. A comprehensive review of telementoring applications in laparoscopic general surgery. Surg Endosc. 2012;26(8):2111–6.
5. Senapati S, Advincula AP. Telemedicine and robotics: paving the way to the globalization of surgery. Int J Gynaecol Obstet. 2005;91:210–6.
6. Cubano M, Poulose BK, Talamini MA, Stewart R, Antosek LE, Lentz R, Nibe R, Kutka MF, Mendoza-Sagaon M. Long distance telementoring. A novel tool for laparoscopy aboard the USS Abraham Lincoln. Surg Endosc. 1999;13:673–8.
7. Parker A, Rubinfeld I, Azuh O, Blyden D, Falvo A, Horst M, Velanovich V, Patton P. What ring tone should be used for patient safety? Early results with a Blackberry-based telementoring safety solution. Am J Surg. 2010;199:336–40. discussion 340–1.
8. Schlachta CM, Lefebvre KL, Sorsdahl AK, Jayaraman S. Mentoring and telementoring leads to effective incorporation of laparoscopic colon surgery. Surg Endosc. 2010;24:841–4.
9. Schlachta CM, Sorsdahl AK, Lefebvre KL, McCune ML, Jayaraman S. A model for longitudinal mentoring and telementoring of laparoscopic colon surgery. Surg Endosc. 2009;23:1634–8.
10. Rosser JC, Wood M, Payne JH, Fullum TM, Lisehora GB, Rosser LE, Barcia PJ, Savalgi RS. Telementoring. A practical option in surgical training. Surg Endosc. 1997;11:852–5.
11. Sebajang H, Trudeau P, Dougall A, Hegge S, McKinley C, Anvari M. Telementoring: an important enabling tool for the community surgeon. Surg Innov. 2005;12:327–31.
12. Bruschi M, Micali S, Porpiglia F, Celia A, De Stefani S, Grande M, Scarpa RM, Bianchi G. Laparoscopic telementored adrenalectomy: the Italian experience. Surg Endosc. 2005;19:836–40.
13. Ushiyama T, Suzuki K, Aoki M, Takayama T, Kageyama S, Ohtawara Y, Fujita K, Uchikubo A. Laparoscopic adrenalectomy using telementoring system. Nihon Hinyokika Gakkai Zasshi. 2003;94:582–6.
14. Smith AL, Krivak TC, Scott EM, Rauh-Hain JA, Sukumvanich P, Olawaiye AB, Richard SD. Dual-console robotic surgery compared to laparoscopic surgery with respect to surgical outcomes in a gynecologic oncology fellowship program. Gynecol Oncol. 2012;126(3):432–6.

Part XIV

Evolving Platforms

Single-Incision Platform

34

Giuseppe Spinoglio

General Overview

In the last 20 years, surgical techniques have moved toward a less invasive approach from open to laparoscopic surgery, to natural orifice transluminal surgery (NOTES) and to single-incision laparoscopic surgery (SILS). The new emerging techniques have been developed to reduce the number of ports in order to limit the invasivity of the surgical access, to improve better cosmesis and to decrease parietal and body image trauma.

The main limitation of NOTES is the lack of instruments for flexible endoscopes, which allows the same performance of laparoscopic ones. Furthermore, this technique necessitates passing through hollow organs with risk of contamination and of dehiscence [1].

SILS

Almost always the SILS technique uses the umbilicus as access: it can be considered as a NOTES with the opening of a naturally closed orifice and truly scarless surgery because an incision is made in a scar that already exists. The first report of single-incision laparoscopic cholecystectomy (SILC) was in 1997 by Navarra et al. [2] followed by others; it showed the feasibility of this approach for cholecystectomy [3, 4]. This technique required the introduction of multiple trocars through separate fascia stabs within the same skin incision.

The evolution was the diffusion of the "multi single-port access devices" that have different shapes and types of embodiment (plastic filled with port holes, glove-form plastic platforms with the outer surface gel, etc.) [5, 6] but have the common feature of allowing the introduction of multiple laparoscopic instruments, simultaneously, through a single fascia and skin incision. The advantage consists of being more similar to laparoscopy but with important conceptual differences.

As known, the founding technical principles of good manipulation in laparoscopic surgery are fulcrum and triangulation.

The fulcrum is placed on the abdominal wall, and the instruments have a favourable or unfavourable leverage depending on their length inside and outside of the abdomen. When the external arm is longer, we get greater precision because a wide movement of the surgeon's hands reflects a short movement of the instrument tip. If the internal arm is long, we get a better ergonomy. The triangulation is obtained with the appropriate distance between the trocars in order to achieve different angles between the instruments. We have to consider three different angles: azimuth angle, elevation angle and the manipulation angle. The azimuth angle is the optimal angle between optical axis and instruments plane

G. Spinoglio, M.D. (✉)
Department of General and Oncological Surgery, City Hospital SS. Antonio e Biagio, Via Venezia 16, Alessandria 15121, Italy
e-mail: gspinoglio@ospedale.al.it

K.C. Kim (ed.), *Robotics in General Surgery*, DOI 10.1007/978-1-4614-8739-5_34,

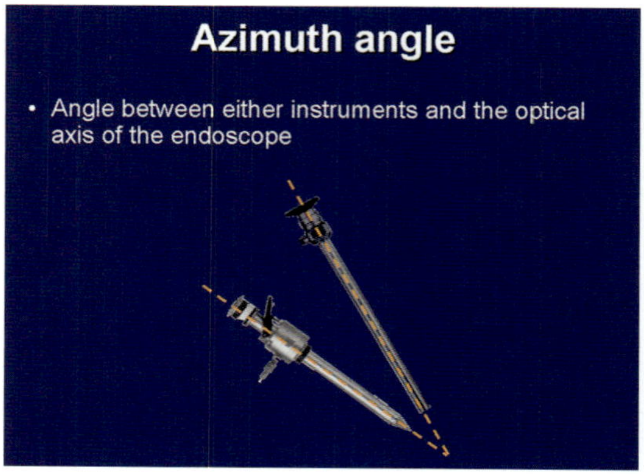

Fig. 34.1 The azimuth angle

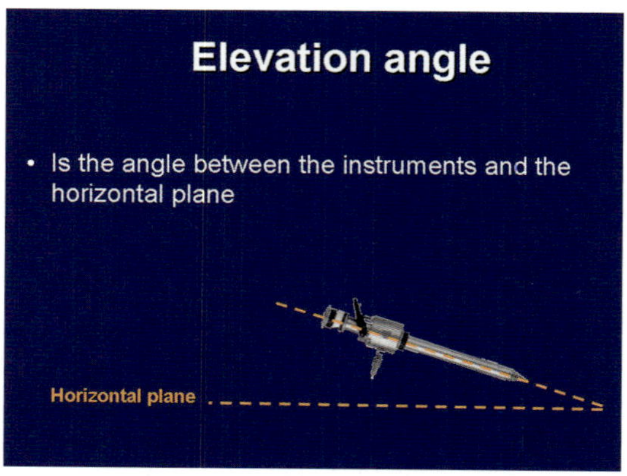

Fig. 34.2 The elevation angle

and has to be between 0° and +15°, with the camera from above (Fig. 34.1).

The elevation angle reflects the optimal elevation angle between the instrument and the horizontal plane and has to be 60° (Fig. 34.2).

The manipulation angle reflects the best ergonomic layout for laparoscopic surgery which is in a range from 45° to 75° between the instruments with equal azimuth angles [7, 8] (Fig. 34.3).

Once obtained, the triangulation allows one to reach the target surgical field correctly, and the ergonomics and accuracy are a function of the length of the lever arms with an optimal ratio between internal and external length of the instruments.

In SILS, there is only one port with the loss of all the correct angles described above. Fixed direction and fulcrum force the parallelism of the

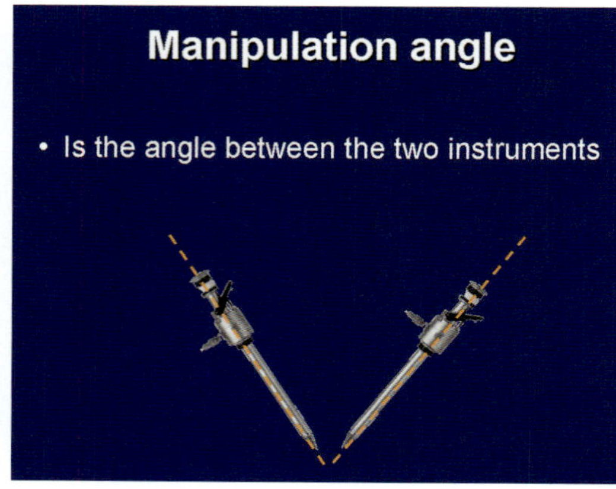

Fig. 34.3 The manipulation angle

instruments: the lateral movements can only be achieved by an inversion of instruments; the tool that comes from the right side can only pull on the left and vice versa. Therefore, the traction is inverted compared to the movement of the hands.

The loss of triangulation results in less accurate manoeuvres. The inversion of the hands causes external crossing of instruments and hands with a consequent internal "sword fighting" and left/right inversion of direction [3, 9].

By using curved, articulated or instruments of different lengths and flexible scopes, we can reduce incidents, but it does not avoid this issue.

For these reasons, SILS is still a demanding technique with manoeuvres that are not easy to do and sometimes inaccurate.

Robotic Assisted SILS

A robotic platform appears to be particularly suitable to overcome some of these limitations with technological advantages such as stable 3D views, tremor filtration, precise and delicate movements, and software that automatically associate the surgeon's hands to the ipsilateral instrument tips to restore intuitive control. First attempts were made using traditional robotic EndoWrist® instruments and homemade or laparoscopic monoport.

The most frequently used was the GelPort/GelPOINT™ (Applied Medical, Rancho Santa

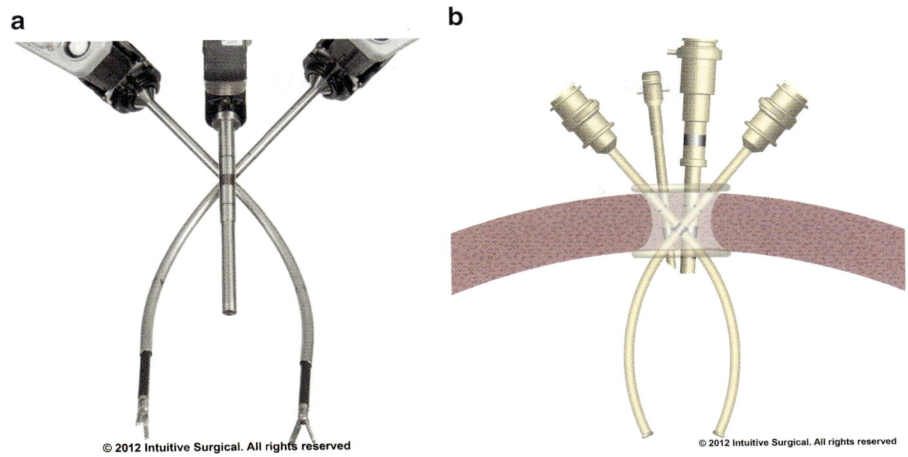

Fig. 34.4 (**a**, **b**) The flexible instruments are introduced through the curved cannulae. The remote centre is at the level of the abdominal wall into the port

Margarita, California, USA) with the possibility of introducing the instruments in more lateral position to reduce external conflict [10, 11]. The robotic software assigns each instrument to the contralateral hand in order to offset their crossing inside the abdomen. The triangulation achieved only by the articulated tips of EndoWrist® is only a few centimetres, whereby the internal and external conflicts of the instruments are not yet resolved. In addition, the force of the robotic arms can displace the port from its seat causing loss of pneumoperitoneum.

The Single-Site™ Platform

The recent new Single-Site Robotic Platform (da Vinci Surgical System, Intuitive Surgical Inc., Sunnyvale, CA) allows one to overcome the issues previously described [12].

The main features of this platform are the use of instruments with flexible shafts, rigid curved cannulae that cross at level of the abdominal wall (remote centre) and restoration of the correct hand/instrument correlation achieved by reassigning control of the instrument arms (Fig. 34.4a, b).

The curvature of the cannulae, crossing inside a dedicate port, increases the distance between the instruments tips allowing each to reach the target anatomy in a convergent way, from the opposite side to the side of introduction, restoring the correct triangulation. The shape of the curved cannulae, externally, keeps the da Vinci arms separated to avoid external collisions and instrument crowding. The intra-abdominal instrument position is reversed: the instrument that enters the abdomen from the left reaches the operative field on the right and vice versa. The da Vinci software automatically reassigns the surgeon's hands to the ipsilateral instrument tips restoring the intuitive control.

Keeping the remote centre at the level of the abdominal wall and the curvature of the cannulae with consequent convergence of the instruments ensures that there is an optimal focal distance of work allowing the instruments to converge correctly on the anatomical target (Fig. 34.5).

If the target is closer or further away with respect to the optimum focus, it will be necessary to advance or retract the cannulae causing an incorrect positioning of the remote centre.

These modifications could cause excessive stress on the port and on the abdominal wall resulting in improper working of the instruments and loss of CO_2. Moreover, if the instruments come out too far from the cannulae to reach a distant target, more of the flexible shaft extends beyond the rigid support of the curved cannulae and loses traction strength. The availability of two sets of robotic curved cannulae of different lengths mitigates this issue.

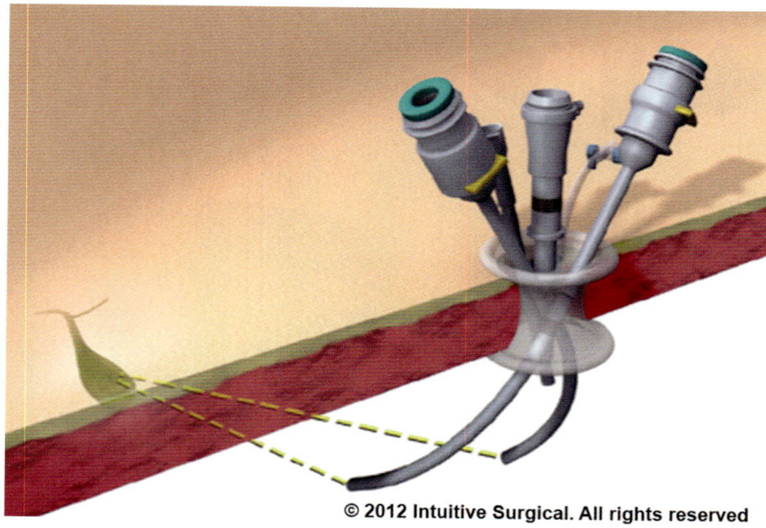

Fig. 34.5 The optimal focal distance of work allows the instruments to converge correctly on the anatomical target

The single-site platform was primarily designed to work in a narrow operative field and with a discrete anatomical target such as during a cholecystectomy; however, recently it has also been used for colonic surgery.

Instruments and Accessories

Single-Site™ Port

The Single-Site™ port is made of silicone and has a target anatomy arrow indicator and five lumens (Fig. 34.6).

Three of these are straight: for the scope, for the insufflation adaptor and for assistant instruments. The two more lateral lumens are curved and cross in the midline of the monoport with the outlet holes on the opposite side of entry. The curved robotic cannulae are inserted into these channels.

Single-Site™ Accessories

5×300-mm curved cannula "1"
5×300-mm curved cannula "2"
5×300-mm flexible blunt obturator
5×250-mm curved cannula "1"
5×250-mm curved cannula "2"
5×250-mm flexible blunt obturator
5-mm straight accessory cannula
10-mm straight accessory cannula
10-mm straight blunt obturator
Dock Assist Tool
8.5-mm endoscope cannula
8-mm blunt obturator
5-mm blunt obturator
Intuitive surgical 30° 8.5-mm endoscope
Intuitive surgical 0° 8.5-mm endoscope

Robotic Flexible Instruments

Maryland dissector
Crocodile grasper
Fundus grasper
Cadiere forceps
Curved scissors
Monopolar cautery hook
Hem-o-Lok® clip applier
Hem-o-Lok ML clips
Suction irrigator
Needle driver

All of the Single-Site™ instruments are flexible in order to allow introduction into the curved cannulae and rotate on their own axis at 360°. The flexibility, however, does not allow, in the current version, the possibility of having EndoWrist® technology, as in traditional robotic instruments.

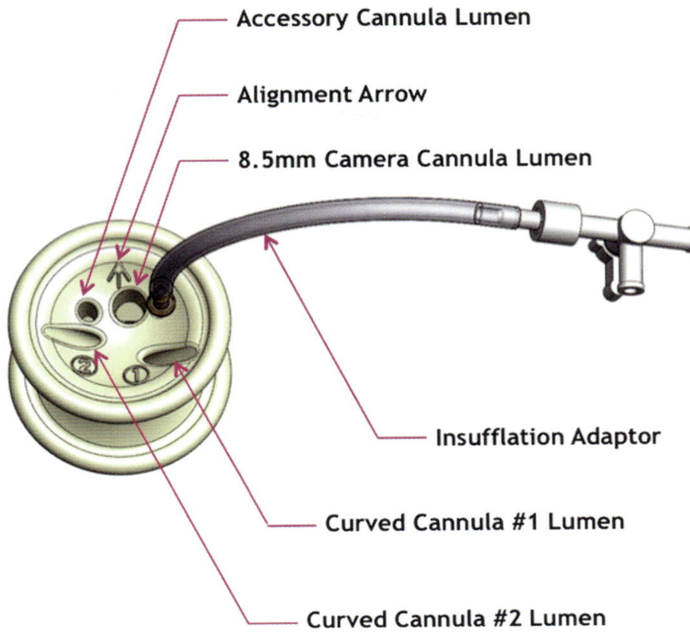

Fig. 34.6 The Single-Site™ port

In this chapter, we described the techniques of robotic Single-Site™ cholecystectomy (SSRC) and robotic Single-Site™ right colectomy.

SSRC Procedure Overview

The patient is placed in a supine position with both arms tucked away as required. The patient cart should approach the patient 45° (from perpendicular) over the right shoulder (Fig. 34.7) ensuring that the target anatomy is in line with the centre column, umbilicus and arrow on the port. Only three robotic arms are used: arms 1, 2 and camera arm. Robotic arm 1 is placed to the left of the patient, and its instruments reach the surgical field from the right (i.e. from the lateral side of the gallbladder); robotic arm 2 is placed to the right of the patient, and its instruments reach the surgical field from the left (i.e. from the medial side of the gallbladder). The camera arm is in line with the centre of the column bent at an angle of 45° (sweet spot). The assistant surgeon is to the left of the patient, and the scrub nurse is positioned at the patient's feet. The main assistant monitor is located at the patient's right within view of the assistant (Fig. 34.8).

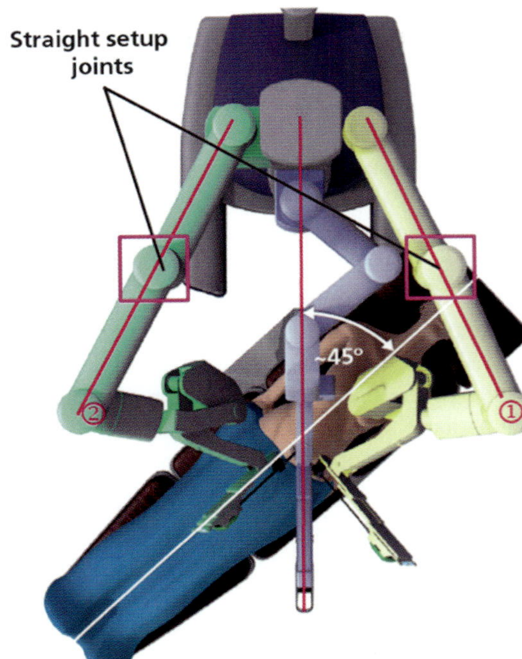

Fig. 34.7 Patient chart set-up

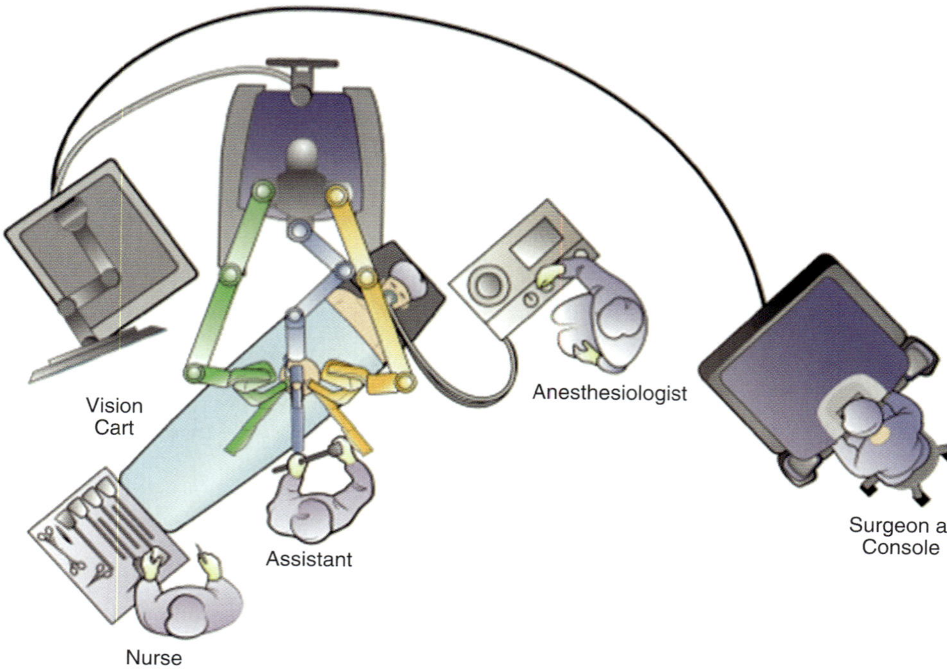

Fig. 34.8 O.R. set-up for Single-Site™ cholecystectomy

Using standard surgical techniques, a 2.5–2.8-cm midline incision is created intraumbilical. After opening the peritoneal cavity, it is necessary to perform a digital exploration of the abdominal wall in order to exclude the presence of adhesions.

The Single-Site™ port can be placed through the umbilical incision using an atraumatic clamp (e.g. Mayo Guyon clamp or Pean forceps) with two different techniques: unfolded or folded clamp technique (Figs. 34.9 and 34.10). In the first technique, it is easier to clamp the port, but it has a larger surface area for entry into the abdomen. The second technique reduces the insertion profile of the port; however, clamping the port can be more challenging. The arrow marking on the port must be aligned with the theoretical anatomical target (gallbladder) (Fig. 34.11). The top port flanges should lay flat against the abdominal wall. If the port seems to be higher than the skin or bulging, the inner rim of the silicone port is likely not completely below the level of the fascia, or the incision may be too small.

The endoscope and the accessory cannulae are inserted (Fig. 34.12). The table is placed in slight reverse Trendelenburg (10–15°) and is rotated to the left (5°) for better exposure of the gallbladder. After abdominal exploration, the assistant retracts the fundus of the gallbladder cephalad with a laparoscopic grasper to expose the infundibulum. This procedure is performed to assess port alignment and to ensure an adequate working space for the cannulae and to assure the cannulae length chosen is the appropriate length. The laparoscopic grasper and accessory cannulae are then removed. Curved cannulae are lubricated by dipping in sterile solution and inserted by sight to avoid visceral injury. The robot is then docked. With the cannulae tips in view, the Cadiere forceps are inserted into the robotic arm 1, and the monopolar cautery hook is inserted into robotic arm 2. The assistant then grasps the fundus of the gallbladder to expose the hepatoduodenal ligament. The scope is retracted, repositioned under the grasper and pushed forward. This lifts the grasper (and the fundus of the gallbladder) upwards (Fig. 34.13). The surgeon at the console retracts the gallbladder infundibulum laterally using the Cadiere forceps to open the Calot's triangle, as in the four-trocar laparoscopy.

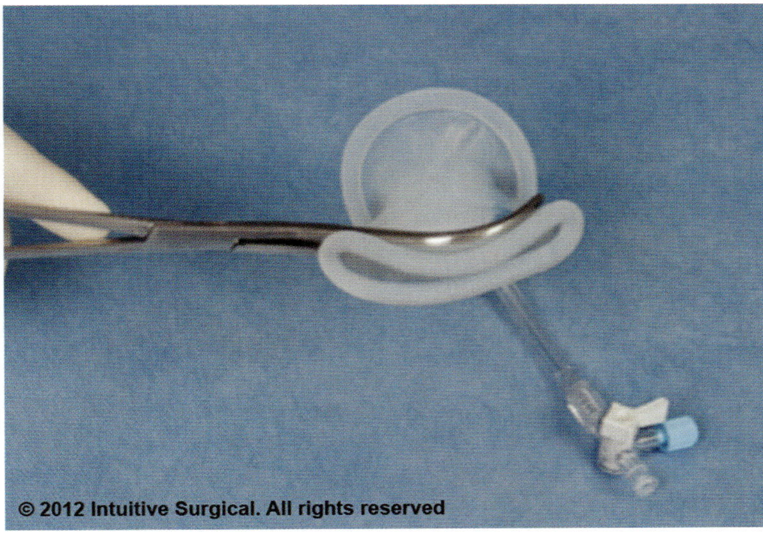

Fig. 34.9 Unfolded clamp technique

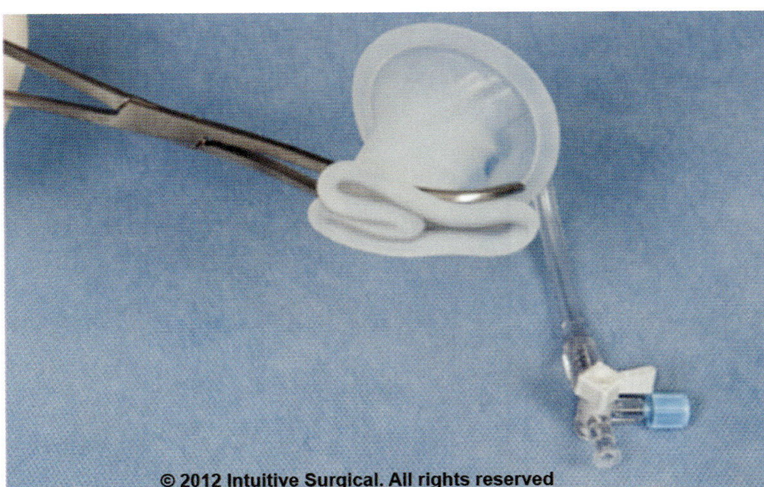

Fig. 34.10 Folded clamp technique

The instrument positions from top to bottom are as follows: the assistant grasper lifting the gallbladder, the 30° scope is in the centre of the operating field and Cadiere forceps and monopolar hook are at the level below the examination scope. The monopolar hook is used to incise the peritoneum close to the gallbladder neck (Fig. 34.14).

The cystic duct and artery are identified and skeletonised (Fig. 34.15). The ligation is performed with Hem-o-Lok ML clips (clip applier arm 2) (Fig. 34.16), and the transection is performed with curved scissors (instrument arm 2). The gallbladder liver bed detachment is performed using the Cadiere forceps (instrument arm 1) and monopolar cautery hook (instrument arm 2) (Fig. 34.17). During this step, the scope is repositioned above the grasper to lift the liver and expose the surgical field. If bleeding requires suction, the cautery instrument is removed and the suction/irrigation instrument is inserted. Before completion of the gallbladder detachment, the liver bed is inspected for evidence of bleeding or bile leaks. After complete dissection of the gallbladder, the specimen extraction is performed by exchanging the 5-mm assistant trocar to a 10-mm trocar and introducing a laparoscopic specimen extraction bag (Fig. 34.18). All the instruments are then removed, including the single-site port and the specimen bag. The fascia defect is closed with adsorbable stitches, and the umbilicus is restored to its physiological position, suturing the dermis at the fascia below. The skin is then closed.

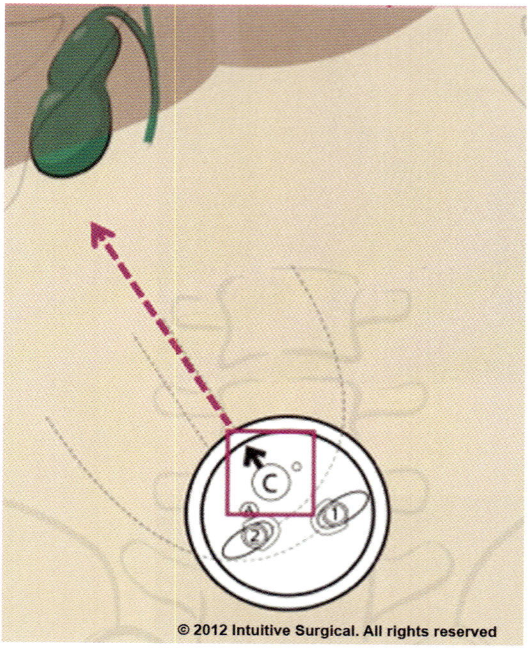

Fig. 34.11 The *arrow* marking on the port is aligned with the anatomical target

If necessary, it is possible to perform an intraoperative cholangiography using a dedicated percutaneous balloon set during the procedure. The catheter is introduced percutaneously in the right upper quadrant of abdomen, so that the robotic instruments can grasp and insert the catheter into the cystic duct. During cholangiography, the instruments and the endoscope are removed, the robotic arms are undocked from the cannulae and the robotic cart is moved away from the patient. The curved cannulae are retracted in a safe position, 3 cm below the remote centre, but left in the port.

After performing the cholangiography, the robot is redocked. The balloon catheter is removed by sight, and the procedure is completed as usual.

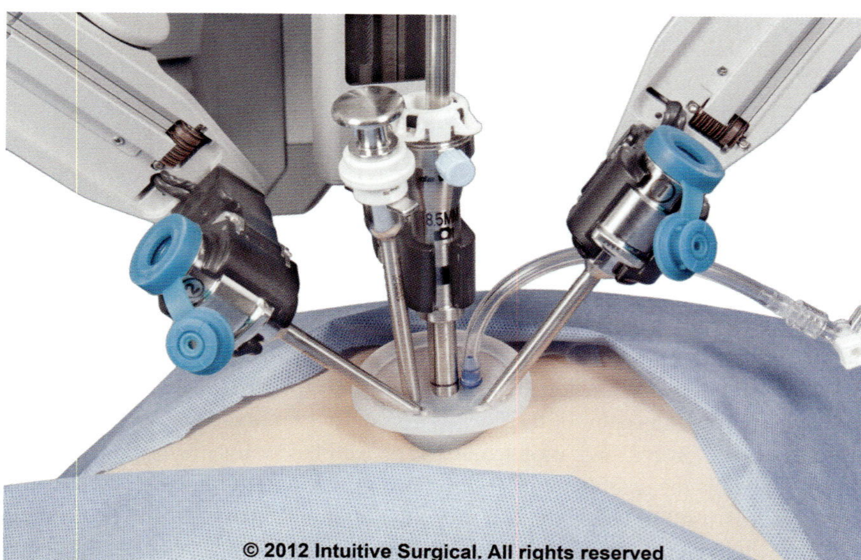

Fig. 34.12 Curved cannulae inserted into the port at the end of docking procedure

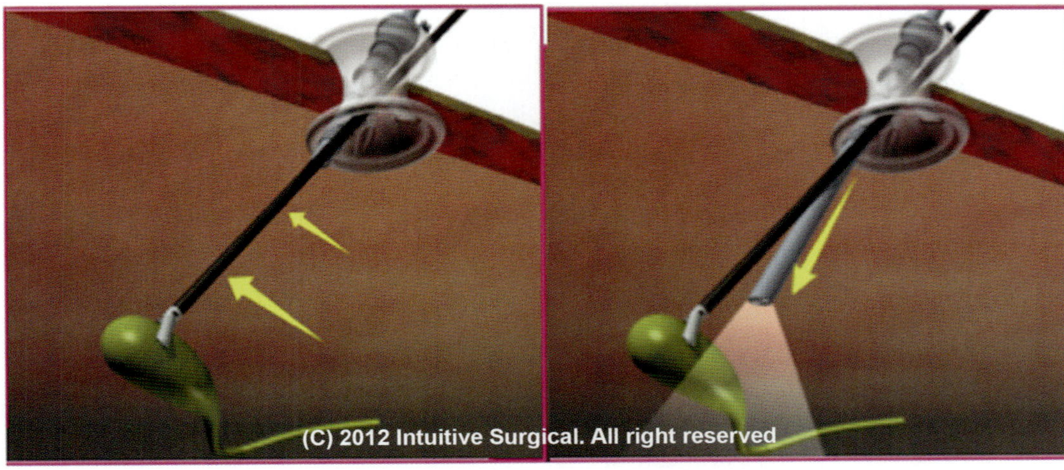

Fig. 34.13 The scope is retracted, repositioned under the grasper and pushed forward

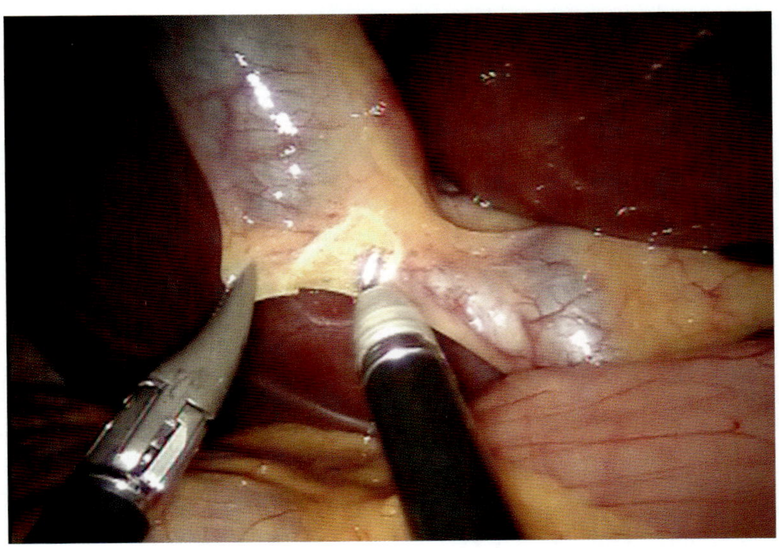

Fig. 34.14 Incision of the peritoneum close to the gallbladder neck

Discussion of Advantages, Limitations and Relative Contraindications

Advantages

The lateral traction of the infundibulum is essential in the four-trocar cholecystectomy to open the Calot's triangle surface, to identify the anatomic landmarks and to avoid biliary and artery damage. The first step for assessment of the biliary tract anatomy toward safer laparoscopic cholecystectomy was the introduction in 1995 by Strasberg et al. [13] of the "critical view of safety" (CVS) [14]. Following this approach, Calot's triangle is dissected to achieve the proximal third of the gallbladder free from the liver bed and the triangle of Calot cleared of fat with the liver segment V visible through the window. Then the cystic artery and

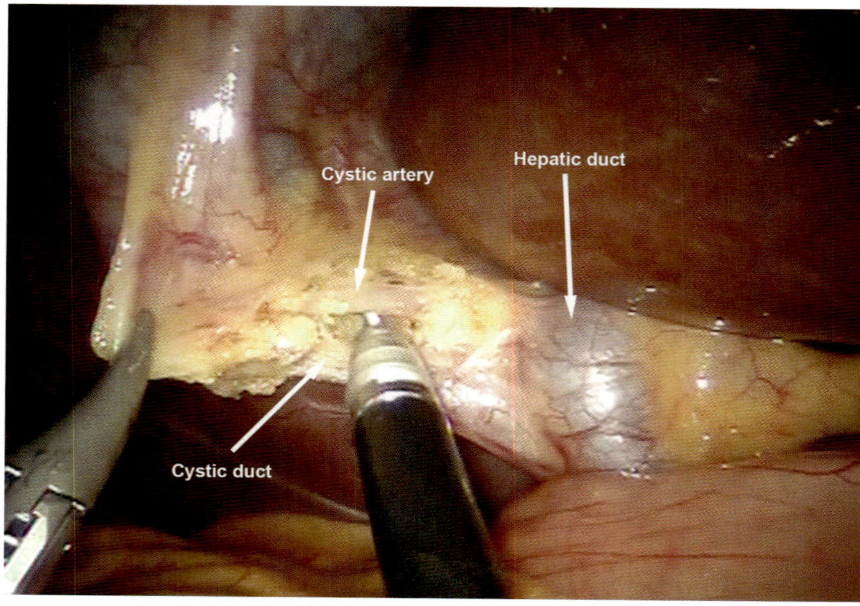

Fig. 34.15 Identification and skeletonisation of cystic duct and artery

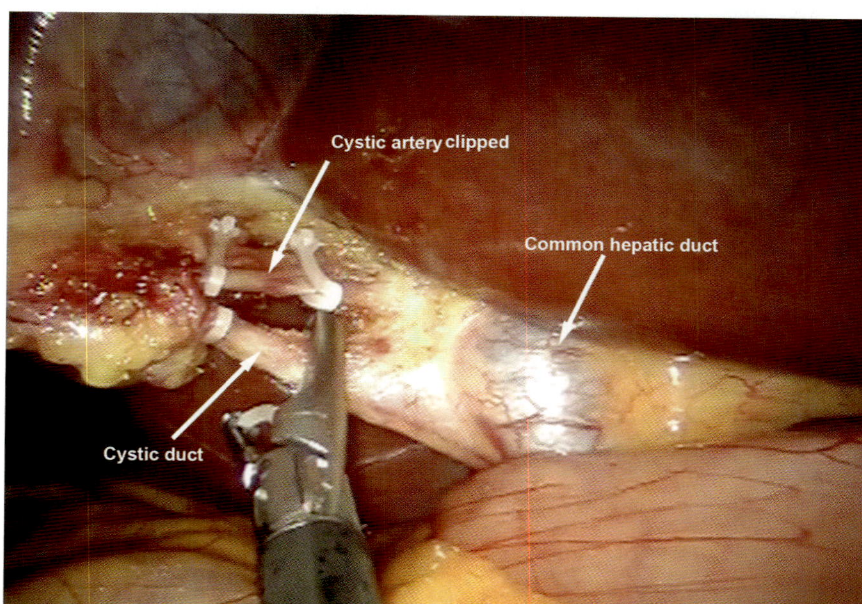

Fig. 34.16 Ligation with Hem-o-Lok ML clips

cystic duct must be the only two tubular structures remaining between the gallbladder and the hepatoduodenal ligament.

During SILS cholecystectomy, because of the parallel alignment of the instruments, lateral traction is achieved by crossing the instruments inside the abdomen and the surgeon's hands outside: thus, the surgical performance decreases and the surgeon fatigue and stress levels increase.

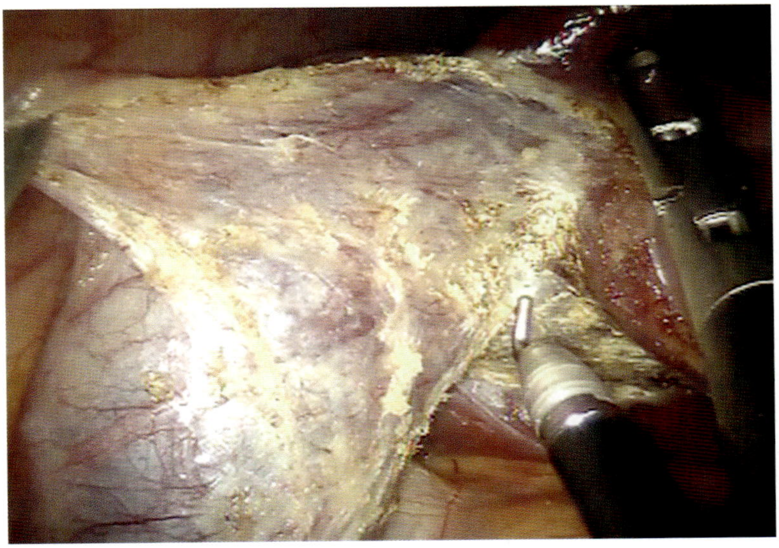

Fig. 34.17 Liver bed detachment

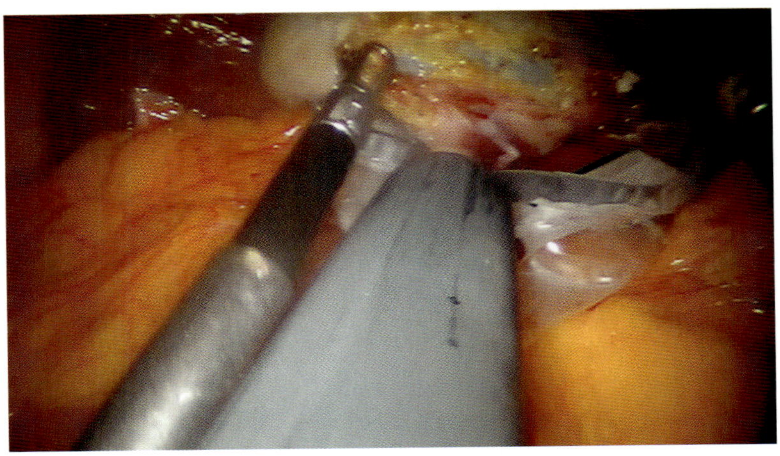

Fig. 34.18 Specimen extraction

The robotic Single-Site™ platform allows a perfect triangulation to open the Calot's triangle as in a four-trocar laparoscopic cholecystectomy to achieve the CVS with the added benefits of stable three-dimensional high-definition view, the added precision and dexterity and the ease and safety in changing instruments. The Cadiere forceps allow a gentle and steady traction on the gallbladder infundibulum, and the monopolar cautery hook enables the surgeon to perform a meticulous skeletonisation of the artery and cystic duct. The Hem-o-Lok® clip applier, with its 360° rotation on its axis, allows for easy and safe ligation of the structures prior to cutting them with the robotic scissor. These manoeuvres require frequent changes of the tools that are easily and safely made possible by the assisted tool change feature enabled by the da Vinci system software that automatically puts the instrument introduced into the same position as that extracted. Moreover, the 3D high-definition vision allows precision in controlling any bleeding and/or bile leaking if needed [15].

Other advantage, recently added to single-site platform for increase safety during a cholecystectomy, is the near-infrared fluorescent vision system [16, 17]. The system components include a surgical 8.5-mm endoscope capable of visible light and near-infrared imaging, a 3DHD stereoscopic camera head that couples to the endoscope and an endoscopic illuminator that provides visible light and near-infrared illumination through the surgical endoscope via a flexible light guide.

The surgeon can quickly switch between normal (visible light or VIS) mode and fluorescence (near-infrared or NIR) mode. A dose of 2.5 mg of indocyanine green (ICG) is administered intravenously during patient preparation to visualise the biliary tree structures switching from white light to fluorescence whilst always keeping an eye fixed on the surgical field. This permits one to obtain an intraoperative dynamic fluorescent cholangiography that could substitute the classic X-ray cholangiography for a safer Calot's dissection [18, 19].

Limitation

A crucial aspect is the correlation of the movements of the assistant instrument and the scope. Because of the close relationship between the scope and the assistant grasper, it is important to consider the reciprocal interactions whenever the grasper or scope is moved (at the beginning of the procedure, the scope is positioned above the assistant grasper and then is retracted and reinserted under the grasper, and during the detachment of the gallbladder, it is repositioned above the grasper). The assistant cannula is close to the camera cannula on the left side of the port and can only be parallel to the scope: for this reason, it is the surgeon at the console that drives the assistant instrument moving the camera.

Moreover, if the instruments protrude too far from the cannulae to reach a distant target, during the lateral traction, they could flex excessively with a potential bullwhip effect and consequent risk of damage to the gallbladder wall. Current limits of the flexible instruments are the lack of EndoWrist® technology and the current absence of monopolar scissors. Bipolar coagulation device has been recently introduced.

Contraindications

There are no absolute contraindications to the technique, but the presence of adhesions and of active inflammatory process could require frequent rotations and realignments of port and cannulae to obtain a proper workspace. For these reasons, the intrinsic limitations of the single-site platform cannot be recommended in cases of acute cholecystitis, biliary pancreatitis and previous upper abdominal surgery.

Outcomes Review

In our experience of 100 SSRC, the indication for surgery was symptomatic gallstones and gallbladder polyposis. Overall, SSRC mean operative time was 68 (range, 35–125) min, mean docking time was 3.8 (range, 3–8) min and mean console time was 23.4 (range, 10–61) min; there were no conversions, and all procedures were performed robotically.

Usually, patients were discharged within 24 h of the surgical procedure. There were no early postoperative complications or readmissions. Two incisional hernias (2 %) were observed.

We compared operative times of first 25 SSRC with operative times of our first 25 SILC performed by the same surgeon to assess the learning curve differences. We report that our average overall operative time for the 25 robotic procedures was significantly lower than the average operative time for our first 25 SILC cases (62.7 vs. 83.2 min, $P=0.001$) [20].

During our experience with the SILC, operating time decreased with increasing number of procedures. In contrast, SSRC operative times were lower than those of SILC since the beginning; robotic technique seems to be more intuitive and does not require a specific learning curve.

A possible explanation is the close analogy of the single-site robotic approach with the four-trocar laparoscopic cholecystectomy; an expert surgeon in four-trocar laparoscopic cholecystectomy might need a very short training period in SSRC to achieve good and steady operative times with no major complications.

SSRC is a safe and feasible option especially for a trained surgeon in four-trocar laparoscopic cholecystectomy [21].

Robotic Single-Site Right Colectomy

Current scientific literature has demonstrated that SILS application in colonic surgery is safe and feasible in selected patients. The main difficulties were related to problems of triangulation, internal and external instrument collision and anatomical exposition. The most frequently reported SILS in colorectal surgery has been the right hemicolectomy with umbilical access [22, 23]. After our experience in SSRC, we decided to use the robotic Single-Site™ platform to test the feasibility and safety also in this surgical procedure, trying to replicate the same techniques we perform with a standard laparoscopic or robotic approach, ready to convert to multiport in case of our inability to maintain the standard of safety and oncological radicality. In our laparoscopic and robotic technique, the overview of mesenteric root, to perform "en bloc" lymphectomy exposing the mesenteric vessel anterior aspect, is achieved by placing the scope in the left iliac fossa in the middle of the line joining the umbilicus and anterior superior iliac spine [24].

The extraction of a specimen is done through a Pfannenstiel incision enlarging the existing access of the suprapubic trocar. The advantages of the Pfannenstiel incision compared to vertical incisions include improved cosmesis and decreased pain and rate of incisional hernia [25].

In our initial experience, we planned to place the Single-Site™ port in Pfannenstiel incision in order to get a correct approach to the mesenteric root, similar to our standardised laparoscopic and robotic approach. The extraction of the specimen, usually really bulky, is performed through the same incision avoiding a median supra- and infraumbilical laparotomy. We describe below our early experience with three robotic single-site right colectomies with suprapubic access and intracorporeal anastomosis.

Procedure Overview

The patient is placed in a supine position with the arms along the body. The robotic cart is positioned at a 40° angle over the patient's right hemithorax, the assistant is at the patient's left side and the scrub nurse at the patient's feet. The main assistant monitor is placed at the patient's right side (Fig. 34.19a, b).

The single port is introduced through a 3-cm transversal left paramedian sovrapubic incision. The last ileocolic loop is then retracted laterally with the Cadiere grasper tenting up the ileocolic vessels (Fig. 34.20). The peritoneum is dissected up to visualise the duodenum creating a window (Figs. 34.21 and 34.22). The ileal branch of ileocolic vessels is clipped and cut (Figs. 34.23 and 34.24).

The ileocolic vessels are followed as a road map to reach the superior mesenteric vessels; they are then clipped and sectioned exposing the superior mesenteric vein surface. Proceeding upward, along this plane, the middle colic vessels are recognised and the right branch is dissected between clips (Fig. 34.25). Mobilisation of the colon is performed in medial to lateral direction in the avascular plane between Gerota's and Toldt's fasciae keeping down the right ureter and the gonadic vessels. The segment of transverse colon chosen for the section is skeletonised, and the vessels of the mesentery are clipped and cut; then the gastrocolic ligament and the omentum are divided.

The hepatic flexure is then mobilised, and the detachment of the right colon is completed by the dissection of the right peritoneal groove.

The ileum and the transverse colon are joined at the point chosen for anastomosis with a 3-0 absorbable monofilament suture. The traction on this stitch keeps vertical and parallel both the intestinal tracts in order to perform an intracorporeal side-to-side termilised anastomosis using a

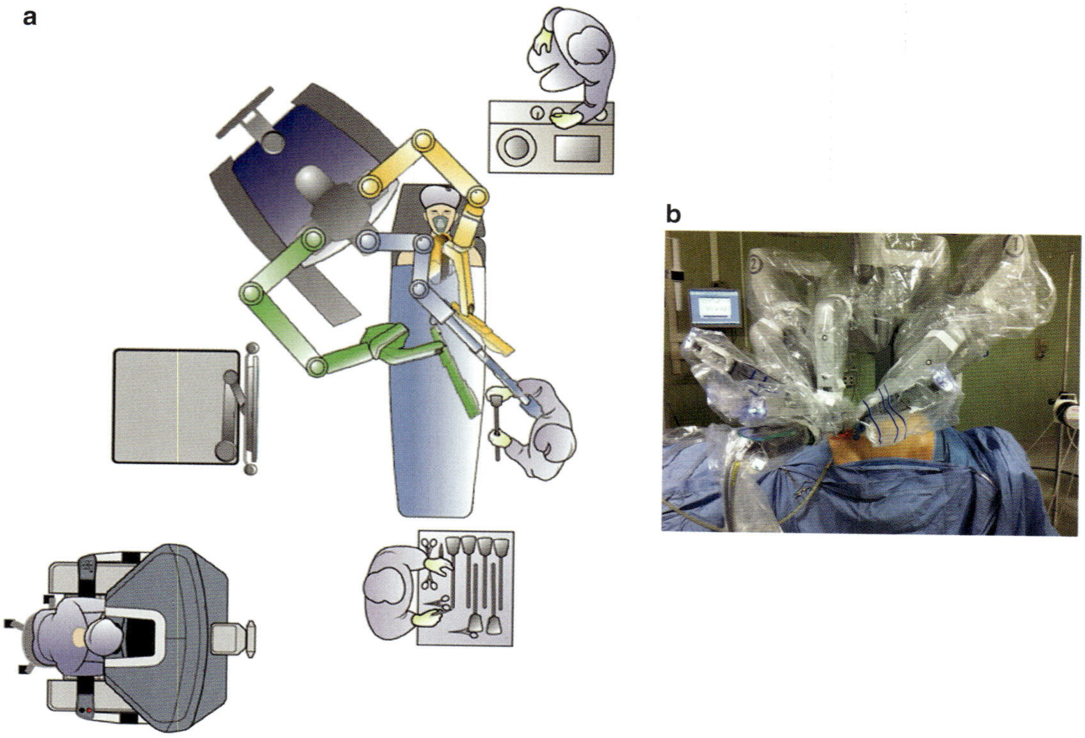

Fig. 34.19 (**a**) O.R. set-up for Single-Site™ right colectomy. (**b**) Patient chart docked for SS right colectomy

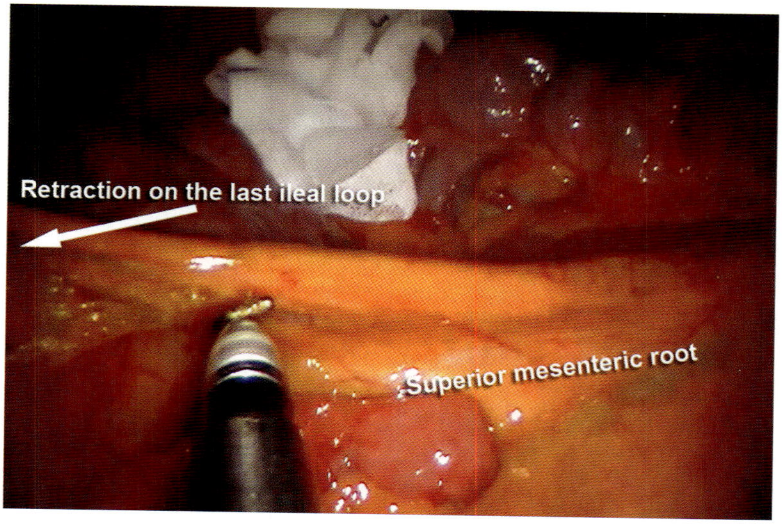

Fig. 34.20 Lateral retraction of the last ileal loop with the Cadiere grasper

flexible stapler (Echelon Flex) 60 blu cartridge. The stapler is introduced by a 15-mm right paramedian sovrapubic trocar, at the side of the robotic port, medially to the rectum muscle without any added incision.

The transverse colon and the last ileal loop, including the bowel defect, are finally transected by stapler performing the classical side-to-side terminalised mechanical anastomosis, with assessment of correct perfusion of the

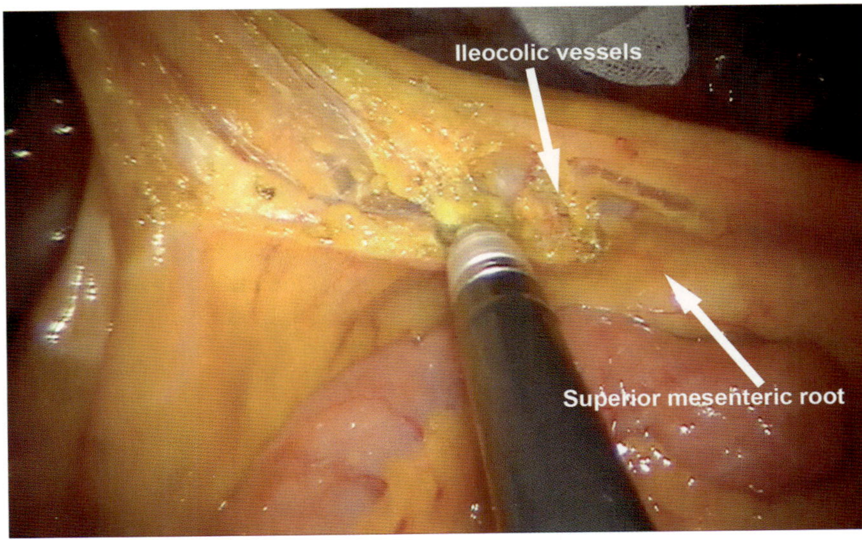

Fig. 34.21 Dissection of the peritoneum visualising the duodenum

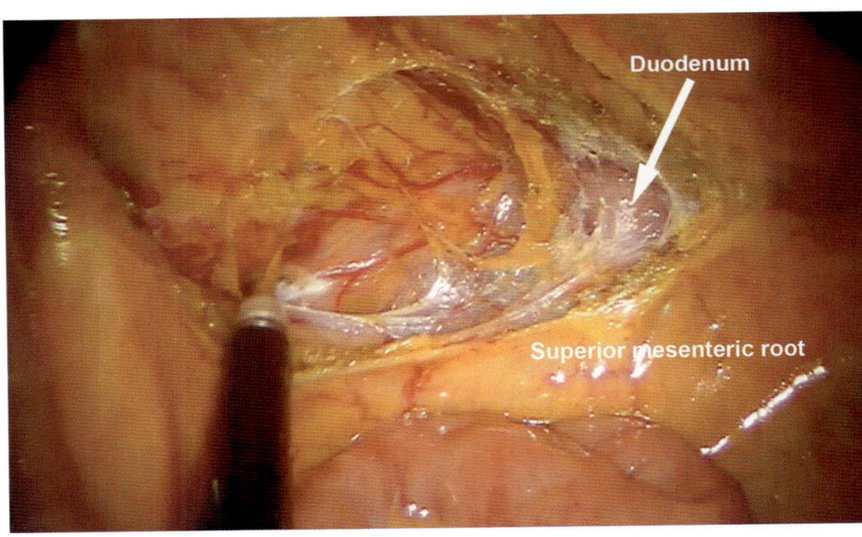

Fig. 34.22 Dissection of the peritoneum visualising the duodenum

stumps by fluorescence imaging (Figs. 34.26, 34.27, 34.28, and 34.29).

Then, the port and the 15-mm trocar are removed, and the specimen is extracted with an endobag through a Pfannenstiel, which is sutured in the standard fashion.

Anastomosis may also be performed extracorporeally through the Pfannenstiel incision.

Outcome Review

Between January 2012 and April 2012, three patients underwent single-site robotic right colectomy. The indication for surgery was caecal carcinoma or severe dysplasia (one case). The mean patient age was 70 years and mean BMI was 21.7. Overall Single-Site robotic right colectomy

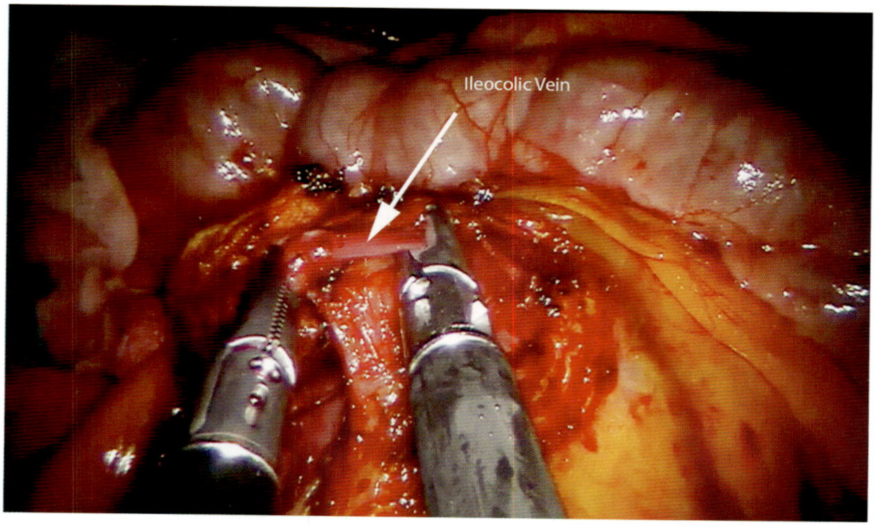

Fig. 34.23 Ileocolic vessels clipped and cut

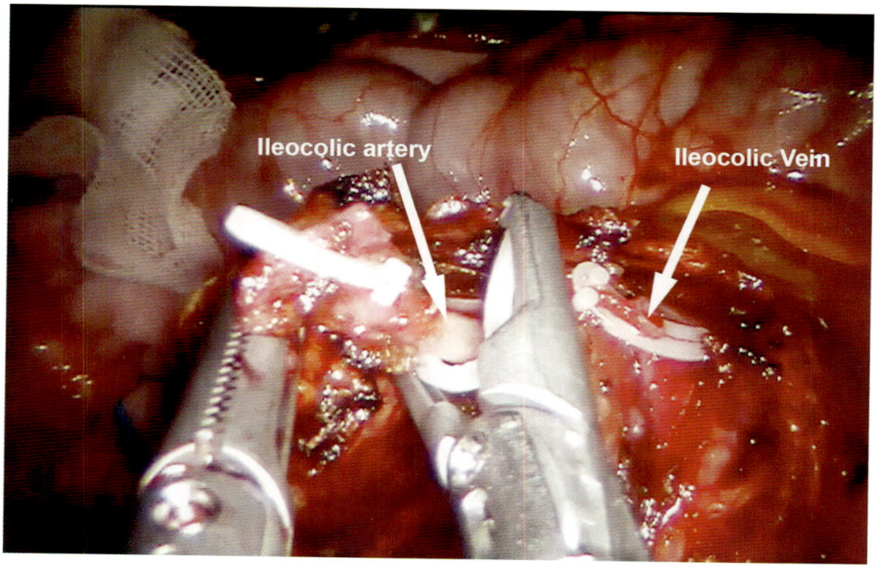

Fig. 34.24 Ileocolic vessels clipped and cut

operative time was 240 min, mean docking time was 6 min and mean console time was 180 min. There were no conversions, and all procedures were performed robotically.

The mean skin incision length was 8 cm. The mean first flatus time was 1.6 days, and all patients resumed feeding in first postoperative day. Patients were discharged within 5 days of the surgical procedure. There were no early postoperative complications or readmissions. Oncological principles have been satisfied, the distal and proximal margins were negative and the mean number of harvested lymph nodes was 24.

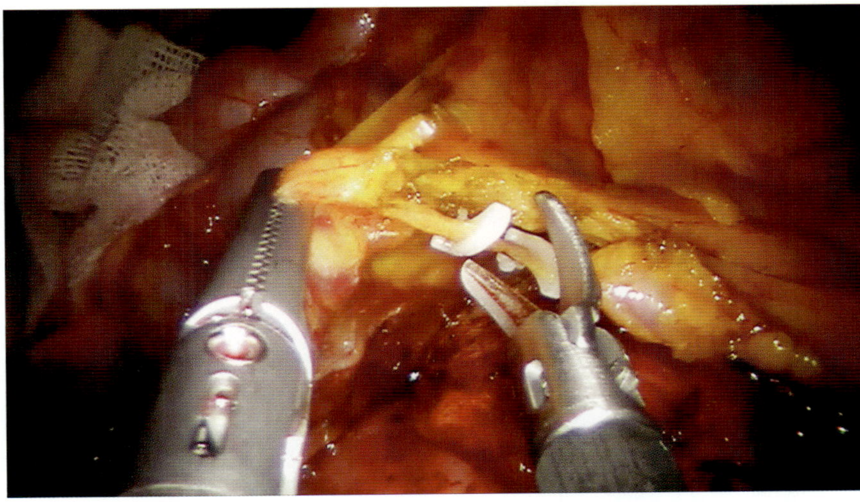

Fig. 34.25 Section of the right branch of middle colic vessels

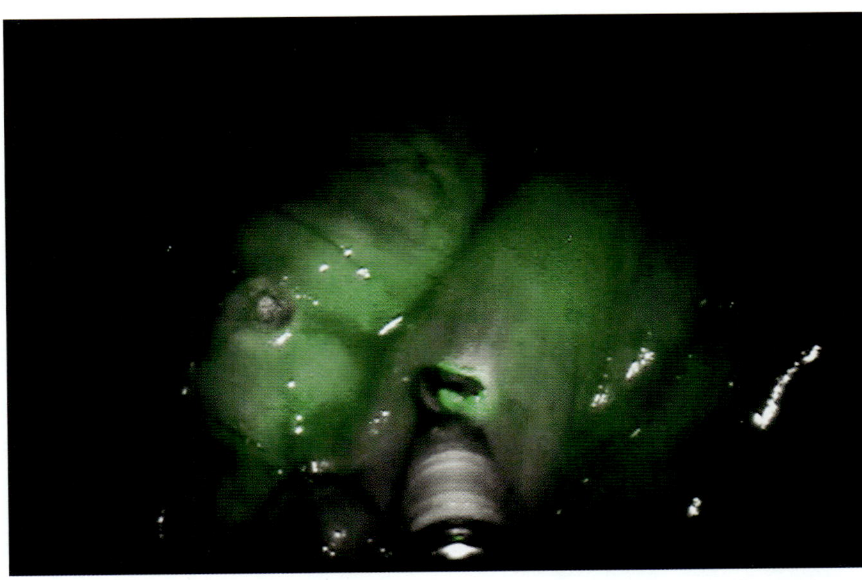

Fig. 34.26 Bowel perfusion assessment by fluorescence imaging

Discussion of Advantages, Limitations and Relative Contraindications

The robotic Single-Site platform allows surgeons to perform an easier and more accurate lymphadenectomy due to a stable 3D vision, absence of tremor and lack of internal and external conflicts compared to the SILS. Monopolar scissors and bipolar forceps, not currently available, will make this technique simpler and safer.

The advantages of the Pfannenstiel incision as the site of single-port insertion include decreased

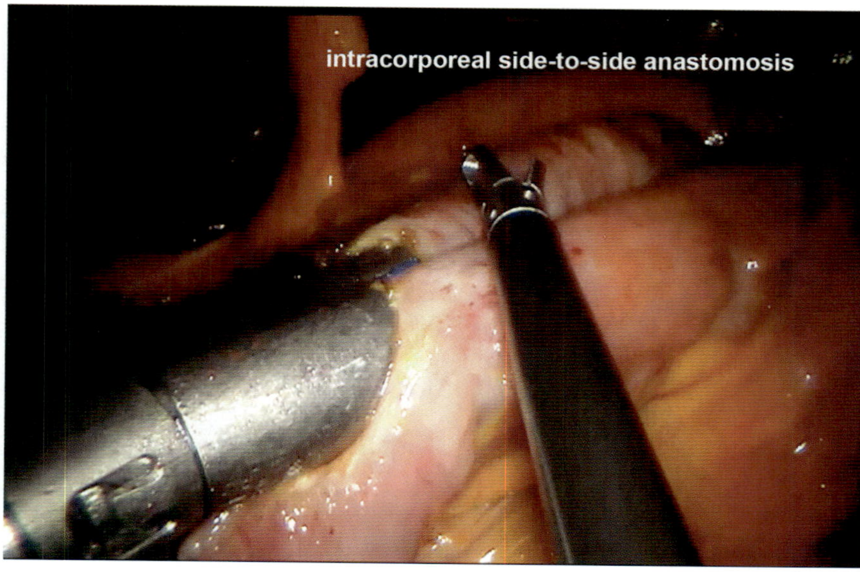

Fig. 34.27 Side-to-side anastomosis

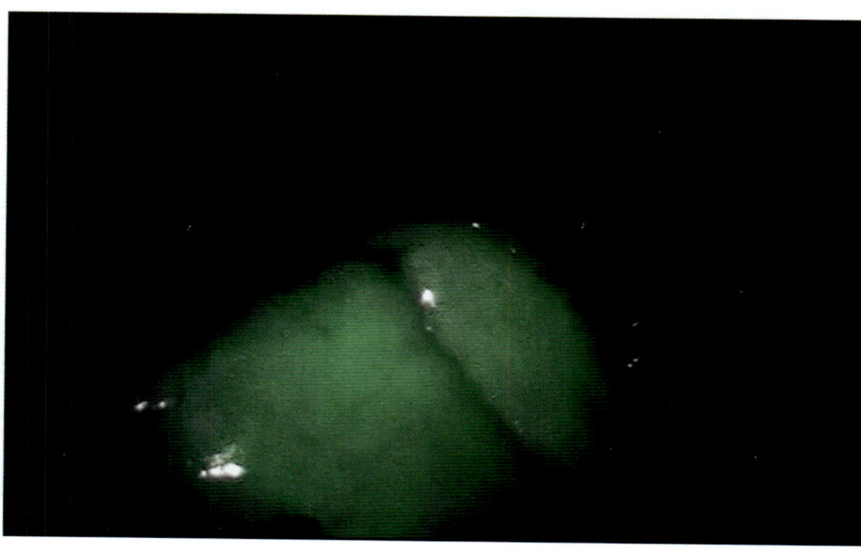

Fig. 34.28 Bowel perfusion assessment by fluorescence imaging

pain, improved cosmesis and optimal view of the mesenteric axis like to that achieved in the multiport technique.

Moreover, it is possible, by this way, to perform an intracorporeal anastomosis using the ICG fluorescence for better evaluation of the stump perfusions [26] (procedure details described in Cap. VIII).

After our initial experience, we believe that the robotic Single-Site right colectomy is a safe and

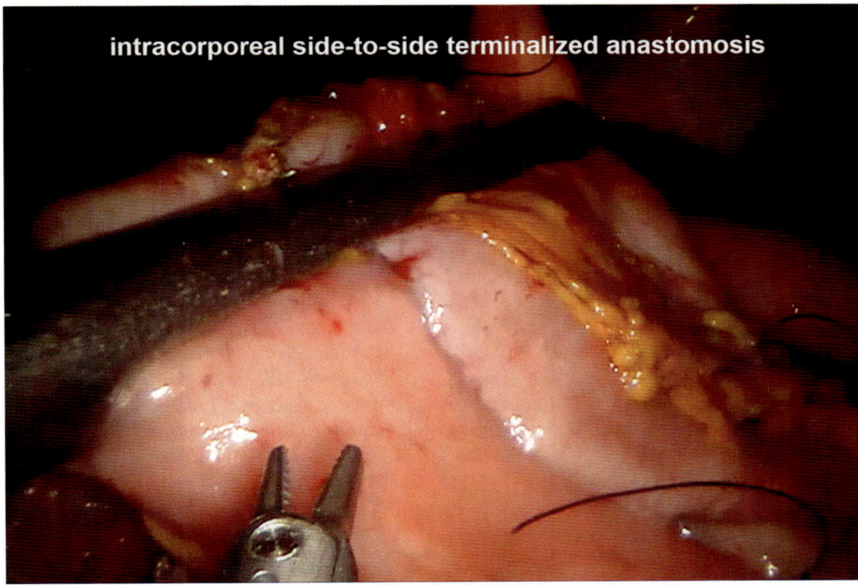

Fig. 34.29 Side-to-side anastomosis terminalised

feasible technique that should be applied in selected patients with low BMI and small tumours.

In the future, prospective, randomised trials will be needed to further evaluate the benefits of this approach compared with SILS right colectomy with regard to potential complications, oncological radicality, patient's quality of life and cosmesis.

References

1. Tomikawa M, Xu H, Hashizume M. Current status and prerequisites for natural orifice translumenal endoscopic surgery (NOTES). Surg Today. 2010;40(10):909–16.
2. Navarra G, Pozza E, Occhionorelli S, Carcoforo P. Donini I One-wound laparoscopic cholecystectomy. Br J Surg. 1997;84:695.
3. Mutter D, Callari C, Diana M, Dallemagne B, Leroy J, Marescaux J. Single port laparoscopic cholecystectomy: which technique, which surgeon, for which patient? A study of the implementation in a teaching hospital. J Hepatobiliary Pancreat Sci. 2011;18:453–7.
4. Prasad A, Mukherjee KA, Kaul S, Kaur M. Postoperative pain after cholecystectomy: conventional laparoscopy versus single-incision laparoscopic surgery. J Minim Access Surg. 2011;7:24–7.
5. Hayashi M, Asakuma M, Komeda K, Miyamoto Y, Hirokawa F, Tanigawa N. Effectiveness of a surgical glove port for single port surgery. World J Surg. 2010;34(10):2487–9.
6. Romanelli JR, Mark L, Omotosho PA. Single port laparoscopic cholecystectomy with the TriPort system: a case report. Surg Innov. 2008;15:223–8.
7. Hanna GB, Shimi S, Cuschieri A. Influence of direction of view, target-to-endoscope distance and manipulation angle on endoscopic knot tying. Br J Surg. 1997;84(10):1460–4.
8. Patil PV, Hanna GB, Cuschieri A. Effect of the angle between the optical axis of the endoscope and instruments' plane on monitor image and surgical performance. Surg Endosc. 2004;18:111–4.
9. Rawlings A, Hodgett SE, Matthews BD, Strasberg SM, Quasebarth M, Brunt LM. Single-incision laparoscopic cholecystectomy: initial experience with critical view of safety dissection and routine intraoperative cholangiography. J Am Coll Surg. 2010; 211:1–7.
10. Ragupathi M, Ramos-Valdes DI, Pedraza R, Haas EM. Robotic assisted single-incision laparoscopic partial cecectomy. Int J Med Robot. 2010;6(3): 362–7.
11. Stein RJ, Wesley WM, RajGoel RK, Irwin BH, Haber GP, Kaouk JH. Robotic laparoendoscopic single –site surgery using GelPort as the access platform. Eur Urol. 2010;57(1):132–6.
12. Kroh M, El-Hayek K, Rosenblatt S, Chand B, Escobar P, Kaouk J, Chalikonda S. First human surgery with a novel single port robotic system: cholecystectomy using the da Vinci Single-Site platform. Surg Endosc. 2011;25:3566–73.
13. Strasberg SM, Hertl M, Soper NJ. An analysis of the problem of biliary injury during laparoscopic cholecystectomy. J Am Coll Surg. 1995;180(1):101–25.

14. Strasberg SM, Brunt M. Rationale and use of the critical view of safety in laparoscopic cholecystectomy. J Am Coll Surg. 2010;211:132–8.
15. Konstantinidis KM, Hirides P, Hirides S, Chrysocheris P, Georgiou M. Cholecystectomy using a novel Single-Site® robotic platform: early experience from 45 consecutive cases. Surg Endosc. 2012;26:2687–94. doi:10.1007/s00464-012-2227-2.
16. Tagaya N, Shimoda M, Kato M, Nakagawa A, Abe A, Iwasaky Y, Oishi H, Shirotani N, Kubota K. Intraoperative exploration of biliary anatomy using fluorescence imaging of indocyanine green in experimental and clinical cholecystectomies. J Hepatobiliary Pancreat Sci. 2010;17:595–600.
17. Ishizawa T, Tamura S, Masuda K, Aoki T, Hasegawa K, Imamura H, Beck Y, Kokudo N. Intraoperative fluorescent cholangiography using indocyanine green: a biliary road map for safe surgery. J Am Coll Surg. 2009;208(1):e1–4.
18. Buchs NC, Hagen ME, Pugin F, Volonte F, Bucher P, Schiffer E, Morel P. Intra-operative fluorescent cholangiography using indocyanine green during robotic single site cholecystectomy. Int J Med Robot. 2012; 8:436–40. doi:10.1002/rcs.
19. Spinoglio G, Marano A. Is the routine use of intraoperative cholangiography during laparoscopic cholecystectomy really the key to lowering bile duct injuries? Surg Endosc. 2013 Aug 14. Epub ahead of print.
20. Spinoglio G, Lenti LM, Maglione V, Lucido FS, Priora F, Bianchi PP, Grosso F, Quarati R. Single-site robotic cholecystectomy (SSRC) versus single-incision laparoscopic cholecystectomy (SILC): comparison of learning curves. First European experience. Surg Endosc. 2012;26:1648–55.
21. Pietrabissa A, Sbrana F, Morelli L, Badessi F, Pugliese L, Vinci A, Klersy C, Spinoglio G. Overcoming the challenger of single-incision cholecystectomy with robotic single-site technology. Arch Surg. 2012;147:709–14. http://archsurg.jamanetwork.com. Accessed April 16, 2012.
22. Patel CB, Ramos-Valadez DI, Ragupathi M, Haas EM. Single incision laparoscopic-assisted right hemicolectomy: technique and application. Surg Laparosc Percutan Tech. 2010;20(5):e146–9.
23. Ostrowits MB, Eschete D, Zemon H, De Noto G. Robotic-assisted single-incision right colectomy: early experience. Int J Med Robotics Comput Assist Surg. 2009;5:465–70.
24. Spinoglio G, Summa M, Priora F, Quarati R, Teasta S. Robotic colorectal surgery: first 50 cases experience. Dis Colon Rectum. 2008;51(11):1627–32.
25. Orcus ST, Ballantine CJ, Marshall CL, Robinson CN, Anaya DA, Arminian SS, Awed SS, Berger DH, Alba D. Use of a Pfannenstiel incision in minimally invasive colorectal cancer surgery is associated with a lower risk of wound complications. Tech Coloproctol. 2012;16(2):127–32.
26. Kudszus S, Roesel C, Schachtrupp A, Hoer JJ. Intraoperative laser fluorescence angiography in colorectal surgery: a noninvasive analysis to reduce the rate of anastomotic leakage. Langenbecks Arch Surg. 2010;395:1025–30.

TilePro

35

Woo Jin Hyung and Yanghee Woo

Introduction

TilePro™ is a multi-input display system of da Vinci surgical system. TilePro™ allows the surgeon and the OR team to view a 3D video of the operative field along with up to two additional video or digital sources. Additional sources can be various types of digital data having information, which can facilitate the operative procedures [1]. Digital data can be images of radiology such as plain radiography, computed tomography (CT), and magnetic resonance images (MRI) as well as video inputs such as ultrasound and endoscopy. Not only radiographic images but any digitalized information can be used such as electrocardiography, vital status of the patient, and hospital electronic medical records [1, 2].

TilePro™ has been suggested as a tool for data integration during robotic surgery. TilePro™ makes it possible to deliver information to the surgeon during the operation without interruption of the operative process. All the information and the view at the console can be shared by all the staff in the OR and outside the OR. Herein, current applications of TilePro during robotic surgery and future perspectives are described.

W.J. Hyung, M.D., Ph.D. (✉)
Department of Surgery, Yonsei University College of Medicine, 50 Yonsei-ro Seodaemun-gu, Seoul 120-752, Republic of Korea
e-mail: wjhyung@gmail.com

Y. Woo, M.D.
Division of GI/Endocrine Surgery, Center for Excellence in Gastric Cancer Care, Columbia University Medical Center, New York, NY, USA

Department of Surgery, Columbia University College of Physicians and Surgeons, New York, NY, USA

Department of Surgery, New York Presbyterian Hospital, New York, NY, USA
e-mail: yw2263@columbia.edu

How to Use TilePro™ System

The setup and use of TilePro are different in da Vinci S and da Vinci Si system. To set up and use the TilePro at da Vinci Si system, digital output of any devices such as ultrasound, endoscopy, and computer systems is connected to the S-video connections or digital video interface (DVI) inputs in the back of the surgeon console (Fig. 35.1).

During the operation, the surgeons can activate the video input by turning on the multi-input TilePro™ system using the touch pad panel at the surgeon's console (Fig. 35.2). Surgeons are able to display the digital input images on the console monitor and other monitors as picture-on-picture mode and to switch on and off the TilePro display by tapping the camera foot pedal. By using the size control bar, the touch pad panel at the surgeon's console, the size of the TilePro image can be adjusted as needed. To control the images of the digital inputs, wireless mouse can be used when the inputs were from the computer systems or a special 3D motion controller was to manipulate the stereoscopic volume-rendered image by the surgeons [3, 4].

K.C. Kim (ed.), *Robotics in General Surgery*, DOI 10.1007/978-1-4614-8739-5_35,

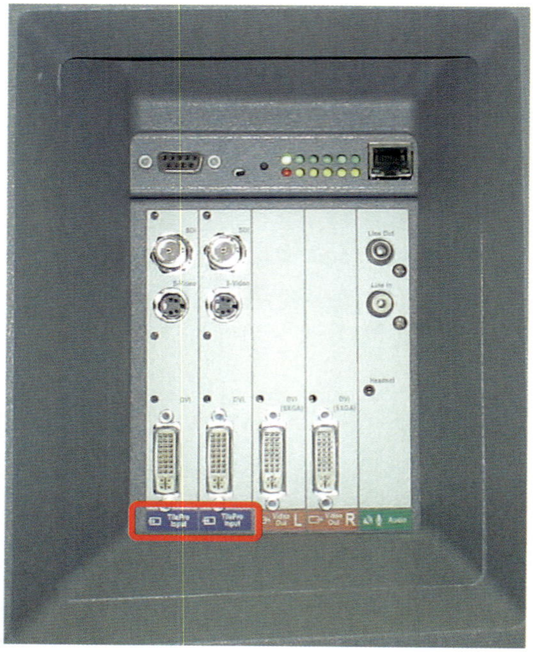

Fig. 35.1 TilePro inputs in the back of the surgeon console

Current Applications of TilePro™ System During Robotic Surgery

Urology Application

The first reported application of TilePro was during an urologic procedure [1–3, 5]. It was used along with a Doppler technology in renal surgery. Laparoscopic ultrasound probe can be controlled by the surgeon as well as an assistant at the patient side. By using Doppler ultrasound, the renal hilum could be identified and aberrant vessels were isolated. It was also useful to confirm ischemia before resection. Surgeons can also correlate the ultrasound images with preoperative CT scan images to localize the tumor by using triple image display.

General Surgery Application

In general surgery, TilePro was used in various types of surgery. During radical gastrectomy for gastric cancer, patient-specific vascular images were reconstructed during operation by the radiologist and transferred to the surgeon console using TilePro (Fig. 35.3).

Reconstructed CT images provide vital information during surgery, in particular, a vascular map that is critical for surgical guidance during lymphadenectomy, and it minimizes the risk of vessel injury, especially of small- or deep-seated vessels. This approach used intraoperative vascular images to depict vasculatures around the stomach (Fig. 35.4), and through it, surgeon could identify important vascular variations [6].

During a totally robotic right colectomy, tumor location and vascular supply were confirmed. During this procedure, surgeon controlled the augmented stereoscopic volume-rendered reconstruction images using 3D mouse. This was the first application of 3D projection of the images via TilePro during surgery. Thus, surgeon can have two 3D images simultaneously: operative view and 3D reconstructed images [4].

Another possible application of TilePro in general surgery area is using various types of intraoperative endoscopy. Intraoperative upper endoscopy is an option for the surgeon to localize a tumor especially for early lesions. Intraoperative colonoscopy can also be used not only for tumor positioning but also for confirming anastomotic line. Intraoperative choledochoscopy may also be a necessary tool for liver and biliary surgery. For liver surgery, laparoscopic ultrasound can be used as was in renal surgery.

Other Applications

Besides urology and general surgery applications, TilePro can be applied in various other areas. For example, echocardiographic images can be transferred during cardiac surgery. Nerve function monitoring may also be a good area of TilePro use.

Limitations

Transmission failure caused by a cabling issue was reported. Testing the system in advance to ensure that all data sources are capable of transmission can prevent this type of failure. Data transmission delay that led to alternative and traditional methods of data integration outside the TilePro system (e.g., audible conveyance of information) was also reported [1]. More importantly,

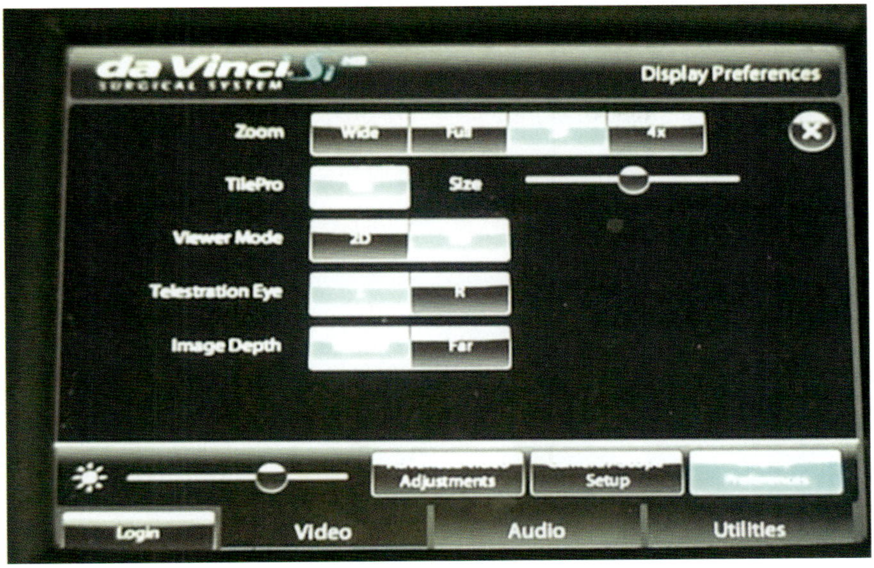

Fig. 35.2 TilePro can be activated by using the touch pad panel at the surgeon console. The surgeon can control the video input on and off by tapping the foot pedal for the camera

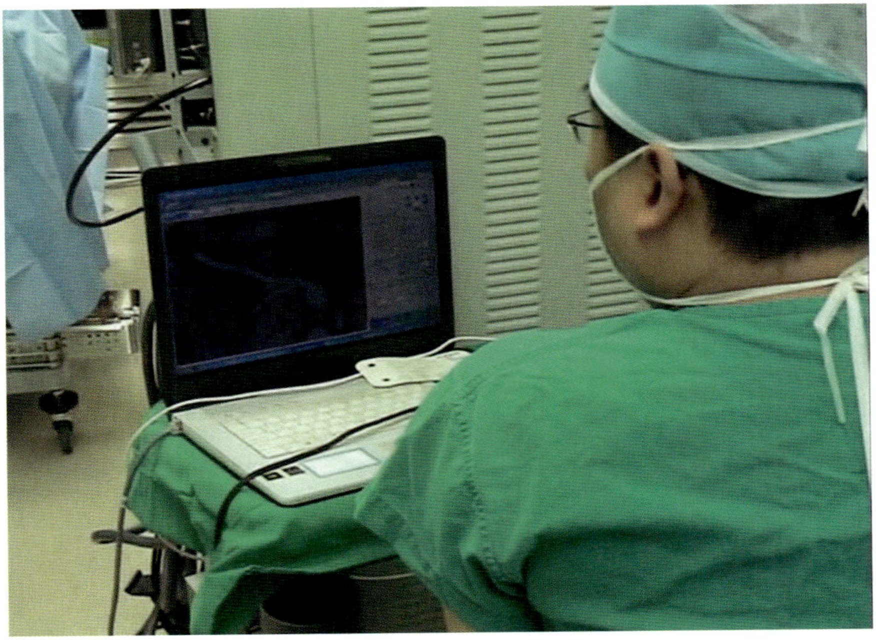

Fig. 35.3 Intraoperative vascular reconstruction by a radiologist during radical gastrectomy for gastric cancer. Reconstructed images are transferred to the surgeon console through TilePro

lack of comparison with and without TilePro application limits the evaluation of clinical impact of TilePro. However, the more information the surgeon has, results of the surgery may improve provided unless TilePro causes trouble to precede the operative procedures.

Another limitation of TilePro is problems related to operating TilePro and manipulating image sources [3]. To manipulate the radiologic images, surgeon has to use mouse. Currently the radiologic images cannot be manipulated on the console. The control of the images are on a device

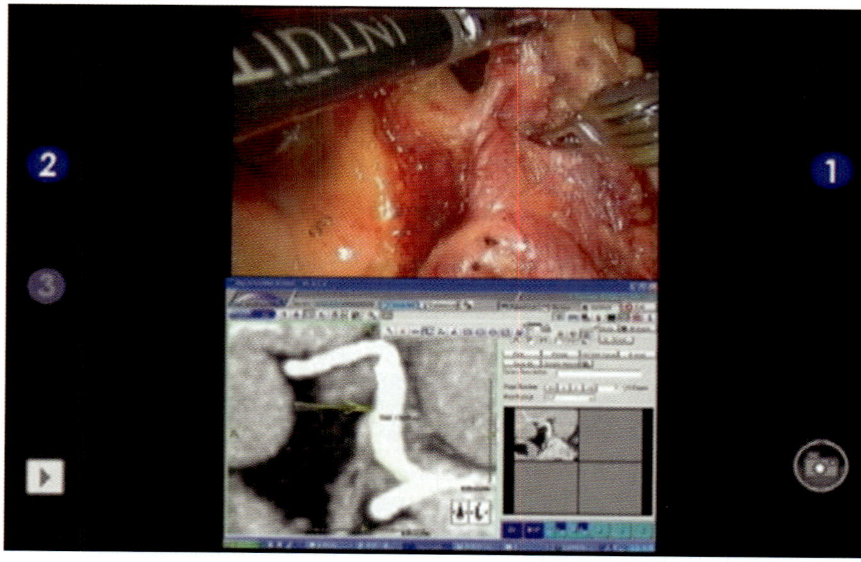

Fig. 35.4 An intraoperative TilePro view at the surgeon console showing operative view and vascular image during radical gastrectomy for gastric cancer

connected to the external image source and requires the surgeon to look away from the operation if any change in the images are necessary. This results in a break in the operation as the surgeon is unable to perform the operation simultaneously. However, this limitation can be overcome by an assistant who can manipulate the images at the surgeons request. In addition, the endoscopy must be performed by another endoscopist.

Conclusions

TilePro is a useful additional tool of the current robotic surgery system. Although currently limited, its applications during robotic surgery have demonstrated satisfactory and favorable outcomes after robotic surgery. In the near future, TilePro may be positioned as an essential tool for surgery. Although it is complicated to use TilePro so far, better surgeon-friendly system will be developed in the near future. The more information we can integrate using TilePro, the better the surgical outcomes will be.

References

1. Bhayani SB, Snow DC. Novel dynamic information integration during da Vinci robotic partial nephrectomy and radical nephrectomy. J Robot Surg. 2008;2:67–9.
2. Hyams ES, Kanofsky JA, Stifelman MD. Laparoscopic Doppler technology: applications in laparoscopic pyeloplasty and radical and partial nephrectomy. Urology. 2008;71(5):952–6.
3. Rogers CG, Laungani R, Bhandari A, Krane LS, Eun D, Patel MN, Boris R, Shrivastava A, Menon M. Maximizing console surgeon independence during robot-assisted renal surgery by using the fourth arm and TilePro™. J Endourol. 2009;23:115–21.
4. Volonté F, Pugin F, Buchs NC, Spaltenstein J, Hagen M, Ratib O, Morel P. Console-integrated stereoscopic OsiriX 3D volume-rendered images for da Vinci colorectal robotic surgery. Surg Innov. 2013;20(2):158–63.
5. Yuh B, Muldrew S, Menchaca A, Yip W, Lau C, Wilson T, Josephson D. Integrating robotic partial nephrectomy to an existing robotic surgery program. Can J Urol. 2012;19(2):6193–200.
6. Kim YM, Baek SE, Lim JS, Hyung WJ. Clinical application of image-enhanced minimally invasive robotic surgery for gastric cancer: a prospective observational study. J Gastrointest Surg. 2013;17(2):304–12.

36 ICG Fluorescence

Giuseppe Spinoglio

For more than 40 years, the technique of fluorescence imaging has been widely used for the study of the blood flows and microcirculation [1]. Indocyanine green (ICG) is a vital dye that binds to plasma proteins when injected into the bloodstream, and conveyed by the proteins, it reaches all the organs and body regions. Its routine use has spread throughout different specialties (cardiac surgery, neurosurgery, ophthalmology, hepatology, etc.), and this has been facilitated by its excellent tolerability, few side effects, extremely low toxicity, and few allergic reactions (1/10,000 as reported by the manufacturer) [1–3]. The dose used for normal diagnostic procedures is between 0.1 and 0.5 mg/kg.

After intravenous injection, in a time interval that lies between 5 and 50 s, the ICG reaches the arterial and venous vessels; after about a minute, it reaches the kidneys where it remains for about 20 min; and after about 2 min, it reaches the liver from where it is eliminated via the bile without being subject to enterohepatic recirculation [4].

The persistence in the liver, before the excretion is complete, is approximately 1–2 h.

When injected intradermally, subcutaneously, subserosally, or submucosally, it is drained through the network of lymphatic vessels; within 15 min, it reaches the first lymph nodes (SLNs); and 1 or 2 h later, it reaches the regional lymph nodes where it remains for about 24–48 h.

The ICG has the ability to absorb light in the near-infrared wavelengths of between 600 and 900 nm. The amplitude of the spectrum depends on the type of solvent used and its concentration. When it binds to plasma proteins, the maximum absorption of infrared light is around 830 nm. If its molecules are excited with infrared laser light at a frequency of 780 nm, they emit a very intense fluorescent signal. At this wavelength, it is possible to suppress the excited laser light through filters and dedicated cameras and detect only the fluorescence signal.

The near-infrared light with wave amplitude of between 700 and 900 nm (NIR) has the ability to penetrate deep into tissue (from several millimeters to several centimeters in depth) with low autofluorescence, thus providing a sufficient contrast [5].

Recently there has been developed and integrated to the da Vinci 3DHD robotic system an optical system that is capable of emitting laser light that is closer to infrared light with the ability to switch between white light and near-infrared (NIR) light view in real time, creating the ability to perform fluorescence-guided surgery. There are many fields of application in general surgery, some still experimental and evolving, ranging from intraoperative cholangiography (IOC) to define biliary anatomy; the study of bowel stump perfusion, especially in colonic resections; and sentinel node and lymph node mapping in cancer surgery. In addition, ICG fluorescence can be

G. Spinoglio, M.D. (✉)
Department of General and Oncological Surgery, City Hospital SS. Antonio e Biagio, Via Venezia 16, Alessandria 15121, Italy
e-mail: gspinoglio@ospedale.al.it

K.C. Kim (ed.), *Robotics in General Surgery*, DOI 10.1007/978-1-4614-8739-5_36,

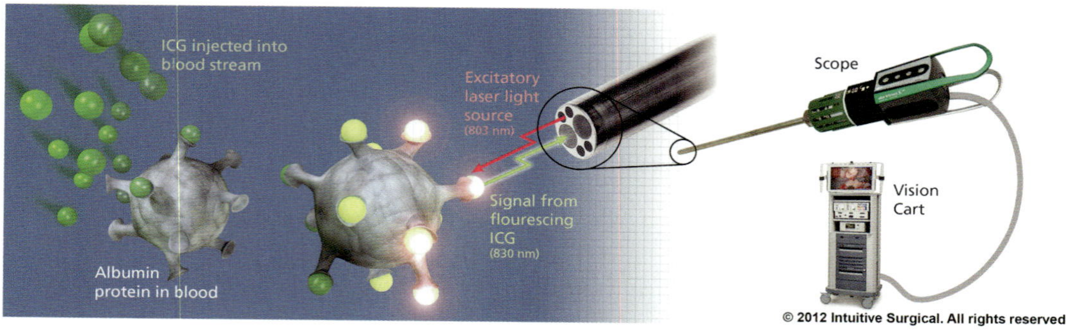

Fig. 36.1 ICG NIR fluorescence explanation

used to endoscopically mark colonic, rectal, and gastric lesions [6–9].

The fluorescence vision system of the da Vinci HD robot comprises an endoscope that is able to provide visible light and near-infrared light images, a 3DHD stereoscopic camera connected to the endoscope, and an endoscopic illuminator that through a flexible cable provides the console surgeon with both near-infrared and visible lighting (Fig. 36.1). The surgeon can quickly switch between normal viewing mode (visible light) and fluorescence (NIR) by pressing the pedal of the surgical console.

In this chapter, we describe current applications in general surgery: fluorescent cholangiography, lymph node mapping, and assessment of the perfusion of the colonic stumps, colorectal, and gastric tattooing.

Cholangiography Fluorescence of Indocyanine Green

Bile duct injury (BDI) is a rare but serious complication of cholecystectomy. The incidence of these lesions increased from 0.1–0.2 % at the time of open cholecystectomy to 0.4–0.7 % in the era of laparoscopic cholecystectomy. The primary cause of BDI is the misinterpretation of biliary anatomy (71–97 % of cases) [10–14].

The single-incision laparoscopic cholecystectomy (SILC) may be associated with an increased risk of bile duct injuries because of insufficient exposure of Calot's triangle compared to traditional multiport cholecystectomy.

Single-site robotic cholecystectomy (SSRC) allows easier and safer surgical procedures, similar to those of multiport laparoscopic cholecystectomy, with good exposure of the Calot's triangle.

However, the difficulty in visualizing the biliary structures can still remain in SSRC, although to a lesser extent with respect to the SILC. This is due to a reduced field of vision and to a forced position of the instruments [15].

Routine IOC to evaluate the biliary anatomy is still recommended by many authors [16], but it has several disadvantages such as a longer operating time, requirement for a multidisciplinary team, staff and patient exposure to radiation, interruption of the workflow, and, in the case of robotic surgery, the need to undock and redock the robot.

ICG NIR cholangiography is a noninvasive method that requires no X-rays or bulky equipment such as the C-arm and permits viewing of the bile duct in real time by alternating between the white light and NIR fluorescent light with a simple switch system.

Recently, several authors have reported the benefits of cholangiography with fluorescence detection of the biliary tract in real time during dissection of the Calot's triangle with no requirement for catheterization of the biliary tract [17, 18].

Technique

The first dose of 2.5 mg of ICG is administered intravenously during the preparation of the patient, about 30–45 min before surgery. A second dose

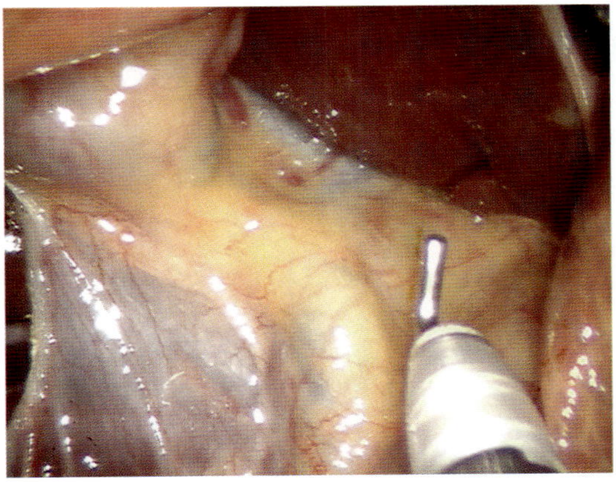

Fig. 36.2 White light view before Calot's dissection

of 2.5 mg ICG is once again administered intravenously if fluorescence is not detected in the liver about 60 min after the injection of the first dose. The surgery begins in the usual manner for SSRC cholecystectomy. Once a view of the Calot's triangle is established, the camera is put into fluorescence mode for an initial attempt to identify the biliary anatomy (Figs. 36.2 and 36.3). Then the dissection of the Calot's triangle begins with the incision of the peritoneum and continues as described in the SSRC chapter, alternatively switching from white to NIR light allowing views of the fluorescent bile ducts in real time. In this way, the surgeon can follow a road map for a safe skeletonization of the cystic duct and cystic artery (Figs. 36.4 and 36.5). The cystic duct may be clipped under fluorescence before sectioning, especially if it is very short and if there are problems in the biliary confluence.

If there are problems with the vascular anatomy during the cystic artery skeletonization, it is possible to proceed with a further injection of 2.5 mg of ICG and, after 10–20 s, obtain a view of the hepatic and cystic arteries and their divisions and avoid any damage to anomalous branches, especially the branch to the sixth hepatic segment.

During the detachment of the gallbladder from the liver bed, use of fluorescence to define the boundary between the gallbladder and liver bed is useful, especially in cases of thin or an intrahepatic gallbladder and to visualize any aberrant ducts of Luschka (Figs. 36.6, 36.7, 36.8, and 36.9).

After the procedure, a final fluorescence view of the operative field may be prudent.

Discussion of Advantages, Limitations, and Relative Contraindications

Advantages

Fluorescent cholangiography, especially during the SSRC, allows safe viewing and immediate and real-time anatomy of the biliary tract and is a further aid to prevent BDI during the procedure.

First, Ishizawa and then Buchs demonstrated the technical feasibility of fluorescent cholangiography during multiport laparoscopic cholecystectomy, SILC, and SSRC [17, 18].

In our experience, 70 patients underwent SSRC with ICG NIR cholangiography (initial data submitted to Surg Endosc).

We visualized at least 1 biliary duct in 100 % of cases before the dissection of the triangle of Calot and two biliary ducts in 97 % of cases after dissection. The operative time of SSRC with fluorescence compared with that of our SSRC experience without fluorescence was not statistically significant.

Mean hospital stay was 1.1 days. There were no conversions, bile duct injuries, other major complications, or adverse events.

The advantages of this method compared to the traditional radiological IOC are many:

- There is no interruption of the workflow in that the images are highlighted on the surgical field during the normal progress of the operation and the surgeon can operate both in white light and fluorescence.
- The interpretation of images is simpler because they appear in real time and can be checked with surgical maneuvers of moving structures whilst they are in view. This is in contrast to the traditional IOC images that are fixed on the screen of the radiology equipment with the surgeon working with static information.

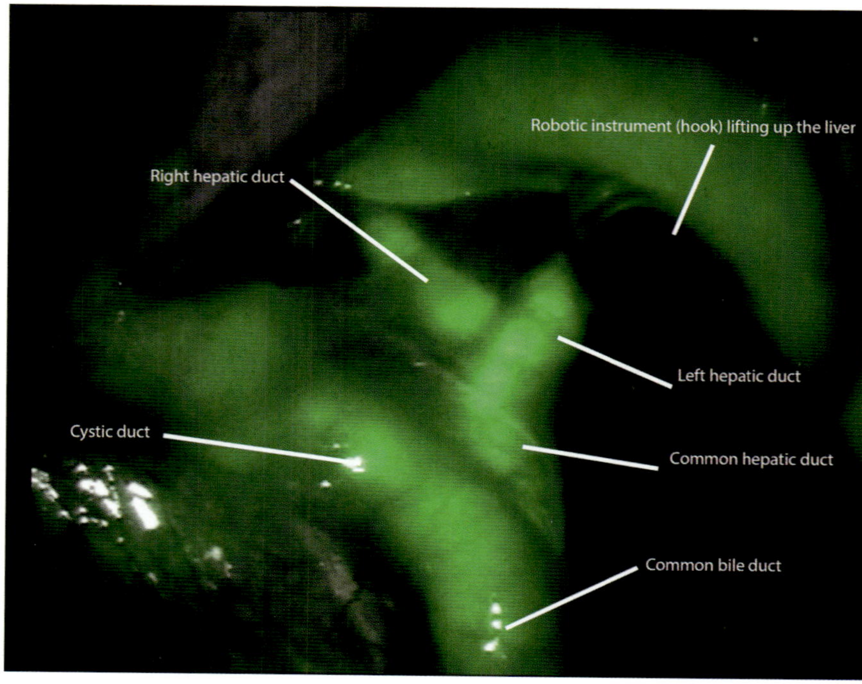

Fig. 36.3 NIR light view before Calot's dissection

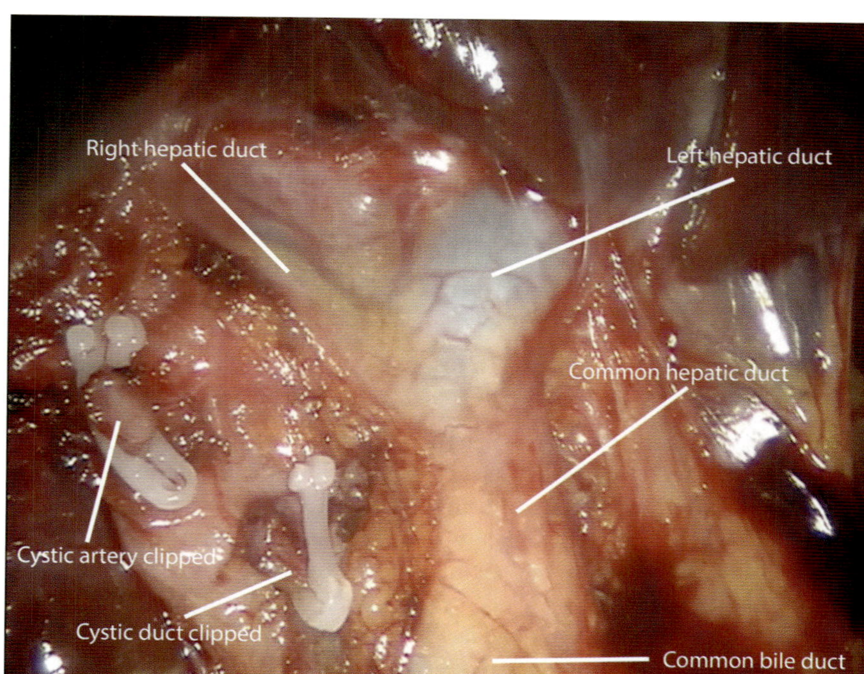

Fig. 36.4 White with light view after Calot's dissection (cyst duct and artery sectioned)

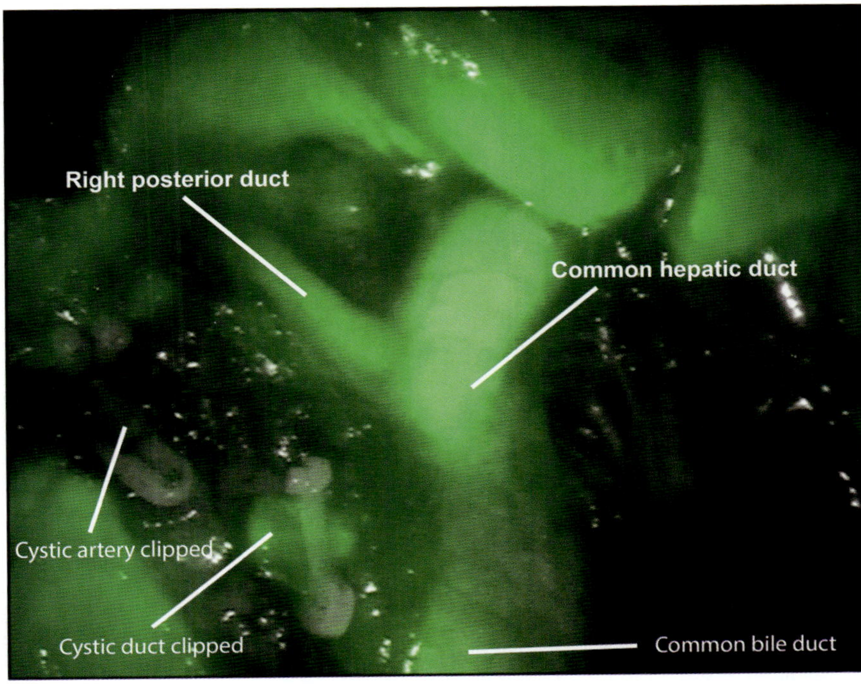

Fig. 36.5 NIR light view after Calot's dissection (cyst duct and artery sectioned)

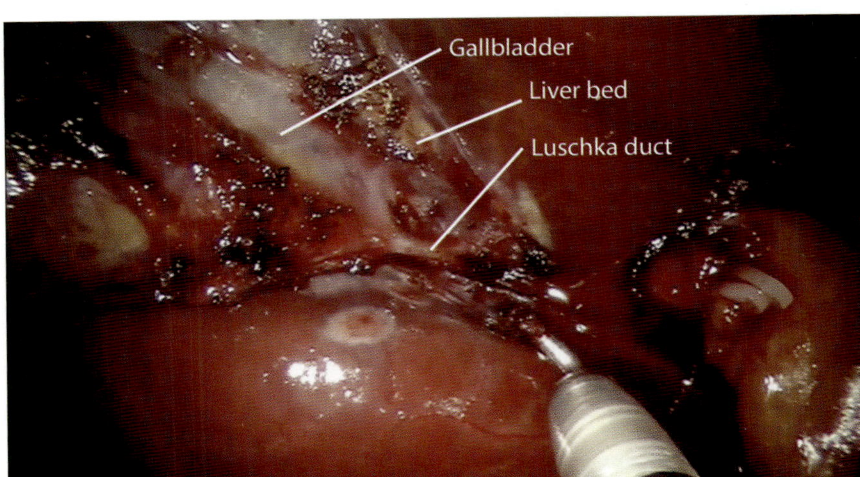

Fig. 36.6 White light view of Luschka duct before sectioning

- It is possible to control the clipping and sectioning of the cystic duct with a clear distinction of the bile ducts.
- During the detachment of the gallbladder from the liver bed, its wall can be better highlighted and any aberrant ducts of Luschka easily found.
- The fluorescent bile that usually comes out of the stump of the cut cystic duct or of the gallbladder in case of perforation is always clearly visible; therefore, the system could potentially highlight any bile leaks. This use of the ICF fluorescence, however, has not yet been reported.

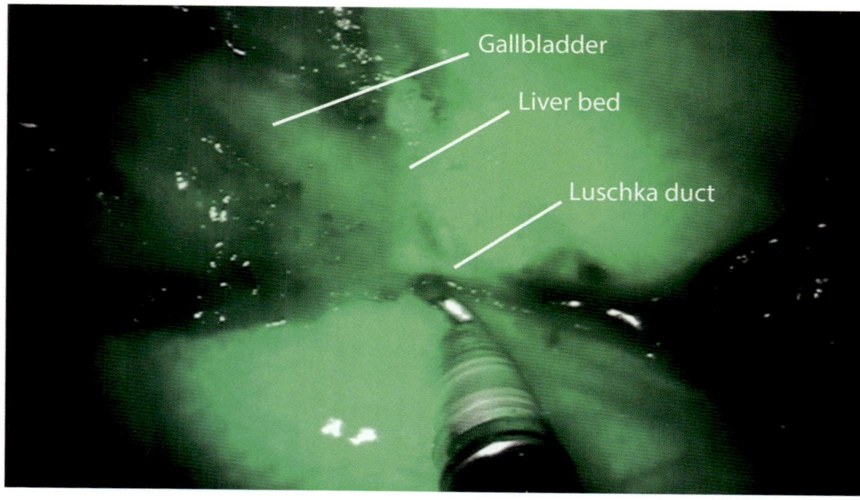

Fig. 36.7 NIR light view of Luschka duct before sectioning

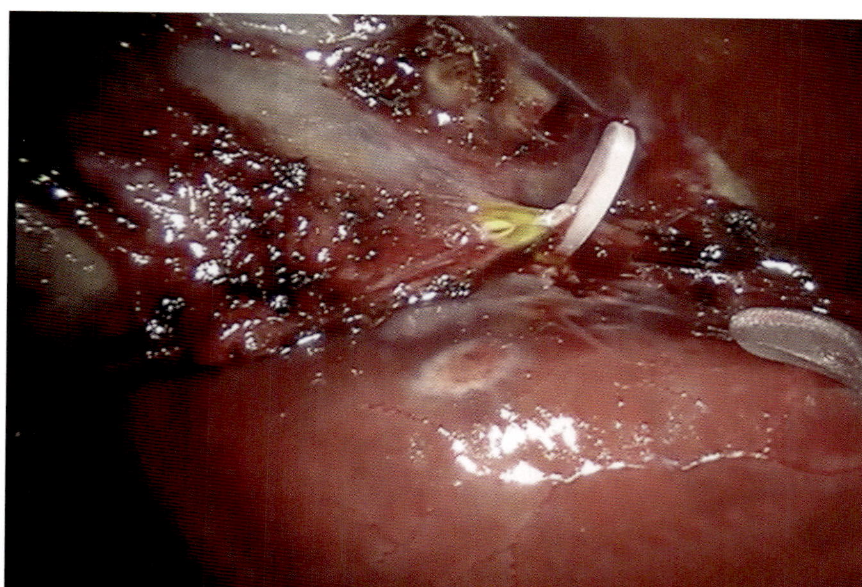

Fig. 36.8 White light view of Luschka duct after sectioning

- When needed, the vascular anatomy of the hepatic artery and cystic artery can be shown.
- C-arm or other equipment is not needed, thus avoiding the undocking and redocking of the robotic system.
- The procedure does not require any additional time compared to normal SSRC.

We can conclude that the procedure is safe and inexpensive; it requires no interaction of multidisciplinary teams, does not expose patients and staff to radiation, and is not burdened by adverse reactions.

Limitations

The current limitations are mainly two:

- So far the procedure has not been tested in cases of an emergency cholecystectomy performed for suppurative cholecystitis or gangrenous

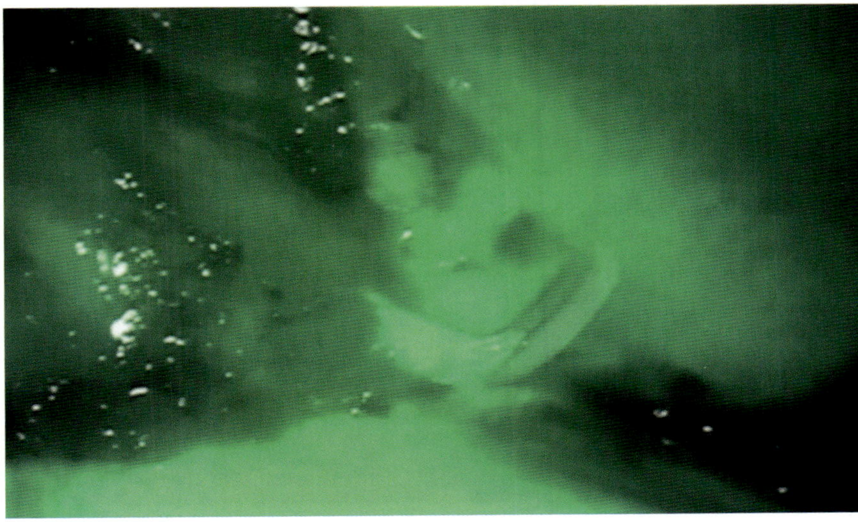

Fig. 36.9 NIR light view of Luschka duct after sectioning

cholecystitis. The ability of NIR light to reach the deeper, edematous, and inflamed tissues must be studied.

- ICG NIR fluorescent cholangiography is optimal for the definition of biliary tree anatomy. The capability of the current system to recognize biliary gallstones or other obstructions has not yet been investigated.

Contraindications

Pregnancy, adverse reaction, or allergy to ICG, iodine, shellfish, or iodine dyes.

Fluorescence for Near-Infrared Imaging During Colorectal Surgery

The advantages of the robotic platform in colorectal cancer surgery have been extensively described in previous chapters. The fluorescence viewing system of the da Vinci HD is able to increase the potential of robot technology in terms of safety and oncologic extent of dissection.

The use of fluorescence in colorectal surgery can be useful for some currently developing applications:

- The evaluation of perfusion of the intestinal stumps
- Real-time identification of vascular anatomy
- Intraoperative lymph node mapping
- Tattooing for the localization of tumors of the colon, rectum, etc.

The Evaluation of Perfusion of the Intestinal Stumps

The anastomotic leakage is one of the most feared complications in colorectal surgery [19, 20]. The causes of and pathogenic mechanisms underlying anastomotic leakages have not been fully clarified, but it is considered that the perfusion of the intestinal stump is an important factor [21]. The evaluation of the adequacy of perfusion of the stumps is usually based on the subjective impression of the surgeon that includes parameters such as active bleeding edge of the section, the pulsatility of the mesentery vessels, and lack of discoloration of bowel segments [22].

The loss of tactile feedback, typical of minimally invasive surgery, can make this assessment more difficult compared to open surgery.

Many different solutions have been proposed: laser Doppler flowmetry, visible light spectroscopy, fluorescence laser angiography, narrow band laser imaging techniques, and near-infrared reflection spectroscopy.

The fluorescence system of the da Vinci robot allows HD viewing in real time both for

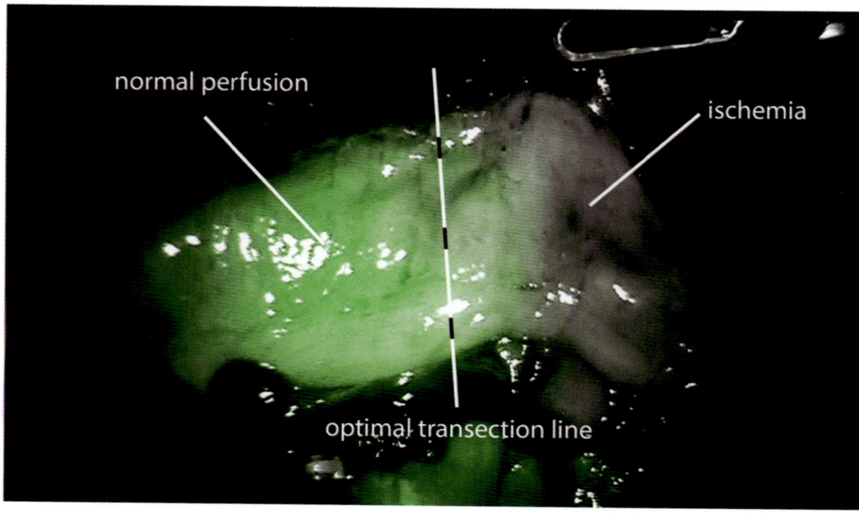

Fig. 36.10 Transection line assessment during left colectomy

macroscopic vascular anatomy of and perfusion of the microcirculation.

This device can be used to assess the intestinal perfusion and reassure the surgeon in their choice of point section of the bowel during left and right hemicolectomies and anterior resection of the rectum. It can also be useful in nonstandardized colic resections such as the resection of the transverse and left colonic angle in which vascular abnormalities can impair the blood supply.

Technique

After having performed surgery with the da Vinci surgical system following the usual technique of vascular control and preparation of intestinal segments, the chosen location for colonic resection is evaluated with white light, and an intravenous dose of 5.0–10 mg mg of ICG is administered.

Approximately 30–45 s after the infusion, the operative field is viewed under fluorescence. Depending on the tissues, the green fluorescent intensity appears different and at different times. With regard to the colonic stumps, the vessels of the epiploic appendices and mesentery turn green first, and then the green spreads across the intestinal wall. The antimesenteric side of the descending colon and transverse colon is always a little paler because the vascularization of the tenia is less intense due to thickness of the muscle tissue.

The perfused segments gradually become green until they assume a bright green color, in contrast with the gray segments that are not well vascularized (Fig. 36.10). The stapler can be placed following a well-perfused transaction line (Fig. 36.11).

If the site chosen for the section does not appear to be sufficiently perfused, the section line can be moved. In case of doubt, the test can be repeated after waiting a few minutes to allow the dye to wash out.

Further checks may be carried out before and after performing the anastomosis (Figs. 36.12 and 36.13).

With regard to the rectal stump, the pelvic wall turns green first (as does the uterus in women) because it is highly vascularized. After a few seconds, the rectal stump colors up allowing the assessment of perfusion at the selected point (Figs. 36.14 and 36.15).

The ends of the section lines of the rectum in Knight-Griffen anastomosis or of the colon in latero-lateral anastomosis are often referred to as critical points of leakage: particular attention should be paid to their perfusion, and today fluorescence is the only tool we have to evaluate it objectively.

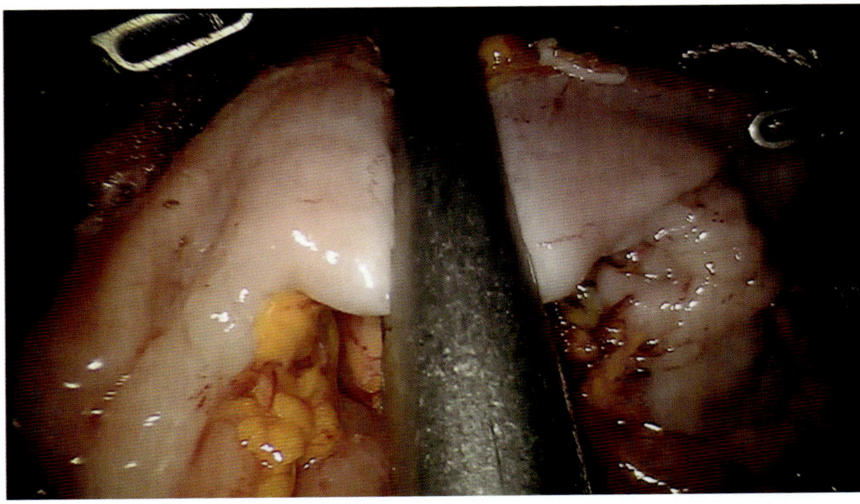

Fig. 36.11 Bowel transection during left colectomy

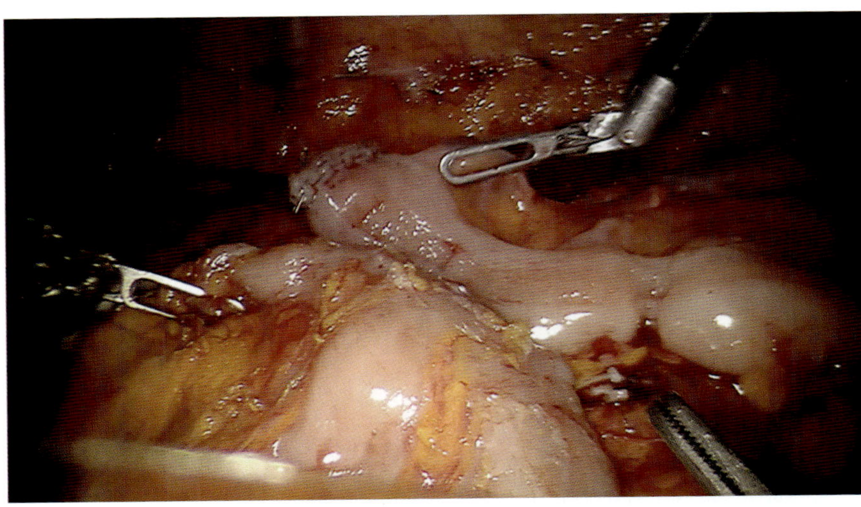

Fig. 36.12 White light view of side-to-side anastomosis during splenic flexure resection

Discussion of Advantages, Limitations, and Relative Contraindications

The potential advantages of bowel perfusion assessment using fluorescence appear interesting and are the subject of several multicenter studies.

Currently there is only one paper regarding this topic. Kudszus et al. reported a 13.9 % rate of change in stapling location after fluorescence perfusion assessment.

This work also demonstrated that the leak rate was reduced from 7.5 to 3.5 %; therefore, it seems this technology might be very impactful for the reduction of anastomotic leaks in colorectal surgery [9].

In most cases, visual inspection, combined with caution, is sufficient to perform a well-vascularized anastomosis, especially for experienced surgeons. However, there are difficult cases, both for patient conditions such as obesity, diabetes, and inflammatory disease and for the types of anastomosis such as in ultra-low rectal

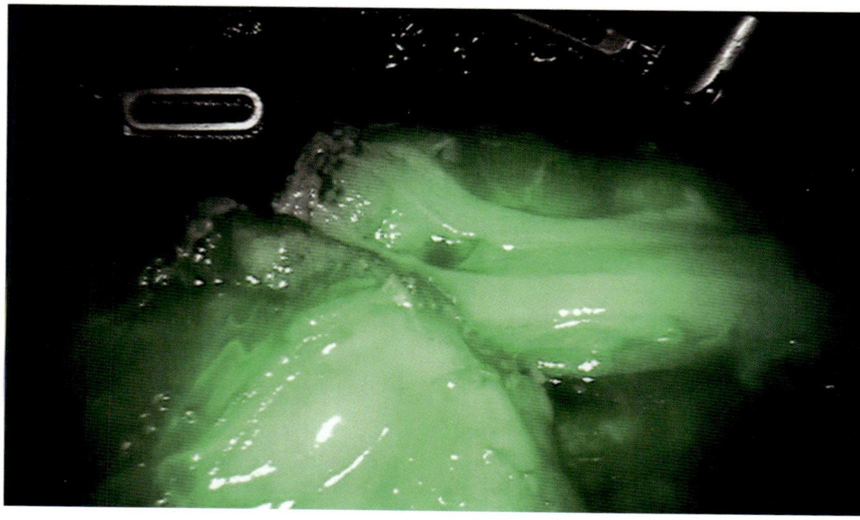

Fig. 36.13 NIR light view of side-to-side anastomosis during splenic flexure resection

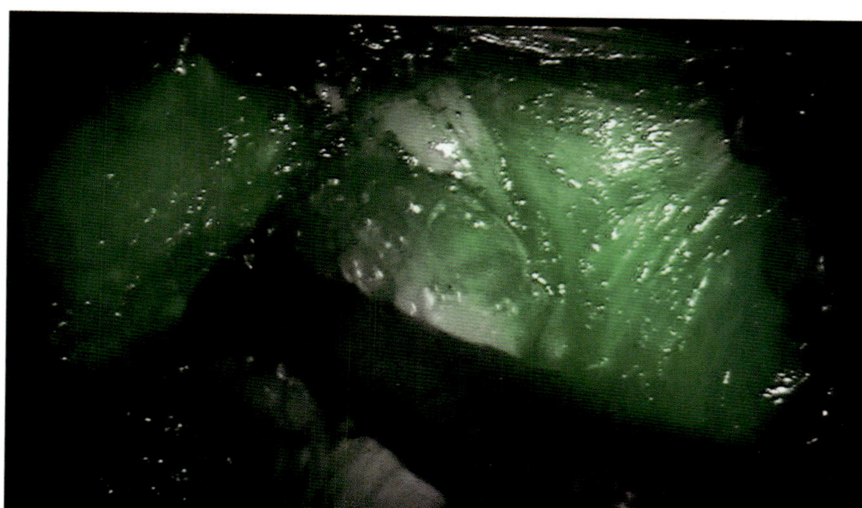

Fig. 36.14 NIR light view of rectal transection

resection, especially in the presence of a thick mesocolon and a short mesentery, and in left angle resections, in which the evaluation of the perfusion is important, even if only as confirmation.

Accidental spillage in the course of injection for tattoo or lymph node mapping may pose a limitation on the use of this method for assessment of perfusion. In this case, it may be difficult to appreciate the fluorescence of the stump associated with perfusion as distinct from the fluorescence resulting from impregnation of the tissue.

The contraindications are those described in general for ICG fluorescence.

Lymph Node Mapping

The prognosis and quality of life of patients with colorectal cancer depend on the extent of the tumor, the characteristics of onset, and the quality of surgical care. In particular, a correct local-regional lymphadenectomy is mandatory for staging and treatment of the tumor.

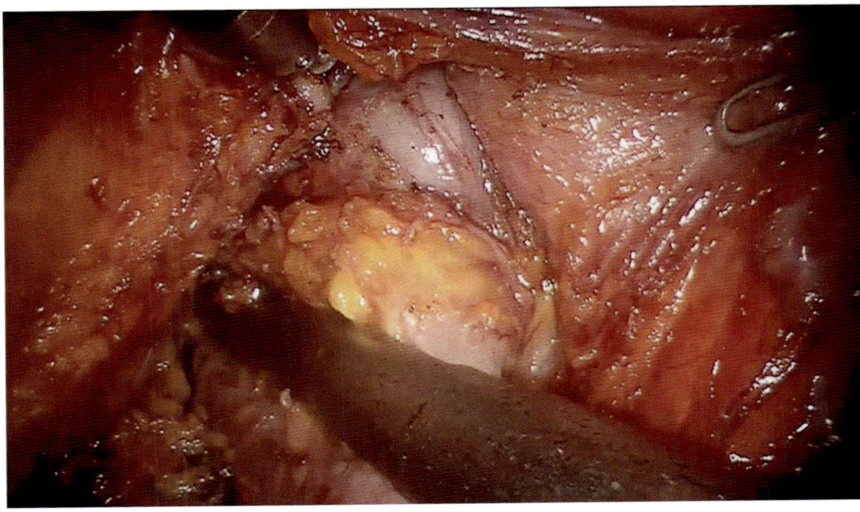

Fig. 36.15 White light view of rectal transection

Colorectal resections (colectomy and partial colectomy and anterior resection of the rectum) are governed by identical pathophysiological principles: cancers and colonic segments are resected en bloc with their relative lymph nodes.

Although in most cases all the lymph nodes of the segment of colon affected by cancer are included in the surgical specimen, in some cases, the lymphatic spread may extend beyond these. Examples of this abnormal extension are represented by lateral pelvic lymph nodes in rectal cancer or by periaortic lymph nodes in left colon cancers. These lymph nodes may be the cause of recurrence and should be removed.

For these reasons, over the years, the indications have often changed from standard lymphadenectomy for cancer of the rectum to extensive lymphadenectomy, such as pelvic lateral lymphadenectomy.

On the other hand, in recent years, surgical oncology is evolving towards less aggressive approaches thanks to early diagnosis, which allows one to perform limited but oncologically correct resections together with the development of techniques for the identification of the sentinel lymph node. The SLN procedure is regarded as standard of care in the treatment of breast cancer and melanoma [23, 24]. Although its value in colorectal cancer has not yet been established, the recent study of Hutteman et al. demonstrated that NIR fluorescent light permits real-time imaging of lymph flow and identification of the SLN in colon and rectal cancer specimens [8].

Technique

When injected intradermally, subcutaneously, subserosally, or submucosally, the ICG is drained through the network of lymphatic vessels; within 15 min, it reaches the first lymph nodes (SLNs); and 1 or 2 h later, it reaches the regional lymph nodes where it remains for about 24–48 h.

The technique differs in the timing of injection of the ICG to assess the lymph node mapping rather than to identify the sentinel lymph node.

In the case lymph node mapping, 1 or 2 cc of a solution of 0.5 % ICG (5–10 mg) is injected endoscopically around the tumor in the submucosa 3–24 h before surgery. The injection should be done by introducing the needle tangentially to the wall and not perpendicularly in order to avoid any risk of perforation of the intestinal wall with consequent diffusion of ICG in the peritoneum or in the surrounding tissues.

Operating in NIR light shows the first lymph node before the peritoneal dissection, and following the dissection, all lymph nodes are highlighted from where the ICG has been drained (Figs. 36.16, 36.17, and 36.18). The lymph nodes are removed

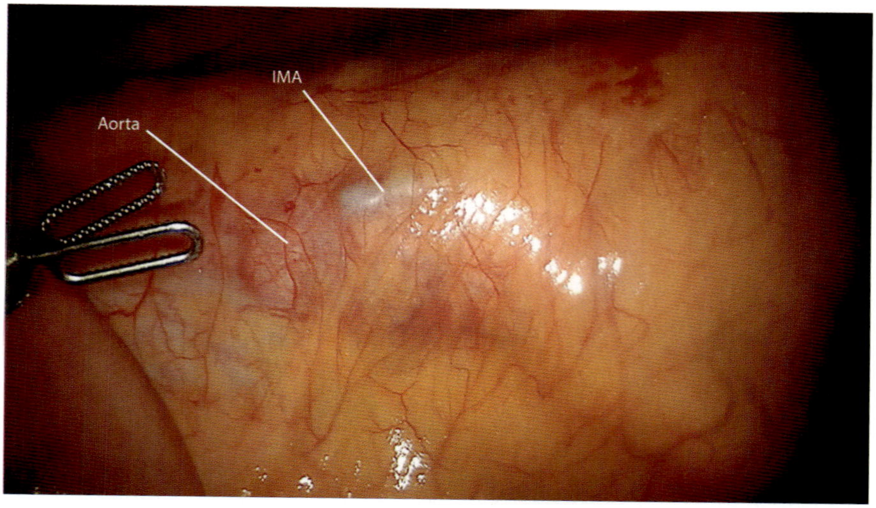

Fig. 36.16 White light view of periaortic lymph nodes during robotic rectal resection

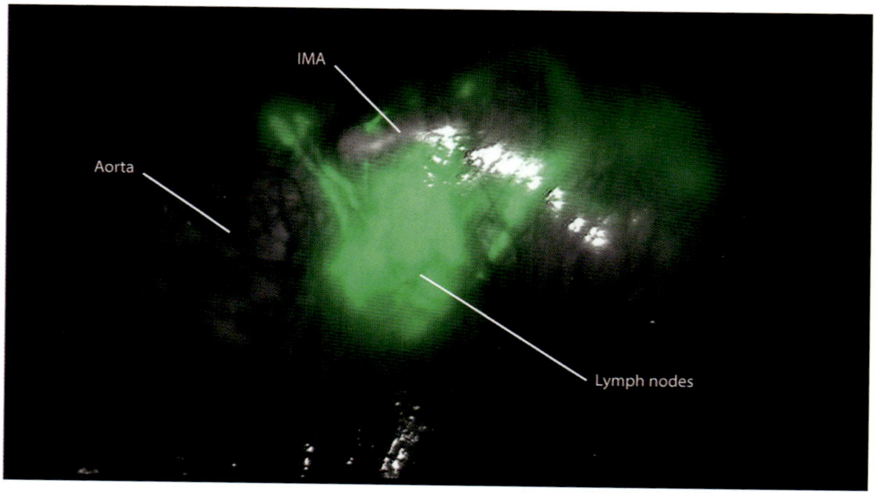

Fig. 36.17 NIR view of periaortic lymph nodes during robotic rectal resection

en bloc if present in typical sites by a standard lymphadenectomy; however, they are removed with the "berry-picking" technique when present in unusual locations (periperiaortic and pericaval in the left colon, pelvic side walls in the rectum).

To locate the sentinel lymph node, the dye is injected intraoperatively into the subserosa. If the location of the tumor cannot be identified laparoscopically, the dye is injected into the submucosa by the endoscopist. The intraoperative technique involves the insertion of a butterfly infusion set connected to a syringe containing the ICG solution of 0.5 % through the trocar by the bedside assistant. The surgeon at the console guides and inserts the needle tangentially into the subserosa or submucosa on 4 sides of the tumor, and the infusion is made by the assistant surgeon at the table (Figs. 36.19 and 36.20). The needle is removed while maintaining suction to prevent leakage of ICG into the peritoneum; the dose of ICG is identical to that injected endoscopically.

After a few minutes after the injection, one or two fluorescent lymphatic channels are displayed which run beneath the serosa and then drain the sentinel lymph node (SLN).

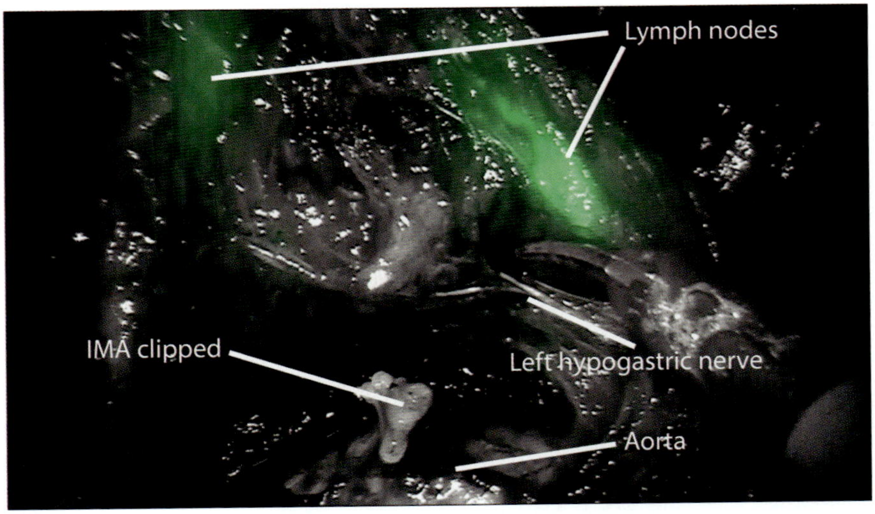

Fig. 36.18 NIR view of dissected periaortic lymph nodes during robotic rectal resection

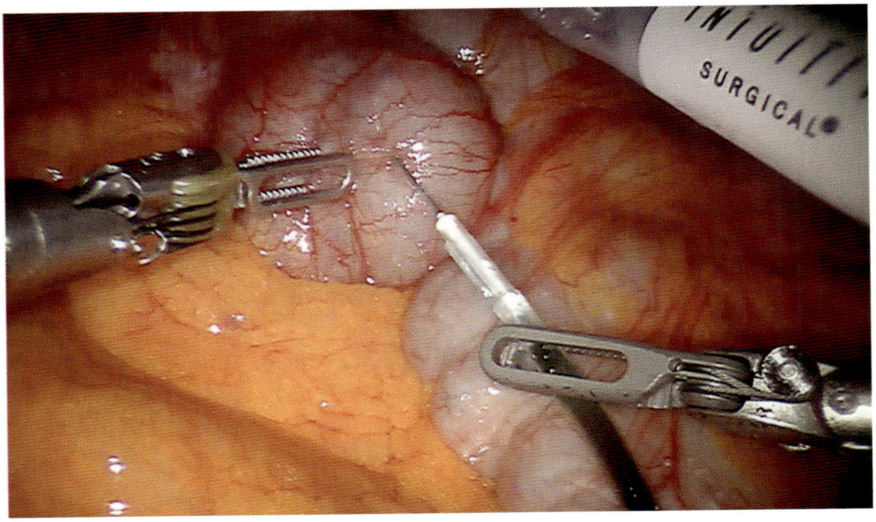

Fig. 36.19 White light view of subserosal ICG injection during right colectomy

Discussion of Advantages, Limitations, and Relative Contraindications

The advantages of the definition of a lymph node map that permits sometimes a more extensive but guided lymphadenectomy could be the compromise solution, based on objective data, between extended and standard lymphectomy with the aim of a "tailored surgery." The removal of lymph nodes outside of the typical sites shown by the fluorescence has an important staging significance rather than surgical therapy and, therefore, may be performed with a "berry-picking" technique that, guided by the fluorescence view, can be more precise, meticulous, and certainly less traumatic than the regional lymphadenectomy.

With regard to the sentinel lymph node, we know that some studies have been published in colorectal surgery, especially with the radioguided technique, but the role of the biopsy for the detection of micrometastases and their

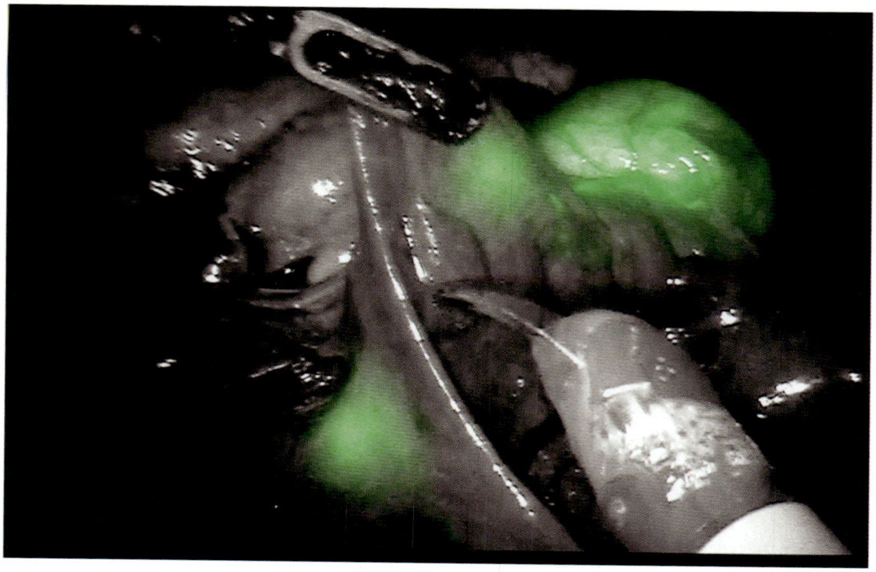

Fig. 36.20 NIR view of subserosal ICG injection during right colectomy

clinical significance has not yet been defined [25–27].

The sentinel node biopsy guided by ICG fluorescence imaging has been shown to increase the detection rate with a low rate of false negatives in breast cancer, melanoma, and cancer of the anus and in the stomach [24, 28–30]. The application of fluorescence in colorectal surgery for sentinel lymph node is still limited to experimental studies. One of the limitations of the application is the rapid diffusion of ICG. For this reason, solutions of ICG with binding protein able to slow down the diffusion such as albumin are under investigation.

In any case, the feasibility of the method during left colonic resections has already been demonstrated [8].

The limit of lymph node visualization techniques with ICG fluorescence is determined by its diffusibility. The peritumoral injection technique must be precise and submucosal, with a small dose. Excessive penetration into the intestinal wall can result in diffusion into the tissues or peritoneum that can cause an extended colorization that masks the lymph nodes. For this reason, the best results are obtained in rectal tumors where the injection can be done directly by the surgeon with a rigid sigmoidoscope and a long spinal needle. On the other hand, the possibility of viewing the sentinel lymph node in subperitoneal rectal neoplasms, even if subjected to neoadjuvant radiotherapy, is limited by the capacity of penetration of the NIR light that decreases drastically with tissue thicknesses >0.5 mm.

Likewise, the intraoperative butterfly needle injection can be difficult and often remains too superficial and spreads the dye into the peritoneum.

An important caveat in the removal of lymph nodes with the “berry-picking” technique is to maneuver the instruments with great delicacy and not to use vigorous movements on the lymph nodes; even without breaking the lymph nodes, the dye can spread easily and stain the robotic forceps and consequently taint neighboring tissues with green fluorescence with each subsequent touch.

Colonic Tattooing

In minimally invasive surgery, the localization of small or flat tumors or those that were removed endoscopically can be difficult to establish. In colorectal robotic surgery, this problem is

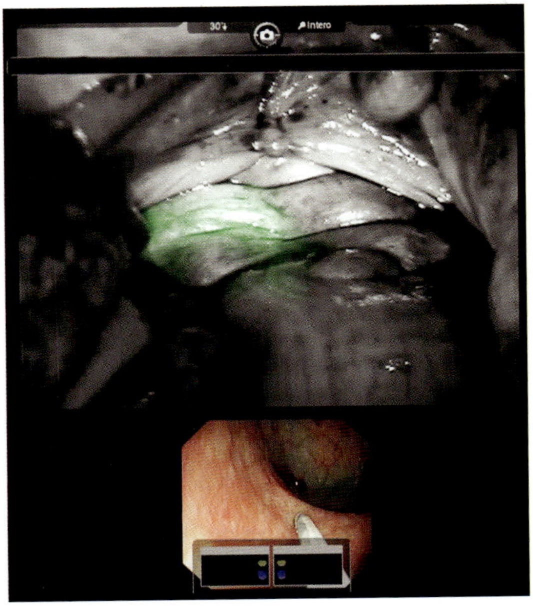

Fig. 36.21 Intraperitoneal NIR view and endoscopic view during rectal tumor tattooing

particularly evident for the lack of tactile feedback from the instruments.

India ink was often used with colonic tattooing, but it has been associated with complications such as perforation of the gut, spread of ink in the peritoneal cavity, paracolic abscesses, and adhesions [31–33].

Some authors have proposed the use of ICG for tattooing before laparoscopic-assisted colectomy. Localization of the tumor with fluorescence is typically accomplished after the exteriorization of the colon through a small laparotomy, using a dedicated vision system. The results of these studies have demonstrated the feasibility of this technique without adverse events [34–36].

The da Vinci fluorescence vision system allows the surgeon to see the tumor in real time during fully robotic surgery for an oncologically safe resection.

The ICG is injected endoscopically, as for lymph node mapping, but the injected dose should be minimal. It must not pass in the peritoneum and must be performed shortly before surgery (Fig. 36.21). This timing is an important limitation, especially in a proximal colonic neoplasia, because an endoscopy can overinflate the colon, making the operation difficult or impossible. An alternative solution could be intraoperative endoscopy, closing the colon upstream with a bowel clamp, so as to perform a tattoo visually guided by the surgeon. This matter is a subject of discussion for the generation of further studies.

References

1. Landsman ML, Kwant G, Mook GA, et al. Light-absorbing properties, stability, and spectral stabilization of indocyanine green. J Appl Physiol. 1976;40:575–83.
2. Alford R, Simpson HM, Duberman J, et al. Toxicity of organic fluorophores used in molecular imaging: literature review. Mol Imaging. 2009;8:341–54.
3. Speich R, Saesseli B, Hoffmann U, et al. Anaphylactoid reactions after indocyanine-green administration. Ann Intern Med. 1988;109:345–6.
4. Shimizu S, Kamiike W, Hatanaka N, et al. New method for measuring ICG Rmax with a clearance meter. World J Surg. 1995;19:113–8.
5. Frangioni JV. New technologies for human cancer imaging. J Clin Oncol. 2008;26:4012–21.
6. Ishizawa T, Bandai Y, Ijichi M, Kaneko J, Hasegawa K, Kokudo N. Fluorescent cholangiography illuminating the biliary tree during laparoscopic cholecystectomy. Br J Surg. 2010;97(9):1369–77.
7. Watanabe M, Tsunoda A, Narita K, Kusano M, Miwa M. Colonic tattooing using fluorescence imaging with light-emitting diode-activated indocyanine green: a feasibility study. Surg Today. 2009;39(3):214–8.
8. Hutteman M, Choi HS, Mieog JS, van der Vorst JR, Ashitate Y, Kuppen PJ, van Groningen MC, Löwik CW, Smit VT, van de Velde CJ, Frangioni JV, Vahrmeijer AL. Clinical translation of ex vivo sentinel lymph node mapping for colorectal cancer using invisible near-infrared fluorescence light. Ann Surg Oncol. 2011;18(4):1006–14.
9. Kudszus S, Roesel C, Schachtrupp A, Höer JJ. Intraoperative laser fluorescence angiography in colorectal surgery: a noninvasive analysis to reduce the rate of anastomotic leakage. Langenbecks Arch Surg. 2010;395(8):1025–30.
10. Adamsen S, Hansen OH, Funch-Jensen P, Schulze S, Stage JG, Wara P. Bile duct injury during laparoscopic cholecystectomy: a prospective nationwide series. J Am Coll Surg. 1997;184:571–8.
11. Flum DR, Cheadle A, Prela C, Dellinger EP, Chan L. Bile duct injury during cholecystectomy and survival in medicare beneficiaries. JAMA. 2003;290:2168–73.
12. Strasberg SM, Hertl M, Soper NJ. An analysis of the problem of biliary injury during laparoscopic cholecystectomy. J Am Coll Surg. 1995;180:101–25.
13. Dolan JP, Diggs BS, Sheppard BC, Hunter JG. 10-year trend in the national volume of bile duct

injuries requiring operative repair. Surg Endosc. 2005;19:967–73.
14. Connor S, Garden OJ. Bile duct injury in the era of laparoscopic cholecystectomy. Br J Surg. 2006;93: 158–68.
15. Spinoglio G, Lenti LM, Maglione V, Lucido FS, Priora F, Bianchi PP, Grosso F, Quarati R. Single-site robotic cholecystectomy (SSRC) versus single-incision laparoscopic cholecystectomy (SILC): comparison of learning curves. First European experience. Surg Endosc. 2012;26(6):1648–55. doi:10.1007/s00464-011-2087-1.
16. MacFadyen BV. Intraoperative cholangiography: past, present, and future. Surg Endosc. 2006;20 Suppl 2:S436–40.
17. Ishizawa T, Tamura S, Masuda K, Aoki T, Hasegawa K, Imamura H, Beck Y, Kokudo N. Intraoperative fluorescent cholangiography using indocyanine green: a biliary road map for safe surgery. J Am Coll Surg. 2009;208(1):e1–4.
18. Buchs NC, Hagen ME, Pugin F, Volonte F, Bucher P, Shiffer E, Morel P. Intra-operative fluorescent cholangiography using indocyanine green during robotic single site cholecystectomy. Int J Med Robot. 2012. doi:10.1002/rcs.1437.
19. Van Geldere D, Fa-Si-Oen P, Noach LA, Rietra PJ, Peterse JL, Boom RP. Complications after colorectal surgery without mechanical bowel preparation. J Am Coll Surg. 2002;194(1):40–4.
20. Grzebieniak Z, Szynglarewicz B. Anastomotic leakage following anterior resection for rectal carcinoma. Przegl Lek. 2006;63(7):543–6.
21. Vignali A, Gianotti L, Braga M, Radaelli G, Malvezzi L, Di Carlo V. Altered microperfusion at the rectal stump is predictive for rectal anastomotic leak. Dis Colon Rectum. 2000;43(1):76–82.
22. Karliczek A, Harlaar NJ, Zeebregts CJ, Wiggers T, Baas PC, van Dam GM. Surgeons lack predictive accuracy for anastomotic leakage in gastrointestinal surgery. Int J Colorectal Dis. 2009;24:569–76.
23. Giuliano AE, Kirgan DM, Guenther JM, Morton DL. Lymphatic mapping and sentinel lymphadenectomy for breast cancer. Ann Surg. 1994;220:391–8.
24. Morton DL, Thompson JF, Essner R, Elashoff R, Stern SL, Nieweg OE, et al. Validation of the accuracy of intraoperative lymphatic mapping and sentinel lymphadenectomy for early stage melanoma: a multicenter trial. Multicenter Selective Lymphadenectomy Trial Group. Ann Surg. 1999;230:453–63.
25. Adell G, Boeryd B, Frånlund B, Sjödahl R, Håkansson L. Occurrence and prognostic importance of micrometastases in regional lymph nodes in Dukes' B colorectal carcinoma: an immunohistochemical study. Eur J Surg. 1996;162:637–42.
26. Noura S, Yamamoto H, Ohnishi T, Masuda N, Matsumoto T, Takayama O, et al. Comparative detection of lymph node micrometastases of stage II colorectal cancer by reverse transcriptase polymerase chain reaction and immunohistochemistry. J Clin Oncol. 2002;20:4232–41.
27. Palma RT, Waisberg J, Bromberg SH, Simão AB, Godoy AC. Micrometastasis in regional lymph nodes of extirpated colorectal carcinoma: immunohistochemical study using anti-cytokeratin antibodies AE1/AE3. Colorectal Dis. 2003;5:164–8.
28. Kitai T, Inomoto T, Miwa M, Shikayama T. Fluorescence navigation with indocyanine green for detecting sentinel lymph nodes in breast cancer. Breast Cancer. 2005;12:211–5.
29. Kusano M, Tajima Y, Yamazaki K, Kato M, Watanabe M, Miwa M. Sentinel node mapping guided by indocyanine green fluorescence imaging: a new method for sentinel node navigation surgery in gastrointestinal cancer. Dig Surg. 2008;25: 103–8.
30. Miyashiro I, Miyoshi N, Hiratsuka M, Kishi K, Yamada T, Ohue M, et al. Detection of sentinel node in gastric cancer surgery by indocyanine green fluorescence imaging: comparison with infrared imaging. Ann Surg Oncol. 2008;15:1640–3.
31. Ponsky JL, King JF. Endoscopic marking of colonic lesions. Gastrointest Endosc. 1975;22:42–7.
32. Gianom D, Hollinger A, Wirth HP. Intestinal perforation after preoperative colonic tattooing with India ink. Swiss Surg. 2003;9:307–10.
33. Yano H, Okada K, Monden T. Adhesion ileus caused by tattoo marking: unusual complication after laparoscopic surgery for early colorectal cancer. Dis Colon Rectum. 2003;46:987.
34. Price N, Gottfried MR, Clary E, Lawson DC, Baillie J, Mergener K, et al. Safety and efficacy of India ink and indocyanine green as colonic tattooing agents. Gastrointest Endosc. 2000;51:438–70.
35. Lane KL, Vallera R, Washington K, Gottfried MR. Endoscopic tattoo agents in the colon; tissue responses and clinical implications. Am J Surg Pathol. 1996;20:1266–70.
36. Lee JG, Low AH, Leung JW. Randomized comparative study of indocyanine green and India ink for colonic tattooing. An animal survival study. J Clin Gastroenterol. 2000;31:233–6.

Part XV

Future

Robotics and Remote Surgery: Next Step

37

Jacques Marescaux and Michele Diana

"All glory comes from daring to begin."

Eugene F. Ware

Introduction

Surgery has been practiced for thousands of years, and there is evidence of some embryonic form of surgery that goes back to prehistory, with clues of rudimental procedures such as skull burr holes. Hippocrates (480–390 BC) defined surgery as the therapeutic activity performed by means of the "hands." As a character, the surgeon has been surrounded by some sort of mysticism since he/she would "touch" the sacred and secret nature of the human body, with his/her bare hands. In the Middle Ages, surgery was banned by medical academies in Europe, and surgical acts were pursued only by men whose activities required craftsmanship (e.g., barbers, butchers, bonesetters) with outstanding manual skills but who were often ignorant about anatomy or physiology. Nineteenth-century discoveries in the fundamental fields of antisepsis and anesthesia enabled the wider use of surgery to treat diseases. The twentieth century has seen the addition of thrilling new technologies to the operating room such as electrocautery. They have enabled the surgeon to perform more complex procedures while concurrently reducing surgical risks. Throughout the evolution of surgery, the physical presence and the real tactile abilities of the operating surgeon have been a constant.

The advent of minimally invasive endoscopic surgery (MIES) techniques in the mid-1980s is considered one of the most groundbreaking surgical innovations. MIES has been the first step towards a successful surgeon-patient distancing process. MIES respects the therapeutic principles of open surgery with reduced surgical trauma since the surgical field is created through small skin incisions and visualized by high-definition cameras and the organs are manipulated with micro-instruments. With the hands of the surgeon away from the patient's body, surgical trauma is reduced, and outcomes are undeniably better with fewer surgical site infections [1, 2], less pain and fewer hernias [3], and improved cosmetic outcome. However, MIES is not straightforward, and the surgeon is faced with some totally new challenges [4] for (1) reduced depth perception due to the 2D vision offered by the flat screen, (2) loss of haptic proprioception due to hand-eye disconnection, (3) limited field of view, and (4) reduced tactile sensation which is possible with laparoscopic instruments. Robotic science offers specific innovations to facilitate MIES. The da Vinci® system (Surgical Intuitive) is a commercial surgical robotic platform equipped with a binocular camera that provides a stereoscopic, tenfold magnified, and high-resolution view. It also offers a haptic interface, which allows the surgeon

J. Marescaux, M.D., F.A.C.S., (Hon.) F.R.C.S., (Hon.) J.S.E.S. (✉) • M. Diana, M.D.
Department of Digestive and Endocrine Surgery, IRCAD (Research Institute against Digestive Cancer), 1, place de l'Hôpital, 67091 Strasbourg, France
e-mail: jacques.marescaux@ircad.fr; Michele.diana@ircad.fr

K.C. Kim (ed.), *Robotics in General Surgery*, DOI 10.1007/978-1-4614-8739-5_37,

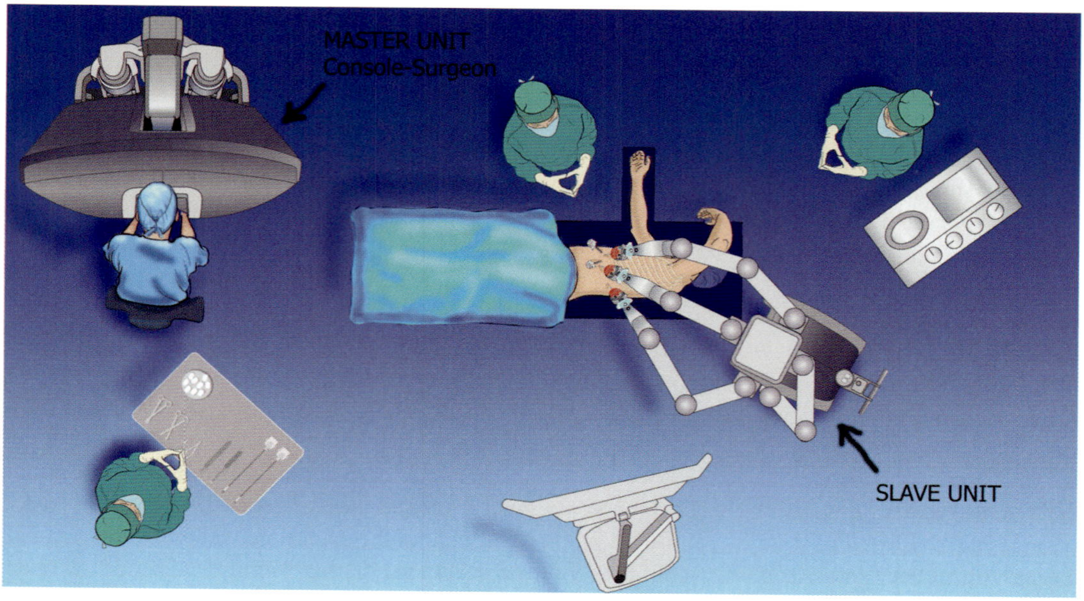

Fig. 37.1 Operative setup with the master–slave surgical robotic platform. The surgeon and control panel (master unit) are separate from patient and robotic arms (slave unit). This is the basic configuration of a surgical robot that enables telesurgery

to be comfortably seated. The surgeon can command the instruments with movements very similar to that of natural hand movement, while effectors exactly replicate the movements into a precise and downscaled fashion, hence eliminating physiological tremors (Fig. 37.1). Additionally, at the turn of the twenty-first century, robotics has yielded technology facilitating surgeon-patient distancing, taking this to extremes, and, as a result, breaking up the frontiers of "telesurgery."

Robotics and Remote Surgery: Expanding Boundaries

The idea to apply robotic technologies to surgery dates back to the 1970s when a military project of the National Aeronautics and Space Administration (NASA) aimed to provide surgical care to astronauts with remotely controlled robots and to replace the surgeon's physical presence in situations of mass casualties in hostile environments such as war or natural catastrophes. The first generation of surgical robots that entered the OR was designed to perform image-guided precision tasks but was limited by basic computer interfaces. Of note is the PUMA 200 industrial robot used since 1985 for CT-guided brain biopsy [5] or the ultrasound-guided PROBOT, introduced in 1988 and used to perform prostate resections [6]. The first commercially available medical robot was manufactured in 1992 and was known as the ROBODOC (Integrated Surgical Systems, Sacramento, CA), which was approved to guide the surgeon during hip prosthetic replacements. The evolution of surgical robots has led to a current generation of real-time telemanipulators where robotic effectors reproduce the surgeon's hand motion in a "master–slave" configuration. In these units, the "master" control console, from which the surgeon operates, is physically separated from the "slave" unit, composed of the robotic arms performing surgery on the patient. Two FDA-approved surgical robots originated from the DARPA (Defense Advanced Research Project Administration)-funded projects: the da Vinci® Surgical System (Intuitive Surgical, Inc., Sunnyvale, CA) and the Zeus® system

(Computer Motion, Goleta, CA). Intuitive Surgery absorbed Computer Motion in 2003, and the only robotic platform available on the market today is the da Vinci® System.

Robotic surgery has been used in a vast array of surgical procedures, and although clinical benefits are not yet clear, the ability to perform remote surgery is certainly unique to the robotic interface.

The data transmission speed is the primary difficulty with teleoperations, especially over large distances or in the presence of insufficient retransmission infrastructures. Early systems, in fact, required the surgeon to be in the same room as the patient. However, with the use of high-speed telecommunications, both telementoring and telemanipulation were attempted from remote locations [7, 8].

Telementoring is the possibility for expert surgeons to mentor local surgeons through telepresence [9]. Telementoring programs that offer rural hospitals the possibility to gain full benefit of specialist advice are being established worldwide. One early report from 1996 demonstrated the ability of a surgeon located in the same city to successfully mentor another surgeon as well as to manipulate an endoscopic camera [10]. Cubano et al. [7] reported the efficacy of telementoring laparoscopic hernia repairs to surgeons operating on the Maryland-USS Abraham Lincoln Aircraft Carrier. Further reports have shown that specialist surgical skills can be disseminated effectively through telementoring [11].

Network latency affects the surgical performance with a longer task completion time of a factor of 1.45 and 2.04 in the presence of delays of data transmission of 250 ms and 500 ms, respectively, when compared to no time delay [12]. However, operators may still perform surgical training with a low error rate even at delays of approximately 1,000 ms [13]. Initially, latency in data transmission limited telemanipulation to a distance of a few 100 km [14].

In September 2001, the first transatlantic surgical procedure (Operation Lindbergh) covering the distance between New York (United States) and Strasbourg (France) was performed by our team. This is considered to be the milestone of global telesurgery [15]. In the Lindbergh operation, a combination of high-speed fiber-optic connection was used with an average delay of 155 ms with advanced asynchronous transfer mode (ATM) along with the Zeus® telemanipulator.

Now that one expert surgeon can operate from across continents, what is the next step?

The ultimate application for robotic telesurgery is probably the one that was initially conceived by the NASA: to provide surgical care to astronauts during long-lasting, extreme distance space explorative missions in which self-sufficiency of the space crew to face surgical emergencies is mandatory.

The challenges that must be overcome to make this possible are still manifold: the ability to perform surgery in reduced gravity conditions, portable and light equipment, and, most importantly, the possibility of cosmic distance data transmission.

The feasibility of Zero-Gravity surgery has been demonstrated with a cyst removal on a human subject onboard the European Space Agency (ESA) Airbus A-300 Zero-G Aircraft. Weightlessness phases were achieved performing parabolic curves [16]. Similarly, experimental laparoscopic surgery on a pig model is feasible in weightlessness [17], with only minor disturbances due to lack of gravity.

In addition, intensive research in miniaturization of surgical telemanipulators is under way, and a number of prototypes have been built with the aim to extend the possibilities for telesurgery, offering a lighter and more practical platform. The Raven (University of Washington, BioRobotics Lab) is a portable 22 kg mass robotic tool with two articulated arms. It has been conceived for both open and MIES [18], and it integrates long-distance remote control links. Another prototype under evaluation is the M7. It is also a light and portable device, developed by Stanford Research International, equipped with two arms with 7 Degrees of Freedom (DOF), and which integrates haptic feedback [19]. The software of the M7 is suitable for teleoperations, and in September 2007, it was successfully tested in the NASA first Zero-Gravity robotic experience during parabolic flights [20].

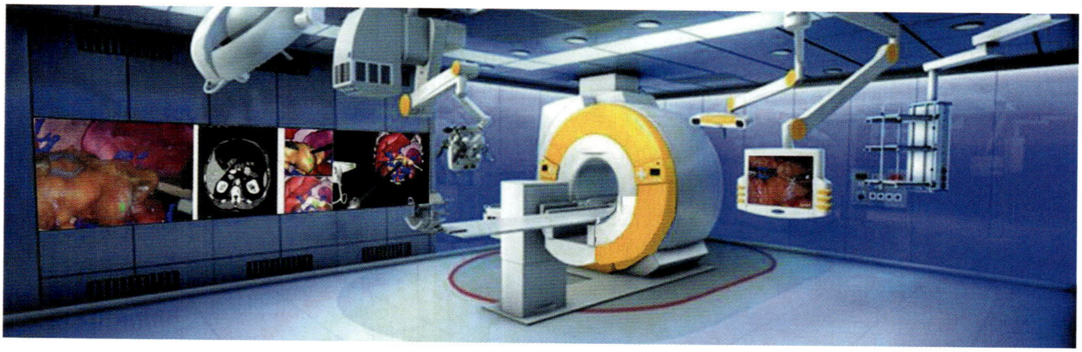

Fig. 37.2 Interactive spacecraft operating room: view of an interactive operating room. The integration of Virtual Reality and Augmented Reality monitors and on-site Medical Imaging facilities offers the remotely located surgeon an immersive and informative environment that enables Image-Guided Telesurgery

Internet-based communication speed and quality are sufficient to practice telesurgery on planet Earth, with reasonable delays of around 400 ms, but it is not suitable for space missions. Telesurgery in extremely remote locations requires more advanced telecommunications [21, 22]. The ability to provide real-time interaction between the spacecraft and the ground is obviously inversely related to distance. Taking advantage of satellite-based transmissions, with signals propagating at light speed (300,000 km/s), approximately 1-s delay would be experienced for an Earth-Moon distance, which is still reasonable for simple remotely controlled procedures. For very large distances, as an example, for an average orbiting distance between the Earth and Mars (72 million km), the delay would be around 6 min, which means that remotely controlling real-time procedures would not be possible, neither would be telementoring. The limitations for effective telementoring are probably below a 60-s delay. Beyond this range, a trained surgeon should be onboard and able to perform "solo."

The development of preoperative simulation using Virtual Reality (VR) patient models, and real-time guidance systems based on Augmented Reality (AR), could well provide invaluable support to solve the issue of semi-real-time monitoring of the surgical act.

VR medical software programs may elaborate a 3D virtual model of the patient from Digital Imaging and Communication in Medicine (DICOM) format images. This 3D virtual model enables to navigate through the human body and to perform a virtual exploration, highlighting anatomical details, which might be underestimated on a customary image [23, 24]. The virtual exploration can assist the preparatory phase of the surgical procedure through interactive and visual planning of the strategy and simulation.

Subsequently, during the intraoperative phase, the 3D VR model may be superimposed onto real-time patient images providing Augmented Reality. This fusion of live images and synthetic computer-generated patient-specific images may provide the surgeon in space with an enhanced navigation tool, highlighting target structures and anatomical variations through a modular virtual organ transparency. Through this computer-assisted surgery, ground-spacecraft communication lag time would be less important (Fig. 37.2).

At the IRCAD, AR guidance was pioneered in a series of laparoscopic adrenal tumor resections [25], using customary software (VR RENDER®) to construct the virtual model of the patient. The system allowed a very accurate navigation with a maximum error of 2 mm. Subsequently, we have applied the same concept to liver surgery [23] and, more recently, to minimally invasive parathyroid surgery [24]. We are currently working on a system to improve "registration," which is the ability to exactly superimpose 3D preoperative model to live images and, secondly, to develop an automatic registration process. Our aim is to establish a blueprint for the ultimate solution for extreme distance surgery: the automation of the surgical procedure via the surgical robotic interface. Although a lot of work is still needed, some of the required technology is already available or under development.

Automation would require the integration of (1) fully automatic Augmented Reality with imaging systems apt to provide real-time refresh and registration, (2) a self-controlled robotic platform through algorithms which implement surgical steps, patient-specific anatomy, and (3) an organ motion prediction.

An elegant demonstration of semiautonomous telesurgical procedure was made in 2006 through a telerobotic atrial fibrillation ablation over a distance between Boston and Milan using an intravascular robot-guided catheter, taking advantage of real-time electromagnetic navigation and preoperative CT-scan images of the patient. The main interest of the system was in that it could create the surgical plane autonomously, using a stochastic model based on an anatomical atlas of 10,000 patients [26].

At our institute, an AR patient-specific surgical simulation is currently under development, using customary medical imaging software (VR RENDER®), which implements the breathing motion and the heart beating of the patient allowing to predict the organ displacement.

Telesurgery is still in its infancy, and significant challenges pervade including technical aspects, surgical robotic platforms, cost-effectiveness, and, mostly, data transfer speed. The potential benefits of telesurgery have become clearer with telementoring programs, but the "niche" applications such as space missions and military projects would be the primer for further developments in the allocation of funds and in the attribution of highly specialized human resources. The maturation of this futuristic field is expected to take place in a stepwise fashion, considering the technology required for this process to occur, but then again, one should remember that the world has not been created in a single day but step by step.

References

1. Diana M, Hubner M, Eisenring MC, Zanetti G, Troillet N, Demartines N. Measures to prevent surgical site infections: what surgeons (should) do. World J Surg. 2011;35:280–8.
2. Hubner M, Diana M, Zanetti G, Eisenring MC, Demartines N, Troillet N. Surgical site infections in colon surgery: the patient, the procedure, the hospital, and the surgeon. Arch Surg. 2011;146:1240–5.
3. Diana M, Dhumane P, Cahill RA, Mortensen N, Leroy J, Marescaux J. Minimal invasive single-site surgery in colorectal procedures: current state of the art. J Minim Access Surg. 2011;7:52–60.
4. Tekkis PP, Senagore AJ, Delaney CP, Fazio VW. Evaluation of the learning curve in laparoscopic colorectal surgery: comparison of right-sided and left-sided resections. Ann Surg. 2005;242:83–91.
5. Kwoh YS, Hou J, Jonckheere EA, Hayati S. A robot with improved absolute positioning accuracy for CT guided stereotactic brain surgery. IEEE Trans Biomed Eng. 1988;35:153–60.
6. Harris SJ, Arambula-Cosio F, Mei Q, et al. The Probot–an active robot for prostate resection. Proc Inst Mech Eng H. 1997;211:317–25.
7. Cubano M, Poulose BK, Talamini MA, et al. Long distance telementoring. A novel tool for laparoscopy aboard the USS Abraham Lincoln. Surg Endosc. 1999;13:673–8.
8. Gagner M, Begin E, Hurteau R, Pomp A. Robotic interactive laparoscopic cholecystectomy. Lancet. 1994;343:596–7.
9. Ballantyne GH. Robotic surgery, telerobotic surgery, telepresence, and telementoring. Review of early clinical results. Surg Endosc. 2002;16:1389–402.
10. Moore RG, Adams JB, Partin AW, Docimo SG, Kavoussi LR. Telementoring of laparoscopic procedures: initial clinical experience. Surg Endosc. 1996;10:107–10.
11. Schlachta CM, Lefebvre KL, Sorsdahl AK, Jayaraman S. Mentoring and telementoring leads to effective incorporation of laparoscopic colon surgery. Surg Endosc. 2010;24:841–4.
12. Lum MJ, Rosen J, King H, et al. Teleoperation in surgical robotics–network latency effects on surgical performance. Conf Proc IEEE Eng Med Biol Soc. 2009;2009:6860–3.
13. Rayman R, Croome K, Galbraith N, et al. Long-distance robotic telesurgery: a feasibility study for care in remote environments. Int J Med Robot. 2006;2:216–24.
14. Satava RM. Emerging technologies for surgery in the 21st century. Arch Surg. 1999;134:1197–202.
15. Marescaux J, Leroy J, Gagner M, et al. Transatlantic robot-assisted telesurgery. Nature. 2001;413:379–80.

16. 'Weightless' surgery performed for first time. The Independent. 2006 Sep 28 [Cited 2012 May 10]. http://www.independent.co.uk/news/world/europe/weightless-surgery-performed-for-first-time-417826.html)
17. Kirkpatrick AW, Keaney M, Kmet L, et al. Intraperitoneal gas insufflation will be required for laparoscopic visualization in space: a comparison of laparoscopic techniques in weightlessness. J Am Coll Surg. 2009;209:233–41.
18. Lum MJ, Rosen J, King H, et al. Telesurgery via Unmanned Aerial Vehicle (UAV) with a field deployable surgical robot. Stud Health Technol Inform. 2007;125:313–5.
19. Doarn CR, Anvari M, Low T, Broderick TJ. Evaluation of teleoperated surgical robots in an enclosed undersea environment. Telemed J E Health. 2009;15:325–35.
20. Haidegger T, Sandor J, Benyo Z. Surgery in space: the future of robotic telesurgery. Surg Endosc. 2011;25:681–90.
21. Rayman R, Croome K, Galbraith N, et al. Robotic telesurgery: a real-world comparison of ground- and satellite-based internet performance. Int J Med Robot. 2007;3:111–6.
22. Ross MD. Medicine in long duration space exploration: the role of virtual reality and broad bandwidth telecommunications networks. Acta Astronaut. 2001;49:441–5.
23. Nicolau S, Soler L, Mutter D, Marescaux J. Augmented reality in laparoscopic surgical oncology. Surg Oncol. 2011;20:189–201.
24. D'Agostino J, Diana M, Soler L, Vix M, Marescaux J. 3D virtual neck exploration prior to parathyroidectomy. N Engl J Med. 2012;367:1072–3.
25. Marescaux J, Rubino F, Arenas M, Mutter D, Soler L. Augmented-reality-assisted laparoscopic adrenalectomy. JAMA. 2004;292:2214–5.
26. Pappone C, Vicedomini G, Manguso F, et al. Robotic magnetic navigation for atrial fibrillation ablation. J Am Coll Cardiol. 2006;47:1390–400.

The Future of Robotic Platforms 38

Mehran Anvari

Introduction

Since its inception, minimally invasive surgery has proven to be advantageous in terms of improved cosmosis, reduced risk of infection, shortened recovery time post-surgery, and reduced pain [1, 2]. These techniques are not without limitations, however, albeit most being technical constraints including a lack of haptic feedback and loss of dexterity (degrees of freedom). Robotic systems have been developed to address these limitations and are continually being advanced to expand on the benefits of minimally invasive surgery and enhance the surgeons' ability. Although robotic-assisted surgery continues to develop and has been shown to reduce hospital stay, pain, and recovery time when compared to conventional surgery [3], the main disadvantages are cost and bulk of current systems, the learning curve associated with the use of current models, and the limited number of cost-effective clinical applications.

Progression in research and design aims to resolve these limitations by reducing the size, improving functionality, and increasing application. As the use of robotics in surgery advances past the investigational stage, and reaches routine practice in many disciplines, the cost will continue to decrease. Technological advances continue to be made with minimized entry ports and improvements in haptic feedback, and visualization with the implementation of magnified imaging, 3D resolution, global positioning and real-time imaging.

There are three distinct architectures of surgical robotics: the master–slave configuration, the image-guided targeted robots, and the micro robots.

Master–Slave Robots

The "master–slave" surgical systems are not a robot in the pure sense of the word, but rather computerized systems, consisting of the console where the surgeon controls the robot (the "master") and the robotic arms holding the instruments being controlled (the "slave"). Major improvements have been made over the years to the master–slave systems since the era of the Zeus and early da Vinci models.

The da Vinci surgical system (Intuitive Surgical, CA, USA) (Fig. 38.1a, b) was the first operative robotic system approved by the US FDA in 2000 [4]. While used in a number of surgical specialties and procedures worldwide, its use in prostatectomy still dominates its application. The most recent version of the surgical system, the da Vinci Si HD (Intuitive Surgical Inc., CA, USA), includes improved features of

M. Anvari, M.B.B.S., Ph.D., F.R.C.S., F.A.C.S. (✉)
Department of Surgery, McMaster University, Hamilton, ON, Canada L8N 4A6

St. Joseph's Healthcare Hamilton, Room G805, 50 Charlton Avenue East, Hamilton, ON, Canada L8N 4A6
e-mail: anvari@mcmaster.ca

K.C. Kim (ed.), *Robotics in General Surgery*, DOI 10.1007/978-1-4614-8739-5_38,

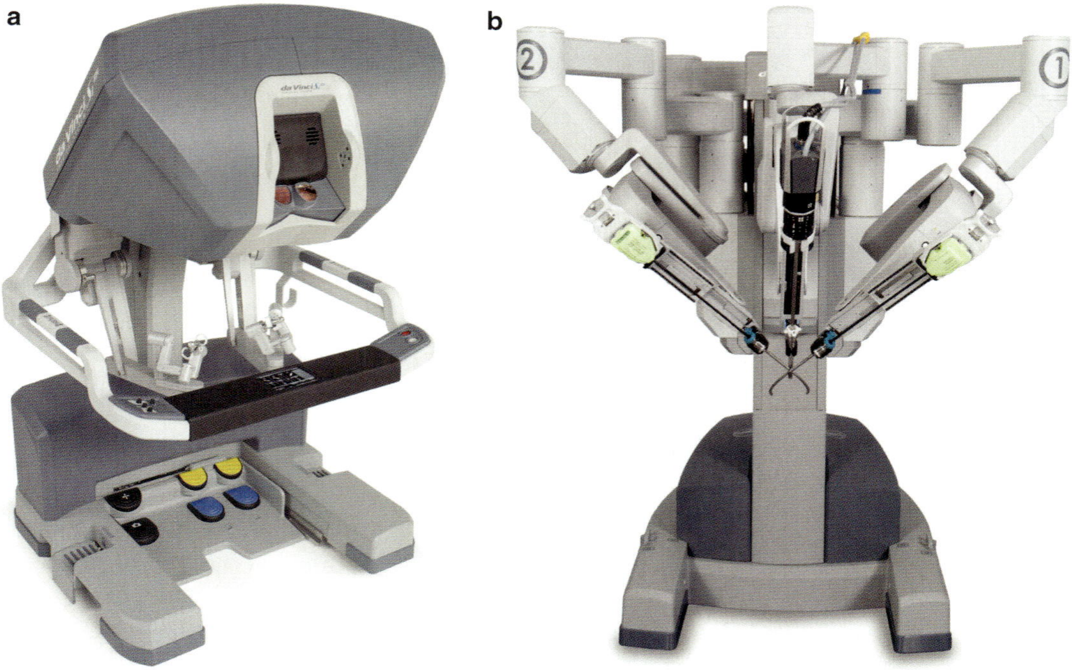

Fig. 38.1 (**a** and **b**) The da Vinci Si HD surgical system: surgeon console and patient cart (© 2009 Intuitive Surgical, Inc., with permission)

3D high-definition visualization, 7 degrees of freedom of movement (DOF), 90 degrees of articulation, intuitive motion finger tip control and tremor, and motion reduction; however, it does not provide haptic feedback, and the system is costly (approximately £1.7 million, 2011 [5]), cumbersome, and bulky. This deficient sense of touch has been explored, with recent developments to restore haptic feedback. The Verro Touch is a device being developed by Kuchenbecker et al. [6] which can be added to the current da Vinci system and emits feedback in the form of high-frequency vibrations and sound in real time.

Other master–slave systems currently being developed include:

The Amadeus by Titan Medical Inc. (Canada) which is a robotic surgical system with multi-articulating arms and single-site and multi-port platform capabilities with infrared and ultrasound imaging and enhanced 3D visualization. Additional features include force feedback and advanced communication technology for patient data, telesurgery, and training [5, 7]. It has been indicated that clinical testing will be initiated in the next 2 years [8]. Titan Medical is also developing a single incision robotic surgical platform with 25 mm access, 3D visualization, and interactive micro-instruments (Fig. 38.2). Projected release of the platform is 2015 [7].

ALF-X (SOFAR S.p.A, Italy) (Fig. 38.3a, b) is a new surgical system undergoing testing in Europe. It enhances surgical dexterity with a realistic tactile-sensing capability due to a patented approach which measures tip/tissue forces, with a sensitivity of 35 g and advanced eye tracking to control view [9]. The robotic system contains four independent arms with adaptable surgical instruments for clinical use in gynecology, urology, and thoracic surgery. With animal trials complete, and indicating significantly reduced procedural time for cholecystectomy compared to the conventional telesurgical system (average of 31.75 min versus 91 min) [10], the ALF-X has now received CE mark and is set to reach market soon [11].

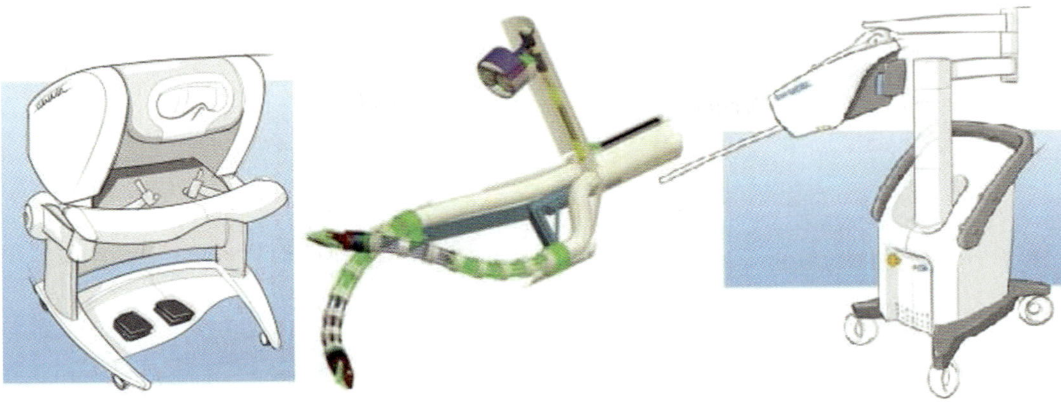

Fig. 38.2 Titan single incision surgery platform, reprinted with permission

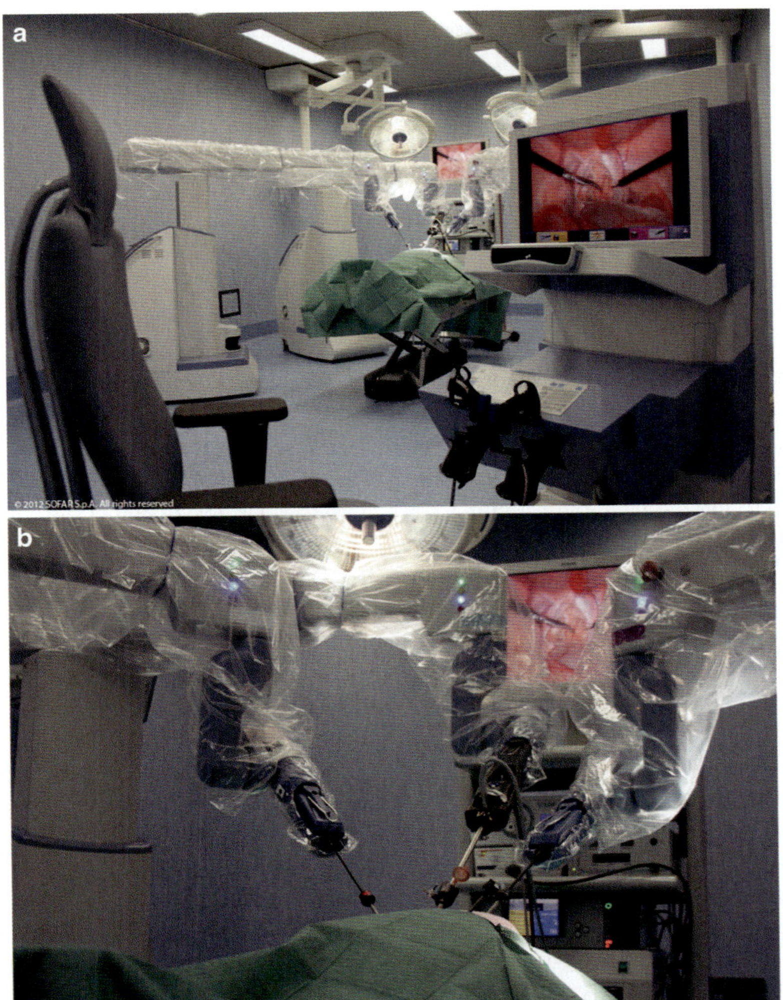

Fig. 38.3 (**a** and **b**) The ALF-X Telelap robot, reprinted with permission

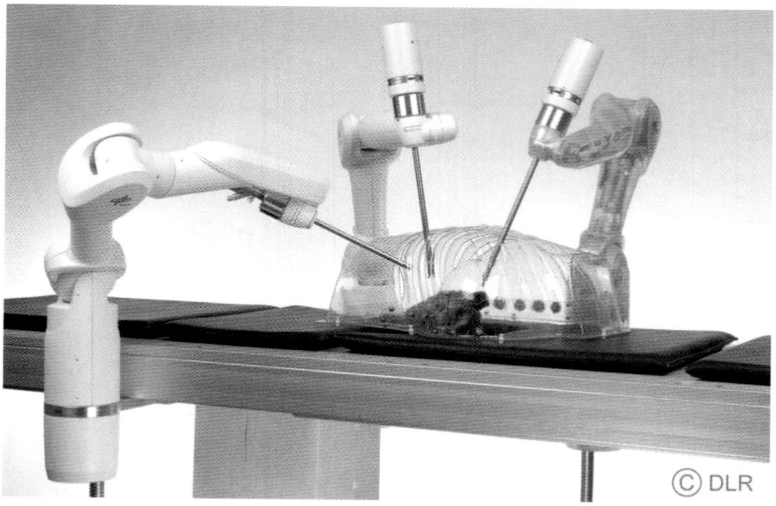

Fig. 38.4 Three DLR MIROs in a setup for minimally invasive surgery (from DLR Institute of Robotics and Mechatronics with permission)

The DLR MIRO system (the Institute for Robotics and Mechatronics, Germany) incorporates haptic feedback through force and tactile feedback or optical tracking [5]. The MiroSurge (Fig. 38.4) is compact and lightweight, consisting of three of the MIRO robotic arms; generally two are used for surgical tools and one for visualization. Each arm has seven torque-controlled joints for flexible movement designed to mimic the human arm. Presently this platform is used for research purposes. Technical advances may include compensation for heartbeat and motion to allow cardiac surgery without stopping the heart [12].

Similarly, developed but not yet available commercially is a remote-operated robotic surgical system named "Sofie": Surgeon's Operating Force-feedback Interface Eindhoven developed by the University of Technology in Eindhoven. The 4D manipulators (surgical arms and a camera) are mounted on the operating table and include a distinctive tactile force feedback system of counter pressure through the joystick controllers [5, 13]. Although this prototype has not yet been released to market, it is anticipated that an advantage of this compact system will be a reduced cost to larger current models [13].

The RAVEN II (the University of Washington and UC Santa Cruz) (Fig. 38.5) consists of two cable-based, articulated aluminum dual arms with 7 DOF, with exterior motors, reducing the size and weight. The robotic prototype is capable of teleoperation and has been released to research labs, with initial application in cardiac surgery, aspiring to include beating heart procedures, with motion compensation and 3D ultrasound imaging capabilities [14, 15].

The NeuroArm (developed at the University of Calgary, AB in collaboration with MacDonald, Dettwiler and Associates Ltd) was one of the first MRI-compatible surgical robotic systems. The master–slave design of this system does not allow freedom of movement by the operating surgeon, but force feedback and real-time imaging combined with preoperative diagnostic images do provide effective tools for reference during the procedure [16]. Used in clinical trial for dissection during microsurgery, successful results were reported with the 34 cases, with one adverse event due to uncontrolled motion of the arm and one conversion to the standard procedure due to reduced access and trouble with positioning during the procedure (Sutherland et al. [17]). The NeuroArm technology was acquired by IMRIS Inc. (NASDAQ: IMRS; TSX: IM) in 2010, after which the SYMBIS neurosurgical robot system was released in 2012 (by IMRIS), pending FDA approval [18].

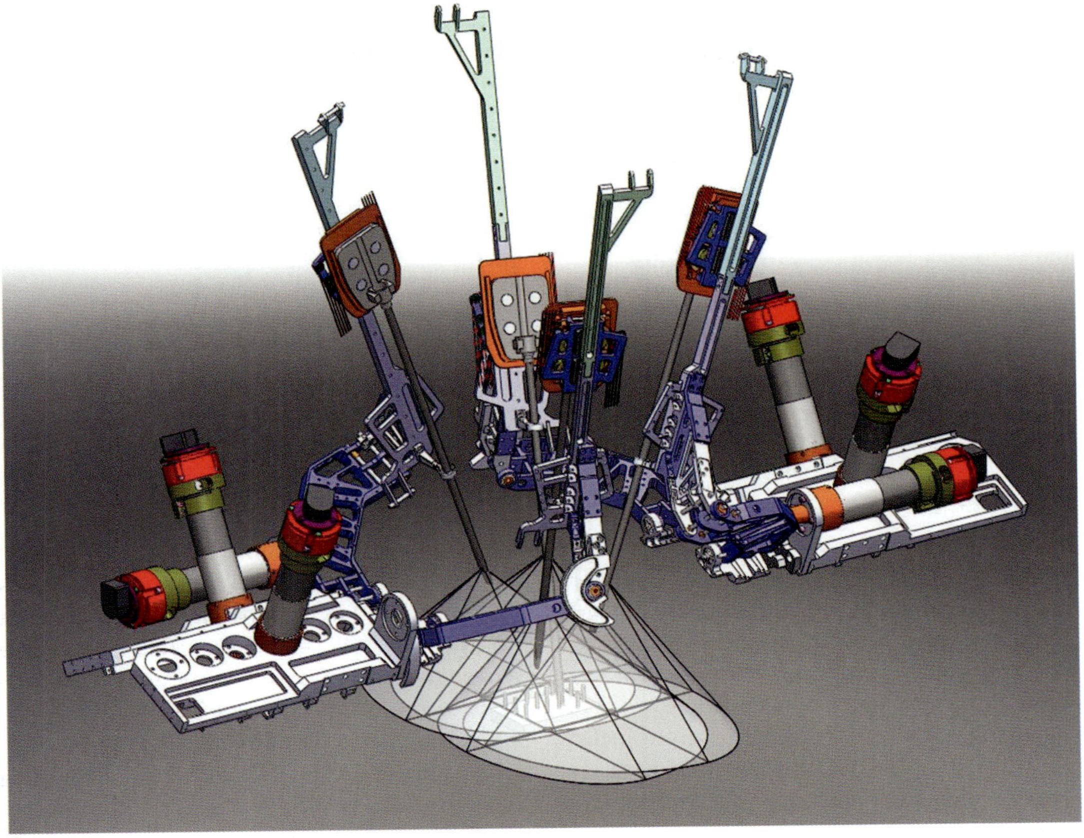

Fig. 38.5 The Raven II, The University of Washington (from: Jacob Rosen, Mika Sinanan, and Blake Hannaford, Objective Assessment of Surgical Skills, Chapter 25 in Surgical Robotics, Systems, Applications, and Visions, Jacob Rosen, Blake Hannaford, Richard M. Satava (Editors), 1 ed. Springer 2011; Zhi Li, Daniel Glozman, Dejan Milutinovic, and Jacob Rosen, Maximizing Dexterous Workspace and Optimal Port Placement of a Multi-Arm Surgical Robot, ICRA 2011, Shanghai, China, May 2011; H. Hawkeye King, Lei Cheng, Philip Roan, Diana Friedman, Sina Nia Kosari, Ji Ma, Daniel Glozman Jacob Rosen, Blake Hannaford, Raven II™: Open Platform for Surgical Robotics Research, The Hamlyn Symposium on Medical Robotics, July 1–2 2012, London, UK; H. Hawkeye King, Blake Hannaford, Ka-Wai Kwok, Guang-Zhong Yang, Paul Griffiths3, Allison Okamura, Ildar Farkhatdinov, Jee-Hwan Ryu, Ganesh Sankaranarayanan, Venkata Arikatla, Suvranu De, Kotaro Tadano, Kenji Kawashima, Angelika Peer, Thomas Schuß, Martin Buss, Levi Miller, Daniel Glozman, Jacob Rosen, Thomas Low, Plugfest 2009: Global Interoperability in Telerobotics and Telemedicine, IEEE International Conference on Robotics and Automation, ICRA May 2010, Alaska, USA with permission)

The Robin Heart 2 robot (developed by the Foundation for Cardiac Surgery Development, Zabrze, Poland) consists of two or more arms for tools and a camera, allowing the surgeon to essentially perform three roles (of two surgeons and an endoscopic assistant) [19]. Future development includes computer simulation and operative planning with application in cardiac surgery for valve repair and replacement, laser revascularization, and possible future utilization in drug delivery and robotic-assisted artificial organ surgery [20].

Continued research and development efforts into the master–slave surgical robotic system and the application of Laparo-Endoscopic Single-Site Surgery (LESS) and Natural Orifice Translumenal Endoscopic Surgery (NOTES) to further reduce surgical invasiveness, and decrease

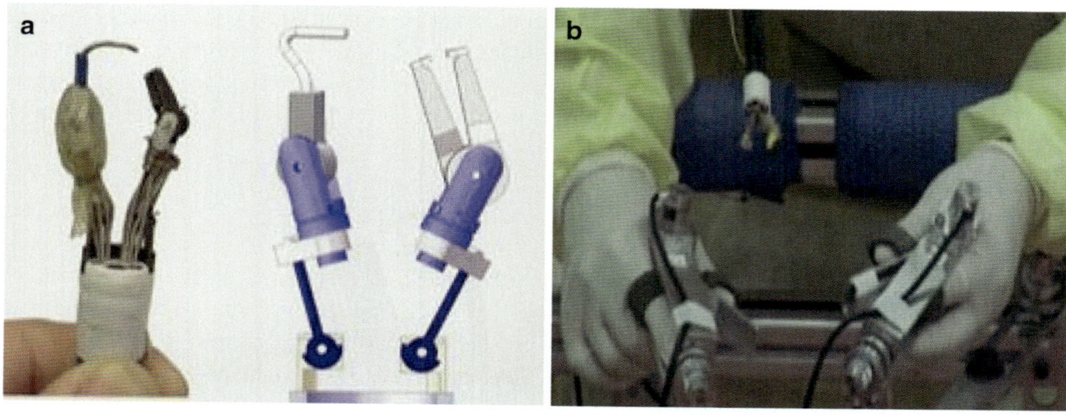

Fig. 38.6 (**a** and **b**) The robotic slave manipulator with two steerable articulating arms and controller (MASTER) (From Felice Cosentino, Emanuele Tumino, Giovanni Rubis Passoni, Antonella Rigante, Roberta Barbera, Antonella Tauro and Philipp Emanuel Cosentino (2011). Robotic Colonoscopy, Colonoscopy, Paul Miskovitz (Ed.), ISBN: 978-953-307-568-6, InTech with permission)

port and trocar access, have brought forth new robotic prototypes. Ideally, robotic platforms for LESS should have the desired instrument maneuverability, dexterity, and freedom of movement and restored triangulation without instrument clashing for precise movement [21]. Designs to current systems have been improved to include pre-bent curved, flexible, and articulating arms to increase maneuverability. Clinical application of robotic-assisted NOTES has been demonstrated in preclinical and clinical study using various approaches. Transgastric, transvesical, and transcolonic approaches have been used in abdominal surgery, colonoscopy, and endoscopy [22].

An agile transluminal endoscopic robot (Master And Slave Transluminal Endoscopic Robot, MASTER) (Fig. 38.6a, b) was developed by Singapore's Nanyang Technological University and National University Hospital to overcome some of the limitations of standard endoscopic devices, including the lack of triangulation [23]. The controller of this system attaches to the wrist and fingers of the operating surgeon, allowing for 9 DOF. Animal trials using the MASTER for endoscopic submucosal dissection (ESD) with NOTES have been conducted with promising results [24], and early results from human trials showed evidence of a shortened procedure time [25]. This system is anticipated to be released to market in the near future.

A computer-assisted robotic technology system, the NeoGuide (NeoGuide Systems Inc., San Jose, CA, USA), has been developed and approved for application during colonoscopy [26]. The system incorporates a tip sensor that continually records the steering commands and an external sensor that records the insertion depth to guide the scope along the natural shape of the colon [27]. A compact endoscopic robot ViKY (EndoControl Medical, France) has been developed, recently obtaining CE mark and FDA approval [28]. The system can be voice controlled or foot switch operated to robotically control the laparoscopic camera with an innovative instrument tracking system [29].

Advances in surgical robotic systems have generated the integration of preoperative and intraoperative imaging for procedural guidance and tracking of tools during surgical intervention while accounting for organ movement [30]. A body-global positioning system for navigation and organ tracking has been pioneered by Ukimura and Gill [30]. This ability to integrate preoperative imaging can also be beneficial in pre-planning, training, and mentoring. Many systems utilize the overlaid images obtained through computerized tomography (CT), magnetic resonance imaging (MRI), or ultrasound for procedural guidance. A system for the 3D imaging of tissue in real time using fluorescence imaging has been developed by Intuitive Surgical Inc. for the da Vinci system and is currently in trial, imaging renal cortical tumors to determine the optimal dose of ICG fluorescence for visualization using the SPY scope [31].

Direct Image-Guided Robots

Robotic systems designed for intervention under image guidance are an exciting development, providing targeted therapy with clinical application in oncology, urology, gynecology, general surgery, neurology, and cardiology.

The Cyberknife system (Accuray, Inc., Sunnyvale, CA) (Fig. 38.7) was the first image-guided robotic technology for noninvasive radiation procedures, receiving FDA approval in October of 2001. The system consists of a large robotic arm that can quickly and accurately deliver targeted radiation with converged beams from multiple angles, reducing radiation exposure to surrounding tissue [32]. A real-time image guidance system and respiratory tracking system identifies the position of the patient, making continual adjustments for movement. Established use in brain tumors as well as lesions of the spine, lung, pancreas, liver, and prostate has been reported [33].

The commercially available, FDA-approved, miniature robot, Spine Assist (Mazor Robotics Ltd, Israel) (Fig. 38.8), is a bone-mounted hexapod robot which assists in navigation and guidance for thoracic and lumbar pedicle screw drilling and implantation, vertebral biopsies, and kypho- and vertebroplasties [34]. Future possible developments may include application in craniocervical surgery and cervical and lumbar total disc replacement [34]. Based on experience with the SpineAssist, Mazor Robotics has introduced the Renaissance platform (Mazor Robotics Ltd) which creates a 3D preoperative blueprint of the procedure, synchronizing with the instrumentation to provide an implant procedure within 1 mm of accuracy [35]. The Renaissance platform received CE mark in 2011 and US FDA marketing clearance in 2012 to be used for application in brain and spinal surgery [35].

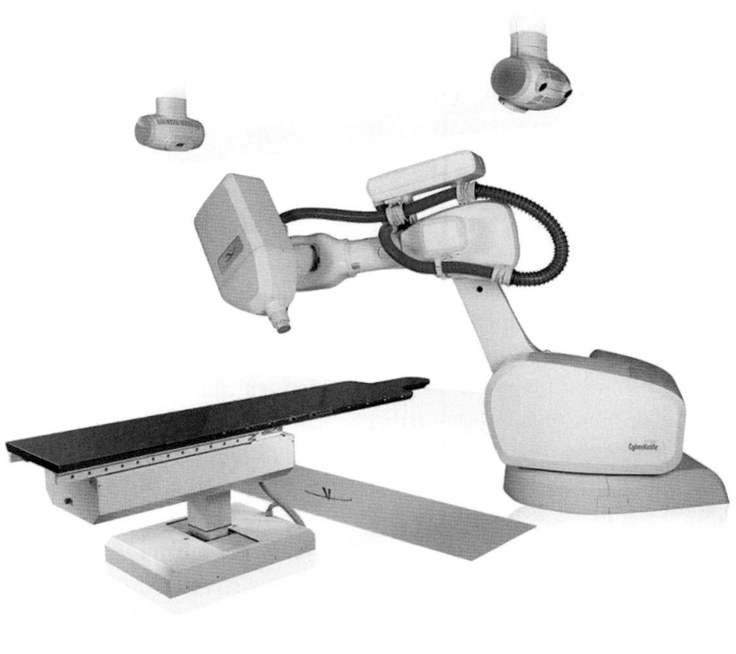

Fig. 38.7 CyberKnife system, Accuray Inc., reprinted with permission

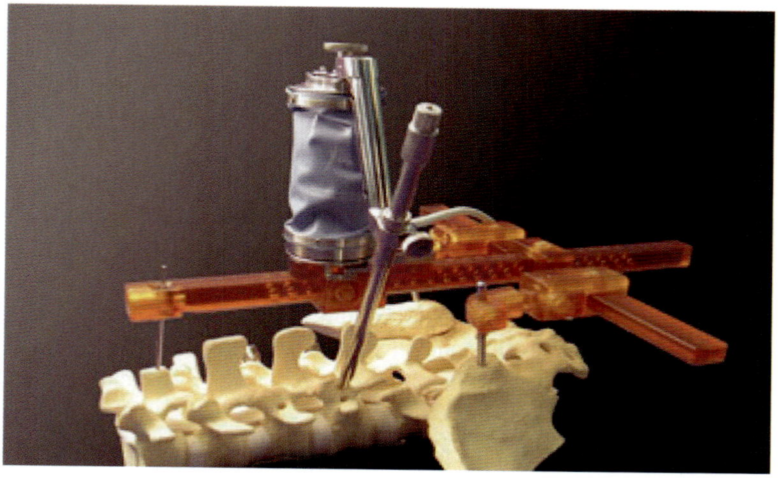

Fig. 38.8 The SpineAssist (Mazor Robotics Ltd, Israel) (From Stüer C, Ringel F, Stoffel M, Reinke A, Behr M, Meyer B. Robotic technology in spine surgery: current applications and future developments. Acta Neurochir Suppl. 2011;109:241–5 with permission)

The RIO (Robotic Arm Interactive Orthopedic System) (MAKO Surgical Corp., USA) received FDA clearance in 2008, for knee joint resurfacing during partial knee and total hip replacement procedures, providing patient-specific pre-planning [36]. The application uses pre-procedure imaging data to create a cutting guide, with integrated digital tracking of the procedure and constant monitoring utilizing visual, tactile, and auditory feedback. The robotic system does not require bone fixation [36], and the feedback resistance system restricts the surgeons' movement to within the planned cutting area [36].

While magnetic resonance (MR)-guided percutaneous interventions, such as biopsies and ablation, have been clinically demonstrated with open-bore systems [37, 38], the closed-bore MR imaging (MRI) scanners provide superior resolution, but offer limited access during imaging and therefore limited feasibility for intervention other than robotic [39]. Innomotion (Innomedic, Herxheim & FZK Karlsruhe Germany & TH Gelsenkir), a CT and MR-compatible robotic instrument-guiding system, was developed to provide precise and reproducible instrument positioning inside the magnet [39]. The Innomotion robotic arm is mounted on specifically designed bed rails, with the transducer attached to the robotic arm guided by the operating surgeon, utilizing MR images and Innomotion software [40].

An MRI-compatible, image-guided, pneumatic, remotely operated robot, the MrBot, has been designed to employ high-precision, image-guided access of the prostate gland, accommodating various needle drivers for different percutaneous interventions such as biopsy, thermal ablations, and brachytherapy [41]. Early results show good accuracy with the image-guided needle and seed placement during testing in a 3 T MRI scanner [42], but no information on commercial availability can be found.

Pfleiderer et al. [43] investigated the feasibility of the ROBITOM II [Institut für Medizintechnik und Biophysik (IMB), Forschungszentrum Karlsruhe und Institut für Diagnostische und Interventionelle Radiologie (IDIR), Jena], a robotic system for MR-guided biopsy and interventional therapy of mammary lesions with the potential to reduce pain, scarring, radiation exposure, as well as time and cost when compared to surgical biopsy. Improvements to the first model were made, including a dedicated double breast coil, which featured an open design for easy access during breast interventions, and a high-speed trocar setting unit [43]. Designed for real-time biopsy procedures within the magnetic bore, with possible future application of therapeutic

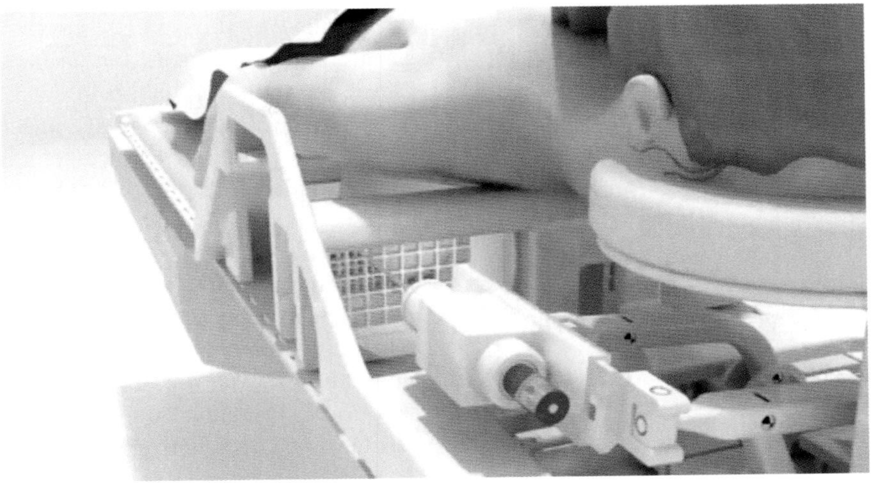

Fig. 38.9 Conceptual rendering of the IGAR system in clinical use with the patient lying prone on a patient support system

treatments during the same procedure, animal and small human feasibility trials have proven successful [43]. No information on commercialization can be found.

MRI-compatible robots continue to be explored in research and development, with promising goals in oncology of improving accuracy and precision for biopsy, radiation, and treatment, with focus on small lesions previously not easily treated. Image-guided robots provide precise, targeted treatment with better cosmosis, reduced pain, and shorter recovery than traditional methods and have future implication in many disciplines including neurosurgery, orthopedics, and urology.

In Hamilton, Ontario, Canada, current development and testing of an image-guided automated robot (IGAR) (Fig. 38.9) for MRI-guided intervention is in progress by the Centre for Surgical Invention and Innovation and MacDonald, Dettwiler and Associates Ltd (MDA). This will be a base technology for image-guided procedures and medical interventions, with the first clinical application of IGAR employed during MRI-guided breast interventions. Future developments will expand to other medical imaging modalities and other clinical applications, including image-guided intervention and ablation of lesions of the lung, liver, kidney, and prostate.

Miniature Robots

Minimizing both the robotic platform and reducing the access needed, while overcoming issues of instrument collision and ergonomic challenge, are important issues facing current surgical platforms. Recent research and development has been focused on the miniaturization of surgical robotics. Miniature robots are either surgically placed or intracorporeally deployed, consisting of fixed-based systems and mobile robots, controlled remotely, performing various tasks. To date, clinical use has been focused on screening for colon cancer, esophageal disorders, and celiac disease [44], with miniature autonomous robots being used for endoscopic imaging and colonoscopy application.

Video capsule endoscopy (VCE) has been developed and used in clinical application for small bowel disease, intestinal disorders, and colon disease. The endoscopic capsule is swallowed by the patient and used to photograph the GI tract. The VCE capsule contains a video camera, a sensing system, a data recorder, and a battery. The capsule moves through the GI tract by visceral peristalsis and gravity; therefore, a major limitation is the lack of control of movement and control of imaging. These limitations have led

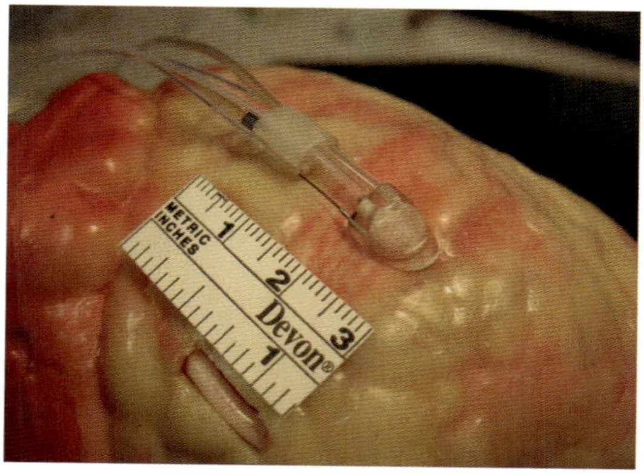

Fig. 38.10 Wire-driven HeartLander model

to exploration of automated, remotely controlled systems.

A miniature in vivo robot developed at the University of Nebraska Medical Center's Center for Advanced Surgical Technology (CAST) is engaged into the abdominal cavity and operated remotely using laparoscopic-type handles. Surgical tasks such as tissue grasping, manipulation, cautery, and intracorporeal suturing are performed with two arms which have been designed to mimic the human arm [45]. The system has been tested successfully in a porcine model, with an intestinal anastomosis procedure and a vessel ligation (Petroni et al. [46]), but has not yet undergone human testing [47].

A similar compact, in vivo prototype, the Insertable Robotic Effectors Platform (IREP), can be folded and deployed into a 15 mm port to perform surgical tasks and consists of two dexterous arms, with eight joints for 7 DOF and 3D stereo vision [19, 48]. The system was developed at Colombia University with the capability of microsurgery, with future development in the application of energy and drug delivery [49]. The technology was acquired by Titan Medical Inc. in early 2012 [7].

Mobile in vivo robots are remotely controlled and are generally propelled with movements based on principles of either the inchworm or the earthworm [50, 51]. A miniature mobile robot for cardiac intervention, the HeartLander (Robotics Institute, Carnegie Mellon University, Pittsburgh, PA) (Fig. 38.10), moves along the epicardium in an inchworm fashion and has proven capability of ambulating and deploying pacing leads and delivering dye injection to the anterior and posterior surfaces of the heart in animal studies [52]. This technology will hopefully be transferable to human interventions, with ablative procedures and regenerative myocardial interventions.

Magnetic anchoring and guidance systems (MAGS) developed by the investigators from University of Texas are micro robots which are fixed to the abdominal wall with external magnets for tissue retraction, cautery, and dissection. Future application may include use in NOTES, as MAGS has proven feasible in animal trials for transvaginal cholecystectomy [53, 54].

Miniature robots address many of the limitations of large master–slave systems used for SILS and NOTES procedures, such as size and the collision of instruments in the limited space (fulcrum effect). The SPRINT (Single-Port lapa-Roscopy bImaNual roboT) (The BioRobotics Institute, Scuola Superiore Sant'Anna, Italy) platform is a teleoperated miniature robot, inserted through the umbilicus. Consisting of two arms with 6 DOF, the handheld manipulators allow translation of the surgeon's hand movements to the end effectors [55].

The technology employed in miniature robotics is under continual development to overcome limitations of function, due to size, and power. Wireless systems, relying on battery life, are limited to an operating time of less than an hour, making their use appropriate in limited situations [56]. Size limitations often result in not being able to implement all desired surgical functions such as visualization, movement, imaging, manipulation, and treatment in the same device. Advancements in propelled movement and biopsy functions are in development [57, 58]. The Korean IMC (Intelligent Microsystems Center) is developing a micro-electro-mechanical systems (MEMS) prototype which integrates micro-optical imaging, physiological sensors, and a micromechanical arm for biopsy, drug delivery, and microsurgery with advanced movement capabilities [59].

Future direction of miniature robotics may include the use of multiple robots to be employed simultaneously, each with a separate function (e.g., one each for imaging, biopsy, resection, and suturing). Micro robots may also incorporate flexible engineering, as has been shown with some current prototypes for VCE, LESS, and NOTES, with more advanced tools for microsurgical intervention (graspers, forceps, scissors, and needledrivers) [22]. VCE may be further developed to allow the control of movement, with the possibility of anchoring the devices, for imaging, sampling of tissue, and target drug delivery [44].

Research and development in the field of nano-robots is an exciting technology, with clinical application perhaps to be seen in the next 5–10 years [60]. Nano-robots have use in target treatment of disease; localizing intravascular cancer cells; providing medication, with future implication in stem cell research; and the treatment of arteriosclerosis, clots, kidney stones, parasites, and gout [61]. The movement and energy systems of these nano-robots continue to be explored, with magnetic fields and biological energy used for targeted drug delivery, cell separation, and manipulation of individual DNA molecules [61–63]. Future applications may include use in the circulatory system, performing targeted drug delivery; removal of plaque or blood clots; and application in neurology, oncology, and urology [32].

Conclusion

The fundamental objective of surgical robotics is to enhance surgical performance beyond human limitations, providing greater quality of care to the patient. As robotic surgical systems and technology become integrated into standard practice, incorporation of robotic training, issues of ethics, and economic feasibility will continue to be explored.

Acknowledgement The author wishes to acknowledge the significant contribution of Ruth Breau in the preparation of this chapter.

Conflict of Interest
This work was not externally funded; the author has not received any financial support.

References

1. Fuchs KH. Minimally invasive surgery. Endoscopy. 2002;34:154–9.
2. Allendorf JD, Bessler M, Whelan RL, et al. Postoperative immune function varies inversely with the degree of surgical trauma in a murine model. Surg Endosc. 1997;11:427–30.
3. Gerhardus D. Robot-assisted surgery: the future is here. J Healthc Manag. 2003;48(4):242–51.
4. Retrieved from http://www.boxchronicles.com/index.php?id=thousands/davinci. The box Chronicles: great moment in technology history: da Vinci Surgical System.
5. Jayne DG, Culmer PR, Barrie J, Hewson R, Neville A. Robotic platforms for general and colorectal surgery. Colorectal Dis. 2011;13 Suppl 7:78–82.
6. Kuchenbecker KJ, Gewirtz J, McMahan W et al. VerroTouch: high-frequency acceleration feedback for telerobotic surgery, haptics: generating and perceiving tangible sensations. In: Proceedings of the EuroHaptics, Part I. Spring; July 2010. p. 189–96.
7. Retrieved from http://www.titanmedicalinc.com.
8. Rippel R. Surgical robotic systems. MetTube Medical jounal. July 14, 2012. Retrieved from http://medtube.net/tribune/surgical-robotic-systems/.
9. Beasley RA. Medical robots: current systems and research directions. J Robot. 2012:1–14.
10. Stark M, Benhidjeb T, Gidaro S, Morales E. The future of telesurgery: a universal system with haptic sensation. J Turkish-German Gynecol Assoc. 2012; 13(1):74–6.
11. Retrieved from http://surgrob.blogspot.ca/2012/01/alf-x-telelap-getting-commercial.html.
12. Tobergte AHP, Hagn U, Rouiller P, Thielmann S, Grange S, Albu-Schäffer A, Conti F, Hirzinger G. The sigma.7 haptic interface for MiroSurge: a new bi-manual surgical console. In: Proceedings of IROS; 2011. p. 3023–3030.
13. Eindhoven University of Technology (2010, September 29). Better surgery with new surgical robot with force feedback. ScienceDaily.
14. Retrieved from http://news.cnet.com/8301-17938_105-57362450-1/paging-raven-ii-the-open-source-surgery-robot/.
15. Retrieved from http://brl.ee.washington.edu/~hawkeye1/documents/r2fs.pdf.
16. Simorov A, Otte RS, Kopietz CM, Oleynikov D. Review of surgical robotics user interface: what is the best way to control robotic surgery? Surg Endosc. 2012;26(8):2117–25.
17. Sutherland GR, Lama S, Gan LS, Wolfsberger S, Zareinia K. Merging machines with microsurgery:

clinical experience with neuroArm. J Neurosurg. 2013;118:521–9.
18. Retrievedfromhttp://www.imris.com/product/evolution-symbis.
19. Nawrat Z. State of the art in medical robotics in Poland: development of the Robin Heart and other robots. Expert Rev Med Devices. 2012;9(4):353–9.
20. Podsedkowski L. RobIn Heart 0, 1, and 3 – mechanical construction development. Bull Pol Acad Sci Tech Sci. 2005;53(1):79–85.
21. Autorino R, Kaouk JH, Stolzenburg JU, Gill IS, Mottrie A, Tewari A, Cadeddu JA. Current status and future directions of robotic single-site surgery: a systematic review. Eur Urol. 2013;63:266–80.
22. Tiwari MM, Reynoso JF, Lehman AC, Tsang AW, Farritor SM, Oleynikov D. In vivo miniature robots for natural orifice surgery: state of the art and future perspectives. World J Gastrointest Surg. 2010; 2(6):217–23.
23. Phee SJ, Ho KY, Lomanto D, Low SC, Huynh VA, Kencana AP, Yang K, Sun ZL, Chung SC. Natural orifice transgastric endoscopic wedge hepatic resection in an experimental model using an intuitively controlled master and slave transluminal endoscopic robot (MASTER). Surg Endosc. 2010; 24(9):2293–8.
24. Phee SJ, Low SC, Huynh VA, Kencana AP, Sun ZL, Yang K. Master and slave transluminal endoscopic robot (MASTER) for natural orifice transluminal endoscopic surgery (NOTES). Conf Proc IEEE Eng Med Biol Soc. 2009;2009:1192–5.
25. Ho K. Robotics in gastrointestinal endoscopy. J Dig Endosc. 2012;3:74–6.
26. Eisenberg D, Storne E, Belson A. Use of a flexible robotic transgastric natural orifice translumenal endoscopic surgery (NOTES) platform in a cadaver to test access, navigation, maneuverability, and stability. Surg Endosc. 2010;24(9):2323.
27. Felice C, Emanuele T, Giovanni RP, Antonella R, Roberta B, Antonella T, Philipp EC. Robotic colonoscopy. In: Paul Miskovitz, editors. Colonoscopy. InTech; 2011. ISBN: 978-953-307-568-6. Available from http://www.intechopen.com/books/colonoscopy/robotic-colonoscopy.
28. Retrieved from http://www.endocontrol-medical.com/viky_ep.php.
29. Mozer P, Troccaz J, Stoianovici D. Urologic robots and future directions. Curr Opin Urol. 2009;19(1): 114–9. Review.
30. Ukimura O, Gills IS. Image-fusion, augmented reality and predictive surgical navigation. Urol Clin North Am. 2009;36:115–23.
31. ClinicalTrials.gov. A service of the United States National Institute of Health. Clinical Trial Identifiers: NCT01281488: Fluorescence imaging in finding tumors in patients with kidney tumors. Accessed 18 July 2012. http://clinicaltrials.gov/ct2/show/NCT01281488?term=NCT01281488&rank=1.
32. Moustris GP, Hiridis SC, Deliparaschos KM, Konstantinidis KM. Evolution of autonomous and semi-autonomous robotic surgical systems: a review of the literature. Int J Med Robot. 2011;7(4): 375–92.
33. Dieterich S, Gibbs IC. The CyberKnife in clinical use: current roles, future expectations. Front Radiat Ther Oncol. 2011;43:181–94. Epub 2011 May 20. Review.
34. Stüer C, Ringel F, Stoffel M, Reinke A, Behr M, Meyer B. Robotic technology in spine surgery: current applications and future developments. Acta Neurochir Suppl. 2011;109:241–5.
35. Retrieved from http://www.mazorrobotics.com/.
36. Pearle AD, O'Loughlin PF, Kendoff DO. Robot-assisted unicompartmental knee arthroplasty. J Arthroplasty. 2010;25(2):230–7.
37. Lewin JS, Nour SG, Duerk JL. Magnetic resonance image-guided biopsy and aspiration. Magn Reson Imaging. 2000;11(3):173–83.
38. Lewin JS, Duerk JL, Jain VR, Petersilge CA, Chao CP, Haaga JR. Needle localization in MR-guided biopsy and aspiration: effects of field strength, sequence design, and magnetic field orientation. AJR Am J Roentgenol. 1996;166(6):1337–45.
39. Melzer A, Gutmann B, Remmele T, Wolf R, Lukoscheck A, Bock M, Bardenheuer H, Fischer H. INNOMOTION for percutaneous image-guided interventions: principles and evaluation of this MR- and CT-compatible robotic system. IEEE Eng Med Biol Mag. 2008;27(3):66–73.
40. Xiao A, Li M, Melzer A. Positioning of focused ultrasound transducer using MR compatible robotic arm (Abstract). San Antonio, TX: SAGES; 2011.
41. Stoianovici D, Song D, Petrisor D, Ursu D, Mazilu D, Muntener M, Schar M, Patriciu A. "MRI Stealth" robot for prostate interventions. Minim Invasive Ther Allied Technol. 2007;16(4):241–8. Erratum in: Minim Invasive Ther Allied Technol. 2007; 16(6):370.
42. Stoianovici D, Song DY, Petrisor D, Mozer P, Armour E, Vigaru B, Muntener M, Patriciu A, Schar M. MRI compatible pneumatic robot MrBot for prostate brachytherapy: preclinical assessment of accuracy and execution of dosimetric plans. Int J Radiat Oncol Biol Phys. 2008;72(1):306–7.
43. Pfleiderer SO, Marx C, Vagner J, Franke RP, Reichenbach JR, Kaiser WA. Magnetic resonance-guided large-core breast biopsy inside a 1.5-T magnetic resonance scanner using an automatic system: in vitro experiments and preliminary clinical experience in four patients. Invest Radiol. 2005;40(7):458–63.
44. Fisher LR, Hasler WL. New vision in video capsule endoscopy: current status and future directions. Nat Rev Gastroenterol Hepatol. 2012;9:392–405.
45. Wortman TD, Strabala KW, Lehman AC, Farritor SM, Oleynikov D. Laparoendoscopic single-site surgery using a multifunctional miniature in vivo robot. Int J Med Robot. 2011;7(1):17–21.
46. Petroni G, Niccolini M, Caccavaro S, Quaglia C, Menciassi A, Schostek S, Basili G, Goletti O, Schurr MO, Dario P. A novel robotic system for single-port laparoscopic surgery: preliminary experience. Surg Endosc. 2013;27:1932–7.

47. Dolghi O, Strabala KW, Wortman TD, Goede MR, Farritor SM, Oleynikov D. Miniature in vivo robot for laparoendoscopic single-site surgery. Surg Endosc. 2011;25(10):3453–8.
48. Sekiguchi Y, Kobayashi Y, Watanabe H, Tomono Y, Noguchi T, Takahashi Y, Toyoda K, Uemura M, Ieiri S, Ohdaira T, Tomikawa M, Hashizume M, Fujie MG. In vivo experiments of a surgical robot with vision field control for single port endoscopic surgery. Conf Proc IEEE Eng Med Biol Soc. 2011; 2011:7045–8.
49. Retrieved from http://engineering.columbia.edu/using-robots-less-invasive-surgery.
50. Peirs J, Reynaerts D, Van Brussel H. Design of miniature parallel manipulators for integration on a self-propelling endoscope. Sens Actuators A: Phys. 2000;85(1):409–17.
51. Zuo J, Yan G, Gao Z. A micro creeping robot for colonoscopy based on the earthworm. J Med Eng Technol. 2005;29(1):1–7.
52. Patronik NA, Ota T, Zenati MA, Riviere CN. A miniature mobile robot for navigation and positioning on the beating heart. IEEE Trans Robot. 2009;25(5): 1109–24.
53. Raman JD, Bergs RA, Fernandez R, Bagrodia A, Scott DJ, Tang SJ, Pearle MS, Cadeddu JA. Complete transvaginal NOTES nephrectomy using magnetically anchored instrumentation. J Endourol. 2009;23(3): 367–71.
54. Scott DJ, Tang SJ, Fernandez R, Bergs R, Goova MT, Zeltser I, Kehdy FJ, Cadeddu JA. Completely transvaginal NOTES cholecystectomy using magnetically anchored instruments. Surg Endosc. 2007; 21(12):2308–16.
55. Petroni G, Niccolini M, Menciassi A, Dario P, Cuschieri A. A novel intracorporeal assembling robotic system for single-port laparoscopic surgery. Surg Endosc. 2013;27:665–70.
56. Canes D, Lehman AC, Farritor SM, Oleynikov D, Desai MM. The future of NOTES instrumentation: flexible robotics and in vivo minirobots. J Endourol. 2009;23(5):787–92.
57. Dario P, Carrozza MC, Pietrabissa A. Development and in vitro testing of a miniature robotic system for computer-assisted colonoscopy. Comput Aided Surg. 1999;4(1):1–14.
58. Wang KD, Yan GZ. An earthworm-like microrobot for colonoscopy. Biomed Instrum Technol. 2006; 40(6):471–8.
59. Pan G, Wang L. Swallowable wireless capsule endoscopy: progress and technical challenges. Gastroenterol Res Pract. 2012;2012:841691.
60. Patel GM, Patel GC, Patel RB, Patel JK, Patel M. Nanorobot: a versatile tool in nanomedicine. J Drug Target. 2006;14(2):63–7.
61. Hill C, Amodeo A, Joseph JV, Patel HR. Nano- and microrobotics: how far is the reality? Expert Rev Anticancer Ther. 2008;8(12):1891–7.
62. Hafeli U, Schutt W, Teller J, Zborowski M. Scientific and clinical applications of magnetic carriers. New York, NY: Plenum; 1997.
63. Holligan DL, Gilles GT, Dailey JP. Magnetic guidance of ferrofluidic nanoparticles in an in vitro model of intraocular retinal repair. IOP Nanotechnol. 2003;14:661–6.

Index

K.C. Kim (ed.), *Robotics in General Surgery*, DOI 10.1007/978-1-4614-8739-5,

N

O

P

R

Printed in the United States of America